Legal and Ethical Issues
in Nursing

third edition

Legal and Ethical Issues
in Nursing

third edition

Ginny Wacker Guido, JD, MSN, RN
Associate Dean and Director, Graduate Studies
College of Nursing
University of North Dakota
Grand Forks, North Dakota

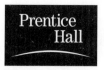 Prentice Hall

Upper Saddle River, New Jersey 07458

Library of Congress Cataloging-in-Publication Data

Guido, Ginny Wacker.
   Legal and ethical issues in nursing / Ginny Wacker
      Guido.—3rd ed.
     p. ; cm.
   Includes bibliographical references and index.
   ISBN 0-8385-5659-0
   1. Nursing—Law and legislation—United States.
  2. Nursing ethics. I. Title.
   [DNLM: 1. Legislation, Nursing—United States—
   Nurses' Instruction. 2. Jurisprudence—United
   States—Nurses' Instruction.]
  KF2915.N8 G85 2000
  344.73'0414—dc21   00–022586

Notice: The author and the publisher of this volume have taken care that the information and recommendations contained herein are accurate and compatible with the standards generally accepted at the time of publication. Nevertheless, it is difficult to ensure that all the information given is entirely accurate for all circumstances. The authors and publisher disclaim any liability, loss, or damage incurred as a consequence, directly or indirectly, of the use and application of any of the contents of this volume.

Publisher: Julie Alexander
Acquisitions Editor: Nancy Anselment
Editorial Assistant: Beth Ann Romph
**Director of Manufacturing
  and Production:** Bruce Johnson
Managing Editor: Patrick Walsh
Production Editor: Linda Begley, Rainbow Graphics
Production Liaison: Cathy O'Connell
Manufacturing Manager: Ilene Sanford
Director of Marketing: Leslie Cavaliere
Marketing Manager: Kristin Walton
Marketing Coordinator: Cindy Frederick
Creative Director: Marianne Frasco
Cover Design: Bruce Kenselaar
Composition and Interior Design: Rainbow Graphics
Printing and Binding: RR Donnelley and Sons

Prentice-Hall International (UK) Limited, *London*
Prentice-Hall of Australia Pty. Limited, *Sydney*
Prentice-Hall Canada Inc., *Toronto*
Prentice-Hall Hispanoamericana, S.A., *Mexico*
Prentice-Hall of India Private Limited, *New Delhi*
Prentice-Hall of Japan, Inc., *Tokyo*
Prentice-Hall Singapore Pte. Ltd.
Editora Prentice-Hall do Brasil, Ltda., *Rio de Janeiro*

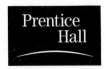

10 9 8 7 6 5 4
ISBN 0-8385-5659-0

As with the first two editions,
this book is dedicated to my family, without whom
it would never have been a reality:

Ed, Jenny, and Joey Guido
and
Cecelia G. Wacker

Contents

Preface

This third edition of *Legal and Ethical Issues in Nursing* (previously titled *Legal Issues in Nursing*) reflects the continuing influence that law, legal issues, and the field of ethics have on the professional practice of nursing. Professional accountability and responsibility are ever increasing, particularly as nurses become more autonomous with the shift from acute care settings to community and ambulatory settings. Professional accountability and responsibility are also enhanced as advanced practice nurses gain more independence through state nurse practice acts and through the entire restructuring of the health care delivery system in the United States.

Consumers continue to become more knowledgeable about their rights within the health care delivery system. Readers familiar with the first and second editions will recognize that much of the content in this text is new, reflecting various changes in the practice of professional nursing. The third edition also combines the field of ethics with legal issues as these two aspects of the professional nurses' practice cannot truly be separated.

This book is, once again, intended for practicing nurses and for nursing students. As with the previous editions, the primary function of this text is to familiarize both nursing students and professional nurses with current legal concepts, allowing the reader to apply legal concepts within an ethical framework, and hopefully providing for improved patient care through the knowledge and understanding of the various means in which these issues affect clinical practice. Additionally, the text is intended to:

1. Educate the beginning nurse, whether in the academic or practice setting, about legal issues, the functions of laws, and ethical application of legal principles.
2. Serve as a resource for practicing nurses, regardless of the clinical practice area.
3. Assist nurses in providing the most competent nursing care possible.

An important caveat is that this book is not meant to take the place of professional advice from practicing attorneys, and nurses are cautioned to seek legal counsel before proceeding with any legal matters. The book is meant to augment the role of legal counsel and assist nurses in understanding the legal process and liability issues as they relate to the ethical practice of nursing.

This edition of *Legal and Ethical Issues in Nursing* differs in several ways, while preserving the unique features of the former editions. The first three chapters acquaint the reader with basic legal knowledge, including sources and types of laws, the role of the court system in legal matters, and the role of case law in determining standards of nursing care. Completely revised, this first part emphasizes the vast impact that law has on the professional practice of nursing, the important role of nurse expert witnesses in defining professional standards of care, and major legal doctrines and rules that underlie nursing practice.

The second part of the book contains a single chapter on ethics in health care. This part was moved from the last part of the book to more fully integrate ethical principles into the entire text. This chapter has been revised to emphasize ethical principles and a usable ethical model for decision making in clinical areas, rather than evaluating various types of ethical issues that could arise in any clinical setting. This revision allows nurses to make realistic, individual decisions in everyday clinical settings, while challenging the reader to become more familiar with ethical decision-making models.

The third part of the book reexplores many of the more basic liability concepts common to all clinical practice areas. Chapters in this part of the book are rewritten, and include expanded sections on patient self-determination, the role of confidentiality and electronic applications in documentation, abuse issues, and the rights of patients in research.

The final part of the book, comprising the bulk of the text, reflects nursing practice in a variety of clinical settings. New chapters in this part emphasize the vital role of ambulatory care nurses and the role managed care is playing in the health care delivery system. Content has been rearranged so that issues pertinent to a specific area of practice flow within a single chapter. Content that has been added include multistate licensure issues, telenursing, alternative therapies, and an entire section on long-term care nursing. Nursing issues are discussed from the perspective of staff nurses in hospital and clinic settings, nurse managers in both inpatient and outpatient settings, community health nurses' roles, and nurses in academic settings.

Some readers may find the content of specific chapters could better have been placed in different chapters in this part. While writing the text, I attempted to find the most natural placement for the various content categories, and some of the material could have been placed in a variety of chapters. For example, telenursing could have been added to the chapter on nursing practice acts and licensure rather than being placed in the chapter on ambulatory care nursing.

Many of the features of the earlier editions have been enhanced. Each chapter opens with a preview of the content to be covered and a listing of the key concepts to be explored. Guidelines are placed throughout the chapters for ease of usage, and many chapters have multiple guidelines. Perhaps the more useful aspect is that current case law has been greatly enhanced, allowing nurses to better understand case examples of application of legal issues to professional nursing practice. Each chapter has several exercises that allow the reader to apply chapter content to actual clinical settings and assist readers in exploring their own state laws. Chapters conclude with a section entitled "After Completing This Chapter, You Should Be Able To" that reinforces the main concepts and goals of the chapter and an "Apply Your Legal Knowledge" section that reflects critical-thinking questions related to the specific chapter content.

Most exciting are the new features of the book, in particular the incorporation of ethical applications in the final 16 chapters of the book. I have been asked by many readers to develop a text that incorporates both legal and ethical issues. Readers are encouraged to address pertinent ethical principles as they complete each chapter. Sections on patient education are incorporated into many of the chapters as nurses continue to assume more of the education and discharge planning aspects of patients' care. With the exception of Chapters 1 and 10, there is also a "You Be the Judge" section in all chapters, allowing the reader to truly incorporate the legal issues addressed in the individual chapter. The two chapters where this new feature is not utilized are the chapters that deal with either complicated contract law (Professional Liability Insurance) or specific procedural law (Legal Concepts).

I am pleased to see this edition of *Legal and Ethical Issues in Nursing* a reality. I have truly learned a tremendous amount about the many aspects of nursing in its writing, and trust that you will learn as much in reading and using this text.

Ginny Wacker Guido, JD, MSN, RN

I INTRODUCTION TO THE LAW AND THE JUDICIAL PROCESS

one

Legal Concepts

■ PREVIEW

The disciplines of law and professional nursing have been officially integrated since the first mandatory nurse practice act was passed by New York in 1938. The profession has continuously relied on statutory law for its right to exist on a licensure basis and toward court decisions for interpretation of statutes. The civil rights movement of the 1960s and the malpractice crisis of the 1970s led to a heightened legal-mindedness of the 1980s and 1990s. With the advent of the third millennium, legal issues continue to escalate in practice settings. No longer can nurses rely on a working ignorance of the law and legal doctrines. Today's professional practitioners must know, understand, and apply legal decisions and doctrines to their everyday nursing practice. This chapter presents an overview of the legal system, including sources and types of laws.

■ KEY CONCEPTS

law	res judicata	misdemeanors
constitutional law	common law	felonies
statutory law	civil law	substantive law
administrative law	specific performance	procedural law
attorney general's opinions	tort law	due process of law
judicial (decisional) law	public law	equal protection of the law
stare decisis (precedent)	criminal law	rational basis test
landmark decision		

DEFINITION OF LAW

Law has been defined in a variety of ways, using simple to complex terms. The word *law* is derived from the Anglo-Saxon term *lagu*, meaning that which is fixed or laid down. Black's *Law Dictionary* defines **law** as "that which is laid down, ordained, or established; a body of rules of action or conduct prescribed by controlling authority and having binding legal force; and that which must be obeyed and followed by citizens subject to sanctions or legal consequences" (1990, pp. 884–885). Perhaps law may be better defined as the sum total of rules and regulations by which a society is governed. Law includes the rules and regulations established and enforced by custom within a given community, state, or nation. As such, law is created by people and exists to regulate all persons.

The actual definition of law is not as important as the impact of law on society. Law is people-made, whether by legislative bodies or by justices of the court. It reflects ever-changing needs and expectations of a given society and is therefore dynamic and fluid. Law is not an exact science, but rather an ongoing and organized system of change in response to current conditions and public expectations.

SOURCES OF LAW

Understanding the various sources of law assists in determining their impact on the nursing profession. Each of the three branches of the government has the authority and right to create laws, and these laws form the basis of the judicial system. Table 1–1 gives an overview of the various sources of law with examples.

Constitutional Law

Constitutional law is a system of fundamental laws or principles for the governance of a nation, society, corporation, or other aggregate of individuals. The purpose of a constitution is to establish the basis of a governing system. The Constitution of the United States establishes the general organization of the federal government, grants specific power to the federal government, and places limitations on the federal government's powers.

The U.S. Constitution establishes the three branches of the federal government and enumerates their powers. Article I establishes the House of Representatives and the Senate. Congress has the power to regulate commerce with foreign nations and among selected states to enact broad and powerful legislation throughout the nation. The Sixteenth Amendment gives Congress the power to collect a national income tax. Article II establishes the presidency and the executive branch of government. While powers of the president are not as clearly enumerated as those of Congress, the president has "executive" power, is the "commander and chief," and has power to grant pardons (except in cases of impeachment) for offenses against the United States. The role and duties of the Supreme Court and the rest of the judicial branch is established by Article III.

The general organization of the U.S. Constitution is, in reality, a grant of power from the states to the federal government, and the federal government has only the power granted it by the Constitution (Article X). The federal government can collect taxes, declare war, and enact laws that are "necessary and proper" for exercising its powers. Federal constitutional law is the supreme law of the land, as federal law takes precedence

TABLE 1–1. SOURCES OF LAW WITH EXAMPLES

Constitutional Law	Statutory Law		Administrative Law	Judicial Law
	Civil Law	*Criminal Law*		
Bill of Rights	Tort law	Penal codes	Boards of	Courts of law
Amendments to	Contract law	City ordinances	nursing	Trial level
the Constitution	Patent law		Regulatory	Appellate level
	Oil and		boards	Supreme Court level
	gas law			

over state and local law. Ideally, state and federal powers should be exercised so as not to interfere with each other, but if there is a conflict, federal laws prevail over state and local laws.

The U.S. Constitution also places limitations on the federal government. Such limitations have been enacted through the Bill of Rights (the first 10 amendments of the Constitution), which protects one's right to freedom of speech, trial by jury, free exercise of religious preference, and freedom from unreasonable search and seizure (U.S. Constitution, Amendments 1–10, 1787). Table 1–2 enumerates these rights and freedoms.

Constitutional law is the highest form of statutory law (defined in the next section). Statutory laws govern and meet existing conditions; constitutional laws govern for the future as well as the present in that the stability of constitutional law protects from frequent and violent fluctuations in public opinion (16 *American Jurisprudence*, 1995).

Each state has its own constitution, establishing the organization of the state government, giving the state certain powers, and placing limits on the state's power. An important difference between federal and state constitutional law is that the federal government derives positive grants of power from the U.S. Constitution, while states enjoy plenary powers subject only to limitations by their individual state constitution, the U.S. Constitution, and any limitations necessary for the successful operation of the federal system.

Statutory Law

Statutory laws are those made by the legislative branch of government. Statutory laws are designed to declare, command, or prohibit. Generally referred to as statutes, these laws are created by the U.S. Congress, state legislative bodies, city councils, or other elected bodies. Statutes are officially enacted (voted on and passed) by legislative bodies and are compiled into codes, collections of statutes, or city ordinances. Examples include the United States Code and Black's Statutes.

The federal and state governments have broad powers to legislate for the general welfare of the public. The federal government's power is granted by the U.S. Constitution, while the states have inherent power to act except where the Constitution restricts the power to the federal government. The states' power to legislate and govern is often referred to as *police power*. This term is generally seen as allowing the states to make laws necessary to maintain public order, health, safety, and welfare.

An example of statutory laws are licensure laws, which regulate health care providers within individual states. Licensure laws are designed to protect the general public from in-

TABLE 1–2. UNITED STATES CONSTITUTION, AMENDMENTS 1–10 AND 14

1. Congress shall make no law respecting an establishment of religion, or prohibiting the free exercise thereof; of abridging the freedom of speech, or of the press; or the right of the people peaceably to assemble, and to petition the Government for a redress of grievances.
2. A well-regulated Militia, being necessary to the security of a free State, the right of the people to keep and bear Arms, shall not be infringed.
3. No Soldier shall, in time of peace, be quartered in any house, without the consent of the Owner, nor in time of war, but in a manner to be prescribed by law.
4. The right of the people to be secure in their persons, houses, papers, and effects, against unreasonable searches and seizures, shall not be violated, and no Warrants shall issue, but upon probable cause, supported by Oath or affirmation, and particularly describing the place to be searched, and the persons or things to be seized.
5. No persons shall be held to answer for a capital, or otherwise infamous crime, unless a presentment or indictment of a Grand Jury, except in cases arising in the land or naval forces, or in the Militia, when in actual service in time of War or public danger; nor shall any person be subject for the same offense twice put in jeopardy of life or limb; nor shall be compelled in any criminal case to be a witness against himself, nor be deprived of life, liberty, or property, without due process of law; nor shall private property be taken for public use, without just compensation.
6. In all criminal prosecutions, the accused shall enjoy the right to a speedy and public trial by an impartial jury of the State and district wherein the crime shall have been committed, which district shall have been previously ascertained by law, and to be informed of the nature and cause of the accusation; to be confronted with the witnesses against him; to have compulsory process for obtaining witnesses in his favor, and to have the Assistance of counsel for his defense.
7. In Suits at common law, where the value in controversy shall exceed twenty dollars, the right of trial by jury shall be preserved, and no fact tried by a jury, shall be otherwise reexamined in any Court of the United States than according to the rules of the common law.
8. Excessive bail shall not be required, nor excessive fines imposed, nor cruel and unusual punishments inflicted.
9. The enumeration in the Constitution, of certain rights, shall not be construed to deny or disparage others retained by the people.
10. The powers not delegated to the United States by the Constitution, nor prohibited by it to the States, are reserved to the States respectively, or to the people.
14. Section 1. All persons born or naturalized in the United States, and subject to the jurisdiction thereof, are citizens of the United States and the State wherein they reside. No State shall make or enforce any law which shall abridge the privileges or immunities of citizens of the United States; nor shall any State deprive any person of life, liberty, or property, without due process of law; nor deny to any person within its jurisdiction the equal protection of the laws.

competent health care providers. Known as *nurse practice acts* or *nursing practice acts* depending on the individual state, these statutory law give authority to qualified and licensed practitioners to practice nursing within a given state, the District of Columbia, or U.S. territories. Other statutory laws that affect the practice of professional nursing include statutes of limitations, protective and reporting laws, natural death acts, and informed consent laws. See Chapter 11 for a more complete discussion of nurse practice acts.

Administrative Law

Administrative laws are enacted by means of decisions and rules of administrative agencies, which are specific governing bodies charged with implementing particular legislation. When statutes are enacted, administrative agencies are given the authority to carry out the specific intentions of the statutes, by creating rules and regulations that enforce the statutory laws. For example, legislative bodies pass the individual nurse practice acts (statutory laws) and create state boards of nursing or state boards of nurse examiners (state administrative agencies). The state boards of nursing implement and enforce the state nurse practice act by writing rules and regulations for the enforcement of the statutory law and by conducting investigations and hearings to ensure the law's continual enforcement.

Such authority is given to administrative agencies by the state legislature, since the elected legislative body has neither the resources nor the needed expertise to ensure that statutory laws are properly enforced. Administrative agencies are normally composed of persons with specific qualifications and experience and are given a single charge to implement and regulate the enforcement of a given statutory law. State boards of nursing are usually composed of predominantly registered nurse members, who are actively employed in educational or practice settings within nursing, and their charge is the enforcement of the state nurse practice act.

■ EXERCISE 1–1

Read the table of contents of your state nurse practice act. Can you distinguish the state administrative body (board of nursing) that is created by the legislature? Which sections of your nurse practice act create the administrative body and which sections serve to distinguish legislative intent?

Administrative rules and regulations have validity only to the extent that they are within the scope of the authority granted by the legislative body. Legislative bodies have some limitations placed on them by state constitutional law. There must be specificity in the charge as given to the administrative agency, and the legislative body remains ultimately responsible for the rules and regulations that the administrative body passes.

There may also be some procedural acts that govern administrative bodies. Such procedural acts delineate how the agency promulgates rules and regulations and provides for comments from the public before the rules and regulations are enforceable. The procedural acts may also provide for publication in a state register prior to the enforcement of the new rules and regulations.

The administrative agency has the initial authority to decide how its rules and regulations are enforced, and the decisions of the administrative agency may be appealed through the state court system. If appealed, the courts limit their review of the agency's actions to one of the following five areas:

1. Was the delegation of power to the specific administrative agency constitutional and proper?
2. Did the specific administrative agency follow proper procedures in enforcing the statutory law?
3. Is there a substantial basis for the decision?
4. Did the administrative agency act in a nondiscriminatory and nonarbitrary manner?
5. Was the issue under review included in the delegation to the agency?

Attorney General's Opinions

A second example of administrative law is the *attorney general's opinion.* Often, the national or state attorney general is requested to give an opinion regarding a specific interpretation of a law. Individuals or agencies may request such an opinion, and the opinion is binding until a subsequent statute, regulation, or court order amends the attorney general's opinion.

The attorney general's opinions provide guidelines based on both statutory and common law principles. Sometimes statutes are written in such vague terms that nurses seek opinions concerning the interpretation of the statute. For example, a board of nursing may request a state attorney general's opinion regarding enforcement of the nurse practice act in agencies that fail to comply with the provision of the act. Such a request would seek guidance on how the board of nursing should proceed to ensure compliance with the nurse practice act.

Opinions can also be formal or informal. The greater the liability risks, the more likely it is that a formal opinion will be issued. If legal issues then arise and the nurse has a formal attorney general's opinion, the court will more likely find that the nurse acted in a reasonable and responsible manner in seeking clarification on the matter.

Judicial Law

Judicial (or *decisional*) *laws* are made by the courts and interpret legal issues that are in dispute. Depending on the type of court involved, the judicial or decisional law may be made by a single justice, with or without the assistance of a jury, or may be made by a panel of justices. As a rule of thumb, the initial trial courts have a single justice or magistrate, intermediary appeal courts have three justices, and the highest appeal courts have a panel of nine justices.

All courts serve to rule on issues in dispute. In deciding cases, the courts interpret statutes and regulations or may decide which of two conflicting statutes or regulations apply to a given fact situation. Courts may also decide if the statute or regulation violates a constitution (federal or state), because all statutes and regulations must be in harmony with the governing constitution. The landmark case of *Marbury v. Madison* (1803) established the power of the judiciary in interpreting constitutional law. For example, a nurse who questions the authority of the state board of nursing may file a court action if the nurse has cause to believe that there has been a legal or procedural error on the part of the board's action against him or her.

Two important legal doctrines, which are directly derived from the U.S. Constitution, guide courts in their decision-making role:

1. The doctrine of *precedent* or *stare decisis* literally means to "let the decision stand." This doctrine is applied by courts of law in cases with similar fact patterns that have been previously decided by the court system. The court looks at the facts of the current case before it reviews previous decisions that applied the same rules and principles with the similar fact situation, and then arrives at a similar decision in the case currently before the court. This doctrine has great implications for nurses, because it gives nurses insight into ways in which the court has previously fixed liability in given fact situations. Nurses must avoid two important pitfalls before deciding if the doctrine of precedent should apply to a given fact situation:

a. The previous case must be within the jurisdiction of the court hearing the current case. For example, a previous New York case decided by an appellate court within New York does not set precedent for a California state court, although the California court may model its decision after the New York case. It is not compelled to do so because two separate jurisdictions are involved. Within the same jurisdiction, the case would set precedent. A New York appellate decision would be relied on by the lower courts in New York State.

b. The court hearing the current case may depart from precedent and set a *landmark decision,* which signifies that precedent is changed by the current court decision. Such a landmark decision is usually arrived at for one of several reasons. Societal needs may have changed, technology may have become more advanced, or to follow the previous decision would further harm an already injured person. A well-known example of a landmark decision was the U.S. Supreme Court holding in *Roe v. Wade* (1973). That court, for the first time in American history, recognized the right of a woman to seek and receive a legal abortion during the first two trimesters of pregnancy.

2. A second doctrine that courts employ in duplication of litigation and seemingly apparent contradiction in decisions is termed *res judicata,* which means literally "a thing or matter settled by judgment." Res judicata applies only when a legal dispute has been decided by a competent court of jurisdiction and no further appeals are possible. This doctrine then prevents the same parties in the original lawsuit from retrying the same issues involved in the first lawsuit. Res judicata prevents multiple litigation by parties who have lost in the original suit in that those parties are prevented from taking the same issues to another court in hopes of persuading a second trial court in their favor.

> Res judicata does not apply to competent appeals to an appellate court, nor does it apply to parties who were not named in the original lawsuit. Res judicata likewise does not apply to issues that were not decided by the original trial court so that a second lawsuit could be filed by the same parties on different specific issues.

All laws, regardless of origin, are fluid and subject to change. Constitutional laws may be amended. Statutory laws may be amended, repealed, or expanded by future legislative action. Administrative bodies may be dissolved, expanded, or redefined. Judicial or decisional laws may be modified or completely altered by new court decisions.

CLASSIFICATIONS (TYPES) OF LAW

Laws may be further classified into several different types. Many nurses may have wondered about classifications such as (1) common law, (2) civil law, (3) public law, (4) criminal law, (5) private law, (6) substantive law, and (7) procedural law.

Common Law

Law may be classified according to the court in which it was first instituted. The federal courts and 49 of the state courts in the United States follow the common law of England. *Common law* is defined as law that derived from principles rather than rules and

regulations, and is based on justice, reason, and common sense. During the colonial period, the English common law was uniformly applied in the 13 original colonies. After
the American Revolution, individual states adopted various parts of the common law,
and differences in interpretation and enforcement began that still exist to this day. Individual state statutory and judicial laws also account for the variation of common law
principles from state to state.

Civil Law

Louisiana elected to adopt civil or Napoleonic laws, because the origins of that state
were of a predominantly French influence. Derived from the civil laws of the French,
Romans, and Spaniards, Napoleonic or *civil law* may be said to be based on rules and
regulations.

Civil law may also be used to distinguish that area of the law concerned with the rights
and duties of private persons and citizens. Civil law is administered between citizen and
citizen (between private persons) and is enforced through the courts as damages or
money compensation. No fine or imprisonment is assessed in civil law, and injured parties usually collect money damages from private citizens who have harmed them.

The court, however, may also decide that an action, known as *specific performance,* be
performed rather than allow money damages, if the court deems that specific performance best aids the injured party. For example, in a contract dispute, the court may force
an employer to reinstate a previously discharged worker and to pay the worker compensation for the time he or she was without employment rather than merely paying the
worker for the time spent without work.

Civil law may be further divided into a variety of legal specialties: contract law, labor
law, patent law, and tort law, among others. Perhaps the most important area of law to
the professional nurse, *tort law* involves compensation to those wrongfully injured by
others' actions. This is the area of law that is normally involved in medical malpractice
claims. Tort law is covered in more depth in Part III of this book.

Public Law

Public law is the branch of law concerned with the state in its political capacity. The relationship of a person to the state is at the crux of public law. Perhaps the best example of
public law is the entire field of criminal law.

Criminal Law

Criminal law refers to conduct that is offensive or harmful to society as a whole. If an act
is expressly forbidden or prohibited by statute or by common law principles, it is referred to as a crime. Most often, crimes are viewed as an offense against the state rather
than as against an individual, and the state, city, or administrative body brings the legal
action against the offender. Examples of crimes include minor traffic violations, theft,
and unlawfully taking another's life. Punishment for the commission of crimes ranges
from simple fines to imprisonment to execution.

Crimes can be classified as either misdemeanors or felonies. *Misdemeanors* are lesser
crimes and may involve fines of less than $1,000 or imprisonment of less than one year.

Felonies are more serious, involve fines of greater than $1,000, and are punishable by prison terms of greater that one year or by death.

The same action by a given individual may be the basis for both a civil lawsuit and a criminal wrong. For example, if a nurse removes a ventilator-dependent patient from a ventilator and the patient subsequently dies, the state board of nursing may remove the nurse's license to practice nursing, and the family may file a wrongful death suit (a civil suit) against the nurse. In the criminal case, the court would consider the intent of the defendant as well as the actual action. In the civil case filed out of the same action, the court only considers the action performed.

There are situations within nursing in which the nurse may be said to have violated criminal laws, and the number of criminal cases against nurses is on the rise. Examples include backdating of records (*Nevada State Board of Nursing v. Merkley,* 1997), mistreatment of patients (*Mississippi Board of Nursing v. Hanson,* 1997), substandard nursing care (*Leahy v. North Carolina Board of Nursing,* 1997), practicing without a license (*People v. Odom,* 1999), and the administration of drugs that cause or hasten a patient's death (*Jones v. State of Texas,* 1986). In the so-called "angel of mercy" line of cases, in which nurses administer fatal doses of lidocaine, insulin, or potassium chloride to elderly patients, nurses have been charged with criminal violations (*The People v. Diaz,* 1992, and *Rachals v. State of Georgia,* 1987).

Other, less common, instances of criminal charges against professional nurses include the rape of patients (*State of North Carolina v. Raines,* 1987), manslaughter (*People of the State of New York v. Simon,* 1990), and attempted murder (*Caretenders v. Commonwealth of Kentucky,* 1991).

■ EXERCISE 1–2

Describe instances in which the conduct of the professional nurse (with regard to the treatment of patients) might be cause for possible criminal charges. For example, the administration of toxic chemotherapeutic agents may place a patient in a more life-threatening condition than the disease process does. How would a court of law distinguish such a case?

Private Law

Private law is synonymous with civil or common law, which has been discussed earlier in this chapter.

Substantive Law

Substantive law, which defines the substance of the law, may be further classified into civil, administrative, and criminal law. Thus, substantive law concerns the specific wrong, harm, or duty that caused the lawsuit or an action to be brought against an individual. Lawsuits brought to remedy violations of these laws must eventually prove the existence of the elements that comprise the actual claims.

Procedural Law

Procedural law, which governs the procedure or rules to create, implement, or enforce substantive law, may vary according to the type of substantive law involved and the jurisdiction in which the lawsuit is brought. Thus, procedural law concerns the process and rights of the individual charged with violating substantive law. Procedural issues that may be contested include admissibility of evidence, the time frame for initiating lawsuits, and the qualifications of expert witnesses.

DUE PROCESS OF LAW AND EQUAL PROTECTION OF THE LAW

Due process of law, a phrase often misquoted, applies only to state actions and not to actions of private citizens. Basically, the due process clause of the U.S. Constitution is intended to prevent a person from being deprived of "life, liberty, or property" by actions of state or local governments (Amendment 14, Section 1, 1787). Although difficult to define, the due process clause is founded on the fundamental principle of justice rather than a rule of law, and its purpose is to ensure the fair and orderly administration of laws (16A *Corpus Juris Secundum,* 1984).

Due process protects the public from arbitrary actions. Laws must operate equally among all persons, and laws must be definite, not vague. Due process is violated if a particular person of a class or community is singled out by the law. A "person of ordinary intelligence who would be law abiding can tell what conduct must be to conform to (the law's) regulation, and the law is susceptible to uniform interpretation and application by those charged with enforcing it" (*State v. Schuster's Express, Inc.,* 1969, at 792).

The two primary elements of due process are (1) the rule as applied must be reasonable and definite, and (2) fair procedures must be followed in enforcing the rule. This latter provision ensures that adequate notice be given before the rule is enforced so that persons who will be affected by it will have time to explain why the rule should or should not be enforced. Nurses become involved in the application of due process when requested to appear before state boards of nursing in that they must be given proper notice of the upcoming hearing and of the charges that the board will be hearing. In the hospital setting, the concept of due process has been interpreted to include a hospital's right to licensure by the state and the right of qualified medical personnel to staff appointments in public hospitals.

A recent case example concerning due process of the law affecting boards of nursing is *Slagle v. Wyoming State Board of Nursing* (1998). In that case, an inmate in the Wyoming correctional system filed a complaint with the Wyoming Board of Nursing claiming an advanced geriatric nurse practitioner was practicing illegally as an advanced practitioner in adult nursing. The board of nursing sent notice to the nurse, requesting that she substantiate her qualifications in adult advanced practice nursing. The nurse sent back numerous materials, including a letter of recommendation from the head of the University of Utah nursing program.

The nurse thought that the board was in the process of updating her qualifications and would be enlarging the scope of her license to include adult advanced practice. In fact, the board of nursing was conducting a disciplinary investigation to see whether the nurse had practiced beyond the scope of her geriatric advanced nurse practitioner standing.

In the subsequent lawsuit, the Supreme Court of Wyoming dismissed the board of nursing sanctions against the nurse, because the notice the board of nursing had sent was so misleading that it violated her Constitutional right to due process of law. The final conclusion was that the board of nursing gave her adult advanced nurse practitioner standing.

Note, however, that minor errors will not be seen as failing to give proper notice. In *Colorado State Board of Nursing v. Geary* (1997), the notice from the board of nursing was mailed to the nurse at an incorrect address. In Colorado, notice had to be sent to the nurse at the last known address and to the attorney, if any, who had notified the board that he or she was representing the nurse. In this case, the attorney received the notice, corrected the incorrect address, and sent the notice to the nurse at her correct address. The nurse received this latter notice from her attorney, but she decided not to appear at her disciplinary hearing. Because she was not at the hearing, the board placed a two-year probation on the nurse's license.

In the subsequent lawsuit, the nurse argued that she had not received notice, as the original notice was misaddressed. The court ruled that when an agency mails out an administrative notice, the law presumes that the notice was properly addressed and was actually received by the person to whom it was addressed. The board does not have to prove that the nurse received its notice. The nurse must prove that she did not receive the notice and, because her attorney had been sent the notice, she had been "duly served." Thus, the court upheld the two-year probation for the underlying charges of professional misconduct.

Like due process, the equal protection clause of the Fourteenth Amendment also restricts state actions and has no reference to private actions. The concept of **equal protection of the law** has become the source of many civil rights (*Words and Phrases,* 1994). More than an abstract right, the equal protection clause guarantees that all similarly situated persons will be affected similarly. Laws need not affect every man, woman, and child alike, but reasonable classifications of persons must be treated similarly (*Dorsey v. Solomon,* 1984). Thus, states may not enforce rules and regulations based solely on classifications as determined by race, religion, and gender. The due process clause does not preclude states from resorting to classifications of persons for the purpose of litigation, but "the classification must be reasonable and not arbitrary and must rest upon some ground of difference having a fair and substantial relationship to the object of legislation so that all persons similarly circumstanced shall be treated alike" (*Ex Parte Tigner,* 1964, at 894–895).

In determining whether equal protection of the law has been achieved, courts use the **rational basis test,** which essentially states that persons in same classes must be treated alike. It also states that reasonable grounds that further legitimate governmental interests exist in making distinction between those persons who fall within the class and those persons who fall outside the class (*Ohio University Faculty Association v. Ohio University,* 1984).

A case decided under the equal protection clause of both the U.S. and Arizona Constitutions held that it was unreasonable to allocate treatment within a service category solely on the criterion of age (*Salgado v. Kirschner,* 1994). In that case, a middle-aged Medicaid recipient was denied a life-saving liver transplant based on an Arizona statue that limits Medicaid coverage for medically necessary transplants to persons under the age of 21. The court found that age was the only criterion used and that age was medically irrelevant to liver transplant outcomes in that no evidence linking age to greater survival rate was shown. This case is significant in that age, if used to set restriction on care, cannot be the sole factor considered nor can it be medically irrelevant.

The distinction between due process and equal protection was perhaps best summarized in a 1983 case, in which the court stated that "the difference between due process and equal protection of the law is that due process emphasizes fairness between state and individual regardless of how other individuals in the same situation are treated while equal protection emphasizes disparity in treatment by a state between classes of individuals whose situations arguably are indistinguishable" (*Peterson v. Garvey Elevators, Inc.*, 1983, at 897).

SUMMARY

A basic understanding of the legal system, though complex, protects nurses against potential litigation while allowing them to be confident in the care they deliver. The legal system is a blend of rules and regulations, contains both federal and state laws, and may seem overwhelming at first glance. An appreciation of the legal system takes time to develop. The subsequent chapters of this book will assist individuals in understanding legal concepts in relationship to professional nursing practice.

AFTER COMPLETING THIS CHAPTER, YOU SHOULD BE ABLE TO

- Define the term *law* and describe four sources from which law is derived, including constitutional, statutory, administrative, and judicial (decisional) law.
- Compare and contrast the doctrines of precedent (stare decisis) and res judicata.
- Define and give an application of jurisdiction and landmark decision.
- List four ways in which laws can be changed.
- Define classifications of law, including common, civil, criminal, public, and private law.
- Distinguish substantive and procedural law, and state why each is important to professional nursing practice.
- Discuss due process and equal protection of the law.

APPLY YOUR LEGAL KNOWLEDGE

- Which classifications of law are more commonly applied to professional nursing?
- How do attorney generals' opinions protect the practice of professional nursing?
- Do all four sources of law protect the practice of nursing? Why or why not?

REFERENCES

Black, H. C. (1990). *Law Dictionary* (6th ed.). St. Paul: West Publishing.
Cartenders v. Commonwealth of Kentucky, 821 S.W.2d 83 (Kentucky, 1991).
Colorado State Board of Nursing v. Geary, 954 P.2d 614 (Colo. App., 1997).

Dorsey v. Solomon, 435 F. Supp. 725 (DC, Md., 1984).

Ex Parte Tigner, 132 S.W.2d 885, 139 Tx. Cr. Rept. 452 (Texas, 1964).

Jones v. State of Texas, 716 S.W.2d 142 (Texas, 1986).

Leahy v. North Carolina Board of Nursing, 488 S.E.2d 245 (North Carolina, 1997).

Marbury v. Madison, 5 U.S. (1 Cranch) 137 (1803).

Mississippi Board of Nursing v. Hanson, 703 So.2d 239 (Mississippi, 1997).

Nevada State Board of Nursing v. Merkley, 940 P.2d 144 (Nevada, 1997).

Ohio University Faculty Association v. Ohio University, 449 N.E.2d 792, 5 Ohio App. 2d 130 (Ohio, 1984).

People v. Odom, 82 Cal. Rptr. 2d 184 (Cal. App., 1999).

People of the State of New York v. Simon, 549 N.Y. Supp. 701 (New York, 1990).

Peterson v. Garvey Elevators, Inc., 850 P.2d 893, 252 Kan. 976 (Kansas, 1983).

Rachals v. State of Georgia, 361 S.E.2d 671 (Georgia, 1987).

Roe v. Wade, 410 U.S. 113 (1973).

Salgado v. Kirschner, 878 P.2d 659 (Arizona, 1994).

Slagle v. Wyoming Board of Nursing, 954 P.2d 979 (Wyoming, 1998).

16 *American Jurisprudence* (2nd ed.). Constitutional Law (1995).

16A *Corpus Juris Secundum,* Constitutional Law, Sec. 1–20, 957 (1984).

State of North Carolina v. Raines, 334 S.E.2d 138 (1987).

State v. Schuster's Express, Inc., 5 Conn. Cir. 472, 256 A.2d 792 (1969).

The People v. Diaz, 834 P.2d 1171 (California, 1992).

Words and Phrases (1994). Equal Protection of the Law. 14A. St. Paul: West Publishing Company.

United States Constitution, Amendments 1–10, 14 (1787).

two

The Judicial Process

■ PREVIEW

To fully appreciate the doctrine of precedent and the vast impact of landmark decisions on the court, nurses must first appreciate the complexities of the American court system. The significance of majority and minority opinions becomes more relevant as one differentiates the court systems, tiers, and jurisdiction issues. This chapter introduces the role of courts, gives a thorough description of the American court system, and concludes with a section on analyzing a legal case.

■ KEY CONCEPTS

questions of fact	state appellate court (court	writ of certiorari
questions of law	of intermediate appeals)	statutes of limitations
fact-finder	state supreme court	discovery rule
jurisdiction	U.S. district court	plaintiff
trial court	U.S. Supreme Court	defendant

QUESTIONS OF LAW OR FACT

Facts are determined by evidence presented by both sides in a legal controversy. *Questions of fact* present a factual dispute that the jury answers. Facts are not necessarily what actually happened, because persons on both sides will have perceived a given incident through their own eyes. Each party to the controversy brings unique perceptions to the trial setting. It is the responsibility of the fact-finder to weigh admissible evidence as presented and to decide where the facts of the case really lie. For example, a question of fact could concern such issues as admission to a hospital. Was the patient formally admitted to a hospital so that a patient–hospital relationship was established? Questions of fact could also include the cost of an operation, the cost of a particular hospital service, or who was involved in a particular incident. To date, questions of fact have concerned practice standards in that juries have decided whether practice standards have set the standard of care for individual patients. If, as Fiesta suggests, practice standards become more widely accepted, they will set the standard of care so that it will become a question of law as to whether the professional practitioner met or violated the standard (1994).

Sometimes facts are agreed on by both sides to the controversy prior to the trial. In these cases, the only questions to be resolved concern *questions of law*, which involve the application or interpretation of laws and are determined by the judge in the court. For example, the judge may rule that a particular provision in a nurse's contract was against public policy and is therefore nonenforceable. Or the judge may rule that a particular provision in the contract is reasonable and thus enforceable. Federal and state statutes, rules and regulations, prior court decisions, new technology, and societal needs may all play a part in determining the law as it applies to a specific trial.

Fact-finders, usually the jurors at trial, determine the facts that are admissible. These selected people are charged with weighing the admitted evidence, while the judge or magistrate determines questions of law. If there is a trial without a jury, then the judge serves as both the fact-finder and the determinator of questions of law.

A case example may help illustrate this distinction. In *Hansen v. Universal Health Services of Nevada, Inc.* (1999), the facts of the case were fairly simple. The patient had surgery to implant a steel spinal fixation device in his back. After the surgery, the wound became severely infected and the patient incurred a series of additional operations on his back, costing over $700,000. There was a serious dispute as to the medical cause of the infection.

In court, the patient's expert witness noted the patient was having episodes of bowel incontinence, which must have resulted in fecal matter being introduced into the wound. The hospital's expert witness related the infection to necrosis of muscle tissue near the surgical site.

The Supreme Court of Nevada agreed that fecal contamination of the surgical wound would be grounds for a negligent lawsuit against the hospital. However, in this case, the jury returned a verdict in favor of the hospital, apparently believing the hospital's expert witness's testimony about muscle necrosis. The court let the jury's verdict stand, as there were two fully plausible competing explanations for the events in question from which the jury made its own choice.

The court ruled that it was proper for the judge to exclude from the jury's attention hospital infection control reports, not connected to this incident, as potentially conflicting and prejudicial to the jury.

JURISDICTION OF THE COURTS

Jurisdiction, the authority by which courts and judicial officers accept and decide cases, is the power and authority of a court to hear and determine a judicial proceeding (Black, 1990). Jurisdiction determines the courts' ability to hear and rule on a given lawsuit. Jurisdiction may be divided into three categories.

Subject matter jurisdiction, sometimes called *res jurisdiction,* refers to the court's competence to hear and to determine a given case within a particular class of cases. For example, a court may have jurisdiction only in cases that involve probate matters (wills, estates, and the like), family matters (adoptions, divorces, and child custody), or criminal matters. Subject matter jurisdiction, along with the nature of the cause of action, may be determined by the amount or value of the claim as pled. For example, some courts have jurisdiction of a given case up to $1,000 or to cases that have a pled-damage figure of between $1,000 and $5,000.

Personal jurisdiction, sometimes referred to as *in personam jurisdiction*, refers to the power of a given court regarding a particular person. Personal jurisdiction is the legal power of a court to render a judgment against a party or parties to the action or proceeding. For example, personal jurisdiction often involves the county of the defendant. A court situated in the county of the defendant would have personal jurisdiction over the defendant. A court situated in the county of the plaintiff's residence can also have personal jurisdiction over the parties to the lawsuit.

The third jurisdictional issue concerns the court's ability to render the particular judgment sought. Any court possesses jurisdiction over matters only to the extent granted it by the constitution or legislation of the sovereignty on behalf of which it functions. *Territorial jurisdiction*, or the court's ability to bind the parties to the action, is a part of this third meaning of jurisdiction. Territorial jurisdiction determines the scope of federal and state court power. State court territorial power is determined by the U.S. Constitution's Fourteenth Amendment, and federal court jurisdiction is determined by the Fifth Amendment.

Courts may be either state or federal in origin. Federal courts seek to ensure that laws created through the U.S. Congress are enforced, and state courts have their sole jurisdiction within the given state. Overseeing the process is the U.S. Supreme Court, which has jurisdiction over all the land.

Overlapping or *concurrent jurisdiction* may occur when more than one court is qualified to hear a given dispute. In some areas of overlapping or concurrent jurisdiction and in some instances of specific subject matter jurisdiction, the federal Constitution gives guidance. For example, the federal courts have original jurisdiction over admiralty cases, crimes involving federal laws, bankruptcy cases, and patent laws. The U.S. Constitution gives the U.S. Supreme Court original jurisdiction (that which is inherent or conferred to the court) over cases "involving ambassadors, other public ministers and consuls and those in which a state is a named party" (Article III, Section 2, 1787).

If there is no mandatory court of jurisdiction, the attorneys representing the party filing the lawsuit will advise their client of the optimal court in which to file the lawsuit. Concurrent jurisdiction frequently occurs in cases with multiple defendants and in cases that involve parties residing in different states. There are many reasons why one court may be more favorable to the party filing the lawsuit, including shorter length of time to trial, more favorable damage awards, and shorter distances for witnesses to travel.

STATE COURTS

Trial Courts

The court of original jurisdiction in most states is the **trial court,** and it is the first court to hear legal disputes. At this level, applicable law is determined, evidence is presented and evaluated to ascertain the facts, and either a judge or a jury (functioning under the guidance of a judge) applies the law to the admissible facts. As stated in the preceding sections, it is the judge who determines questions of law and then guides the jury in applying this law to the questions of fact.

Even though the jury's tasks are to determine facts and, after proper instructions, to apply the law to the facts, the judge retains control over the entire trial process. The judge may find that the evidence is inadmissible or that the evidence as presented is insufficient to establish a factual issue for the jury to resolve. The judge may dismiss the case or may overrule a jury decision if he or she finds that justice has not been served.

Most state courts operate on a three-tier system. Sometimes called *inferior courts,* trial courts are the courts with original jurisdiction in most states with three-tier systems. Other names for this first court in which the lawsuit is filed include *circuit courts, superior courts, supreme courts* (New York), *courts of common pleas, chancery courts,* and *district courts.*

State Appellate Courts

The side that loses the case at trial level may decide to pursue the case to appellate level if there are procedural or legal grounds on which to base an appeal. In a three-tier system, these **state appellate courts,** or **courts of intermediate appeal,** do not rehear the entire trial but base their decisions on evidence as presented in a record of the trial hearing. There are no witnesses, new evidence, or jurors. The intermediate court may concur (agree) with the previous decision, reverse the prior decision, or remand (send the case back to the trial level) and reorder a new trial.

Intermediate courts of appeal have different names throughout the states. They may be called *courts of appeal, intermediate appellate courts* (Hawaii), *appellate divisions of the supreme court* (New York), *superior courts, courts of special appeals* (Maryland), *courts of civil appeals,* and *courts of criminal appeals.* States that have a two-tier system, such as North Dakota, Rhode Island, and Maine, have no intermediate appellate courts.

State Supreme Courts

The ultimate court of appeal in the state is usually named the **state supreme court.** This court hears appeals from the intermediate appellate courts and also serves to adopt rules of procedure for the state and to license attorneys within the individual state. This court is the final authority for state issues, unless a federal issue or constitutional right is involved. The state supreme court may hear cases directly from the trial level. For example, if the trial court case concerned the interpretation of the state constitution or a state statute, the case can be appealed directly to the state supreme court. An example of such a direct appeal involving the interpretation of the Missouri nurse practice act occurred in *Sermchief v. Gonzales* (1983).

Other names for this highest court of appeals within the state include *state court of last resort* (West Virginia), *supreme judicial court* (Maine and Massachusetts), and *court of appeals* (New York and Maryland). Some states may also have a separate supreme court of criminal appeals (Texas and Oklahoma).

■ EXERCISE 2–1

Explore your own state court system. What types of trial courts exist and what is their jurisdiction? Which court would most likely hear nursing malpractice cases?

FEDERAL COURTS

The structure of the federal court system has varied a great deal throughout the history of the United States. The Constitution provides merely that the judicial power of the United States be "vested in one Supreme Court, and in inferior courts as Congress may from time to time ordain and establish" (U.S. Constitution, Article III, Section 8, 1787). Thus, the only indispensable court is the Supreme Court. Congress has established and abolished other U.S. courts as national needs have changed over time.

Courts are presided over by judicial officers. In the Supreme Court, the judicial officers are called *justices.* In the courts of appeals, district courts, and specialty courts, most of the judicial officers are called *judges.* The authority, duties, and benefits assigned judicial officers are enacted and amended by the U.S. Congress.

District Courts

The federal court system mimics the majority of state court systems. The original trial courts in the federal three-tier system are the **U.S. district courts** and the specialty courts such as the U.S. court of claims, the U.S. bankruptcy courts, and the U.S. patent courts. There are currently 94 district courts, as well as specialized courts, including the Tax Court, Court of Federal Claims, Court of Veterans Appeals, and the Court of International Trade. The district courts normally hear cases in which a *federal question* (questioning a federal statute or violations of the rights and privileges granted by the U.S. Constitution) is involved or in which the parties to the suit have citizenship in different states (*diversity of citizenship*). In cases involving diverse citizenship, the federal court system applies rules of federal procedure in deciding applicable state law.

Courts of Appeal

The intermediary courts are the U.S. courts of appeal. These courts were known as the circuit courts of appeal prior to June 25, 1948. There are currently 13 courts of appeal, not including the U.S. Court of Appeals for the Armed Forces, and they are frequently called U.S. circuit courts even today. These courts are located in 13 areas (or circuits) of the country. The U.S. courts of appeal are numbered 1 through 12, with the District of Columbia Court of Appeals being the 13th court. Each of the first 12 courts of appeal consist of one to five state regions. These courts serve to correct potential errors that have been made in the decisions of the trial courts.

Supreme Court

The highest level of the federal court system is the **U.S. Supreme Court,** and its decisions are binding in all state and federal courts. This nine-justice court hears appeals from the U.S. courts of appeal and from the various state supreme courts when state court decisions involve federal laws or constitutional questions based on a **writ of certiorari,** or written petition to hear the case. The Supreme Court ensures the uniformity of decisions by reviewing cases in which constitutional issues have been decided or in which two or more lower courts have reached different conclusions.

Because most cases involving nursing practice concern tort law or state licensure issues, it is rare for lawsuits involving nurses as primary defendants to be heard in the federal court system. Exceptions to this rule are nurses working in the military and veterans' hospitals or other federally funded health care centers. Cases involving these nurses are frequently settled in federal courts.

■ **EXERCISE 2–2**

Find out which district court and federal court of appeals have jurisdiction over your city and state. What types of nursing malpractice cases have these courts heard in the past? How did the courts rule on those issues? How did their decisions affect the professional practice of nursing in your state?

STATUTES OF LIMITATIONS

Statutes of limitations, procedural law time frames, are essentially time intervals during which a case must be filed or the injured party is *barred* (prevented legally) from bringing the lawsuit. Statutes of limitation establish a time frame within which a suit must be brought. Set by the state legislature, most states allow one to two years for the filing of a personal injury lawsuit. The majority of the states do not begin measuring time until the injured party has actually discovered the injury that will become the basis of the ensuing lawsuit. According to the often-termed *discovery rule,* patients have two years from the time that they knew or should have known of the injury to file a personal injury lawsuit in the majority of states. This can differ, and some states, such as California and Ohio, adhere to a one-year statute of limitation.

Because of the malpractice crisis of the mid-1970s, many states have moved away from open-ended discovery statutes. Some courts have distinguished between traumatic injury cases and disease cases. In *traumatic injury cases,* the injury is normally of the type that the patient knows or should have known of immediately. For example, the patient who has an operation on the opposite extremity or wrong area of the body will immediately know that an injury has occurred. In traumatic injury cases, the one- or two-year statute of limitations is strictly applied.

In *disease cases,* the statute of limitations may be less strictly applied, because it may be some time before the patient becomes aware of the possible malpractice event. The statute of limitations would begin to measure time when the patient did become aware of the injury (event) or when the reasonable patient would have become aware of the injury. For example, in *Melendez v. Beal* (1985), the patient had entered the hospital for gallbladder surgery in May 1968. She had no complications following the surgery and was discharged. Late in 1981, she began experiencing abdominal pain and entered the hospital for tests. The tests revealed an abscess under her liver caused by a surgical sponge that had been retained in the abdomen following the 1968 surgery. Additionally, the retained sponge was found to be eroded into the small intestine at the time of surgery, thus necessitating extensive repair to the small intestine.

The patient filed a lawsuit for the retained sponge against the surgeon, nurses, and hospital. The trial court ruled in favor of the defendants because of the 14-year gap from the time of the original surgery to the time that the tests revealed the retained sponge.

The court of appeals reversed and remanded the case for a new trial. The court concluded that the "two-year limitation period could not be applied constitutionally to this patient, who had no way of discovering the negligent act within the two years from the date of the medical treatment. The filing of the action within two years after the patient's discovery of the negligence was, in fact, timely" (*Melendez v. Beal*, 1985, at 873). The court further concluded that a two-year limitation may be appropriate, but that it should not be used when the results would be "unreasonable, absurd, or unjust" (at 877).

A similar outcome occurred in *Playford v. Phelps Memorial Hospital Center* (1997). In this case, a patient had routine blood work in October 1992 as part of a prenatal visit. She was told that she was human immunodeficiency virus (HIV) negative. In December 1995, a later-born child was tested at one year of age and tested positive for HIV. The 5-year-old child was then tested, and he too was HIV positive. At that point, the original patient was retested and she learned for the first time that she was HIV positive. She then sued the hospital.

The hospital filed a pretrial motion to dismiss, citing that the statute of limitations barred the lawsuit. The New York Supreme Court ruled that the time period for the statute of limitations would not begin running when the patient was given another person's results, but would begin running when the patient discovered the mix-up and the correct test results.

Note, however, that courts apply the statute of limitation and dismiss causes of action if the facts support such conclusions. For example, in *Blackburn v. Blue Mountain Women's Clinic* (1997), the patient was given negligent advice by the clinic nurse and, believing her child to be HIV positive and capable of passing the disease to the patient in utero, had an abortion. Complications followed the abortion, including a hospitalization for severe depression.

The patient filed a lawsuit against the clinic for negligence. She claimed damages for her own physical and mental suffering and for the wrongful death of her unborn child. The court, in dismissing the suit, relied on the Montana five-year time limit for filing such a case, stating that a malpractice suit was not valid more than five years after the events in question.

Similar conclusions were reached by the Ohio Appellate Court in *Scott v. Borelli* (1996) and in *Long v. Warren General Hospital* (1997). In the first case, the patient sued her psychotherapist for sexual assault and professional malpractice that had occurred during her therapy 25 years earlier. The court even said that the patient could rely on memories recovered during Eye Movement and Desensitization and Reprocessing Therapy in bringing such a suit. However, once the patient's memory of past abuse is recovered, the statute of limitations begins to run and this case was filed after the applicable time limit.

In *Long*, the court ruled that when a patient falls, is seriously injured, and files a lawsuit, even the simplest aspects of the patient's care can come under scrutiny. The patient was taken into an examination room in preparation for a colonoscopy. Because it was cold, the nurse told the patient to keep his socks on, rather than getting for him the non-skid slippers that the hospital used for patients.

When the orderly came for the patient, he told the patient just to walk to the gurney.

Two feet from the gurney, the orderly told the patient to turn around and go back and get his pillow for the ride on the gurney. In turning around, the patient slipped, lost his balance, and fell, hitting his head on the wall and his elbow on the floor. He sustained a comminuted fracture of his elbow, requiring surgery and extensive physical therapy.

The patient filed suit against the hospital. The court was highly critical of the care that this patient had received. However, because the lapses in judgment that led to this patient's injuries occurred in a health care setting, the court believed that the case should be considered under the rules for medical malpractice. In Ohio, there was a one-year statute of limitations for such suits, and the case was dismissed.

Parties cannot be added to an already-filed lawsuit after the statute of limitations has expired. In *Reynolds v. Thomas Jefferson University Hosptial* (1996), the patient reported hoarseness and a sore throat to her family practice physician almost immediately after her emergency cesarean section. The physician said he would wait two weeks to see what happened. Although there was some improvement in the patient's voice, her persistent hoarseness did not improve. After four months, he sent her to an Eye, Ear, Nose, and Throat specialist, who diagnosed and repaired a dislocated right arythenoid cartilage. The surgical procedure was considered a success but left the patient, a semiprofessional singer, with a residual "airy" quality in her voice.

The patient first sued the anesthesiologist for faulty intubation and extubation. The anesthesiologist prevailed, because the court held that some cartilage damage can occur even with the best intubations. She then sued the family practice physician for his failure to refer her to a specialist more promptly. Although the allegations of malpractice against the family practice physician were valid, he was not added to the lawsuit until after the statute of limitation had run. Thus, the case was dismissed.

Some states have begun to view a *continuous treatment time frame doctrine*, which states that the time limit for filing a medical malpractice case is calculated not from the date of the alleged malpractice but from the date that the patient was last treated for the condition. The treatment for the same condition must have been continuous, not sporadic, for this doctrine to apply.

In *Stilloe v. Contini* (1993), a New York appellate court unanimously ruled that if there was no personal contact between the patient and the physician, where the two parties intend for their professional relationship to continue and the patient continues to rely on the doctor for care and treatment, there is continuous care and treatment for the purpose of satisfying the statute of limitations. Under this doctrine, the time in which to file a medical malpractice suit is extended when the course of treatments that includes the alleged wrongful acts or omissions has run continuously and is related to the same original medical condition or complaint. Thus, patients have an extended time period during which they may file lawsuits for medical malpractice.

The rationale behind statutes of limitations is that potential defendants should have the opportunity to defend themselves within a reasonable time period. The purpose of statutes of limitations is to suppress fraudulent claims after the facts concerning them have become obscured from lapse of time, defective memory, or death or removal of witnesses (*Noll v. City of Bozeman*, 1975). If too much time has lapsed between the occurrence and the lawsuit, facts become stale and witnesses cannot be identified or found.

At one time, courts uniformly allowed one major exception, in the case of minors, to the prompt filing of a lawsuit for personal injury. Because parents may not always seek what is in the best interest of their child, the court allowed minors to reach their majority before the statute of limitations began to be measured. In most states, this meant that the statute begins to be counted when the child reaches the 18th birthday. The lawsuit must be filed by the time the injured minor reaches his or her 20th birthday or the suit is barred by law. Today, a minority of states have become more restrictive, and have opted to disallow the right of a minor to bring suit upon reaching adulthood (majority).

ANALYZING LEGAL CASES

The introduction of the study of law would hardly be complete without an understanding of case-law analysis. The entire legal system seems to be organized around such interpretation. Laws are enacted by legislative and administrative bodies, and disputes are settled in courts. It seemingly follows that if one is able to analyze the decisions the courts hand down, then one truly understands the law. Although nurses need not fully comprehend every procedural tactic to appreciate the doctrine of precedent and its mandate to nursing practice, the nurse needs a working knowledge of case-law interpretation.

CASE CITATIONS

Perhaps a starting point is the understanding of case citations. A case citation is written as follows: *Darling v. Charleston Community Memorial Hospital*, 211 N.E.2d 53 (Illinois, 1965). All cases give the names of the plaintiff and defendant, as in *Darling v. Charleston Community Memorial Hospital*. The first listed name is the **plaintiff**, or the party bringing the lawsuit. At trial level, the plaintiff is synonymous with the injured party. The second named party is the **defendant**, or the party against whom the case is filed. Named parties may be individuals, corporations, states, or partnerships. The formal case citation lists the primary plaintiff and defendant. Multiple parties may be included in a single suit, but such multiple plaintiffs and defendants are listed only on the original petition as filed with the court hearing the case.

The order of listing is crucial. At any level of hearing, the party seeking restitution is named first, and the defending party is always named second. After the named parties to the suit is a string of numbers and abbreviations, for example, 211 N.E.2d 53. These abbreviations refer to a specific set of law reporters. Law reporters are published volumes containing the decisions and opinions of state and federal courts. The nation is divided geographically into regions such as the northeast (N.E.), northwest (N.W.), south (So.), southwest (S.W.) and Pacific (P.) regions. Additionally, some of the courts in a minority of states hear so many cases per year that one state may have its own reporter, as with California and New York. The "2d" or "3d" reference refers to the second and third series of the given reporter. Most state reporters are now in the third series. If no series reference is given, the first series of the reporter is indicated.

The abbreviations may also refer to a set of federal reporters, as in 381 Fed.2d 811. The number listed before the reference to a specific reporter is the volume of the reporter, and the number listed after the reporter is the starting page of the case within that volume of the reporter. In the last example, the case would be found in volume 381 of the Federal Reporter, second series, on page 811.

Some cases will refer to different sets of reporters, indicating that the case is located in more than one set of reporters. For example, in *Schloendorf v. Society of New York Hospital,* 211 N.Y. 125, 105 N.E. 92 (1914):

211 is the volume number.
N.Y. stands for the New York Reporter, first series.
125 is page 125.
105 is the volume number.
N.E. stands for the Northeast Reporter, first series.
92 is page 92.
1914 is the year that the decision was published.

Many federal cases are found in more than one set of reporters, and some states have a recording system as well as the national service of reporting cases.

Case citations also list the specific court hearing the case and the year that the decision was decided. A state listed in the citation indicates that the highest court within the state heard the case. Examples include *Wyatt v. Stickney,* 344 F. Supp. 387 (Alabama, 1972) and *Castillo v. United States,* 406 F. Supp. 585 (DC, N.M., 1975). Understanding the state references is crucial, because the references indicate the jurisdiction of the ruling. References to U.S. Supreme Court decisions never list the state in which the case originated, because the jurisdiction of that court is nationwide.

ELEMENTS OF A CASE

The format used to report lawsuits is fairly standardized, and most cases have the following elements. Refer to the sample case for clarification of these basic elements.

1. A brief paragraph sets forth a synopsis of the case with the rulings by this specific court. The synopsis lists: (a) the judicial panel; (b) from which court the case was appealed; and (c) the final holding (finding) of this specific court. In the sample case, the justice is named and the final holding of the court is identified.
2. Key concepts are identified by the reporting system and numbered according to appearance in the case. Usually, these concepts concern broad fields of law, as constitutional or contract law, and key points as they are developed by the given decision. These key concepts are known as *headnotes.*
3. An opinion follows the headnotes, stating why the plaintiff is appealing a lower court case and the ultimate decision of this court. In the sample case, this opinion section outlines eight grounds of appeal and the final decision of this court. Here, the previous court decision was upheld.
4. All cases begin with a review of the facts of the case. The more elaborate and complicated the fact situation, the more developed is this first section. It is crucial that the specific facts be understood, because even a slight variation in facts may lead to wide discrepancies in the rulings. This sample case has a fairly simple fact pattern, and those facts are stated in a single paragraph.
5. Usually, the court next considers a legal question. This specific question is the issue of the case. The issue will never be a global question, such as "Is the defendant at fault?" Instead the issue will be more narrow and specific to the case at hand. Here, the legal issue could be phrased as "Could there be significant apprehension to warrant a finding of an assault when the injured party is struck from behind?"

6. The court then answers the question. This is the substance of the case. Included in this section are cites to other cases, quotations from recognized authorities in various fields of law, and an analysis of the issue. The reporters divide this section according to the headnotes that were used at the beginning of the case. This is done for the convenience of a reader who may be scanning for a particular concept. In the sample case, the court addressed some headnotes in a single section, while addressing others collectively.
7. The ruling of the court follows the analysis of the case. The court may affirm the lower court findings, abandon the lower court findings, or partially concur with the lower court findings.
8. Sometimes, a dissent section follows the court's findings and is included with this case. This section allows justices who do not concur (either totally or in part) to express their individual views. While absent in the sample case, such a dissent section allows for equally important opinions on the same issues, and dissents may give insight into future arguments and may be the basis for future landmark decisions.

■ EXERCISE 2-2

Which district courts and federal court have jurisdiction over your city and state? What types of nursing malpractice cases have these courts heard in the past? How did the courts rule on the issues? How did their decision affect the professional practice of nursing in your state?

NURSING CONSIDERATIONS

To fully appreciate and incorporate legal principles into an individual nurse's practice, the nurse must know how to analyze court determinations and must be able to base future nursing actions on that analysis. Several benefits may be derived from a critical analysis of a crucial lawsuit.

1. The profession of nursing is forced to examine its practice through impartial and, hopefully, unbiased eyes.
2. The profession is given tested legal principles on which to base future nursing actions and interventions.
3. Nurses and their employers are given an acceptable standard of care that must be matched or exceeded to avoid future litigation.
4. Nursing faculty and health care instructors are provided a core of legal content for integration through their various programs.
5. The health care consumers' rights to quality and competent health care delivery is defined for the practitioner.

A caveat to nurses: Do not rely on your analysis of a case too completely. The intent of this chapter is to aid nurses in interpreting case law. However, it is important that individual nurses continue to seek further legal assistance in understanding all the pertinent ramifications of the case analyzed. Before acting on one's own interpretation of the case,

SAMPLE CASE

114 N.M. 13
Dawna Charlene Baca,
Plaintiff-Appellant,
v.
Dr. Jose VELEZ, Defendant-Appellee.
No. 11540.
Court of Appeals of New Mexico.
May 13, 1992.
Certiorari Denied June 18, 1992.

Nurse brought tort action against surgeon, alleging assault and battery. The District Court, Curry County, Peggy J. Nelson, D.J., entered judgment on jury verdict in favor of surgeon, and nurse appealed. The Court of Appeals, Chavez, J., held that: (1) there were no evidence of assault, and (2) trial court's evidentiary rulings were proper.

Affirmed.

1. Appeal and Err 863,934 (1)

In reviewing motion for summary judgment, Court of Appeals looks to whole record and views matter in light most favorable to support trial on merits.

2. Assault and Battery 2

Not all batteries include assaults; to be assault, there must have been act, threat or menacing conduct which caused another person to reasonably believe that he is in danger of receiving immediate battery. NMSA 1978, § 30-3-1, subd. B.

3. Assault and Battery 2

Physician who allegedly jabbed nurse in course of argument over surgical instruments was not liable for assault absent evidence that nurse felt scared before touching took place.

4. Appeal and Error 970(2)

Admission of character evidence is within discretion of trial court and will not be disturbed on appeal in absence of abuse of discretion.

5. Evidence 106(1)

Exclusion of evidence on defendant's character, in civil suit to recover for battery, was not abuse of discretion; defendant did not put his character into issue and such evidence was offered by plaintiff expressly on issue of propensity. SCRA 1986, Rule 11-404, subd. B.

6. Evidence 146

Exclusion of testimony of size or strength differences between plaintiff and battery defendant was not abuse of discretion; comparison would have been more prejudicial than probative and in any event, jury was able, by their own in-court observations, to view differences between parties.

7. Pretrial Procedure 45

Trial court properly allowed testimony from three lay witnesses disclosed near date of trial; defendant disclosed identity of witnesses within time frame allowed by pretrial order and there was no evidence that defendant knew he would be calling witnesses at earlier point in time and chose not to disclose their identities until it would be too late for plaintiff to depose them.

8. Pretrial Procedure 202

Unsigned deposition testimony of witness was properly excluded upon defendant's reasonably prompt objection, absent showing that defendant had waived signature requirement. SCRA 1986, Rule 1-030, subd. E.

9. Estoppel 68(2)

Party who offers deposition in support of motion for partial summary judgment effectively vouches for accuracy of that deposition and is thereafter judicially estopped from objecting to its admission when offered by opposing party.

10. Pretrial Procedure 202

Tape recording of deposition was properly excluded absent evidence that any stipulation or order regarding recording of deposition was made, or that any measures were taken to assure that recording was accurate and trustworthy. SCRA 1986, Rule 1-030, subd. B(4).

11. Evidence 150

Polygraph interview tape was properly excluded; rules of evidence concerned themselves only with admission of results of polygraph examination, which required professional skill of trained polygraph examiner. SCRA 1986, Rule 11-707.

12. Appeal and Error 1060.1(11)

Any conclusory arguments made by battery defendant's counsel in his opening statement did not warrant reversal of defense verdict absent showing that statement, in all probability, must have produced some effect on final results of trial.

OPINION

CHAVEZ, Judge.

Plaintiff appeals a jury verdict in favor of Defendant on her assault and battery claim. She raises eight issues on appeal: (1) whether the trial court erred in granting summary judgment on the assault claim; (2) whether the trial court erred in excluding evidence of the character of Defendant; (3) whether the trial court erred in excluding testimony of size and strength differences between Plaintiff and Defendant; (4) whether the trial court erred in allowing the testimony of three witnesses disclosed near the date of trial; (5) whether the trial court erred in refusing to allow the admission of the deposition or the taped testimony of a witness; (6) whether the trial court erred in refusing to allow a polygraph tape to be played to the jury; (7) whether the trial court erred in allowing Defendant to make conclusive remarks in his opening statement; and (8) whether the trial court erred in refusing to instruct the jury on assault. We affirm.

FACTS

This cause of action arose as a result of an incident alleged by Plaintiff to have occurred at Clovis High Plains Hospital in July 1986. Defendant is an orthopedic surgeon and a member of the staff of the hospital. Plaintiff, a nurse at the hospital at the time of the incident, worked with and was in charge of instruments. A disagreement occurred between Plaintiff and Defendant regarding certain instruments, including an osteotome, also known as a bone chisel. During the disagreement, Plaintiff alleges that Defendant jabbed Plaintiff in the back with the sharp end of the osteotome.

DISCUSSION

[1] Plaintiff's first issue is whether the trial court erred in granting partial summary judgement on her cause of action for assault. In reviewing a motion for summary judgment, this court looks to the whole record and views matters in the light most fa-

vorable to support a trial on the merits. *North v. Public Serv. Co.,* 97 N.M. 406, 640 P.2d 512 (Ct. App. 1982). Defendant's motion for partial summary judgment was supported by excerpts from the depositions of Mary Jane Petty and Plaintiff. Plaintiff did not file affidavits or other material opposing the motion, but argued at the hearing, as she does on appeal, that she felt afraid "after the initial jabbing." In her deposition, when asked if she felt "any anticipation that he might injure [her] further," Plaintiff answered "I wasn't sure. I was scared then." She also stated that she left immediately after the alleged touching.

[2, 3] We determine this evidence to be sufficient to sustain the trial court's grant of partial summary judgment on the issue of assault. While assault and battery are closely related, one may exist without the other. See W. Page Keeton et al., Prosser and Keeton on the Law of Torts § 10, at 46 (5th ed. 1984). All batteries do not include an assault. For there to be an assault, there must have been an "act, threat or menacing conduct which causes another person to reasonably believe that he is in danger of receiving an immediate battery." NMSA 1978, § 30-3-1(B) (Repl. Pamp. 1984). There was no evidence that Plaintiff felt scared before the touching took place. Therefore, there was no genuine issue of material fact whether, under these circumstances, an assault actually occurred.

[4, 5] Plaintiff's second issue is whether the trial court erred in excluding character evidence of Defendant. Admission of character evidence is within the discretion to the trial court and will not be disturbed on appeal in the absence of an abuse of discretion. *State v. Allen,* 19 N.M. 759, 581 P.2d 22 (Ct. App. 1978). Plaintiff cites several cases that allowed character evidence when character itself was at issue. In this case, however, Defendant did not put his character into issue. Also, Plaintiff's counsel argued to the trial court that the evidence in question was probative of Defendant's character and his propensity to be aggressive and domineering over women. SCRA 1986, 11-404(B) prohibits the use of evidence of other acts "to prove the character of a person in order to show that he acted in conformity therewith." Refusal to admit this evidence was not an abuse of discretion.

[6] Plaintiff's third issue is whether the trial court erred in refusing to admit testimony of size or strength differences between Plaintiff and Defendant. The determination of relevancy and materiality rests largely within the discretion of the trial court. *Wilson v. Hayner,* 98 N.M. 514, 650 P.2d 36 (Ct. App. 1982). In light of the nature of the charges against Defendant, we do not consider it an abuse of discretion for the trial court, under these circumstances, to have ruled that comparisons of the size and strength of the parties would be more prejudicial than probative. In addition the jury was able, by their own in-court observations, to view the differences between the parties.

[7] Plaintiff's fourth issue is whether the trial court erred in allowing testimony from three witnesses disclosed near the date of trial. In reference to the lay witnesses, SCRA 1986, 1-026(E)(1) places a duty on a party to seasonably supplement his response to a request to identify each of the persons expected to be called as a witness at trial. Plaintiff failed to provide us with facts indicating that the time frame in which Defendant informed her of the lay witnesses was not seasonable. See SCRA 1986, 12-208(B)(3). There is nothing to indicate that Defendant knew he would be calling the two new lay witnesses at an earlier point in time and chose not to disclose their identities until it would be too late for Plaintiff to depose them. ID. Also, Defendant dis-

closed the identity of the witnesses within the time frame allowed by the pre-trial order. The pre-trial order states that both counsel for Plaintiff and Defendant presented argument on Defendant's motion for a pre-trial order, which only asked that time deadlines be set by the court and did not specify what deadlines were desired. Therefore, counsel for Plaintiff could have anticipated such problems arising and argued against the deadlines that were set.

The case of *Beverly v. Conquistadores, Inc.*, 88 N.M. 119, 537 P.2d 1015 (Ct. App. 1975), is distinguishable from the case at hand. In *Beverly*, counsel for one of the parties indicated he had knowledge of an additional witness whom he might call to testify at the trial and refused to name the witness when ordered to do so by the trial court. This is not the situation here.

With regard to the expert witness, SCRA 1986, 11-707(D) requires any party who intends to use polygraph evidence at trial to serve written notice of such intention on the opposing party, not less than ten days before trial. Plaintiff admits Defendant complied with this rule. Under these circumstances, we cannot say the trial court abused its discretion in not granting Plaintiff a continuance and in allowing the expert witness to testify.

[8] Plaintiff's fifth issue is whether the trial court erred in refusing to allow the admission of the unsigned deposition or the taped testimony of witness Mary Petty. SCRA 1986, 1-030(E) states in pertinent part:

> Unless examination and reading of a deposition are waived by the witness and the parties, or unless the party requesting that a witness sign his deposition make[s] other arrangements for submitting a deposition to the witness, the court reporter shall advise the witness and the parties, in writing, when the transcript is ready for examination. Any changes in form or substance which the witness desires to make shall be entered. . . The deposition shall then be signed by the witness.

Additionally, SCRA 1986, 1-032(C)(4), which here should be read in conjunction with Rule 1-030(E), provides that "[E]rrors and irregularities in the manner in which the . . . deposition is . . . signed . . . under Rules 1-030 and 1-031 are waived unless a motion to suppress the deposition or some part thereof is made with reasonable promptness after such defect is, or with due diligence might have been, ascertained."

In this case, Defendant's objection was made with reasonable promptness upon discovery that the deposition was unsigned and Plaintiff did not claim that Defendant had waived the signature requirement. We hold that the trial court did not err in refusing to allow the unsigned deposition testimony of the witness into evidence. See *Garcia v. Co-Con, Inc.*, 96 N.M. 308, 629 P.2d 1237 (Ct. App. 1981).

[9] We note that Defendant offered the Petty deposition in support of his motion for partial summary judgment. When Defendant did so he in effect vouched for the accuracy of that deposition. We believe that having offered the deposition, Defendant should not thereafter be allowed, under the doctrine of judicial estoppel, to object to the admission of the same deposition when offered by the opposing party. See, e.g., *Citizens Bank v. S & H Constr. & Paving Co.*, 89 N.M. 360, 366, 552 P.2d 796, 802 (Ct. App. 1975) (" 'Judicial estoppel' simply means that a party is not permitted to maintain inconsistent position in judicial proceedings."); *Eads Hide & Wool Co. v. Merrill*, 252 F.2d 80, 84 (10th Cir. 1958) ("Where a party assumes a certain position in a

legale proceeding and succeeds in maintaining that position, he may not thereafter, simply because his interests have changed, assume a contrary position, especially if it be to the prejudice of the party who has acquiesced in the position formerly taken by him."). Had Plaintiff argued that the first deposition should have been admitted, notwithstanding the lack of the witness's signature or express waiver of same, on the basis that defendant himself had utilized that same deposition in support of his successful motion for partial summary judgment, we would have favored reversal and remand for new trial. Plaintiff, however, has not advanced a judicial estoppel argument on appeal, nor did she invoke a ruling on this issue by the trial court. See SCRA 1986, 12-216 (party must invoke a ruling by the trial court to preserve issue for review). Because Plaintiff has not raised or preserved this issue, we cannot address it on appeal.

[10] With regard to the tape recording of the deposition, SCRA 1986, 1-030(B)(4) states:

> The parties may stipulate in writing or the court may upon motion order that the testimony at a deposition be recorded by other than stenographic means. The stipulation or order shall designate the person before whom the deposition shall be taken, the manner of recording, preserving and filing the deposition, and may include other provisions to assure that the recorded testimony will be accurate and trustworthy.

There is no evidence in the record that any stipulation or order was made, or that any measures were taken to assure that the recording was accurate and trustworthy. The trial court did not err in refusing to allow the tape recording of the deposition.

[11] Plaintiff's sixth issue is whether the trial court erred in not allowing the polygraph interview tape to be played to the jury. SCRA 1986, 11-707 specifically deals with the use of polygraph examinations. Polygraph examinations are defined as "test[s] using a polygraph instrument which at a minimum simultaneously graphically records on a chart the physiological changes in human respiration, cardiovascular activity, galvanic skin resistance or reflex for the purpose of lie detection." SCRA 1986, 11-707(A)(2). A polygraph examiner is a licensed professional who uses his skills and training to read, interpret, and score the responses to the examination. *Lewis v. Rodriguez*, 107 N.M. 430, 759 P.2d 1012 (Ct. App. 1988). Therefore, the specific rule concerns itself with the admission of the results of the polygraph examination, which requires the professional skill of a trained polygraph examiner. See SCRA 1986, 11-707(C). In light of this, we cannot say the trial court erred in refusing to allow the tape of the examination to be played.

[12] Plaintiff's seventh issue is whether the trial court erred in allowing Defendant's counsel to make conclusory arguments in his opening statement. "The burden is on the plaintiff to establish that the opening statements made by defendant, in all probability must have produced some effect upon the final results of the trial." *Proper v. Mowry*, 90 N.M. 710, 716, 568 P.2d 236 252 (Ct. App. 1977). Our examination of the record shows Plaintiff failed to make such a showing to the trial court or this court.

Plaintiff's eighth issue is whether the trial court erred in refusing to instruct the jury on assault. Having previously decided that the trial court did not err in granting summary judgment on the assault issue, the jury did not need to be instructed on the assault, because that claim was not properly before them. We affirm.

IT IS SO ORDERED.

consult a legal expert or a practicing attorney for an interpretation of the same case. This is especially true if the facts of the case are complicated or if the decision is lengthy and complicated by numerous legal doctrines and procedural issues.

It is also important to recognize that judicial rules and holdings vary greatly from one jurisdiction to another. What constitutes the law in one state may be quite different from what constitutes the law in a different state.

Some practical suggestions on how to consult with an attorney and use case-law analysis to improve quality nursing practice include:

1. Ask the hospital attorney to meet with a concerned group of hospital nurses to discuss the legal implications of a given case.
2. Request that a professional organization (either general, such as the State Nurses' Association, or specific, such as the American Association of Critical-Care Nurses) present an in-depth program on a given case of interest to the membership.
3. Form an interest group and ask for legal assistance from attorneys within the geographic area. This latter suggestion would be a good opportunity to involve the nurse attorneys within the area.

■ EXERCISE 2–3

Invite a hospital staff attorney, or an attorney familiar with the health care industry, to a staff meeting. Prepare two sets of questions to ask the attorney:

1. Those concerning practice in an acute care setting.
2. Those concerning a home health or community setting.

SUMMARY

Understanding the court system allows nurses to appreciate which decisions more greatly affect nursing practice and how nursing practice changes based on decisional law. Federal cases affect nursing in a variety of states, whereas local trial court decisions may affect nurses in only a small portion of a given state. Similarly, being able to appreciate case law also allows nurses a greater appreciation of legal issues that affect the professional practice of nursing.

AFTER COMPLETING THIS CHAPTER, YOU SHOULD BE ABLE TO

- Differentiate between questions of law and questions of fact in trial settings, and give an example of both.
- List two types of jurisdictions, giving the definition and an example of both.
- Explain the functions of the trial courts, appellate courts, and supreme courts at both the state and federal levels.

GUIDELINES: HOW TO READ REPORTED CASES

1. Recognize that you cannot answer all the questions surrounding the case for yourself; consult a licensed attorney as needed for clarification.
2. Read the case carefully, especially the facts of the case. Make sure that you are clear on the given sequence of events and pertinent fact situations.
3. Identify the issue(s) as addressed by the case. Read the court's decision and analyze how the court answers the issue(s) and the reasoning given by the court. This is one instance in which a yes or no answer is not sufficient; the reasoning behind the answer is crucial for one's understanding of the law.
4. Research doctrines that are used by the court, especially if you are unfamiliar with the quoted doctrines.
5. Read any dissent very carefully. Dissents often help to clarify the majority opinion by recanting significant facts and applicable doctrines.
6. Incorporate lessons learned from the case into your nursing practice. Ensure that those with whom you work also incorporate lessons learned from case law.

- Describe statutes of limitation, their significance, and their purpose at law.
- Describe the process and significance for analyzing a court case.

APPLY YOUR LEGAL KNOWLEDGE

- Does the court in which a case is filed affect the ability of the injured party to have a more favorable or less favorable verdict?
- How do statutes of limitation favor defendants in a lawsuit?
- How does being able to analyze a court case enhance the professional practice of nursing?

YOU BE THE JUDGE

In March 1983, the plaintiff, Donna Harden Wilsman, filed suit against Dr. Sloniewicz, alleging that he negligently performed a tubal ligation. Wilsman alleged that she suffered severe abdominal pain following the surgery for four years and had damages of $350,000. The hospital was subsequently dismissed from the case by the plaintiff.

Dr. Sloniewicz testified that when he admitted Wilsman to the hospital, she was suffering from severe headaches and abdominal pain. The procedure used by the defendant during the operation was the removal of a section of the fallopian tube and placement of hemoclips on the tube close to the opening. This procedure was used on both fallopian tubes. After the procedure, Wilsman saw the physician for removal of her sutures on June 20 and 27, 1977. Wilsman had no complaints at that time, and Dr. Sloniewicz did not treat her again, according to testimony that Dr. Sloniewicz gave at court. In fact, after the June 27 visit, Wilsman owed the physician $215 that was not paid, and Dr. Sloniewicz testified that his practice was not to see patients—except on emergency bases—who owed outstanding amounts unless they asked for special arrangements on their bill. Dr. Sloniewicz stated that Wilsman never asked for any special arrangements.

Wilsman testified that she continued to have pain after the tubal ligation and that she saw the surgeon three or four times in 1978 and 1979. She testified that she was billed for those subsequent visits by Dr. Sloniewicz, but her divorce decree listed only an outstanding debt to the physician for $215. She said that an antacid was prescribed for her by Dr. Sloniewicz.

In 1981, she had a hysterectomy, which was performed by another surgeon, and learned that hemoclips had been used in 1982. Expert testimony was presented at trial level that the use of hemoclips deviated from the prevailing standard of care, and that the clips used by Dr. Sloniewicz were too large. There was additional testimony to show that hemoclips were appropriate and that their usage did not violate a standard of care.

Wilsman had a subsequent surgery in 1985, when scar tissue was removed from her abdomen that, a medical expert testified, may have accounted for her continuing pain.

Findings at the trial court level centered on the applicable standard of care and on a statute of limitations claim by the defendant. The court ruled in favor of the defendant physician, and the patient appealed.

Legal Questions

1. How does the statute of limitations affect this case?
2. Is there evidence to support the physician's claim that the statute of limitations barred the cause of action?
3. Is there evidence to support the plaintiff's claim that the statute of limitations should not bar this action?
4. How would you decide this case?

REFERENCES

Baca v. Velez, 833 P.2d 1194, 114 N.M. 13 (Ct. App. N.M., 1992).

Black, H. C. (1990). *Law Dictionary* (6th. ed.). St. Paul: West Publishing Company.

Blackburn v. Blue Mountain Women's Clinic, 951 P.2d 1 (Montana, 1997).

Fiesta, J. (1994). Legal aspects standards of care: Part II. *Nursing Management* 24(8), 16–17.

Hansen v. Universal Services of Nevada, Inc., 947 P.2d 1158 (Nevada, 1999).

Long v. Warren General Hospital, 700 N.E.2d 364 (Ohio App., 1997).

Melendez v. Beal, 683 S.W.2d 869 (Texas, 1985).

Noll v. City of Bozeman, 534 P.2d 880, 166 Mont. 504 (Montana, 1975).

Playford v. Phelps Memorial Hospital Center, 665 N.Y. Supp.2d 1017 (N.Y. Super., 1997).
Reynolds v. Thomas Jefferson University Hospital, 676 A.2d 1205 (Pa. Super., 1996).
Scott v. Borelli, 666 N.E.2d 322 (Ohio App., 1996).
Sermchief v. Gonzales, 600 S.W.2d 683 (Mo. en banc, 1983).
Stilloe v. Contini, WL 233404 (N.Y.A.D. 3 Dept, 1993).
U.S. Constitution, Article III, Sections 2 and 8 (1787).

three

Anatomy of a Lawsuit

■ PREVIEW

The ultimate goal of any court system is to resolve, in an orderly and fair process, a controversy that exists between two or more parties. To reach this orderly and fair conclusion, the trial process has evolved. This chapter presents all aspects of the trial process, from initiation of the complaint to appeals, and highlights nursing's role—with special emphasis on the role as an expert witness—in the process.

■ KEY CONCEPTS

complaint	counterclaim	opening statements
default judgment	right of discovery	cross-examination
alternative dispute resolution (ADR)	interrogatories	verdict (decision)
mediation	deposition	injunction
arbitration	pretrial conference (hearing)	lay witness
prelitigation panel	settlement	expert witness
pleadings	trial	legal counsultant
motion to dismiss	voir dire	

THE TRIAL PROCESS

Essentially there are six procedural steps to any given lawsuit. (See Table 3–1.) Each step, with its special application to nursing, is discussed in the following sections.

Step One: Initiation of the Lawsuit

A party, the plaintiff, who believes he or she may have a valid cause of action against another person initiates a lawsuit. The answering party or parties, the defendant(s) in the lawsuit, may then respond. (In reality, the attorneys carry out the intentions of their

TABLE 3–1. PROCEDURAL STEPS IN THE TRIAL PROCESS

Initiation of the Lawsuit
1. Complaint or summons is initiated by the plaintiff.
2. Service of the complaint is made to the defendant.
3. Health care provider contacts insurance carrier for attorney or provider attains independent attorney.
4. Answer or response is filed by the defendant.
5. If no response is made within the legal time frame, a default judgment is entered by the court against the defendant.
6. Prelitigation panel is held if state has such a medical review panel.

Pleadings and Pretrial Motions
1. Plaintiff makes initial complaint.
2. Defendant files original pleadings or answer.
3. Motion to dismiss is initiated by either plaintiff or defendant.
4. Counterclaims are filed with the court.
5. Amended and/or supplemental pleadings are entered.
6. Motion for judgment is based on the pleadings.

Discovery of Evidence
1. Interrogatories are served to both plaintiff and defendant.
2. Depositions of witness and named parties are taken.
3. Request to produce documents is made.
4. Requests for an independent medical examination of the plaintiff are made.
5. Subpoena of witnesses are issued as needed.
6. Pretrial conference or hearing is held.
7. Settlements are initiated and may be accepted.

Trial Process
1. Jury is selected (voir dire).
2. Opening statements are made, first by plaintiff, then by defendant.
3. Plaintiff's case is presented with cross-examination by defendant.
4. Defendant's case is presented with cross-examination by plaintiff.
5. Motion is made by defendant for directed verdict against plaintiff.
6. Closing statements are made, first by defendant, then by plaintiff.
7. Jury instructions are given.
8. Jury deliberates.
9. Verdict is brought in.

Appeals
1. Appellate level or state intermediate level court
2. State supreme court or highest state court
3. Federal court

Execution of Judgment
1. Payment of damages
2. Specific performance or injunction
3. Imprisonment or fining of defaulting party

clients, but the parties to the suit are always referenced as though they are the ones controlling and instigating the proper motions, claims, forms, and the like.)

In most instances, it is rare to have a single plaintiff versus a single defendant. More commonly, there are multiple parties on either or both sides to the lawsuit. In medical malpractice suits, a single plaintiff typically sues multiple defendants, including physicians, the hospital's board of directors, and various members of the nursing staff. Naming as defendants all possible persons or entities involved in the cause of action may be a wise strategy for the plaintiff, since the plaintiff could be barred by the statute of limitations from later adding defendants to the lawsuit. Should plaintiffs subsequently discover that a named defendant has been incorrectly named as a party to the suit, that defendant may be *nonsuited* (sometimes called *dismissed*) and removed from the case entirely.

Once the plaintiff's cause of action is well identified, a **complaint** is filed in a court with competent jurisdiction to hear the case. Upon filing the complaint, the court serves the defendant(s) with a summons to appear before the court at a specified time. This process, known as *service* in both state and federal court systems, alerts the named defendants that a lawsuit is now pending against them. The complaint outlines the names of the parties to the suit, the allegations of the breaches of standards of care, injuries or damages, and the demand for an award. In some states, the demand for damages is a specified amount, whereas other states determine the amount of the award based on the evidence as presented at court.

Once served, the defendants must respond to the complaint within a specified period of time or forfeit their right to defend the suit. The time frame for answering is determined by state or federal law and may vary according to the jurisdiction. When served, each defendant should promptly notify his or her liability insurance carrier for representation by one of the retained attorneys or procure a personal attorney. Never ignore the complaint because complaints do not merely go away when ignored. If not properly answered within the time period allotted by law, a default judgment will be entered in the court against the defendant. A **default judgment** means that the defendants automatically lose the lawsuit, whether they had any liability or not. Each defendant should act promptly, because each jurisdiction sets specific time periods for each phase of the pretrial procedures and motions.

Nurse-defendants should remember the following two points: First, after notifying their insurance carrier and arranging to be represented by an attorney in the impending suit, they should also notify the hospital administrative staff of the lawsuit (assuming that they are still employed at the institution named in the lawsuit). This notification allows the hospital attorney to better represent the hospital's and the nurses' interests. Second, nurse-defendants should not discuss the impending suit with anyone except their attorney and the hospital attorney. The less said, the less likely are nurse-defendants to be misquoted, and the less likely are their comments to be introduced into evidence.

Mandated by law in some states, **alternative dispute resolution (ADR)** refers to any means of settling disputes outside of the courtroom setting. Typically, ADR includes arbitration, mediation, early neutral evaluation, and conciliation. Although all of these processes are somewhat different in application, all serve to provide ways for parties to legal disputes to avoid formal lawsuits and costly trials. Other advantages of ADR include time savings (since most disputes take between three and six years from actual cause to resolution through the nation's court systems) and privacy (since the details of the disagreement and its resolution are private). Thus, institutions and health care providers can avoid public disclosure and adverse publicity. A major disadvantage to ADR is possible compromise of fairness and due process.

Two of the more common approaches to ADR include mediation and arbitration. *Mediation* involves one or more professional mediators, usually experts in the discipline, listening to both sides of the dispute and helping each side see the other side's position. Hopefully, the two sides to the dispute will be able to solve their differences. Although this approach frequently is helpful in contract disputes, it has rarely been effective in medical malpractice issues because emotions tend to dominate and health professionals have their careers at stake. Additionally, agreements reached through mediation may not be enforceable unless both sides agree to a binding decision before initiating the process.

Arbitration is a more formal process and is often seen as a "mini-trial." Attorneys are present at arbitration, questioning the parties to the arbitration and witnesses. Testimony is given under oath, so that the process does look like a trial. The differences are that there are no rules of evidence, no court reporter, and no formal record made of the arbitration process. The arbitrator's judgments are legally binding, as agreed to before the process is initiated.

Arbitration in malpractice cases is problematic because neither party typically wants to give up the ability to be heard in court. Also, because no rules of evidence apply, testimony that is inadmissible in courts of law may be freely asked in arbitration sessions. For example, a health care provider may be asked about substance abuse if that issue is relevant to the case. Finally, there is no appeal process with arbitration, unless one can show that the arbitrator was biased in favor of or against one of the parties.

Courts usually will uphold the arbitration decision. Two California cases illustrate this fact. In *Michaelis v. Schori* (1993), the California Court of Appeals held that a minor was bound to an arbitration agreement that involved claims arising from treatment she had received during her pregnancy. The same court, in *Coon v. Nicola* (1993), had previously ruled that a retroactive arbitration agreement between a physician and his patient did not violate California law and was binding. The court in the latter case also emphasized expanding utilization of ADR (*Coon v. Nicola*, 1993, at 1233).

A separate mechanism for ensuring the appropriateness of causes of actions is the prelitigation panel. *Prelitigation panels* ensure that there is an actual controversy or fact question before the case is presented at court. At the prelitigation hearings, evidence concerning the injury, its cause, and the extent of the injury are reviewed by a panel of medical and legal experts. Evidence presented may include medical records, expert reports, photographs, x-rays, authoritarian texts, medical journal articles, and medical or legal memoranda.

Not all states employ prelitigation panels because arguments abound as to whether they should exist. Defendants' attorneys argue that such panels reduce frivolous lawsuits and expedite the trial process, whereas plaintiffs' attorneys contend that they merely prolong the legal process and increase the overall expense of the trial. Most malpractice cases take three to six years from the time of injury to a decision, and in states with prelitigation panels, the time is increased by six to twelve months.

■ EXERCISE 3–1

List four reasons why nurse-defendants might not seek the hospital attorney as the attorney to represent their impending case and four reasons why they might.

Step Two: Pleadings and Pretrial Motions

Pleadings, written documents setting forth the contentions of the parties, are statements of facts as perceived by the opposing sides to the lawsuit. Pleadings give the basis of the legal claim to opposing parties and to prevent unfair surprise to either side. In actuality, the *initial complaint* or *petition* is also a pleading to the court setting out the plaintiff's facts and declaring that an injustice or wrong has been done. Each defendant responds with a pleading, giving his or her version of the facts to the court. In the defendants' *original pleadings,* the defendants set forth objections to the plaintiff's complaint. These objections cite *possible errors* in the plaintiff's case. Possible errors may be *procedural* (e.g., the process of service was incorrectly performed or the lawsuit is filed in a court that lacks personal jurisdiction over the defendant). Possible errors may also be *factual* (e.g., the defendant named in the suit was in reality on vacation or scheduled off at the time of the occurrence and thus has no liability in the matter before the court).

The defendant may also file a ***motion to dismiss,*** stating that there is no valid cause of action on which a claim may be made. The judge may either dismiss the suit upon such a filing or decline to dismiss. If the case is dismissed, the plaintiff may appeal the dismissal. If the motion to dismiss is declined, the defendant must answer the complaint.

A third alternative for the defendant is to file a counterclaim. A ***counterclaim*** states a cause of action that the defendant has against the plaintiff, such as failure to timely pay a hospital bill or comparative negligence on the part of the injured party. For example, if the plaintiff is suing for the improper casting of a broken arm but failed to keep scheduled appointments to check the alignment of the fracture, the plaintiff could have contributed to the purported negligence.

Either side may then file amended or supplemental pleadings as needed. *Amended pleadings* correct or add new material to the original pleadings before the court; *supplemental pleadings* add to the statement of facts already before the court. For example, an amended pleading would be filed to correct a deficiency in the original pleading. Instead of stating that one injection had been negligently given to the plaintiff by the nurse-defendant, the amended pleading might state that two injections, at two separate times, were administered by the nurse-defendant and that both injections resulted in injury to the plaintiff. A supplemental pleading allows the original pleading to stand while supplying additional facts. For example, a supplemental pleading might be filed to bring a third party into the lawsuit.

Pleadings may raise questions of fact or law. If there are no questions of fact, the case may be decided by the judge merely upon the pleadings. Usually, there are a variety of questions of fact and law, necessitating a full trial with or without a jury.

Once the pleadings have been completed, either or both parties may move for a judgment based on the pleadings. Some state courts allow the party seeking a judgment based on the pleadings to introduce sworn statements as evidence showing that the claim or defense is false. Normally, a substantial controversy is involved, and the motion for a judgment based on the pleadings is denied.

Motions, formal requests by one of the parties asking the court to grant its request, may also be filed. Motions may include the need for a speedy trial date owing to the elderly status of the plaintiff or a major witness, the need for a later trial date owing to the length of time needed to obtain necessary documents, or the need for additional documents. Motions are supported with a written narrative, known as a *brief,* which contains legal arguments for the granting of the motion. Motions are then argued before the judge, who issues a ruling regarding the motion.

Step Three: Pretrial Discovery of Evidence

Many state courts and the federal courts allow parties the *right of discovery,* which permits:

1. Witnesses to be questioned by the opposing side prior to the trial itself.
2. The uncovering of relevant written materials.
3. Possible additional examinations of the plaintiff.

Because of the right of discovery, this step of the trial process may take up to two or three years to complete.

There are several methods of allowable pretrial questioning of witnesses. *Interrogatories* are written questionnaires mailed to opposing parties that ask specific questions concerning the facts of the case. Most states limit the number of questions on the questionnaire that a given party may be required to complete. Interrogatories must be answered under oath, within a time period set by state law.

Parties should not attempt to answer interrogatories on their own. Most attorneys instruct their clients to answer the questions as completely as possible on a separate sheet of paper. The attorneys then complete the interrogatory for their clients, appropriately objecting to objectionable questions, and wording answers so as not to suggest or admit liability. Clients should read the answers as completed carefully before signing, and, because they are given under oath, make sure that the answers are true as stated.

A second means of obtaining witness testimony is through *deposition,* which is a witness's sworn statement, made outside the court, that is admissible as evidence in a court of law. Depositions are taken of a witness, who is questioned by the attorney representing the opposing side of the controversy. The deposition's purpose is to assist opposing counsel in preparing for the court case by revealing potential testimony from witnesses before the actual trial.

One must not be fooled by the fact that a deposition is taken at an attorney's office and that there are few persons present. A deposition is a crucial part of the discovery phase, and one must be alert to the questions being asked and their answers. The deposing witness is under oath during the entire deposition. The attorney representing the person deposed normally does not ask any questions during the deposition or take an active part in the deposition. The attorney for the deposing party already knows the extent of the testimony and does not need to reveal strategy to the opposing side.

Also present at the deposition is a court reporter, who records all questions and answers verbatim. The deposing party will be allowed to see and read the final written document before signing it, and the deposition becomes sworn testimony. When reviewing the final copy, the deposing witness may correct typographical errors, such as the misspelling of a name, but may make no substantive change to the record.

Deposing witnesses should give their attorneys sufficient time to object to the various questions, and time should be taken when answering each question. The witness may bring medical records, notes, and literature sources to the deposition, and may refer to them as needed during the deposition. Information should not be guessed at, but the witness should ensure its accuracy before responding. This same information will be given in court.

An error that physicians and nurses frequently make during depositions is in giving too much information. Often, such information is given because the health care provider knows the right questions to ask and the essential information to elicit. Opposing counsel may not be as well versed and may have ignored an entire area of pertinent information during questioning. Do not assist opposing counsel by giving them the answers needed to pursue the case. That is the domain of attorneys, who have the ultimate responsibility to their clients.

A newer concept in taking depositions is to videotape the witness during the entire deposition rather than to record the deposition through a court reporter. If the witness giving the deposition has a pleasing personality and appears to be caring and compassionate on tape, playing of this type of deposition in court mimics the personal effect of a live appearance. It is the option of deposing parties (and their counsel) to choose this type of deposition.

A recent case, however, illustrates the danger of videotaped depositions. In *Parkway Hospital, Inc. v. Lee* (1997), the hospital's attorneys objected vigorously during the trial that the plaintiff's attorneys were trying to embarrass the hospital and prejudice the jury against the hospital by playing back pretrial videotaped depositions of the nurses who had cared for the injured patient.

A nurse gave Pitocin to a patient in labor, causing the uterus to quickly rupture; the child was born with severe neurological injuries. The obstetrician claimed he had never ordered Pitocin. One nurse gave a videotaped deposition saying that there had been no order for Pitocin, but that the physician's routine orders were to be followed. This same nurse testified that she told the oncoming nurse at the change of shift that the physician's routine orders were to be followed. She also testified that she had never said anything about Pitocin or that it had been ordered.

The second nurse testified in her taped deposition that the first nurse told her to administer Pitocin, so she proceeded with the administration. These two depositions were played back to back at trial. The depositions were dramatic proof that the nurses were confused about the physician's orders. The jury was led to conclude that negligence by the hospital's nursing staff caused a nurse to give Pitocin to a patient on the labor and delivery unit, especially since the medication had not been ordered by the patient's physician. The jury found that the physician had no liability in the case but found liability against both the hospital and its nursing staff.

The court, however, said it was a perfectly acceptable trial tactic to place into evidence the conflicting testimony of two different agents of the same defendant. The court also upheld the showing to the jury of an 11-minute videotape that showed the child attempting to walk forward and backward, draw on a piece of paper, and talk, to demonstrate graphically the profound limitation in the child's motor control and functional abilities.

Taped depositions are frequently reserved for witnesses who will not be present for the actual trial. For example, witnesses who are outside the jurisdiction of the court or who may be unavailable during the time of the trial hearing may choose to have their depositions videotaped. Although the same evidence could be read at trial from a traditional deposition, the impact of having the witness in the courtroom setting via a taped deposition carries much more weight with the jury.

Depositions serve to uncover facts for the opposing side and to perpetuate the testimony of witnesses. Elderly witnesses or very ill witnesses may actually have their testimony preserved for trial through pretrial depositions.

Either side in the controversy may also obtain and examine copies of the medical records, business records, x-ray films, and the like through a *request to produce documents.* The court may also require a physical or mental examination of a party through a *request for an independent medical examination of the plaintiff,* if the medical information so obtained is pertinent to the case. Either party may object to these requests based on grounds that they are unduly burdensome, seek confidential or privileged information, or are protected as part of the attorney's work product. Generally, the scope of discovery is large, and parties are allowed to discover all relevant materials that would be admissible in the subsequent trial.

During the discovery phase, both sides decide on their strategy for the ensuing trial and interview the witnesses they need to testify in court. Both sides also obtain evidence to submit at trial in the form of x-ray films, medical records, consultation reports, and other tangible items that affect the case.

The final phase of the pretrial discovery of evidence is a **pretrial conference,** or **pretrial hearing.** This is a fairly informal session during which the judge and the representing attorneys agree on the issues to be decided and settle procedural matters. The pretrial conference may result in a finalization of a **settlement,** which is favored by the judicial system because it allows for a quick resolution. A settlement is not synonymous with the admission of guilt or liability but is a means of allowing the parties to forgo the trial process and to settle for an agreed-upon dollar figure. Included among the many reasons for settling a case prior to trial are the expense of the trial process, lengthy delays in reaching a trial date, emotional and physical drain on an already injured plaintiff, uncertainty of the jury trial process, and the nature of the harm complained of and its potential ability to shock a jury.

Step Four: The Trial

At the **trial,** the evidence is presented, facts are determined by the jury, principles of law are applied to determined facts, and a solution is formally reached. Evidence is usually presented through various witnesses' answers to specific questions. The jury relies on the testimony and credibility of the witness in determining the facts of the case.

If a jury trial has been requested, the trial begins with the selection of the jury, or **voir dire.** A panel of qualified persons is questioned by the attorneys representing both sides, and a four-, six-, or twelve-person jury is selected and sworn in by the judge. In some jurisdictions, a panel of six may be stipulated by the parties to the lawsuit. If no jury is requested or mandated by law, the judge serves as both judge and jury.

After jury selection, both sides make their opening statements. **Opening statements** generally indicate for the jury what each side intends to show by the evidence to be presented. Because the plaintiff has the legal burden of proof to show not only that an incident occurred but that the incident did in fact cause the plaintiff's injury, the plaintiff's attorney has the first opening statement.

Witnesses are then called, one by one, to answer specific questions. The witnesses are directly questioned first by the attorney calling the witness. The opposing side then has the opportunity for **cross-examination,** during which the questioning attorney attempts to discredit or negate the witness's testimony. The attorney originally calling the witness may then ask additional questions in an attempt to reestablish the credibility of the witness.

The plaintiff calls all of his or her witnesses in presenting the entire case. The plaintiff's side then *rests the case,* meaning that they have attempted to meet the burden of proof and have legally established their cause of action. At that point, the defendants' attorneys may *petition for a directed verdict,* indicating from their perspective that the plaintiff has failed to present sufficient facts on which to decide the case in the plaintiff's favor. This motion for a directed verdict is typically overruled, and the defendants then call their witnesses one by one to present their case to the jury.

At the conclusion of the defendant's entire case, both sides or either side may again move for a directed verdict. If these attempts are overruled (and they traditionally are), the attorneys make their final arguments, and the judge instructs the jury as to their charge and the principles of law involved. This last step varies greatly from jurisdiction to jurisdiction. The jury then retires to deliberate and to reach a ***verdict (decision).***

Once the verdict is known, the losing side may move for a new trial. If the motion is granted, the entire trial is repeated before a new jury panel. If it is denied, the judgment becomes final, and the losing side may appeal to the proper appellate court if there are legal grounds for such an appeal.

A case example illustrating legal grounds for an appeal is *Pivar v. Baptist Hospital of Miami, Inc.* (1997). In that case, an elderly patient had been hospitalized for several days following hip replacement surgery. The patient was known by the nursing staff to waken several times during the night with the urgent need to arise and go to the bathroom. On the night of the patient's fall, she awoke, feeling the urgency to urinate, and rang her call bell. When no one responded to the call bell, the patient got out of bed by herself and used her walker to get to the bathroom. She placed the walker next to the toilet and transferred herself to the toilet. When she finished urinating, the patient rose, took a step toward the walker, and fell on the water that still remained in the bathroom from an earlier shower.

Detailed for the court was the institution's procedure for showering a patient who had a recent hip replacement. The last part of the procedure is that the nurse assisting the patient is to return to the bathroom once the patient is safely back in bed and clean up any water that may be on the floor from the shower.

In the patient's civil lawsuit against the hospital, the trial judge exercised his prerogative to dismiss the lawsuit without submitting the issues to the jury. The District Court of Appeals held that the trial judge was guilty of a legal error, because there were valid grounds for a civil negligence suit against the institution.

Specifically, the Court of Appeals held that a hospital is "legally bound to exercise such reasonable care as the patient's condition may require, the degree of care in proportion to the patient's known physical and mental impairments" (*Pivar v. Baptist Hospital of Miami, Inc.,* 1997, at 277). Applying this concept to the current case, the court held that it was the nurse's responsibility, given the patient's unsteadiness on her feet and her propensity to use the bathroom unaided when she felt an urgency to urinate, to ascertain that the water had been wiped up after the evening shower and to document that fact in the nursing notes.

■ EXERCISE 3–2

Plaintiff Monroe has sued Nurse Smith for malpractice, stating that she was given an oral medication by Nurse Smith and that she then suffered a severe allergic reaction to the medication. What additional information might cause the court to enter a directed verdict for the plaintiff?

Step Five: Appeals

The appropriate appellate court reviews the case based on (1) the trial record, (2) written summaries of the principles of law applied, and, in many states, (3) short oral arguments by the representing attorneys. Depending on the outcome at the intermediate appellate level, the case may be eventually appealed to the state supreme court. Once decided at this highest level, the judgment typically becomes final, and the matter is closed. A few cases may be appealed to the U.S. Supreme Court, but this is a rarity in medical malpractice cases today.

Step Six: Execution of Judgment

Most lawsuits involving nurses result in one of two possible conclusions: the awarding of money damages against the nurse-defendant or the dismissal of all causes of action against the nurse-defendant. Nothing can return plaintiffs to their original, pretrial status, and the American judicial system attempts to compensate plaintiffs (if the evidence supports compensation) with money damages. Other forms of conclusion include an *injunction* requiring the nurse-defendant to either perform or refrain from performing a certain action.

After all appeals, the plaintiff will ask that the judgment as provided for by the court be executed. This procedure gives legal relief to the plaintiff if a losing defendant chooses to ignore a court order. If an injunction has been mandated by the court, the defendant may be fined or imprisoned. For a default judgment or money damages award, the defendant's wages may be garnished (i.e., a certain amount of money is taken from the defendant's earnings and given to the winning plaintiff on a weekly or monthly basis) or property may be confiscated and sold to pay the amount of the award. Not all states apply garnishment laws in the same manner, and some states have restrictions on the type of property that may be confiscated; therefore, there will be some differences from state to state in the *execution of judgment.*

EXPERT AND LAY WITNESSES

Lay Witness

Most nurses are aware of the expert witness status. Equally important in the judicial system is the *lay witness,* who establishes facts at the trial level, stating for the judge and jury exactly what transpired. The lay witness is allowed to testify only to facts and may not draw conclusions or form opinions. Lay witnesses define for the jury what happened. Both sides to the controversy will have lay witnesses who attempt to describe for the jury what, when, and how a particular event occurred. The lay witness thus has a direct connection with the case in controversy. Lay witnesses at trial may be the patient, patient's family members, nurses not named in the lawsuit, or other interdisciplinary staff members.

Expert Witness

The second type of witness, the *expert witness,* explains highly specialized technology or skilled nursing care to the jurors, who typically have little or no exposure to medicine and nursing. Expert testimony is admissible when conclusions by a jury depend on facts and scientific information that is more than common knowledge.

The use of nurses as expert witnesses has evolved since the late 1970s and early 1980s. Before then, physicians served as nursing's voice and testified at court regarding the role and accountability of professional nurses. Two court cases in 1980, one in North Carolina and one in Georgia, set the stage for acceptance by the court of nurses serving as expert witnesses in defining the role of nursing (*Maloney v. Wake Hospital Systems* and *Avet v. McCormick*). In *Maloney,* the court held that "the role of the nurse is critical to providing a high standard of health care in modern medicine. Her expertise is different from, but no less exalted, than that of the physician" (1980, at 683). Other courts have concluded that physicians may not establish the nursing standards of care. In *Young v. Board of Hospital Directors, Lee County* (1984), the court held that a psychiatrist was not familiar with the daily practices of psychiatric nursing and therefore could not testify to a deviation from nursing standards.

The courts have continued to define qualifications and expectations of nurse expert witnesses. In *Kent v. Pioneer Valley Hospital* (1997), the court allowed a nurse to testify about the legal standard of care for nursing but held that the nurse was not qualified to state an opinion making a cause-and-effect connection between a departure from accepted nursing standards and the injury that the patient had incurred. In two cases, *Stryczek v. Methodist Hospital, Inc.* (1998) and *Taplin v. Lupin* (1997), the court ruled that a nurse is not legally qualified to render an opinion about a medial diagnosis. There is, in the words of the *Stryczek* court, "a significant difference in the scope of nurses' and physicians' legal authority with respect to diagnosis and treatment" (1998, at 697).

The courts have also helped to establish when expert witness testimony is necessary. Two cases, *Peete v. Shelby County Health Care Corporation* (1996) and *Prairie v. University of Chicago Hospital* (1998), both discounted the need for expert testimony. In *Peete,* a patient recovering from abdominal surgery was still confined to his bed when a hospital technician attempted to remove an orthopedic structure from the bed. A piece of the orthopedic hardware struck the patient's head. The court said this was "simple" negligence, and no expert testimony was needed.

In *Prairie,* the facts are a little more complicated. A patient who was recovering from back surgery was ordered to be up in a chair on the second postoperative day. That was the same day that the nurse, without a physician's order, reduced the patient-controlled analgesic to one-tenth of the previous dosage. When informed that she was to get up, the patient told the nurse that she was in great pain and was "not getting up." The nurse tugged at the patient's arm and moved the patient's feet so that they were dangling off the bed. The patient pleaded with the nurse to leave her alone, but the nurse forced the patient to a standing position and "shoved" her into a straight-back chair. The nurse moved the patient's call bell out of her reach before leaving the room.

The court ruled that this type of behavior was not malpractice but gross negligence. The legal significance of gross negligence is that no expert witness is required. When a patient is crying out in pain, concluded the court, "any lay person can tell the patient is not tolerating the activity and that the activity must be discontinued for the patient's sake" (*Prairie v. University of Chicago Hospital,* 1998, at 616).

The minimum credential for a nurse expert witness is current licensure to practice professional nursing within a state. Other criteria for selection include total lack of involvement with the defendants either as an employee or consultant, clinical expertise in the area of nursing at issue, certification in the clinical area if possible, and recent continuing or formal education relevant to the specialty of nursing at issue. Ideally, the expert witness should also have earned graduate degrees and authored publications in nursing. Some attorneys will substitute status as a nurse manager, nurse educator, or preceptor for advanced degrees.

The purpose of these criteria for the nurse expert witness is to display for the jury that the nurse is well qualified to be an expert witness. Therefore, credentials that speak to the highest level of nursing expertise and knowledge of the appropriate standard of care weigh favorably with judges and jurors. Such criteria also further ensure the objectivity of the nurse expert. Expert witnesses who have either worked for the defendant institution or who are associated with defendant nurses on a personal level may be seen as giving subjective testimony. Such subjective testimony is most likely to be seen as a verdict for the plaintiff and against the defendants.

When nurses are first contacted about the possibility of serving as expert witnesses, they should consider some guidelines. First, is the case of interest to them and is it in the area of their expertise? Second, all materials sent should be reviewed carefully and a determination made whether a standard of care has been upheld or breached. Do not put thoughts and opinions in writing at this stage because such writings may be viewed by both sides to the controversy. Formal writings can be done once the position of expert witness has been confirmed. Third, decide on the fee schedule before proceeding. Acceptable fee schedules can be determined by the geographic area and whether the nurse will appear at trial. Finally, know the time frames for discovery and the actual court trial, so that the expert witness can be available for an extended period of time, if that is foreseen.

An expert witness may also serve as a *legal consultant,* one whose name is not revealed to the opposing side and whose reports or comments are not disclosed. When nurses are named as expert witnesses, their reports and comments are discoverable by opposing counsel only on request (Quigley, 1991).

When the need for an expert witness arises, both sides in the controversy retain their own. Testimony is generally in the form of opinions and answers to hypothetical questions. This practice has evolved because expert witnesses have the ability to analyze facts presented and to draw inferences from those facts, something the lay witness is not allowed to do.

Once selected as an expert witness, the nurse is prepared for this role by the attorney. Legal doctrine or state procedural rules that pertain to the individual case are discussed. The following should also be reviewed:

1. The facility or area where the incident occurred, to identify special environmental factors and the location of the patient in relation to needed equipment, medications, and staff
2. The state nurse practice act and any relevant rules that the board of nursing may have promulgated
3. Relevant nursing literature to ensure the status of acceptable practice at the time of the occurrence

4. The applicable nursing process of the institution during the time of the occurrence
5. All written records pertaining to the incident or that may have implications for assessment, planned actions, implementation, and evaluation of the incident
6. Supportive management records and/or patient classification acuity records
7. Support functions provided by the institution for nursing

Each of these has implications for the applicable standard of care during the incident.

Unfortunately, the number of lawsuits naming nurses as defendants is currently on the rise. The role of the expert nurse is therefore becoming more vital. Some experts estimate that the role of expert nurse witnesses will increase in importance as nurses are expected to testify not only in malpractice cases, but in custody and criminal cases, especially where nurses have been managing the care of either defendants or plaintiffs (Josberger and Ries, 1995).

Nurses are the only professionals with the competency, credentials, and right to define nursing or to judge whether the appropriate standard of care has been delivered. As nurses come forward to assume this role, the system will adjust not only to incorporate them, but to actively solicit their professional testimonies.

■ EXERCISE 3–3

List three possible instances in which no expert witness testimony is needed to assist the jury in their deliberations. Here is an example: Patient P is an elderly man, admitted 30 minutes previously from the postanesthesia care unit. Earlier in the day, he had surgery to remove his gallbladder. Patient P fell out of bed, breaking his knee and right wrist, and Nurse N admits leaving both siderails down and the bed in its highest position.

SUMMARY

The court system and the trial process have evolved to resolve disputes between two or more parties in an orderly and fair manner. There are essentially six steps to the trial process, all of which are important in the final outcome of the case. Nurses may be most involved as expert witnesses, presenting complicated facts and explaining standards of nursing care to the judge and jury.

AFTER COMPLETING THIS CHAPTER, YOU SHOULD BE ABLE TO

- List and explain the purpose of the six procedural steps in the trial process.
- Distinguish between traditional depositions, court reporter–recorded depositions, and the more modern videotaped depositions, stating the pros and cons of both methods.
- Distinguish between lay and expert witnesses and their roles in the trial process.

GUIDELINES FOR TESTIFYING AS AN EXPERT WITNESS

1. Personal characteristics are important. Be attentive and alert. Look at the person asking the question, showing that you are giving great thought to what is being asked. Do not try to impress anyone. Use normal, conversational language, and refrain from using jargon or "hospital talk." The judge and jury must be able to understand your answers.

2. Time must be taken when considering the answer to each question. Once spoken, an answer cannot be retracted. Understand the question or ask that it be repeated or rephrased. Give your attorney time to object to the question. Objections after an answer is given serve little value in jurors' minds.

3. A favorite ploy of opposing counsel is to either fluster, confuse, or anger an expert witness. Such ploys may prevent a clear and concise answer and may cause you to blurt out the first thought that enters your mind. All answers must be carefully considered, giving only the information that answers the questions. The battle being played out in court is about the facts of the case, not about people and personalities. Remain as objective as possible, take a deep breath if needed, and answer objectively, not defensively. Strive to be like a popular teacher to whom the judge and jury will want to listen.

4. Remember that there are several ways to accomplish any given intervention. The selection of an alternative approach does not equate with substandard care. Do not allow yourself to be backed into a corner where only one means of implementing an intervention is correct. Keep your options open, and reiterate that any of these approaches could have been selected.

5. Ensure that interventions as presented were appropriate at the time of the occurrence, not at the time of the court case. The expert witness should not be manipulated into discussing current practice standards, because they are most likely not reflective of the standard at the time the incident occurred.

6. Testimony previously given during a deposition is sworn testimony and cannot be changed at trial. If you are unsure of your previous testimony, such as quoting the patient's blood pressure or pulmonary wedge pressure, verify the information before speaking. You may refer back to your deposition or to the patient record before responding. If the answers are different, the next question by opposing counsel will inevitably be "Tell me, nurse, are you lying now or were you lying before?" Either answer destroys all credibility with the jury.

7. The expert witness should answer only what pertains to nursing, a nursing role, or standards of nursing care. If you cannot answer the attorney's questions without testifying to medical standards, then say that it is outside of the scope of nursing and that you cannot answer. The attorney can also be asked to rephrase the question so that it pertains to nursing standards of care.

8. Remember to dress appropriately, in a suit or more conservative dress, because appearance does make a valuable first impression with the jury. Look at the jury as you give your answers, thus showing your sincerity and knowledge.

9. Give only enough information to answer the question. If a simple yes or no will suffice, stop after stating yes or no. Frequently, nursing experts damage their credibility by trying too hard to ensure that the jury is aware of their knowledge base. The jury will already know that the expert is knowledgeable by the introduction of your credentials.

10. If opposing counsel asks if you are being paid to appear and testify, the answer is yes. However, stress that the payment is not for testimony, but for any provisions or inconveniences you had to make to be in court, such as travel to a distant court, lost work hours, child care, and review of pertinent facts and standards. The difference is subtle but extremely important.

11. Expect opposing counsel to question your credentials. Remember, they are trying in every way possible to lessen the weight of your testimony in the eyes of the jurors. Rather than credentials, it may be ethics that are attacked, such as a question asking if you had solicited the attorney of record for the opportunity to testify.
12. Be positive in your answers. Do not predicate your answers with "I believe," "I think," or "in my opinion." These are words of equivocation that impair your credibility as a witness.
13. Remember the three "C"s when testifying: Be calm, courteous, and consistent in your demeanor.

APPLY YOUR LEGAL KNOWLEDGE

- Does the trial process ensure that both plaintiffs and defendants have equal opportunity to present their case?
- When is it advisable to settle a case rather than persist with a long and lengthy trial?
- How does understanding the trial process aid the professional nurse?

YOU BE THE JUDGE

Patricia Ann Dooley, the plaintiff, was under the care of Dr. Skodnek, a psychiatrist. Dooley had been hospitalized following an unsuccessful suicide attempt. She remained under the care of Dr. Skodnek for three years, during which time she was prescribed Mellaril, an antipsychotic drug. It was undisputed at trial that the Mellaril caused her to suffer pigmentary retinopathy, causing her to be rendered legally blind. At trial, Dooley presented evidence of both negligence on the part of the defendant and lack of her informed consent.

During the trial, the defendant testified consistently that he recognized that Mellaril could cause pigmentary retinopathy, a condition that could result in diminished vision and blindness. Indeed, his knowledge was demonstrated by his very actions in discontinuing the patient's medication upon learning of the patient's vision difficulties and referring the patient to an ophthalmologist. Critical in the evaluation of the defendant's testimony is the opinion of Dr. Halpern, a board-certified psychiatrist who testified that Dr. Skodnek had in all aspects followed good and accepted medical practice. The expert witness even testified to the appropriate discontinuance of the medication when vision is first impaired, stating, "You have to stop the Mellaril long before pigmentary retinitis goes to blindness."

There was testimony that the patient was already taking Mellaril when she was first treated by Dr. Skodnek and that he refrained from advising her about the more serious side effects because of her emotional problems and suicidal state. However, Dr. Skodnek testified that he had informed the patient, when she was in a condition to comprehend, that there were some adverse side effects associated with the medication and that she was to notify him immediately if she experienced vision changes. This failure to warn immediately was also supported by Dr. Halpern, who stated that it was inadvisable while

Dooley was so acutely depressed to recount to her all the detailed horrors of this medication and its side effects.

After the presentation of all the evidence in the case, the trial court granted the plaintiff's motion for judgment as a matter of law on both theories. Dr. Skodnek appealed.

Legal Questions

1. Was there a sufficient controversy on which to try this lawsuit in a court of law?
2. Was an expert witness needed for the jury to understand the issues being tried?
3. Was Dr. Skodnek correct in appealing the lower court's decision?
4. How would you rule in such a case as presented by these facts?

REFERENCES

Avet v. McCormick, 271 S.E.2d. 833 (Georgia, 1980).
Coon v. Nicola, 17 Cal. App. 4th 1225, 21 Cal. Rptr. 2d 846 (Cal. Ct. App., 1993).
Josberger, M. C. and Ries, D. T. (1995). Nurse experts. *Trial* 21(6) 68–71.
Kent v. Pioneer Valley Hospital, 930 P.2d 904 (Utah App., 1997).
Maloney v. Wake Hospital Systems, 262 S.E.2d. 680 (North Carolina, 1980).
Michaelis v. Schori, 20 Cal. App. 4th 133, 24 Cal. Rptr. 2d 380 (Cal. Ct. App., 1993).
Parkway Hospital, Inc. v. Lee, 946 S.W.2d 580 (Tex. App., 1997).
Peete v. Shelby County Health Care Corporation, 938 S.W.2d 693 (Tenn. App., 1996).
Pivar v. Baptist Hospital of Miami, Inc., 699 So.2d 273 (Fla. App., 1997).
Prairie v. University of Chicago Hospital, 698 N.E.2d 611 (Ill. App., 1998).
Quigley, F. M. (1991). Responsibilities of the consultant and expert witness. *Focus on Critical Care* 18, 238–239.
Stryczek v. Methodist Hospital, Inc., 694 N.E.2d 1186 (Ind. App., 1998).
Taplin v. Lupin, 700 So.2d 1160 (La. App., 1997).
Young v. Board of Hospital Directors, Lee County, #82-429 (Florida, 1984).

II INTRODUCTION TO ETHICS

four

Ethics

■ PREVIEW

Every day, nurses make ethical decisions in their professional practice. Some of the decisions are clear-cut and easily made, such as when all health care deliverers agree that lifesaving measures will not be initiated for a terminal patient. Often, however, nurses find themselves trapped in the midst of ethical dilemmas among physician, patients, family members, and even their own peer group, such as when a patient refuses treatment. This chapter explores the distinction between law and ethics, various ethical theories and principles, and gives the nurse an ethical framework on which to base ethical decisions.

■ KEY CONCEPTS

ethics	rule utilitarianism	paternalism (parentialism)
normative theories	act utilitarianism	standard of best interest
deontological theories	principalism	justice
situation ethics	autonomy	respect for others
act deontology	beneficence	ethical committees
rule deontology	nonmaleficence	autonomy model
teleological theories	veracity	patient benefit model
utilitarianism	fidelity	social justice model

DEFINITIONS OF ETHICS AND VALUES

Ethics is the science relating to moral actions and moral values. Ethics encompasses "principles of right or good conduct" or "a body of such principles" (Boyer et al., 1991,

51

p. 253). A broader conceptual definition is that ethics is concerned with motives and attitudes and the relationship of these attitudes to the good of the individual. "Ethics has to do with actions we wish people would take, not actions they must take" (Hall, 1990, p. 37). Many people envision ethics as dealing solely with principles of morality—that which is good or desirable as opposed to that which is bad or undesirable. The problem faced by such a right or wrong definition is who decides what is good and what is evil: individuals, communities, professionals, or cultures?

A broader conceptual definition of ethics is concerned with motives and attitudes and their relationship to the good of the individual. Thus, values become interwoven with ethics. Values are personal beliefs about the truths and worth of thoughts, objects, or behavior. With values comes value clarification, a process aimed at understanding the nature of one's own value system and its vast impact on the individual nurse's delivery of health care services.

DISTINCTION BETWEEN ETHICS AND THE LAW

The *legal system* is founded on rules and regulations that guide society in a formal and binding manner. Although made by individuals and capable of being changed by the judiciary or legislative enactments, the legal system is a general foundation that gives continuing guidance to health care providers, regardless of their personal views and value system. For example, the law recognizes the competent patient's right to refuse therapy. The patient retains this right whether health care deliverers agree or disagree with the choice.

This right, however, is not absolute. If there are overriding state interests, treatment may be mandated against a patient's or parent's wishes. Cases concerning Jehovah's Witnesses, mandatory immunization statutes, and fluoridation of water enactments are three examples of overriding state interests.

Ethical values are subject to philosophical, moral, and individual interpretations. Both the health care provider and the health care recipient have a system of rights and values. Can one justify allowing competent adult patients to refuse therapy if the cost is their lives? Does ethics allow the refusal of health care therapies and treatments based on one's religious convictions that all medications and therapies are against God's law?

Most health care providers have difficulty in areas that transect both the law and ethics, such as the issues of death and dying, genetics, abuse of others, and futility of health care. Table 4–1 attempts to distinguish these two opposing concepts.

Ethics and legal issues often become entwined, and it becomes difficult to separate ethics from legal concerns. Both legal and ethical issues assist nurses in decision making and in the delivery of competent, quality curing care. Thus, nurses must be cognizant of both areas in clinical settings.

ETHICAL THEORIES

A variety of different ethical theories have evolved to justify moral principles. These *normative theories* are universally applicable, involve questions and dilemmas requiring a

TABLE 4–1. DISTINCTION BETWEEN LAW AND ETHICS

	Law	Ethics
Source	External to oneself; rules and regulations of society	Internal to oneself; values and beliefs, and individual interpretations
Concerns	Conduct and actions; what a person did or failed to do	Motives, attitudes and culture; why one acted as he or she did
Interests	Society as a whole as opposed to the individualy	Good of the individual within society
Enforcement	Courts, statutes, and boards of nursing	Ethics committees, and professional organizations

Source: Guido, G. W. *Legal Issues in Nursing: A Source Book for Practice.* Norwalk, CT: Appleton & Lange, 1988, p. 264.

choice of action, and entail a conflict of rights and obligations on the part of the nurse/decision maker. Most normative approaches to ethics fall into two broad categories, although a third category has recently evolved.

Deontological (from the Greek *deon* or "duty") *theories* derive norms and rules from the duties human beings owe one another by virtue of commitments that are made and roles that are assumed. Generally, deontologists hold that a sense of duty consists of ra-

GUIDELINES: MAINTAINING LEGAL RIGHTS WITHIN ETHICAL DILEMMAS

1. Recognize the difference between legal rights and ethical views. While both concepts are important, legal rights must be afforded the patient. For example, consent may be obtained for an abortion within the first trimester from both prospective parents, but only the prospective mother must sign the consent form.
2. Nurses must realize that their ethical views and values may differ greatly from the patient's value system. Such an understanding allows nurses to remain objective when caring for patients and when serving as consultants for decision making by the patient.
3. Nurses must remain current about recent judicial decisions in their jurisdiction and incorporate these standards and rights into their nursing care.
4. If the courts have not reviewed a case involving a particular ethical issue, then a legal standard may not exist. In such an instance, nurses are guided by the ethics of the profession and by personal moral values.
5. It is recommended that nurses remove themselves from patients' nursing care if values come into major conflict, for example, when a terminally ill patient is kept alive by life-support measures solely because the family cannot bear to let the patient die. If the nurse feels that the patient should be allowed to die without further resuscitation efforts, the best solution may be to remove oneself from this patient's care.
6. Ethical dilemmas have no perfect answers, just better answers. Legal questions have right and wrong answers. When in conflict, follow the established legal principles.

tional respect for the fulfilling of one's obligations to other human beings. The greatest strength of this theory is its emphasis on the dignity of human beings.

Deontological ethics look not to the consequences of an action, but to the intention of the action. It is one's good intentions that ultimately determine the praiseworthiness of the action.

A branch of deontological ethics is commonly referred to as *situation ethics,* wherein the decision making takes into account the unique characteristics of each individual, the caring relationship between the person and the caregiver, and the most humanistic course of action given the circumstances. Situation ethics is frequently relied on when the nurse has cared for a particular patient over a long time frame. Sometimes situation ethics is referred to as *love ethics,* conveying the deep respect for the human person.

Deontological theories can be subdivided into act and rule deontology. *Act deontology* is based on the personal moral values of the person making the ethical decision, whereas *rule deontology* is based on the belief that certain standards for ethical decisions transcend the individual's moral values. An example of such a universal rule could be "all human life has value" or "one should always tell the truth."

Teleological (from the Greek *telos* or "end") *theories* derive norms or rules for conduct from the consequences of actions. Right consists of actions that have good consequences, and wrong consists of actions that have bad consequences. Teleologists disagree, though, about how to determine the rightness or wrongness of an action.

This theory is often referred to as *utilitarianism;* what makes an action right or wrong is its utility, with useful actions bringing about the greatest good for the greatest number of people. An alternate way of viewing this theory is that the usefulness of an action is determined by the amount of happiness it brings.

Utilitarian ethics can then be subdivided into rule and act utilitarianism. *Rule utilitarianism* seeks the greatest happiness for all. It appeals to public agreement as a basis for objective judgment about the nature of happiness. *Act utilitarianism* attempts to determine, in a given situation, which course of action will bring about the greatest happiness, or the least harm and suffering, to a single individual. As such, utilitarianism makes happiness subjective.

An emerging theory is that of *principalism,* which incorporates various existing ethical principles and attempts to resolve conflicts by applying one or more of these principles. Ethical principles actually control professional decision making much more than do ethical theories. Principles encompass basic premises from which rules are developed. Principles are the moral norms that nurses both demand and strive to implement daily in clinical practice. Each of the principles can be used solely, although it is much more common to see the principles used in combination.

APPLYING ETHICAL THEORIES IN CLINICAL DECISION MAKING

Although ethical theories do not provide easy, straightforward answers, they do form an essential base of knowledge from which to proceed. Without ethical theories, the decision revolves solely on personal emotions and values. Because most nurses do not ascribe to either deontology or teleology exclusively, but to a combination of the two theories, principalism is growing in popularity.

■ EXERCISE 4–1

In a clinical setting, a patient refuses surgical intervention in favor of medical management for coronary artery disease. The health care delivery team and the patient's family favor surgical intervention. Can this dilemma be resolved solely on the theories of deontology and teleology? Why or why not? How would you resolve the issue?

ETHICAL PRINCIPLES

Nurses apply eight ethical principles in everyday clinical practice, some to a greater degree than others. Each principle is discussed separately.

Autonomy addresses personal freedom and self-determination—the right to choose what will happen to one's own person. The legal doctrine of informed consent is a direct reflection of this principle. Autonomy involves health care deliverers' respect for patients' rights to make decisions affecting care and treatment, even if the health care deliverers do not agree with the decisions made. Because autonomy is not an absolute right, restrictions may be placed on a person's right to endanger others, as in the case of communicable diseases.

The *beneficence* principle states that the actions one takes should promote good. In caring for patients, good can be defined in a variety of ways, including allowing a patient to die without advanced life support. Good can also prompt nurses to encourage the patient to undergo extensive, painful treatment procedures if these procedures will increase both the quality and quantity of the patient's life. Nurses frequently consider this principle when viewing the long-term outcomes of invasive and noninvasive procedures. The difficulty with this principle is in defining *good*.

The corollary of beneficence, *nonmaleficence* states that one should do no harm. Many nurses find it difficult to follow this principle when performing treatments and procedures that bring pain to patients. Even the act of giving an intramuscular injection to relieve postoperative pain brings some immediate pain to most patients. Nurses frequently choose to follow the principle of beneficence rather than nonmaleficence. Ethicists frequently reserve this principle for issues of major impact, such as "Can one preserve the life of anencephalic infants merely as a source for organ transplantation?" Today, ethicists are concerning themselves with the issue of cloning, particularly cloning of human beings.

Veracity concerns truth telling and incorporates the concept that individuals should always tell the truth. This principle also compels that the whole truth be told. This principle is followed when one completely answers patients' questions, giving as much information as possible, and telling the patient when information is not available or known.

Fidelity is keeping one's promises or commitments. Staff members know not to promise patients what they cannot deliver or what they do not control, such as when the patient asks that nothing be done should he or she stop breathing, before consulting the patient's physician for such an order. Keeping one's promises may become an issue in that patients are assured that they will be kept comfortable in the postoperative period, but complications may occur that prevent their being medicated (e.g., when the patient is hemodynamically unstable following surgery).

Paternalism (also known as *parentialism*) allows one to make decisions for another and is often seen as an undesirable principle. By definition, paternalism allows no collaboration on the decision, but totally removes the decision making from the patient or patient's family members. Called the *standard of best interest* by many ethics professors, this principle may be used to assist patients in making a decision about their health care when they are unable to have full or complete knowledge on which to base the decision (Aiken and Catalano, 1994). Derived from the best interest test, this principle allows health care personnel to assist in decision making when patients lack the expertise or data to make decisions. When the entire decision is taken from the patient, the principle is to be avoided.

Justice states that people should be treated fairly and equally. This principle frequently arises in times of short supplies or when there is competition for resources or benefits, such as when two patients require intensive care beds and only one bed is available.

Respect for others, seen by many as the highest principle, incorporates all other principles. Respect for others acknowledges the right of individuals to make decisions and to live or die by those decisions. Respect for others transcends cultural differences, gender issues, religious differences, and racial concerns. This principle is the core value underlying the Americans with Disabilities Act and several discrimination statutes. Nurses positively reinforce this principle daily in actions with peers, interdisciplinary health team members, patients, and family members.

■ EXERCISE 4–2

Give examples of how the eight principles just discussed are used daily among nurses. How does the incorporation of all the principles strengthen the health care delivery system and further ensure quality, competent nursing care?

ETHICAL DECISION-MAKING FRAMEWORK

In clinical practice, nurses seldom rely on a single ethical principle when caring for patients. Often, the ethical principles that nurses employ every day in practice settings come into conflict with each other. For example, envision the scenario of an elderly but independent patient who cherishes his independence. As a caregiver, one must balance the need to preserve this independence (autonomy) while discussing with his family alternative living situations (beneficence).

One way to begin resolving such issues is through ethical decision-making frameworks. Ethical decision making involves reflection on the following questions:

1. Who should make the choice?
2. What are the possible options or courses of action?
3. What are the available options or alternatives?
4. What are the consequences, both good and bad, of all possible options?
5. Which rules, obligations, and values should direct choices?
6. What are the desired goals and outcomes?

When making ethical decisions, nurses need to combine all the elements using an orderly, systematic, and objective method. Ethical decision-making models assist toward this end.

The various models for ethical decision making typically have five to fourteen ordered steps that begin with fully comprehending the ethical dilemma and conclude with the evaluation of the implemented decision. Perhaps the easiest model to use at the bedside is the MORAL model, developed by Thiroux (1977) and refined for nursing by Halloran (1982). Many nurses prefer this model as the letters of the acronym remind nurses of the subsequent steps of the model, and thus the model can easily be used in all patient care settings.

The model includes the following steps:

M **Massage the dilemma.** Identify and define issues in the dilemma. Consider the opinions of the major players—patients, family members, nurses, physicians, clergy, and other interdisciplinary health care members—as well as their value systems.

O **Outline the options.** Examine all options fully, including the less realistic and conflicting ones. Make two lists, identifying the pros and cons of all the options identified. This stage is designed to fully comprehend the options and alternatives available, not to make a final decision.

R **Resolve the dilemma.** Review the issues and options, applying basic ethical principles to each option. Decide the best option based on the views of all those concerned in the dilemma.

A **Act by applying the chosen option.** This step is usually the most difficult because it requires actual implementation, whereas the previous steps had allowed for only dialogue and discussion.

L **Look back and evaluate the entire process, including the implementation.** No process is complete without a thorough evaluation. Ensure that all those involved are able to follow through on the final option. If not, a second decision may be required and the process must start again at the initial step.

■ EXERCISE 4–3

Jody Smith, a retired nurse with three adult children and numerous adult grandchildren, lives in a small rural area. Her income is limited. Two months ago, she fell and broke her left hip. After surgery for an artificial hip replacement, she was transferred to a rehabilitation center, where she had a left-sided cerebrovascular accident (CVA). She was then readmitted to the acute care facility, where she has received aggressive therapy for the CVA.

Completely paralyzed on her left side, Mrs. Smith has decided that she no longer desires aggressive therapy and frequently asks the staff why she cannot die in peace. "The rehabilitation is so painful and I'll never walk again. What's the use?"

Both the doctors and her family are much more optimistic. The orthopedic surgeon is convinced that she will walk again, and the neurologist believes that she will make a full recovery and be able to return home and care for herself. Both doctors have excluded Mrs. Smith from their conversations, assuring her children that she will be "as good as new" and ignoring her requests to discontinue anticoagulant and rehabilitative therapy.

While not in a life-threatening condition, Mrs. Smith refuses to cooperate with the physical and occupational therapists and to take her medications. She also refuses to perform simple tasks, relying on staff to meet her activities of daily living.

Using the MORAL model, how would you resolve this dilemma?

Ethical decision making is always a process. To facilitate the process, use all available resources, including the ethics committee if the institution has one, and communicate with and support all involved in the process. Some decisions are easier to reach and support. It is important to allow sufficient time for the process so that a supportable option can be reached.

HOSPITAL ETHICS COMMITTEES

With the increasing numbers of legal and ethical dilemmas in patient situations today, health care providers are considering guidance with decision making. Perhaps one of the best solutions for both long-term and short-term issues is the creation and use of an institution ethics committee. *Ethical committees* can (1) provide structure and guidelines for potential problems, (2) serve as an open forum for discussion, and (3) function as a true patient advocate by placing the patient at the core of the committee discussions.

To form such a group, if one does not already exist, the proposed committee should first begin as a bioethical study group so that ethical principles and theories as well as current issues can be explored by members of the group. The committee should be composed of nurses, physicians, clergy, clinical social workers, nutritional experts, pharmacists, administrative personnel, and legal experts. Once the committee has become active, individual patients or patients' family members may also be invited to the committee deliberations.

Ethics committees generally follow one of three distinct structures, though some institution ethics committees blend the three structures, and others differ in their approach depending on the individual case:

1. The *autonomy model* facilitates decision making for the competent patient.
2. The *patient benefit model* uses substituted judgment and facilitates decision making for the incompetent patient.
3. The *social justice model* considers broad social issues and is accountable to the institution.

In most settings, ethics committees are a reality, in part because of the complex issues in health care. In 1992, the Joint Commission for the Accreditation of Healthcare Organizations (JCAHO) mandated ethics committees or, in the alternative, other vehicles for addressing ethical concerns. Included in the 1992 manual was a chapter on patient rights, further clarifying the important role of ethics committees.

The three-page chapter includes standards that address the issues of a patient's participation in health care decisions, the creation of advanced directives, and the enactment of do-not-resuscitate orders and policies. The chapter's premise is that the hospital supports the rights of each patient and that the hospital's policies and procedures describe the means by which those rights are protected and exercised. The policies must also include a means for resolving conflicts in decision making and a description of the respective roles of physicians, nurses, and family members in decisions involving do-not-resuscitate orders or the withholding of treatment (JCAHO, 1992).

In many medical centers, *ethical rounds*, which are conducted on a weekly or monthly schedule, allow staff members who may be involved in later ethical dilemmas to begin viewing all the issues and in becoming more comfortable with ethical issues and their resolutions. These ethical rounds serve as an alternative to ethics committees. Other institutions, to meet the requirements of JCAHO, employ a bioethics consultant or pastoral staff care member rather than having the more traditional ethics committee.

Perhaps the more relevant ethical questions are yet to be addressed, though at some point they must be addressed, and nursing must be among those addressing the issues. Health care providers continue to debate the ethics of individual patients but reject the need to look at the ethics of the social system itself. Untold amounts of time and resources are spent on debating informed consent, autonomy, and discontinuance of life support systems, while seemingly nothing is done about debating the ethics of the entire system—the oversupply of acute care beds, continual duplication of revenue-generating procedures, and overproduction of medical specialists, to name but a few of the more pressing issues. As Richard Lamm so aptly states, "The sum total of much of our ethical thinking about individuals has given us an unethical health care system" (1999, p. 14).

■ EXERCISE 4–4

If your health care institution has an active ethics committee, attend one of their sessions. Who is on the committee? Were family members or patients allowed to attend? Which structural model was used in the deliberations? Was their final recommendation consistent with your expectations? Would you have changed the outcome based on your use of the MORAL model?

SUMMARY

In ethics, unlike legal concerns, there are frequently no easy answers. Sometimes there are no definable answers and nurses must explore new issues and develop novel solutions. The more nurses are versed in ethical principles and everyday ethical issues, the more confidence they will have in working with more difficult situations. Nurses should be encouraged to attend ethics committee hearings and ethical grand rounds as a starting point in developing their own ethical values and positions.

AFTER COMPLETING THIS CHAPTER, YOU SHOULD BE ABLE TO

- Distinguish law from ethics.
- Compare and contrast the three different ethical theories of deontology, teleology, and principalism.

GUIDELINES: HOSPITAL ETHICS COMMITTEES

1. The hospital ethics committee should consist of a core group of health care professionals who are knowledgeable about legal and ethical issues within the institution.
2. The patient is the focus of ethical dilemmas. Decisions are made based on patient values, desires, needs, and capabilities.
3. The hospital ethics committee serves as an objective body to provide assistance to those in need during difficult decision-making times. Hospital ethics committees are supportive of patients and patients' families, staff, and physicians.
4. The hospital ethics committee projects a positive public image through its committees and decisions. Such committee meetings aid in closing the gap between unrealistic societal expectations and the reality of everyday health care delivery.
5. The hospital ethics committee serves in a preventive capacity against potential litigation by being knowledgeable of current court decisions and by incorporating the same into its deliberations. This is especially true in the broad area of risk management.
6. The hospital ethics committee must guard against breaching patient privacy by ensuring that confidential matters are discussed only when vital and with only those staff members and medical personnel who are directly concerned with the patient's care.

- Define and apply to nursing practice the eight ethical principles of autonomy, beneficence, nonmaleficence, veracity, fidelity, justice, paternalism, and respect for others.
- Analyze the MORAL model in ethical decision making.
- Discuss the importance and role of hospital ethics committees and ethics grand rounds.

APPLY YOUR ETHICAL KNOWLEDGE

- How can the professional nurse employ the concepts of ethics and law in clinical practice settings?
- Do professional nurses use ethical theories or ethical principles in clinical practice settings?
- Can the MORAL model be used truly at the bedside?
- What types of ethical dilemmas do professional nurses face on a daily basis?
- What types of ethical dilemmas will we face in the new millennium?

YOU BE THE ETHICIST

Until last April, Tyrell Dueck was a normal eighth-grader in Canada, hoping that his favorite team would win the Stanley Cup for the third time. Then, early in the school year, he slipped climbing out of the shower and discovered a lump on his leg. He was then diagnosed with bone cancer.

After receiving two rounds of chemotherapy and being told that further therapy would mean the amputation of his leg, he announced that he wanted therapy stopped. He and his parents, devout fundamentalist Christians, decided to leave his health in God's hands and seek alternative therapy. The decision sparked a court battle between his parents, who supported Tyrell's decision, and the health care team, who sought to compel continued medical treatment and the planned amputation. The battle ultimately ended when doctors said that his cancer had spread to his lungs and that there was little more that could be done for Tyrell.

Ethical Questions

1. What are the compelling rights that this case addresses?
2. Whose rights should take precedence?
3. Does a child (here, a competent 14 year old) have the right to determine what will happen to him? Should he ethically have this right?
4. How would you have decided the outcome if his disease state had not intervened?

REFERENCES

Aiken, T. D., and Catalano, J. T. (1994). *Legal, Ethical, and Political Issues in Nursing.* Philadelphia, PA: F. A. Davis Company.

Boyer, M., Ellis, K., Harris, D. R., and Soukhanov, A. H., eds. (1991). *The American Heritage Dictionary.* (2nd ed.). Boston: Houghton Mifflin Company.

Guido, G. W. (1988). *Legal Issues in Nursing: A Source Book for Practice.* Norwalk, CT: Appleton & Lange.

Hall, J. K. (1990). Understanding the fine line between law and ethics. *Nursing 90* 20(10), 37.

Halloran, M. C. (1982). Rational ethical judgments utilizing a decision-making tool. *Heart and Lung* 11(6), 566–570.

Joint Commission for Accreditation of Healthcare Organizations. (1992). *Accreditation Manual for Hospitals.* Oakbrook Terrace, IL: Author.

Lamm, R. (1999). The ethics of excess. *Hastings Center Report* 24(6), 14.

Thiroux, J. (1977). *Ethics: Theory and Practice.* Philadelphia: Macmillan.

III LIABILITY ISSUES

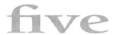

Standards of Care

■ PREVIEW

Standards of care are implemented daily in all aspects of health care delivery and in all practice settings, forming the basis for quality, competent health care. Standards of care are the criteria for determining if less than adequate care was delivered to health care consumers. This chapter explores the foundations of standards of care, describing how they are derived and defined within courts of law.

■ KEY CONCEPTS

standards of care	external standards	error in judgment rule
internal standards	locality rule	two schools of thought doctrine

DEFINITION OF STANDARDS OF CARE

Standards of care may be viewed as the level or degree of quality considered adequate by a given profession. Standards of care are the skills and learning commonly possessed by members of a profession. Created by the duty undertaken, standards of care describe the minimal requirements that define an acceptable level of care, which is to exercise ordinary and reasonable care to see that no unnecessary harm comes to the patient. The court, in *King v. State of Louisiana* (1999), further defined standards of care as "legal duty of care or standards of care means a nurse must have and use the knowledge and skill or-

63

dinarily possessed and used by nurses actively practicing in the nurse's speciality area" (at 1029).

The basic purposes of standards of care are to protect and safeguard the public as a whole. Were there no standards of care, consumers would open themselves to varying levels of care and varying degrees of quality of care, and the consumers would eventually be the persons who suffered. Standards of care have evolved to help the health care recipient avoid substandard health care, and to give guidance to health care providers.

Standards of care may easily be differentiated from objectives, philosophies, and guidelines. *Objectives* are goals that give direction to what must be accomplished. For example, a goal may be to ambulate the patient 20 steps. *Philosophies* state why an action is performed. Ambulation of the postoperative patient helps to prevent complications due to thrombus formation and orthostatic hypotension. *Guidelines* describe recommended courses of action. For example, patients should be ambulated more than once per day, preferably when they are most rested and steady on their feet.

Standards are authoritative statements promulgated by a profession by which the quality of practice, service, or education can be evaluated (American Nurses Association, 1998). A standard of care may be written as "The early postoperative patient must be ambulated pursuant to a valid order with two nurses or assistants in attendance, and vital signs will be taken and recorded both before and after ambulation."

■ EXERCISE 5–1

Review your current institution policy and procedure manual. Randomly select a policy and procedure and show how the language used makes this a standard as opposed to an objective, philosophy, or guideline. Then rewrite the policy so that it is an objective, a philosophy, and a guideline. Why do standards give the most guidance to nurses for effective patient care?

ESTABLISHMENT OF NURSING STANDARDS OF CARE

Nursing standards of care may be established in a variety of ways and often are classified into two broad categories: internal and external standards.

Internal Standards

Internal standards are those set by the role and education of the nurse or by individual institutions. These include the professional nurse's job description, education, and expertise as well as individual institution's policies and procedures.

In court cases, institutional policies and procedures are presented and evaluated to determine if a nurse defendant has met the standards of care for that given institution. In *Beck v. Director, Arkansas Employment Security Department* (1999), a clearly written policy existed for the dispensing and charting of medications. The nurse in this case admitted that she made it a practice to wait until the end of her shift to chart all medications that she had given during the shift. She further admitted that at the end of the day in question she could not remember what she had given or to whom it was given. The nurse also admitted on one occasion that she had given Darvocet without looking at the patient's record and that the patient had received the medication earlier than it should have been administered. The court upheld the termination of this nurse because she was guilty of misconduct by intentionally violating a policy that was established for the patients' well-being and safety.

Horton v. Carolina Medicorp, Inc. (1996) and *Donaldson v. Sanders* (1995) illustrate the importance of adhering to written policies and procedures in avoiding potential liability. *Horton* concerned a 24-hour period in which a patient failed to void following removal of an indwelling catheter. Although written policy and procedures existed, the physician was not notified of the patient's failure to void; in fact, the nurses were not aware of the fact because they failed to appropriately assess and monitor the patient during the same time period. In *Donaldson,* a patient who had been hospitalized for deep vein thrombosis superimposed on underlying peripheral vascular disease, hypertension, and congestive heart failure, had a greatly diminished pedal pulse sometime during the night shift. His lower extremity was cool to the touch, pale, and the foot had a bluish discoloration. The nurse attending the patient did not notify the physician, but rather elected to wait until the morning report to inform other nurses of her findings, requesting that they notify the physician when he came in to see the patient.

Santa Rosa Medical Center v. Robinson (1977), which remains the leading case in its area, extended internal standards to include hospital in-service films as policy and procedure. In that case, the standard of care for closed-head injuries was reduced to an in-service film, and the viewing of the film was mandatory for all staff members. When members of the staff violated the standard of care as outlined in the film, the court allowed the jury to view the film to show what the hospital's standard of care should have been.

Courts have routinely allowed policy and procedure manuals to be introduced as criteria for the acceptable standard of care. Policies and procedures need not be in writing to be considered legally enforceable. Unwritten policies may potentiate liability because not all employees are aware of the policy's existence. In *Hartman v. Riverside Methodist Hospital* (1989), the patient had undergone emergency surgery after eating a full meal. The nurses in the postanesthesia care unit were informed that the patient had received Fentanyl and that she "had a full stomach." Precautions should have been taken to ensure that Mrs. Hartman did not aspirate. Instead, the patient was given a pain medication and died of aspiration. The unwritten policy of the attending anesthesiologist was that no medications were to be given his patients unless he was first consulted and ordered such medication directly. The other attending anesthesiologists had no such unwritten policy and nurses could give pain medications without prior approval. Because some of the nurses did not know this unwritten policy, this particular patient was medicated, and the court found in favor of her family and against the hospital and employees.

External Standards

External standards are those set by the state boards of nursing, professional organizations, specialty nursing organizations, federal organizations, and federal guidelines. These standards are seen as external as they transcend individual practitioners and single institutions. In many instances, external standards are synonymous with national standards.

State boards of nursing publish acceptable standards in the state nurse practice act or in rules and regulations promulgated to enforce the state nurse practice act. These rules and regulations have the force of law because they are created to carry out the law. Courts consider whether standards of care were met or violated based on the evidence presented.

Professional organizations add to the body of acceptable standards of care for professional nursing. The profession has the inherent right to direct and control its activities. The most active professional organization in this area is the American Nurses Association (ANA) with its state components. The ANA Congress for Nursing Practice set eight basic standards of care in 1973. Based on the nursing process, these eight standards are applicable to all nurses, regardless of clinical specialty. These standards of care for nursing practice represent the first step in unifying standards of care throughout all jurisdictions.

The ANA and the state nurses associations have lobbied to encourage enactment of these generic standards of care through state legislative processes. One of the basic arguments for such generalized standards of care is to upgrade the standards set by individual hospitals and institutions that were traditionally based on a local standard of acceptability.

In 1974, the ANA's publication of specialty standards of care was first published. These specialty standards of care were published for various clinical specialties, including (1) community health nursing, (2) geriatric nursing, (3) maternal–child health nursing, (4) mental health nursing, and (5) medical–surgical nursing. Standards published in the past few years have greatly expanded clinical applications to areas outside acute care settings, including standards for advanced nurse practitioners, standards of college health nursing practice, standards for professional development, standards of diabetic nursing, standards of genetics clinical nursing practice, and standards of parish nursing practice. Today, ANA publishes some 22 standards that pertain to specialty practice areas (ANA, 1999).

In 1991, the ANA Congress of Nursing Practice adopted the Standards of Clinical Nursing Practice. The second edition was published in 1998. This document is divided into standards of care and standards of professional performance. The standards of performance section outlines professional activities such as formal and continuing education, research, ethics, peer review, and continuous quality improvement. The language of this document has been broadened so that standards of care and standards of performance are described in terms of competency as opposed to reasonable or acceptable level of performance (ANA, 1998). This broadened language has been incorporated so that criteria used to measure compliance may change as needed with technological advances and alternative delivery sites.

Standards of care are also set by the National League for Nursing (NLN). The NLN evaluates the quality of nursing education and accredits schools of nursing, both on the undergraduate and graduate levels. Directly and indirectly, these standards of education influence the quality of acceptable nursing standards within a community.

Individual nursing specialty-practice organizations also publish standards of care to upgrade and generalize the standards for patients within a given clinical setting or within a given category. For example:

1. The American Association of Critical-Care Nurses (AACN) publishes standards of care for the critically ill patient.

2. The Emergency Nurses Association (ENA) publishes standards of care for trauma and urgent care patients.
3. The Oncology Nursing Society (ONS) publishes standards for cancer patient care.
4. The Association of Operating Room Nurses (AORN) publishes standards of care for patients in the perioperative setting.
5. On an international perspective, the International Council of Nursing (ICN) has published its standards through an ethical code (1973).

Federal organizations and federal guidelines are other examples of external standards. The Joint Commission for Accreditation of Healthcare Organizations (JCAHO) sets nursing standards by publishing the *Accreditation Manual for Hospitals* on a yearly basis (1999). Their requirements for individualized nursing care plans set a standard of care. For example, one of their standards states that patients must be assessed and individualized care plans written. Such a requirement may actually assist nurses if a subsequent lawsuit is filed. The individualized care plan may indeed show that the nursing staff did meet the standard of care for safety by innovative measures aimed at preventing an individual patient's injury or further injury.

In *Pugh v. Mayeaux* (1998), a patient had intermittent labor contractions and was slightly dilated on admission to the acute care setting. Pancreatitis, not explained by her history, developed in the hospital. The physicians determined that the pancreatitis did not threaten the fetus, but the patient was continuously assessed for signs of fetal distress. When signs of distress occurred, an emergency cesarean section was performed, but not quickly enough to prevent permanent damage due to hypoxia.

The nurses were applauded by the court for their individualization of this patient's care. When the patient was admitted, the nurses were alert to the possibility that another medical condition could manifest itself. In fact, it was the nursing staff who first assessed signs of pancreatitis and alerted the physicians. The patient was transferred to the intensive care unit after the nurse notified the physician of the patient's worsening condition and called to recommend such a transfer. In the intensive care unit, labor and delivery nurses were available to check the fetal monitor and assess the infant's condition.

Although there were catastrophic complications to the baby, the court indicated in their final summary the respect that the justices had for the nurses and how competently they both cared for the patient and communicated all aspects of that care with the physicians.

A similar conclusion was reached in *Barnett v. University of Cincinnati Hospital* (1998). In that case, a home health care patient became increasingly more forgetful and irrational. The social worker who saw her determined that these were signs of her inability to live independently and arranged for admission to an acute care geriatric psychiatric unit of the hospital.

At the hospital, the patient was diagnosed with dementia and agitation, for which Ativan was prescribed. The nurses assisted the patient out of bed and into a "geri chair," where the patient slept for a few hours. They repositioned her in bed, where she slept for the majority of the morning. She was awaked for meals and medications, and the nurses assisted in feeding the patient.

She was assessed on a routine basis and was later found on the floor after she fell trying to get out of bed. The resulting lawsuit was dismissed by the Court of Claims of

---

INTERNATIONAL CODE FOR NURSES

The fundamental responsibility of the nurse is fourfold: to promote health, to prevent illness, to restore health, and to alleviate suffering.

The need for nursing is universal. Inherent in nursing is respect for life, dignity, and rights of man. It is unrestricted by considerations of nationality, race, creed, color, age, sex, politics, or social status.

Nurses render health services to the individual, the family, and the community and coordinate their services with those of related groups.

NURSES AND PEOPLE
The nurse's primary responsibility is to those people who require nursing care.

The nurse, in providing care, promotes an environment in which the values, customs, and spiritual beliefs of the individual are respected.

The nurse holds in confidence personal information and uses judgment in sharing this information.

NURSES AND PRACTICE
The nurse carries personal responsibility for nursing practice and for maintaining competence by continual learning. The nurse maintains the highest standards of nursing care possible within the reality of a specific situation.

The nurse uses judgment in relation to individual competence when accepting and delegating responsibilities.

The nurse when acting in a professional capacity should at all times maintain standards of personal conduct which reflect credit upon the profession.

NURSES AND SOCIETY
The nurse shares with other citizens the responsibility for initiating and supporting action to meet the health and social needs of the public.

NURSES AND CO-WORKERS
The nurse sustains a cooperative relationship with co-workers in nursing and other fields. The nurse takes appropriate action to safeguard the individual when his care is endangered by a co-worker or any other person.

NURSES AND THE PROFESSION
The nurse plays the major role in determining and implementing desirable standards of nursing practice and nursing education.

The nurse is active in developing a core of professional knowledge.

The nurse, acting through the professional organization, participates in establishing and maintaining equitable social and economic working conditions in nursing.

From International Council of Nurses. (1973). *Code for Nurses*. Geneva, Switzerland: Author. Used by permission.

Ohio. They ruled that close supervision of a dementia patient sedated with Ativan requires periodic checks to ensure the patient's safety. But close supervision does not mean one-to-one in-room supervision. The court praised the nurses for placing this patient in a room next to the nurses' station so that they could keep a closer watch on her, and in maintaining the frequent periodic checks that were done and documented. They also did not fault the nurses for not restraining the patient while she was asleep in her room.

Other federal agencies, such as the Social Security Administration (overseeing Medicare and Medicaid funding, nursing home qualifications, and maternal and child health programs), also are directly responsible for setting nursing standards of care. These agencies serve a vital role in setting standards of care as they periodically publish rules and regulations regarding the care of patients, and in setting minimum qualifications for those who care for patients receiving their support. For example, the requirement that a registered nurse perform and record complete physical assessment data on hospitalized patients on a 24-hour basis was initially introduced by federal funding agencies as a Medicare and Medicaid requirement.

The court has also seemed to create a new source of external standards in *Hall v. Huff* (1997). In that case, a patient's care providers were having difficulty managing his end-stage renal disease. Peripheral venous access sites had been damaged by repeated dialysis, and a central venous catheter was inserted for medications. During insertion, the catheter was advanced too far, perforating the heart muscle, and the patient subsequently died. The family brought a lawsuit for the patient's wrongful death.

In holding both the physician and the nurses accountable for the death, the court noted that despite several warnings printed on the manufacturer's label insert for the central venous catheter, cautioning health care personnel to be alert for signs and symptoms of cardiac tamponade, neither the attending physician nor the nurses caring for this patient discovered the condition until after the patient died. The court noted that the nurses' notes, charted on the days following the insertion of the catheter, reflected that the nurses were seeing signs and symptoms of cardiac tamponade, though none of the nurses recognized the signs and symptoms for what they were. The court ruled that it was within the standard of care for the competent nurse to detect such a complication following the insertion of a central venous catheter.

■ EXERCISE 5–2

Obtain copies of standards of care from two specialty organizations, such as AACN, AORN, ENA, or ONS. Compare and contrast the written standards against your institution's policies and procedures. Do your internal standards compare with the national standards? How would one begin to rewrite standards of care?

What are the nurse's ethical duties regarding standards of care? Are there instances in which the nurse might ethically feel obligated to relax a standard of care? For example, do you always awaken patients at night for routine vital signs, in particular patients who have finally had their pain relieved and are now sleeping for the first time in 20 hours? When, if ever, do ethical principles become equally important?

NATIONAL AND LOCAL STANDARDS OF CARE

Appropriate standards of care may be decided based on a national versus local standard. *National standards* are based on reasonableness and are the average degree of skill, care, and diligence exercised by members of the same profession. Such a national standard means that nurses in rural settings must meet the same standards as those members of the profession practicing in large urban areas.

In areas of specialty practice, courts are almost universally holding health care providers to a national standard of care. An older case, *Brune v. Belinkoff* (1968), illustrates this point. In that case, it was ruled that a person holding himself out as a specialist should be held to the same standard of skill and care as the average member of that specialty, not merely the skill and ability of specialists practicing in a particular city.

There are two important reasons for national standards of care, and both are fairly obvious. With the advent of educational programs, educational videos, and the ability to transport specialists across the nation, all areas with health care delivery systems have access to the same information and educational opportunities. This is increasingly true today as advancing technology allows patient data and test results to be reviewed by consultants worldwide. A second—and perhaps more important—reason is that all patients have the right to quality health care, whether hospitalized in a small community or a large, university institution.

Some states still follow a *locality rule,* which allows standards of care to be viewed from the perspective of care within a given geographic area or a "similar community." Under this perspective, health care is judged by the skill, care, and diligence of members of the profession within that geographic area. The trend today is toward a total national standard.

 ## GUIDELINES: STANDARDS OF CARE

1. Recognize that all professions have standards of care. Standards are the minimal level of expertise that must be delivered to the patient. Standards of care are the starting point for greater expectations.
2. Standards of care may be either externally or internally set. The nurse is responsible for both categories of standards: those set on a national bases and those set by the role of nursing.
3. Standards of care may be found in:
   a. The state nurse practice act
   b. Published standards of professional organizations and specialty practice groups such as the American Association of Critical-Care Nurses or the Association of Operating Room Nurses
   c. Federal agency guidelines and regulations
   d. Hospital policy and procedure manuals
   e. The individual nurse's job description
4. Nurses are accountable for all standards of care as they pertain to their profession. To remain competent and skillful, the nurse is encouraged to read professional journals and to attend pertinent continuing education and in-service programs.
5. Standards of care are determined for the judicial system by expert witnesses. Such persons testify to the prevailing standards in the community—standards that all nurses are accountable for matching and exceeding. Adherence to such standards ensures that patients receive quality, competent nursing care.

IMPORTANCE OF STANDARDS OF CARE TO THE INDIVIDUAL NURSE

Standards of care are referenced in malpractice cases against nurses to show that they breached the duty of care owed the patient. *Duty of care* has frequently been defined to mean the applicable standard of care. The test for the court to apply is what a reasonable, prudent nurse, with like experience and education, would do under similar conditions in the same community (*King v. State of Louisiana*, 1999).

A recent case example that distinguishes the acceptable standard of care for various services within a health care setting is *Sabol v. Richmond Heights General Hospital* (1996). In that case, the patient was admitted to the intensive care unit of a general acute care hospital following an attempt to commit suicide with a medication overdose. The attending physician wanted to stabilize the patient's condition while his family made arrangements for transfer to a psychiatric facility. There was a delay in obtaining the patient's transfer because of lack of insurance coverage.

At the time of admission, the institution agreed to the patient's hospitalization, even though the institution had no inpatient psychiatric unit. After admission, the patient became more paranoid and delusional. A nurse sat at his bedside and tried to calm him. The nursing staff deliberated whether to restrain the patient, but decided against it, fearing that it would only compound the situation by making him more agitated and increasing his level of paranoia. The patient got out of bed, knocked down the nurse in his room, fought his way past two other nurses who were trying to corral him, and ran off the unit. Once away from the unit, he kicked out a third-story window and jumped, fracturing his arm and sustaining other relatively minor injuries.

The Court of Appeals of Ohio ruled that the nurses were not negligent. The nurses realized that the patient was a danger to himself, and they acted reasonably under the circumstances. Their actions were fully consistent with basic professional standards of practice for medical–surgical nurses in an acute care facility. They did not have, nor were they expected to have, specialized psychiatric nursing education and would not be judged as though they did.

When deciding which standards of care apply, courts also consider the error in judgment rule and a two schools of thought doctrine. The honest *error in judgment rule* allows the court to evaluate the standards of care given a patient even if there was an honest error in judgment, including an error in the diagnosis. What the court evaluates is the care given and whether that care met the prevailing standards, not whether the judgment was correct. *Fraijo v. Hartland* (1979) is the landmark case in this matter. In that case, the court stated that a nurse is not bound to do exactly what another nurse would do, only to select one approach among several that exists at the time and is reasonable.

The second consideration by courts is the *two schools of thought doctrine,* which supports the nurse who chooses among alternative means of delivering quality health care. In this instance, the court evaluates the standards of care given when the nurse chooses among the alternative modes of treatment. Were standards of care met in the chosen mode of treatment? If the answer is yes, courts support the quality of care as delivered, even though other nurses would choose a different course of action. *Fury v. Thomas Jefferson University,* (1984) remains the leading case illustrating this doctrine.

Standards of care provide the criterion for determining if a nurse has violated the state

EXAMPLE OF A STATE'S STANDARDS OF NURSING PRACTICE

The registered professional nurse shall:

1. Be responsible for knowing and conforming to the law governing the practice of professional nursing.
2. Be responsible and accountable for his or her actions commensurate with educational preparation and experience in nursing.
3. Assess and evaluate the health status of the patient or client based upon objective and subjective data as it relates to the physiological, psychological, and social processes of the particular individual.
4. Make nursing judgments and decisions about the nursing care for the patient or client by using assessment data to formulate and implement a plan of goals and objectives; and to evaluate the patient or client response(s) to the nursing care.
5. Be responsible for accurate reporting and documentation of the patient's or client's symptoms, responses, and progress.
6. Evaluate a patient's or client's status and institute appropriate nursing intervention that might be required to stabilize a patient's or client's condition or prevent complications.
7. Promote and participate in patient or client education and counseling based on the individual's health needs and illness status and involve the individual and significant others for a better understanding and implementation of immediate and long-term health goals.
8. Provide patient or client and significant others with information needed by them to make decisions and choices about promoting, maintaining, and restoring health.
9. Collaborate with members of related health disciplines in the interest of the patient's or client's health care.
10. Consult and utilize community agencies as resources for continuity of patient or client care.
11. Be responsible for the knowledge of the rationale for the effects thereof in the administration of medications or treatments as prescribed by a licensed physician or dentist.
12. Be responsible and accountable for the quality and the quantity of nursing care rendered under his or her supervision. Assignment and delegation of duties to other nursing personnel shall be commensurate with their educational preparation and demonstrated proficiency.
13. Assist personnel under his or her supervision to develop the necessary skills needed for continued competence in providing patient or client care, comfort, and safety.
14. Be responsible for individual professional growth.

Source: Texas Register. *Licensure and Practice.* Rule 217.13.

nurse practice act. The court in *Botehlo v. Bycura* (1984) held that when patients choose a practitioner of a recognized branch of the health care professions, they elect to undergo the care and treatment common to that profession. Thus, nurses must meet the standards of care of the profession. Each state publishes acceptable standards of care as part of the nurse practice act or through the rules and regulations promulgated by the state board of nursing. Violations of those standards open the nurse to possible disciplinary action by the board. See Chapter 11 for a full explanation of nurse practice acts and the board of nursing.

Standards of care may be used by the state criminal system to decide if the nurse has violated the state or city criminal codes. In *State of Louisiana v. Brenner* (1986), standards of care were examined to show that the nursing home staff had failed to properly train staff members, to supply an adequate staff, and to adequately maintain patients' records, among other charges of cruelty, neglect, and mistreatment of the infirm.

Finally, standards of care provide the criterion for placing nursing practice on a professional level. Standards of care both increase the status of the nursing profession and, at the same time, set minimal standards for nursing practice. National standards of care

---

ANA CODE OF ETHICS

1. The nurse provides services with respect for human dignity and the uniqueness of the client unrestricted by considerations of social or economic status, personal attributes, or nature of health problems.
2. The nurse safeguards the client's right to privacy by judiciously protecting information of a confidential nature.
3. The nurse acts to safeguard the client and the public when health care and safety are affected by the incompetent, unethical, or illegal practice of any person.
4. The nurse assumes responsibility and accountability for individual nursing judgments and actions.
5. The nurse maintains competence in nursing.
6. The nurse exercises informed judgment and uses individual competence and qualifications as criteria in seeking consultation, accepting responsibilities, and delegating nursing activities to others.
7. The nurse participates in activities that contribute to the ongoing development of the profession's body of knowledge.
8. The nurse participates in the profession's efforts to implement and improve standards of nursing.
9. The nurse participates in the profession's efforts to establish and maintain conditions of employment conducive to high quality nursing care.
10. The nurse participates in the profession's efforts to protect the public from misinformation and misrepresentation and to maintain the integrity of nursing.
11. The nurse collaborates with members of the health professions and other citizens in promoting community and national efforts to meet the health needs of the public.

Reprinted by permission from *Code for Nurses with Interpretive Statements*. Kansas City, MO, 1985.

have further increased this acceptance of professional status. National standards dictate that all patients receive the same expert nursing care, whether they are cared for in a major medical center or in a small community hospital. All professions have standards. The ANA, through its *Code of Ethics,* has delineated standards promoting professionalism and quality nursing care.

EXPERT TESTIMONY

In courts of law, the deviation of the standard of care is shown through the use of expert witnesses. See Chapter 3 for a review of this concept.

EXPANDED NURSING ROLES

With the advent of expanded roles in nursing and the rewriting of several state nurse practice acts to accommodate these expanded roles, the standard of care that is owed the patient by advanced nurse practitioners is frequently that of a medical (physician) standard of care or a "nurse practitioner" standard of care. Chapter 12 discusses the expanded nursing role and further clarifies this concept.

■ EXERCISE 5–3

Read the "Example of a State's Standards of Nursing Practice" in this chapter. Give examples of how these standards are met in your clinical practice and how these standards support the standards of care of your institution.

SUMMARY

Standards of care, derived from a variety of sources, are crucial in ensuring that patients are provided quality, competent nursing care. Standards of care form the basis of the professional duty owed to patient.

AFTER COMPLETING THIS CHAPTER, YOU SHOULD BE ABLE TO

- Define standards of care from both a legal and a nursing perspective.
- Compare and contrast internal versus external standards of care.
- Discuss the concept of the reasonably prudent nurse in defining standards of care.
- Describe the role of the nurse expert witness in determining standards of care in court cases.

APPLY YOUR LEGAL KNOWLEDGE

- How do standards differ from objectives, philosophies, and guidelines?
- How can the professional nurse ensure that he or she is practicing according to standards of care?
- Why are there both internal and external standards when the "national" standard of care is favored over the locality rule? Are these separate concepts?
- How would one prepare to be an expert witness for the purpose of defining standards of care?

YOU BE THE JUDGE

On April 17, 1993, Wendy Smedes, a registered nurse, was caring for Leon Bayless on the evening shift (2:15 to 10:45 P.M.). Mr. Bayless had peripheral vascular disease, was in a terminal condition, and had chosen a do-not-resuscitate policy. He was ischemic below the waist. Smedes and the nursing staff were instructed to make the patient as comfortable as possible. The patient's son, Dr. Joseph Bayless, an anesthesiologist at the hospital, visited his father during this time.

At 5:00 P.M., Smedes administered Percocet to the patient. It soon became apparent that the Percocet was doing little to relieve Mr. Bayless's pain. Smedes called Dr. Shapiro, the physician in charge of Mr. Bayless's care, and a morphine drip, at 10 mg/hr, with a 3-mg loading dose, was started. According to Dr. Bayless, Dr. Shapiro asked him if the dosage was adequate, and it was understood that this order was a "starting point" and that the dosage was less important than controlling the patient's pain.

Thomas Merkley was the clinical leader that afternoon. While Smedes was occupied with other patients, Merkley picked up a solution containing 125 mg of morphine from the pharmacy. Dr. Bayless testified that he hung the bag at 6:20 P.M. and "let it run wide open" until his father said that he was feeling better. About 30 minutes later, Smedes reassessed the patient and noted that the intravenous (IV) drip was being administered correctly. She checked on the patient again at 9:30 P.M., and she charted that the patient had a normal respiratory rate and that the IV solution was running correctly. The IV was timed to run over a 12-hour period.

At 11:30 P.M., Merkley went into the patient's room because the IV pump was alarming and found the bag of morphine empty. Dr. Bayless, noting that his father was restless and uncomfortable, ordered Merkley to begin a second bag of morphine. On his way to the pharmacy, Merkley saw his nursing supervisor, informed her of the situation, and was told to fill out a variance report.

Dr. Bayless offered to write an order for the second bag of morphine, but Merkley refused to accept an order from a family member. Therefore, Dr. Bayless phoned a second anesthesiologist and had him order the morphine. This telephone order occurred at 12:20 A.M., but Merkley backdated it to appear as if it were written at 9:00 P.M. the previous evening. Mr. Bayless received approximately 100 mg of the second bag of morphine before he died at 1:00 A.M.. The death certificate listed his cause of death as cardiorespiratory failure due to gangrene of the left lower extremity secondary to severe arteriosclerosis.

A variance report was completed, and the hospital subsequently fired both Merkley and Smedes. When the hospital notified the board of the investigation against Merkley, the board filed an administrative complaint, charging him with gross negligence and unprofessional conduct. The board concluded that Merkley has committed four acts of unprofessional conduct:

1. Inaccurate recording, falsifying narcotic or otherwise destroying records
2. Failing to collaborate with other members of a health care team as necessary to meet the health needs of a patient
3. Failing to observe the conditions, signs, and symptoms of a patient; to record the information; or to report significant changes to the appropriate persons
4. Failing to perform nursing functions in a manner consistent with established or customary standards

The board suspended his license for one year, then stayed the suspension, placing Merkley on probation for one year.

Legal Questions

1. Did Merkley fall below the standards of care? If yes, which standards of care did he fail to uphold?
2. Should Merkley be cited for failing to collaborate with other members of the health team?
3. Did the nurse fail to record and report the patient's condition to appropriate persons?
4. How would you decide the outcome of this case?

REFERENCES

American Nurses Association (1999). *Catalogue of Publications.* Washington, DC: Author.
American Nurses Association (1985). *Code of Ethics with Interpretive Statements.* Kansas City, MO: Author.
American Nurses Association (1998). *Standards of Clinical Nursing Practice* (2nd ed.). Washington, DC: Author.
American Nurses Association (1973). *Standards of Nursing Practice.* Kansas City, MO: Author.
Barnett v. University of Cincinnati Hospital, 702 N.E.2d 979 (Ohio Ct. Cl., 1998).
Beck v. Director, Arkansas Employment Security Department, 987 S.W.2d 733 (Ark. App., 1999).
Botehlo v. Bycura, 320 S.E.2d 59 (Pa. Super., 1984).
Brune v. Belinkoff, 354 Mass. 102, 235 N.E.2d 793 (1968).
Donaldson v. Sanders, 661 So.2d 1010 (La. App., 1995).
Fraijo v. Hartland Hospital, 99 Cal. Rptr. 3d 331, 160 Calif. Rptr. 848 (1979).
Fury v. Thomas Jefferson University, 472 A.2d 101 (Louisiana, 1984).
Hall v. Huff, 957 S.W.2d 90 (Tex. App., 1997).
Hartman v. Riverside Methodist Hospital, 577 N.E.2d 112 (Ohio, 1989).
Horton v. Carolina Medicorp, Inc., 472 S.E.2d 778 (North Carolina, 1996).
International Council of Nursing (1973). *Code for Nurses.* Geneva: Author.

Joint Commission for Accreditation of Healthcare Organizations (1999). *Accreditation Manual for Hospitals.* Oakbrook Terrace, IL: Author.

King v. State of Louisiana, 728 So.2d 1027 (La. App., 1999).

Pugh v. Mayeaux, 702 So.2d 988 (La. App., 1998).

Santa Rosa Medical Center v. Robinson, 560 S.W.2d 751 (Tex. Civ. App.–San Antonio, 1977).

Sobol v. Richmond Heights General Hospital, 676 N.E.2d 958 (Ohio App., 1996).

State of Louisiana v. Brenner, 486 So.2d 101 (Louisiana, 1986).

Texas Register. *Licensure and Practice.* Rule 217.13.

six

Tort Law

■ PREVIEW

Intentional wrongdoings and negligence/malpractice have their origins in tort law. Although most cases that are filed against nurse-defendants concern negligence and malpractice, nurses may be held equally accountable for intentional and quasi-intentional actions. Health care providers and the general public frequently interchange the terms *malpractice* and *negligence*. While the distinction is technical, nurses should be able to distinguish between the two terms and to apply both in the provision of quality nursing care. This chapter discusses the elements of negligence, malpractice, and intentional torts, and presents guidelines for nurses practicing in all practice settings for preventing potential lawsuits in this area of the law.

■ KEY CONCEPTS

tort	injury or harm	false imprisonment
negligence	damages	conversion of property
malpractice	res ipsa loquitor	trespass to land
tortfeasor	locality rule	intentional infliction of emotional
duty of care	intentional tort	distress
breach of duty	quasi-intentional tort	invasion of privacy
foreseeability	assault	defamation
causation	battery	

DEFINITION OF TORTS

A *tort* is a civil wrong committed against a person or the person's property. Torts, derived from the French, are "acts or omissions which unlawfully violate a person's rights by law and for which the appropriate remedy is a common law action for damages by the injured party" (Keeton, 1984, p. 2). Tort law is based on fault. The accountable person either failed to meet his or her responsibility or performed an action below the allowable standard of care. Tort law is distinguishable from contract law. Because torts are civil wrongs, they are not based on contracts. Tort law may also be said to be based on personal transgressions in that the responsible person performed an action incorrectly or omitted a necessary action. Review Chapter 1 for a more thorough discussion of tort law.

NEGLIGENCE VERSUS MALPRACTICE

Of primary importance to health care providers is the area of negligence or malpractice. Used interchangeably, there is a fine distinction between the two terms.

Negligence is a general term that denotes conduct lacking in due care. Thus, negligence equates with carelessness, a deviation from the standard of care that a reasonable person would use in a particular set of circumstances. Negligence may also include doing something that the reasonable and prudent person would not do. As such, anyone—including nonmedical persons—can be liable for negligence. An example is a fall by an elderly person who is being cared for by a sitter. The reasonable person in the place of the sitter has a standard of care to prevent such a fall.

A case that illustrates the concept of negligence is *Dent v. Memorial Hospital of Adel* (1998). In this case, a hospitalized child had an episode of apnea and was brought to the facility's emergency center by her parents. The emergency center physician admitted the child for observation and ordered a pediatric apnea monitor.

After admission to the pediatric unit, the child again suffered an apneic episode, which was not discovered for several minutes, despite the fact that the apnea monitor had been placed on the child by the nursing staff. The reason for the delay was that the monitor was never turned to its "on" position. A code was called, but it too was delayed because the items appropriate for pediatric patients (airways, endotracheal tubes, and laryngoscope blades) were not on the unit's crash cart and had to be retrieved from other areas of the facility.

Simple acts, the court held, are not exercises in professional judgment. "It is ordinary negligence for nurses not to check that the on/off switch on a pediatric apnea monitor is on . . . . It is ordinary negligence for nurses not to make sure that a crash cart is stocked with items for pediatric patients" (*Dent v. Memorial Hospital of Adel*, 1998, at 514). Interestingly, the court did hold that the selection of items appropriate for placement on a crash cart does involve professional judgment, but the restocking or validation of whether those items are on the cart does not involve professional judgment.

Malpractice is a more specific term and looks at a professional standard of care as well as the professional status of the caregiver. To be liable for malpractice, the *tortfeasor* (person committing the civil wrong) must be a professional—physician, nurse, accountant, lawyer, or other type of professional. Courts have continually defined malpractice as any professional misconduct or unreasonable lack of skill or fidelity in professional or judiciary duties. Moreover, this wrong or injudicious treatment results in injury, unnecessary suffering, or death to the patient, and proceeds from ignorance, carelessness, want of proper professional skill, disregard of established rules and principles, neglect, or a malicious or criminal intent. In a more modern definition, malpractice is the failure of a professional person to act in accordance with the prevailing professional standards or failure to foresee consequences that a professional person, having the necessary skills and education, should foresee.

The same types of acts may form the basis for negligence or malpractice. If the action is performed by a nonprofessional person, the result is negligence. When the same action is performed by a professional person, the acts form the basis for a malpractice lawsuit. In the earlier example, an elderly person fell while being watched by a sitter. The result was negligence on the part of the sitter. Had a professional nurse failed to raise the siderails and the elderly patient had then fallen, the nurse could have been liable for malpractice. Some actions will almost always constitute malpractice because only a professional person would be performing the actions. These include the drawing of arterial blood gases via a direct arterial stick or the initiation of blood transfusions.

Is the distinction important? Many authorities have concluded that the general public has a right to expect and receive a higher standard of care from a professional person than from a nonprofessional worker. Courts have likewise concluded that this increased expectation of duty exists and, as a result, substantially higher awards have been given to injured parties.

■ EXERCISE 6–1

List the types of nursing actions that you perform on a daily basis in your clinical setting. Could all types of nursing actions be the basis for both negligence and malpractice? Why or why not?

ELEMENTS OF MALPRACTICE OR NEGLIGENCE

To be successful in either a malpractice or negligence cause of action in court in most jurisdictions, the plaintiff (injured party) must prove the following elements to establish liability on the part of the defendant(s):

1. Duty owed the patient
2. Breach of the duty owed the patient
3. Foreseeability
4. Causation
5. Injury
6. Damages

Remember, malpractice is negligence as it pertains to a professional person. Therefore, the elements are the same. The only difference is the status of the person committing the action or failing to act when legally required to act. (See Table 6–1.)

Duty Owed the Patient

Duty of care is owed to others and involves how one conducts oneself. When engaging in an activity, an individual is under a legal duty to act as an ordinary, prudent, reasonable person would act. The ordinary, prudent, reasonable person will take precautions against creating unreasonable risks of injury to other persons. The duty of care that is owed has two distinct aspects: (1) It must first be shown that a duty was indeed owed the patient,

TABLE 6–1. NEGLIGENT TORTS

Elements	Examples of Nursing Actions
Duty owed	Failing to monitor the patient
Breach of the duty owed the patient	Failing to report a change in patient status
Foreseeability	Failing to report another health care provider's incompetence
Causation	Failing to provide for the patient's safety
Cause-in-fact	Restraining a patient improperly
Proximate cause	Improper medication administration
Injury	Allowing a patient to be burned
Damages	Failing to question an inappropriate medical order
General	Using equipment incorrectly
Special	Failing to follow ordered treatments
Emotional	Failing to provide patient education and discharge instructions
Punitive/exemplary	Giving the patient incorrect information

and (2) the scope of that duty must be proven. The first aspect may be the easier to prove.

The duty of care owed to a given patient is usually fairly easily established, especially if the nurse is employed by a hospital or clinic. Once the nurse–employer and patient–hospital contractual entities are established, the doctrine of duty arises. The patient has a right to rely on the fact that the nursing staff has a clear-cut duty to act in the patient's best interest.

Duty, however, is created by a relationship and not merely by an employment status. More important than employment is the concept of a nurse–patient relationship or a patient–provider relationship. This *reliance relationship*—of one person depending on another for quality, competent care—actually forms the basis of the duty-owed concept.

Today's primary nursing easily creates a concept of reliance in that the nurse is assigned the entire nursing care of a given patient. Thus, the duty of care and the establishment of a nurse–patient relationship are readily seen. But even the more traditional, team nursing approach creates such a duty of care. In that functional mode, several nurses were assigned a particular group of patients, and both reliance and a nurse–patient relationship existed.

Even if the nurse is not assigned to a particular patient, a general duty of care arises if the patient presents with an emergency or is in need of instant help. For example, a general duty of care would exist if the nurse was on the way to another part of the hospital and happened to pass the open door of a patient about to fall out of bed. Although not assigned to that given patient or even to the nursing unit, the nurse has a limited duty to assist patients in times of crisis and imminent harm.

Most cases have not concerned themselves with this portion of the nursing duty element because a showing of hospital employment usually is considered sufficient in proving that a duty is owed to the patient. An exception to this rule is *Lunsford v. Board of Nurse Examiners* (1983), a landmark decision concerning when the nurse–patient relationship arises. There the nurse attempted to show that, because the patient was never formally admitted to the hospital and there was no physician–patient relationship, a nurse–patient relationship had never been formed. Thus, according to her argument, there was no duty owed the patient. The court refused this argument, stating that by virtue of licensure, a nurse–patient relationship automatically existed when the patient presented at the hospital's admitting office for emergency care and was met by the nurse.

The second aspect of duty is the *scope of care* that must be delivered. The standard of care owed is that of the reasonably prudent nurse under similar circumstances as determined by expert testimony, published standards, and common sense. The test for the court to apply is what a reasonable, prudent nurse, with like experience and education, would do under similar conditions in the same community (*Fraijo v. Hartland Hospital,* 1979). See Chapter 5 for a more extensive discussion of the standards of care that must be delivered to a particular patient.

Breach of Duty Owed the Patient

Breach of duty owed naturally follows as the second element of malpractice and negligence. This element involves showing a deviation from the standard of care owed the patient; that is, something was done that should not have been done or nothing was done when it should have been done. For example, an incorrect medication was administered to a patient or a scheduled medication was omitted. Omissions entail as much potential liability as commissions.

A case that illustrates this breach of duty owed the patient is *Glassman v. St. Joseph Hospital* (1994), in which a patient's temperature rose to 106°F, and he had a grand mal seizure. His surgeon, after having been notified by the staff nurse of the patient's condition, requested a consultation with a neurologist. Shortly after the neurologist arrived on the unit, the patient had a second seizure. The neurologist ordered two doses of Dilantin. The patient then had a third seizure and a third dose of Dilantin was administered. The neurologist left the unit after this third dose of Dilantin.

The patient then had two more seizures (numbers four and five). The nurse called the neurologist after the second of these later seizures and obtained an order for phenobarbital, which was to be given if the patient had any more seizures. When the patient had his sixth seizure, the phenobarbital was given as ordered. Neither she nor the nurse on the next shift gave the patient any medication after his next four seizures (numbers seven through ten), and neither one notified the physician that the seizures were continuing. The second nurse did give the patient phenobarbital after the patient's eleventh seizure, and again she did not notify the physician.

The patient suffered severe, permanent, diffuse brain damage. The patient's expert witness testified that the nurses breached the standard of care by failing to notify the physician after each of the subsequent seizures. The jury also concluded that this conduct was a breach of the duty owed the patient.

Foreseeability

Foreseeability involves the concept that certain events may reasonably be expected to cause specific results. For example, the omission of an ordered insulin injection to a known diabetic patient will foreseeably result in an abnormally high serum glucose level. The challenge is to show that one could reasonably foresee a certain result based on the facts as they existed at the time of the occurrence rather than what could be said based on retrospective thinking and results. In the preceding example, could one foresee, at the time of omission of the ordered insulin, that the patient would lapse into a diabetic coma and arrest?

A case example illustrating forseeability is *Niece v. Elmview Group Home* (1997). Courts find liability when patients are harmed in a manner that is foreseeable. In this case, a female resident in a group home for the developmentally disabled reported being raped by a male caregiver who was employed by the home. The home had investigated his background prior to hiring the caregiver and found that he had no criminal record or prior history of abuse or sexually inappropriate conduct. However, because of previous problems, the home had initiated a policy that stated the male staff could not work alone when caring for the vulnerable female residents. This policy was not followed and thus the court found liability against the home in this case. They concluded that it was foreseeable that such an incidence could occur and that was the purpose of creating and implementing the policy.

Some of the more common cases concerning foreseeability include those involving medication errors and patient falls. The questions of when and how to provide siderails, restraints, and other protections have been addressed by most jurisdictions in the United States (*Delaune v. Medical Center of Baton Rouge*, 1996; *Hardman v. Long Island Urological Associates, P.C.*, 1998; *Crane v. Lakewood Hospital*, 1995; *Dickerson v. Fatehi*, 1997; *Lane v. Tift County Hospital Authority*, 1997; and *McGraw v. St. Joseph's Hospital*, 1997). In *Delaune*, the hospital had equipped a bathroom with a wheelchair ramp, and the patient, who was using a walker rather than a wheelchair, fell when she exited the shower unassisted. In *Hardman*, the patient was allowed to fall from an examining table, and in *Crane*, a visitor to the hospital fell from a chair that was lightweight and unstable. *Dickerson* concerned an operating room case in which the final needle count was incorrect because a marker needle was not included in the final count. In *Lane*, an elderly patient, confused from medications, was allowed to fall while in the radiology department for x-rays, and in *McGraw*, a patient was dropped during transfer from a wheelchair to his bed.

Note that in none of these cases was there any high technology involved or what could be considered advanced nursing skills. These cases represent the most commonly occurring injuries to patients—injuries that occur because of lack of foresight, common sense, and adherence to standards of care.

For example, in *Kadyszewgki v. Ellis Hospital Association* (1993), the court found liability when a 67-year-old patient, having received a combination of Demerol, phenobarbital, Vistaril, and Motrin, fell when she attempted to get to the bathroom. At court, she stated that she had been trying unsuccessfully for over 30 minutes to get someone to come help her to the bathroom and that she had no trouble getting out of bed because the siderails were not raised. The court focused their conclusion more on the lack of siderails (a direct violation of the hospital policy and procedure manual) than on the failure of staff to respond to the patient's bell.

Note, however, that foreseeability is important in imputing liability. Two cases illustrate this fact clearly. In *Hesler v. Osawatomie State Hospital* (1999), the court concluded that there was no foreseeability and thus no liability. In that case, the patient was being treated at a psychiatric facility. During the 24-hour period before his weekend pass with his parents, the patient appeared to be appropriate and was demonstrating no behavior that would prevent his weekend pass. The patient was talking and interacting with others, was not pacing, did not seem overly anxious about going home with his parents, and verbalized that he was excited about going home. He had also handled a four-hour pass with his parents appropriately five days earlier.

The evening before his pass, he asked for medication. This was seen by staff members as a sign that the patient understood his need for medication to control his mental illness and that he wanted to take care of himself.

While on the weekend pass, he was riding with his parents when he suddenly grabbed the steering wheel of the car, forcing it into a head-on collision with an oncoming car, causing the death of one occupant and injuring several other occupants in the oncoming car. The injured parties and the estate of the deceased party sued the nurse, physician, and facility.

The Supreme Court of Kansas upheld the lower court's dismissal of the case, stating that there was no solid basis to foresee that this patient posed a risk of harm to another person. The court held that, although diagnosed as a paranoid schizophrenic, he had never been assessed as a danger to others and there was no basis for anyone on the treatment team to anticipate he could or would commit a sudden violent or self-destructive act.

Swift v. Northeastern Hospital of Philadelphia (1997) concerned a patient who had fallen off a ladder at home and presented herself to the emergency center with a compression fracture and myasthenia gravis. While hospitalized, she fell while using the bathroom. Her statement at the time of the hospital fall was that her "legs had given out," but in her lawsuit she contended that there had been water on the floor of the bathroom, causing her fall.

The Superior Court of Pennsylvania ruled that without proof from the injured party that the hospital knew about the water, the chance of the patient falling was not foreseeable, and the court applied to the hospital the same traditional rule that applies to retail and other business establishments in slip-and-fall cases.

Causation

Somewhat more difficult to prove is *causation,* which means that the injury must have been incurred directly by the breach of duty owed the patient. Causation is frequently subdivided into the concepts of (1) cause-in-fact and (2) proximate cause.

Cause-in-fact denotes that the breach of duty owed caused the injury. If it were not for the breach of duty, no injury would have resulted. For example, a medication is incorrectly administered in the wrong dosage, and the patient subsequently suffers direct consequences due to the medication. In *Brown v. Southern Baptist Hospital* (1998), a patient received Bunnell's irrigation solution following surgery for a severely infected finger. The irrigating solution was to be dripped on the patient's surgical wound for 24 hours. A pharmacy student extern mixed the solution at about 100 times the ordered strength, creating a 47% glacial acetic acid solution rather than the ordered 0.49% solution. The patient suffered serious complications to the surgical site, had to have numerous follow-up surgeries, and ultimately lost the finger.

In assessing blame, the court concluded that the majority of the liability fell on the nursing staff. Even though they did not know of the pharmacy error, they did know that the patient repeatedly complained of the burning pain in his arm, and they should have known that Bunnell's solution is supposed to have a soothing effect and should not cause pain and burning. Thus, they were negligent for not listening to the patient's repeated complaints of pain and for not discontinuing the solution and notifying the patient's physician.

Several tests have been established to determine cause-in-fact. The *but for* test answers the question if the act or omission is a direct cause of the injury or harm sustained. Would the injury have occurred but for the act or omission by the defendant? Would the patient have developed complications, such as an abscess, but for the sponge that was inadvertently left in the abdomen during surgery?

The *substantial factor* test has been developed to aid in pinpointing liability when several causes occur to bring about a given injury. With several possible causes, the but for test is inadequate, because the answer to each defendant's liability would be that no defendant caused the entire set of circumstances, and therefore the entire result could not have been foreseen. Rather than allow such a result, the substantial factor test is used, not to determine certainty but to establish a causal link between actions and injury. This test asks if the defendant's act or omission was a substantial factor in causing the ultimate harm or injury. If the answer is yes, there is cause-in-fact. For example, in the above-cited case, the court had to determine which of the multiple defendants was most responsible for the patient's ultimate loss of his finger—the student pharmacist, her university, her pharmacy preceptor at the hospital, the hospital, the physician, or the nursing staff.

An equally complex example of substantial factor is *Depesa v. Westchester Square Medical Center* (1997). In this case, a 49-year-old patient entered the emergency center with severe abdominal pain. Physicians prescribed Mylanta and sent her home, advising her to contact her personal physician if her condition worsened.

She took the medication but continued to experience increasing abdominal pain. After 20 days, the patient visited a different hospital's emergency center. Tests revealed a perforated bowel and peritonitis. Following surgery, the personnel at this second hospital administered almost double the prescribed fluids, and the patient died of acute heart failure. The court was left to determine the exact cause of the patient's death—the initial failure to diagnose the perforated bowel or the substandard care at the second hospital. In addition, the court had to decide to what degree each of the defendants shared responsibility—the physicians, nurses, and individual institutions. Ultimately, the court apportioned liability between the two hospitals and their employees.

The *alternate causes* approach also addresses the problem in which two or more persons have been accused of negligence. Under this test, the plaintiff must show that the harm or injury was caused by one of the multiple defendants, and the burden of proof then shifts to the defendants to show who actually caused the harm or injury that is at issue. In *Donahue v. Port* (1994), a 32-year-old male lost his leg due to failure to diagnose vascular problems associated with a dislocated knee. At trial, the defendant orthopedic surgeon claimed that the nurses were negligent in not reporting vascular problems until it was too late to save the leg. An expert witness for the nurses testified that, if there was an initial popliteal artery injury, there was only a 12-hour window in which to successfully repair the artery and that the 12-hour window had expired before the patient was treated. The patient has the burden of proof to show that the harm was caused by one of the defendants, and the defendants have to show which one of them did (or did not) cause the harm. If neither defendant could establish his or her own innocence or the other's negligence, they may both be liable.

The alternate causes approach is frequently seen in a negative light by juries. Defendants blaming each other have often resulted in large malpractice awards for the injured plaintiff (Fiesta, 1994), and thus is not often used at trial.

Proximate cause attempts to determine how far the liability of the defendant extends for consequences following negligent activity. Thus, proximate cause builds on foreseeability. Could one foresee the extent to which consequences will follow a negligent action? For example, in *Moore v. Willis-Knighton Medical Center* (1998), the court held that when a hospital staff knows that a patient will be using a medical appliance at home, the hospital and its staff can be ruled at fault due to inadequate discharge instructions for the use of the specific device. In this case, the patient was discharged home with a walker following hip replacement surgery. Before discharge, the physician also prescribed an elevated toilet seat for use at her home, the same type and model that she was using in the hospital. Seventy days after her discharge, the patient fell off her toilet seat and reinjured the hip. She sued for failure to provide adequate discharge instructions for using an elevated toilet seat in conjuction with a walker.

In finding for the nursing staff and hospital, the court noted that the longer a patient has been living independently, with limitations but without problems, the more responsibility that patient has for his or her own safety, and the less an accident should be blamed on the hospital's discharge instructions.

A second case that illustrates proximate cause is *Silves v. King* (1999). Donald Silves presented to the hospital, complaining of a sore and swollen toe. Because of a history of blood clots, Silves feared he might be experiencing another one. Dr. King, the emergency center physician, took his medical history, performed a physical examination, diagnosed gouty arthritis, and prescribed indomethacin. She instructed Silves to follow up with his regular physician within five days. She testified she knew that Silves was currently taking heparin for his history of blood clots.

The emergency center nurse gave Silves two pages of discharge instructions, which included a list of warnings concerning indomethacin, including a caution not to take the medication if the patient has problems with blood clotting or bleeding. Silves signed the discharge instruction sheet, which contained a statement that he had received and could read the instructions. At trial, he testified that he did not read the discharge instructions prior to taking the indomethacin. Approximately two weeks after he started the indomethacin, he suffered a pulmonary hemorrhage that left him permanently disabled.

Silves sued the physician, her employer, the hospital, and its staff. The trial court entered summary judgment in favor of the hospital and its staff and found that Dr. King had not violated the standard of care, but did fail to obtain Silves's informed consent prior to the use of the indomethacin. However, the jury found that the failure to obtain informed consent was not a proximate cause of Silves's injury.

In the finding against liability on the part of the nursing staff, the court rejected Silves's claim that the discharge nurse had a duty to inform him of possible drug interactions. The nurse does not need to review the medication discharge instructions with the patient if the patient has read and signed the form. Assuming the patient can read and understand the medication instructions, there is no reason to require nurses to read these same instructions to the patient. This too, said the court, was not a proximate cause of his injury.

Proximate cause is fairly clear as long as the result is directly related. Proximate cause becomes less clear when intervening variables are present. Intervening forces may combine with the original negligent action to cause injury to the patient. As a rule of thumb, in medical malpractice cases, the health care provider is frequently liable for intervening forces when they are foreseeable. For example, a patient, hurt in an automobile accident, could sue the driver's physician, alleging that the driver was given an excessive amount of Valium by the physician and that the physician failed to adequately evaluate his patient's psychiatric and drinking history before prescribing Valium. The court could conclude that a foreseeable consequence of prescribing Valium under such circumstances is that the patient with psychiatric problems will drink, and such a patient, high on alcohol and Valium, may injure others.

But often intervening factors are not foreseeable. In *Van Horn v. Chambers* (1998), a patient admitted for seizures and alcohol withdrawal was sedated, given antiseizure medications, and restrained. He was admitted to the neurological intensive care unit. The following day, the attending neurologist determined that the restraints were no longer indicated and transferred the patient to a private room on a medical–surgical unit.

The patient decided to leave against medical advice. Three individuals, a patient care technician, a medical student, and a food service worker attempted to prevent his leaving. In the subsequent fight that occurred, two of the hospital personnel were injured and one was killed.

The Supreme Court of Texas ruled that each had acted at their own risk and could not sue the neurologist for malpractice. The neurologist did not misdiagnose the patient and had no duty to control the patient. Thus, proximate cause did not exist.

Injury

The fifth element that must be shown is an actual *injury* or *harm*. The plaintiff must demonstrate that some type of physical, financial, or emotional injury resulted from the breach of duty owed the patient. Generally speaking, courts do not allow lawsuits based solely on negligently inflicted emotional injuries. Such emotional injuries are actionable only when they accompany physical injuries.

Pain and suffering are allowed if they accompany a physical injury but not by themselves (*Jones v. Department of Health*, 1995, and *Majca v. Beekil*, 1998). *Jones* involved the potential damages for pain and suffering, loss of capacity for the enjoyment of life, and the reasonable expectation for life following a false-positive test result for human immunodeficiency virus (HIV), and *Majca* concerned the fear of contracting acquired immune deficiency syndrome (AIDS) without evidence of exposure to HIV. This contrasts with intentional infliction of emotional harm, an intentional tort, which is covered later in this chapter.

Note, however, that negligent actions coupled with pain and suffering may provoke the court to find that psychological harm is sufficient to sustain a cause of action against defendants. The court in *Curtis v. MRI Imaging Services II* (1998) acknowledged that, as a general rule, the law does not allow lawsuits for damages for emotional distress in negligence cases unless the victim had sustained some type of physical harm. Having noted such, the court concluded that there is a major exception to the rule: the relationship that exists between patients and their health care providers. Health care professionals, said the court, are held to a legal standard of care that includes the specific duty to be aware of and guard against particular adverse psychological reactions or consequences of medical procedures.

There are certain specific interventions that carry with them known foreseeable risks of adverse psychological reactions. Steps must be taken to assess the particular patient's susceptibility to foreseeable adverse reactions and steps must be taken to minimize or avoid them. In this case, the patient had a magnetic resonance imaging (MRI) scan, but no explanation of the potential for claustrophobic effects were explained to the patient before the examination. No adequate history was taken, which would have made known the patient's preexisting asthmatic condition and his propensity to panic reactions and breathing difficulties. During the MRI, the patient was not closely monitored, and the caregivers could not terminate the procedure quickly and extract the patient from the MRI device once he did begin having difficulty breathing and respiratory distress.

A second exception to the nonrecovery for emotional harm concerns instances in which a parent views an injury to his or her child. In these types of cases, the courts have frequently allowed damages for a purely emotional injury (*Bond v. Sacred Heart Medical Center*, 1991).

Damages

Unlike intentional torts, *damages* are not presumed. Nominal (e.g., a $1 or $2 award) damages do not exist for negligent torts. The basic purpose of awarding damages is compensatory, with the law attempting to restore the injured party to his or her original position so far as is financially possible. The goal of awarding damages is not to punish the defendants but to assist the injured party.

There are essentially four types of damages that may be compensated:

1. *General damages* are those that are inherent to the injury itself. Included in general damages are pain and suffering (past, present, and future) and any permanent disability or disfigurement because of the injury.
2. *Special damages* account for all losses and expenses incurred as a result of the injury. These include medical bills, lost wages (past, present, and future), cost of future medical care, and cost of converting current living areas to more easily accommodate the injured party.
3. *Emotional damages* may be compensated if there is apparent physical harm as well. A very limited number of cases, such as *Curtis v. MRI Imaging Services II* (1998) do allow for such emotional damages without evidence of physical injury.
4. *Punitive* or *exemplary damages* may be awarded if there is malicious, willful, or wanton misconduct. The plaintiff must show that the defendant acted with conscious disregard for his or her safety. *Luby v. St. John's Episcopal Hospital* (1995) expanded this definition to include "conduct which is wanton, malicious, or activated by evil or reprehensible motives" (at 776). Punitive damages are usually considerable and are awarded to deter similar conduct in the future. This type of damage award is usually not covered by professional liability insurance coverage, because the harm is with malice aforethought. In one of the few cases in which punitive damages were awarded against nurse-defendants, a decision was made to move a patient to another room on the same unit, without supplemental oxygen. The patient was terminal, with less than 24 hours to live, and the family begged that supplemental oxygen be given during the move. The nurses declined, and the patient—a "no-code" patient—arrested about 15 feet from his original room and was pronounced dead by the attending physician. The court found that punitive damages were appropriate because the nurses' action was extreme deviation from the standard of care (*Manning v. Twin Falls Clinic and Hospital*, 1992).

Sometimes general and special damages are grouped into one category called *compensatory damages*. The last two classifications are retained, and thus there are three categories for damage awards.

With multiple defendants, courts apportion the harm caused the plaintiff according to each defendant's portion or percentage of the actual harm. Harm is seen as a total percentage of 100% and each defendant's part in the harm is calculated, with all the defendants' portions equaling the original 100%. Then the court multiples the total damage award by each defendant's percentage. *Estate of Chin v. St. Barnabas Medical Center* (1998) illustrates the concept. In that case, the patient died following a hysteroscopy. The total damages awarded by the jury were $200,000. Five defendants were involved:

1. The circulating nurse was 20% at fault and was assessed $40,000.
2. One scrub nurse was 25% at fault and was assessed $50,000.
3. Another scrub nurse was 0% at fault and was assessed no dollar amount.
4. The hospital was 35% at fault and was assessed $70,000.
5. The physician was 20% at fault and was assessed $40,000.

■ EXERCISE 6–2

A nurse administers a medication to a patient as ordered by the patient's physician. Can the nurse be found liable if the patient suffers an allergic reaction? Does liability depend on whether it was a fatal allergic response or merely a mild allergic response to the medication?

DOCTRINE OF RES IPSA LOQUITOR

The doctrine of **res ipsa loquitor** allows a negligence cause of action without requiring that all six elements of malpractice or negligence be proven. Essentially, res ipsa loquitor allows the jury to find the defendant negligent without any showing of expert testimony on the plaintiff's part.

Res ipsa loquitor—"the thing speaks for itself"—is a rule of evidence that emerges when plaintiffs are injured in such a way that they cannot prove how the injury occurred or who was responsible for its occurrence. The negligence of the alleged wrongdoer may be inferred from the mere fact that an accident or incident happened. The proviso is that the nature of the incident and the circumstances surrounding the incident lead reasonably to the belief that, in the absence of negligence, it would not have occurred. The instrument that caused the injury must be shown to have been under the management and control of the alleged wrongdoer, not the injured party.

This doctrine is used by the courts in cases in which the person injured has an insurmountable burden in proving the facts of the case. For example, the landmark case for this doctrine is a California case in which the injured party underwent a routine appendectomy and suffered a permanent loss of neuromuscular control of the right shoulder and arm as a result of the surgery (*Ybarra v. Spangard*, 1944). The injured party had no means of accurately showing how or when this permanent injury occurred. All the patient could show was that this was not the type of complication normally incurred with

GUIDELINES: AVOIDING NEGLIGENT TORTS

1. Treat patients and their families with respect and honesty. Communicating in a truthful, open, and professional manner may well prevent a negligence cause of action.
2. Use your nursing knowledge to make appropriate nursing diagnoses and to implement necessary nursing interventions. You have an affirmative duty not only to make correct nursing diagnoses, but to take the actions required to implement your diagnoses.
3. Remember that the first line of duty is to the patient. If the physician is hesitant to order necessary therapy or to respond to a change in the patient condition, call your supervisor or another physician. Question orders if they are (a) ambiguous or unclear, (b) questioned or refused by the patient, (c) telephone orders, or (d) inappropriate, such as when a major change occurs in the patient's status and the orders remain unchanged. For telephone orders, reread the orders to the physician and clarify them prior to hanging up the phone.
4. Remain current and up-to-date in your skills and education. Take advantage of continuing education programs and in-service programs on a regular basis. Read your professional journals. Refuse to perform skills and procedures if you are unfamiliar with them, have never performed them before, or lack the necessary materials and equipment to perform them safely.
5. Base your nursing care on the nursing process model. Using all five steps of the model prevents the inadvertent overlooking of a vital part(s) of required nursing care for a given patient.
6. Document completely every step of the nursing care plan and the patient's responses to interventions. Express yourself clearly and completely. Chart all entries as soon as possible while the facts and observations are still clear in your mind.
7. Respect the patient's right to education about his or her illness, and ensure that the patient and family are taught about the disease entity, therapy, and possible complications prior to discharge. Chart any discharge instruction in the medical record.
8. Delegate patient care wisely, and know the scope of practice for yourself and those whom you supervise. Never accept or allow others to accept more responsibility than they can handle or than they are allowed to accept by law.
9. Know and adhere to your hospital policies and procedures. Help to update those that are outdated, and ensure that the personnel you supervise are also aware of hospital policies and procedures. All personnel should reread the manual periodically.
10. Keep your malpractice liability insurance policy current, and know the limits of coverage. This may not help you to give better care, but it will help you if a patient should name you in a malpractice cause of action.

an appendectomy and that he had full range and movement of the affected arm prior to the surgical procedure.

To prevent injured parties from an unfair disadvantage and to prevent wrongdoers from benefiting by their silence, the court enacted the doctrine of res ipsa loquitor. The injured party must prove three elements for this doctrine to apply:

1. The accident must be the kind that ordinarily does not occur in the absence of someone's negligence.
2. The accident must be caused by an agency or instrumentality within exclusive control of the defendant.

3. The accident must not have been due to any voluntary action or contribution on the part of the plaintiff (*Ybarra v. Spangard*, 1944, at 687).

Once these three elements are shown, the defendant must disprove them. The courts view the defendants as being in a better position to actually explain what happened, because they had exclusive control during the time the incident occurred.

The doctrine of res ipsa loquitor is normally applied in medical malpractice cases in which the injured party is unconscious, was in surgery, or was an infant. Typical examples of cases for which the courts have allowed the doctrine of res ipsa loquitor to be applied include those in which a foreign object has been left in the patient during surgery, infection was caused by unsterile instruments, neuromuscular injury occurred due to the improper positioning of an unconscious patient, burns occurred during surgery, or a surgical procedure was performed on the wrong limb or part of the body.

Not all states apply the doctrine of res ipsa loquitor in the same manner. Some states have actually expanded the doctrine through recent court cases. Other states have tended to limit the application of the doctrine, especially in areas where more than common knowledge is needed to ensure the jury's understanding of the facts, such as in the area of secondary infections.

Two recent cases illustrate the application of res ipsa loquitor. In *Harder v. F. C. Clinton, Inc.* (1997), a resident required transfer from a nursing home to an acute care facility for treatment of hypoglycemic coma. An IV was placed in the dorsum of her foot, which later became gangrenous, and an above-the-knee amputation was performed. She filed a civil suit against the nursing home for their administration of an overdose of tolbutamide, a medication that had never been prescribed for her. The administration of the tolbutamide was established at court from the physician's note on the hospital record of the patient.

The Supreme Court of Oklahoma ruled that the doctrine of res ipsa loquitor applied in this instance. An overdose of medication is not a usual or expected outcome in administering medications in a nursing home. The nursing home had complete control and management of the medications that the residents received. At trial, testimony was presented about the medication system at the nursing home. All residents' medications were stored in a locked medication cart at the nurses' station and were administered to residents only by licensed nurses. The final element, the court ruled, was that an overdose of medication is an occurrence that would not have happened if those in control of the medication had exercised due care.

A similar finding was upheld in *Lane v. Tift County Hospital Authority* (1997). In that case, an elderly patient, recently sedated with Demerol, was allowed to fall while in the radiology department. The court held that carrying out the hospital's legal duty is not the sole prerogative of the professional staff, but also extends to nonlicensed personnel.

Note, however, that res ipsa loquitor may also be invoked on behalf of the nursing staff and health care facility. In *Slease v. Hughbanks* (1997), a patient was admitted following an industrial mishap for orthopedic ankle surgery. One or two days after the surgery, he noticed a burn on his thigh and filed a malpractice suit. In court, the plaintiff's attorney did not produce expert witnesses to show that the burn was the type consistent with an electrical burn from a bovie pad, but rested the case solely on the doctrine of res ipsa loquitor.

In finding for the hospital and against the plaintiff, the court relied on the admission note as charted when the patient first came to the hospital. The admission nurse had noted that there was a burn on the patient's thigh as one of the multiple traumas he had incurred in the industrial accident. Thus, res ipsa loquitor did not apply.

A third trend by states is to deny the injured party the use of the doctrine through statutory or decisional law. This latter denial of the doctrine is based on the fact that negligence must be proven, not presumed (67 ALR 4th, 1989).

LOCALITY RULE

Whenever the legal system refers to the reasonable, prudent practitioner, there is a statement to the effect that the professional is viewed by a prevailing community standard, "in a similar community" or "under the same circumstances." Known as the *locality rule,* such a statement attempts to hold the standard of the professional to that of other professionals practicing in the same geographic area of the country.

The locality rule arose because there were wide variations in the care that the particular patient received, depending on the type of setting in which the hospital was situated—rural or urban. Rural hospitals and health care providers did not have the same sophistication and means of technology that were available within large medical centers.

In most jurisdictions, the locality rule has been abolished either by statute or by judicial rulings. Today, a *national standard* is emerging that offers to all persons an acceptable minimal standard of care.

Several factors arose to help abolish the locality rule. First, because of mass media, national conferences, and improved transportation, health care providers were no longer able to defend the acceptance of a lower standard of care for rural areas. The practitioner has available all the teaching aids and continuing education programs needed to stay informed about new and innovative therapeutic approaches as well as to understand new technological advances. The patient may, fairly readily, be transported to a larger, metropolitan area, or the needed equipment and personnel can be transported to the patient.

Second, professional organizations (e.g., the Joint Commission for the Accreditation of Healthcare Organizations or the American Association of Critical-Care Nurses) have moved toward the creation of an acceptable standard for given patients by publishing national standards of care. Additionally, state nurse practice acts have enacted standards of nursing practice for all nurses within the jurisdiction, not just for nurses within large medical centers.

Third, standards for accreditation of hospitals should be the same no matter where the hospital is located geographically.

AVOIDING MALPRACTICE CLAIMS

Nurses frequently inquire about the impact that the medical malpractice crisis will have on the professional practice of nursing. This is especially true as more and more nurses are being sued along with physicians or hospitals. Can anything be done to stop the increased litigation? What should nurses do to protect themselves?

They can limit their potential liability in several ways. Possibly the first and most important concept to remember is that patients and their families who are treated honestly, openly, and respectfully and who are apprised of all facets of treatment and prognosis are not likely to sue. Communications done in a caring and professional manner have been shown time and time again to be a major reason why more people do not sue, despite adequate grounds for a successful lawsuit. Even given untoward results and a major setback, the patient is less likely to file suit if there has been an open and trusting nurse–patient relationship or physician–patient relationship. Remember, it is people who sue, not the action or event that triggered a bad outcome.

Second, nurses should know relevant law and legal doctrines and combine these concepts with the biological, psychological, and social sciences that form part of the basis of all rational nursing decisions. The law can and should be incorporated into everyday practice as a safeguard for the health care provider as well as the health care recipient.

Third, nurses should stay well within their areas of individual competence. To remain competent, nurses should upgrade technical skills consistently, continuously attend pertinent continuing education and in-service programs on a regular basis, and undertake only those actual skills that they can perform competently.

Fourth, joining and actively supporting professional organizations allow nurses to take advantage of their excellent educational programs and to become active in organizations' lobbying efforts, especially if it means a stronger nurse practice act or the creation or expansion of advanced nursing roles. Far too many nurses are afraid to become politically involved; yet, as a unified profession, nursing could have a very strong voice, particularly in upgrading and strengthening nurse practice acts.

Fifth, recognize the concept of the *suit-prone patient*. This type of patient is more likely than other patients to initiate malpractice action in the event that something untoward happens during the treatment process. Because the psychological makeup of these persons breeds resentment and dissatisfaction in all phases of their lives, they are much more apt to initiate a lawsuit.

Suit-prone patients tend to be immature, overly dependent, hostile, and uncooperative, often failing to follow a designated plan of care. They are unable to be self-critical and shift blame to others as a way of coping with their own inadequacies. Suit-prone patients actually project their fear, insecurity, and anxiety to health care providers, overreacting to any perceived slight in an exaggerated manner.

Recognizing such patients is the first step in avoiding potential lawsuits. The nurse should then attempt to react on a more human or personal basis, such as expressing satisfaction with the patients' cooperation, showing empathy and concern with their suffering and setbacks, and repeating needed information to keep patients less fearful of unknown treatments and procedures. An atmosphere of attentiveness, caring, and patience will help prevent the suit-prone patient from filing future lawsuits.

Sixth, recognize that nurses' personality traits and behaviors may also trigger lawsuits. *Suit-prone nurses* are those who (1) have difficulty establishing close relationships with others, (2) are insecure and shift blame to others, (3) tend to be insensitive to patients' complaints or fail to take the complaints seriously, (4) have a tendency to be aloof and more concerned with the mechanics of nursing as opposed to establishing meaningful human interactions with patients, and (5) inappropriately delegate responsibilities to peers to avoid personal contact with patients. These nurses need counseling and education to change these behaviors into more positive attitudes and behaviors toward patients and staff. Such positive changes lessen future potential lawsuits.

Seventh, while it may not prevent lawsuits, nurses are encouraged to investigate having professional liability insurance. This will better protect them should a lawsuit be filed.

Eighth, it seems inevitable that at some point the consumer of health care must begin to accept some responsibility for risks along with the health care providers. One of the reasons cited for high medical malpractice claims against obstetricians is the fact that consumers want total assurance that they will have only healthy, perfectly formed children. Perhaps part of nursing's imminent tasks is in helping to educate consumers. All health care entails some risks, no matter how remote or far-fetched.

Finally, remember that many of the malpractice claims that arise today involve patient education and discharge planning issues. All patients and/or significant others must be taught before discharge from any health care setting, acute care and community-based, and this education may include both formal and informal education. Instructions that are given and information that is learned must become part of the patient record.

■ EXERCISE 6—3

Review all the patients that you have cared for in the past seven to ten days. Were any or all of the patients classifiable as suit-prone patients? What can nurses do to lessen the potential of future lawsuits?

Do the nurses' ethical principles affect such patients? Which ethical principles should the nurse consider when caring for these suit-prone patients? Do remaining firm and insisting that patients learn to care for themselves fall under any of the ethical principles?

PATIENT EDUCATION AND TORT LAW

Patient education, especially through discharge planning and instruction information, is one of the more visible ways of preventing malpractice claims. As health care providers have become more aware of standards of care and are delivering quality, competent care in the acute care setting, there are fewer malpractice cases being filed against nurses. But the same is not true of the outpatient setting and the home setting. Patients are now returning to their homes, failing to follow instructions or claiming that no instructions were given, and filing suits for injuries that arose in the home setting. For example, the newly diagnosed diabetic patient is able to properly do a blood test for his blood sugar content, give himself the necessary dose of insulin, and correctly pick his foods and prepare healthy meals. But what happens when he decides to replant his flowerbed and sustains an open foot injury? Unfortunately, that is the exact scenario being played out across the nation. The patient received excellent acute care but is unable to follow the medication regime or does not know when to seek emergency medical care after returning to the community.

Because of such instances, acute care settings as well as outpatient settings are developing more formalized discharge instructions. These instructions may be in English or other languages, they are usually one to two pages and printed in larger fonts, and they are geared toward an eighth-grade educational level. When using these discharge instruction forms, remember to evaluate the patients' and families' understanding of the content. Did they ask pertinent questions? Were they able to perform a repeat demonstration of the skill? Were they able to answer simple questions about the skill? Did they know possible side effects and what to do if such side effects occurred? Retain a copy of the discharge instruction form for the medical record and carefully chart what was taught, how it was evaluated, and what printed information the patient and family were given. More information on legally defensive charting is discussed in Chapter 9.

DEFINITION OF INTENTIONAL TORTS

Intentional torts share three common elements (see Table 6–2):

1. There must be a volitional or willful act by the defendant.
2. The person so acting must intend to bring about the consequences or appear to have intended to bring about the consequences.
3. There must be causation. The act must be a substantial factor in bringing about the injury or consequences.

Intentional torts may be differentiated from negligence in the following manner:

1. Intent is necessary in proving intentional torts. The nurse must have intended an action. For example, the nurse must have intended to hold the patient so that an injection might be given to the patient or so that a nasogastric tube might be inserted into the patient's stomach.
2. There must be a volitional or willful action against the injured person. In intentional torts, there cannot be the omission of a duty owed as with negligence. In the preceding example, the nurse held the patient so that the injection could be given or the nasogastric tube inserted.
3. Damages are not an issue with intentional torts. The injured party need not show that damages were incurred. Whether the patient encounters out-of-pocket expenses or not, the patient could still show that an intentional tort had occurred.

INTENTIONAL TORTS

The more commonly seen intentional torts within the health care arena are assault, battery, false imprisonment, conversion of property, trespass to land, and intentional infliction of emotional distress (see Table 6–3). Defamation and invasion of privacy are usually discussed with intentional torts, although these two wrongs are more correctly classified as quasi-intentional torts.

Assault

An *assault* is any action that places another person in apprehension of being touched in a manner that is offensive, insulting, or physically injurious without consent or author-

TABLE 6–2. SHARED ELEMENTS OF INTENTIONAL TORTS

1. There must be a volitional (voluntary and willful) act by the defendant.
2. The person so acting must intend to bring about the consequences.
3. There must be causation—the act must be a substantial factor in bringing about the injury or consequences.

TABLE 6–3. INTENTIONAL TORTS

Tort	Elements	Examples of Nursing Actions
Assault	Shared elements, plus places another in apprehension of being touched in an offensive, insulting, or physically injurious manner	Threatening patients with an injection or with starting an intravenous line
Battery	Shared elements, plus the actual contact with another person or the person's clothing without valid consent	Forcing patients to ambulate against their will Holding a patient so that a nasogastric tube can be inserted
False imprisonment	Shared elements, plus unjustified detention of a person without legal warrant to so confine the person	Refusing to allow patients to leave against medical advice Restraining competent patients against their wishes
Conversion of property	Shared elements, plus interference with the patient's right of possession in his/her property	Searching patients' belongings and taking medications or removing patients' clothing
Trespass to land	Shared elements, plus unlawful interference with another's possession of land	Patient refusing to leave the hospital after being discharged Visitor's refusal to leave the hospital when so requested
Intentional infliction of emotional distress	Shared elements, plus conduct that goes beyond that allowed by society, conduct that is calculated and causes mental distress	Handing a mother her stillborn child in a gallon jar of formalin

ity. No actual touching of the person is required. The action or motion must create a "reasonable apprehension in the other person of immediate harmful or offensive contact to the plaintiff-person" (*Words and Phrases,* 1995).

Usually thought of as a violent, angry, or unwarranted contact with the patient, knowledge is the prerequisite to assault. For example, the nurse cannot assault a patient who is sleeping or unconscious because, no matter how angry or violent the nurse might be or how irrational his or her actions, the patient has no knowledge of the potential contact and is therefore not apprehensive of the potential contact. In *Baca v. Valez* (1992), an operating room nurse sued for assault and battery when an orthopedic surgeon struck her on the back with a bone chisel. In finding that there was no assault (although a battery had occurred), the court concluded that since she was struck in the back, there was "no act, threat or menacing conduct that causes another person to reasonably believe that he is in danger of receiving an immediate battery" (at 1197).

Words alone are not enough for assault to occur, although the addition of words may accompany the overt act. For example, the nurse moves toward the patient with a syringe in one hand while telling the patient why the injection is necessary or while telling the patient to "lie still or this will really hurt!" Either example is an assault if the patient is apprehensive of an offensive touching of his or her body.

Assault also requires a present ability to commit harm. For example, if someone is threatened over a telephone, there is no present ability to commit a harm, and thus no tort has been committed.

Two important reminders: (1) The actual touching of the person (battery) does not have to follow an assault; and (2) either the nurse or the patient may be the *tortfeasor* (person committing the tort). Assault is apprehension of an unwarranted touching, and the apprehension is all that is needed to prove that a tort has occurred. The nurse may approach the patient or the patient may approach the nurse.

Battery

A *battery*, the most common intentional tort within the practice of nursing and medicine, involves a harmful or unwarranted contact with the patient-plaintiff. Liability for such an unwarranted contact is based on the individual's right to be free from unconsented invasions of the person.

The legal system recognizes several factors regarding battery:

1. A single touch, however fleeting and faint, is sufficient for the tort to have occurred. Everyday examples include brushing against another person in a crowded elevator or auditorium or placing one's hand on the patient's shoulder for reassurance. It is the touching, not the manner of the touch, that creates the tort.
2. No harm, injury, or pain need befall the patient. The unwarranted contact frequently will not harm or physically hurt the patient.
3. The patient need not be aware of the battery for the tort to have occurred. Unlike assault, in which knowledge is a key factor, taking a pulse of a sleeping patient could be considered a battery at law.
4. Causation is an important factor, and the nurse may be liable for direct as well as indirect contact. For example, the nurse, intending to restrain a patient for the purpose of starting an intravenous infusion, accidentally drops the intravenous tray on the patient. Even though the nurse has not directly touched the patient, a battery has occurred because the nurse put the scenario into motion.
5. The nurse may also commit a battery by the unwarranted touching of the patient's clothes or of an article held by the patient, such as a purse or a suitcase. For purposes of a battery, anything that is connected with the patient's person is viewed as part of the person.

Most health care–related lawsuits in this area have focused on consent for medical or surgical procedures. Lack of consent always sets the stage for a potential assault and battery lawsuit. The classic and landmark case of *Schloendorff v. Society of New York Hospitals* (1914) held that the medical practitioner had committed a battery when he removed a tumor from a patient who had authorized merely an examination. *Mohr v. Williams* (1905) had reached a similar previous conclusion when that court found the practitioner liable for performing surgery without prior consent. That court also limited damages because of the good faith of the practitioner and the beneficial results of the surgery to the patient.

More recent examples of such unwarranted treatment are *Loungbury v. Capel* (1992), *Foflygen v. R. Zemel* (1992), and *Anderson v. St. Francis-St. George Hospital* (1992). Each of these cases held that treatment without prior consent by the patient resulted in a battery.

Nurses may also be the plaintiffs in assault and battery cases, rather than the patient, because the rules of law apply to all persons. In *Creasy v. Rusk* (1998), a certified nursing assistant filed a civil personal injury case against a patient who had hurt him. The Court of Appeals of Indiana acknowledged, as a general rule, that health care workers can sue patients for personal injuries if the worker is harmed by the patient.

False Imprisonment

False imprisonment is the unjustifiable detention of a person without legal warrant to confine the person. Nurses falsely imprison the patient when they confine the patient or restrain the patient in a confined, bounded area with the intent to prevent the patient from freedom and nonrestraint. The confined area may be the patient's room or bed. False imprisonment may also occur if the act is directed at the patient's family or possessions. For example, one has effectively been confined if the nurse refuses to give the patient her purse, car keys, or clothing, or refuses to allow the patient to see his family members unless the patient stays in bed.

There must be knowledge of the restraint for false imprisonment to occur. Sedated patients who are incapable of realizing their confinement do not have a suit for false imprisonment. Likewise, future threats are not enough to sustain the tort of false imprisonment. Threatening a patient who is about to leave against medical advice with "if you leave now, no physician will ever take your case in the future" does not constitute false imprisonment, though it may be unadvisable from a nursing perspective. Detaining the patient who wishes to leave against medical advice until the supervisor can be located or until the patient's physician can be contacted to come and see the patient is false imprisonment.

Some of the more recent cases involving false imprisonment in the health care setting concern the area of mental health. In *Arthur v. Lutheran General Hospital, Inc.* (1998), the patient prevailed when he was held against his will after refusing voluntary admission to an inpatient psychiatric facility. The court noted that the patient could be held if there had been a physician's certification to show why the patient was a grave danger to others. State law must be followed, the court held, "to the letter when a citizen's liberty is at stake, and if not, the citizen can sue for false imprisonment" (at 1242).

A second case, *Wingate v. Ridgeview Institute, Inc.* (1998), centered around a patient who was held against his will in an alcohol rehabilitation program. The patient had voluntarily admitted himself and then changed his mind and desired to leave. Again, the court held that the legal standard for involuntary mental health treatment is grave danger of serious harm or death of the person or another.

A third case, *Remmers v. DeBuono* (1997), was decided as a case of mistreatment of a patient, rather than false imprisonment of the patient, because of the patient's inability to understand he had been imprisoned. Here, a nurse's aide was assigned to a patient in a nursing home setting. The patient was confined to a wheelchair but was highly mobile because he could wheel himself about easily. He was labeled a "wanderer" by the staff, because he frequently roamed away from the nursing unit and could be found in other patients' rooms.

One evening, he wheeled himself off the unit and into other patients' rooms four times. After the fourth time, the aide requested permission to put the patient to bed early. The charge nurse said no, but to keep the patient under watch and go get him when he wandered off the unit. The aide then wheeled the patient into his room, slammed the door closed, and moved the bed into such a position that the door barely opened. There was no way that the patient could exit the room in his wheelchair. The court found the aide had mistreated the patient by barricading him in his room and fined her $1,500.

Some circumstances, however, justify detainment. Hospitals have a common law duty to detain persons who are confused or disoriented. Most states have laws authorizing the detainment of mentally ill persons or persons with a contagious disease who would be a threat to society. In *Blackman for Blackman v. Rifkin* (1988), the hospital was allowed to detain a highly intoxicated, head trauma patient in the emergency center despite her insistence that she be allowed to leave.

As a rule of thumb, mentally ill persons may be detained only if they are a grave threat to themselves or are capable of jeopardizing others. The only force that may be used to detain such persons is that necessary under the circumstances; otherwise, the patient may be able to show battery and false imprisonment.

Restraints are an interference with the patient's liberty, but relatively few cases exist in which a patient has filed for false imprisonment due to use of restraints. Care, caution, and reasonableness are the prerequisites to use of restraints.

Conversion of Property

The tort of *conversion of property* arises when the health care practitioner interferes with the right to possession of the patient's property, either by intermeddling or by dispossessing the person of the property. Examples include searching a patient's suitcase and removing prescription drugs from the patient's possession or taking the patient's car keys or clothing without just cause. This tort is often seen in combination with other torts. Taking a patient's car keys to prevent the patient from leaving the hospital could also be termed false imprisonment. As with the other intentional torts, however, the practitioner may be free from liability if there is adequate justification for the action. For example, taking the car keys to prevent the confused, disoriented person from driving is permissible.

Trespass to Land

Trespass to land is the tort of unlawful interference with another's possession of land, and may occur either intentionally or as the result of a negligent action. This tort occurs when a person (1) intrudes onto another's property, (2) fails to leave the property when so requested, (3) throws or places something on the property, or (4) causes a third person to enter the property.

Institutions and health care facilities, including parking areas, are private property and people do not have an absolute right to remain on the property. Trespass to land thus occurs when a patient refuses to leave the institution after having been properly discharged or when visitors refuse to leave the area. Trespass may also occur when protestors enter the health care facility as part of a dispute.

Saucier v. Biloxi Regional Medical Center (1998) raised the issue of trespass to land. A group of teenage boys broke into an abandoned hospital to hide and smoke marijuana and to see if ghosts really inhabited morgues as rumored. They found that the pharmacy in the abandoned hospital still had medications on several of the shelves. They returned the next night and looted pills from the pharmacy shelves. They then went to one of the boys' homes to look in a copy of the *Physician's Desk Reference* to identify the pills before consuming them. One of the boys overdosed on amphetamines and barbiturates. The boy's mother sued the hospital on her son's behalf.

The Supreme Court of Mississippi ruled that the boys who had broken into the hospital were trespassers. They knew the hospital was not open for business, that they were not entering the building for a purpose associated with the owner's business, and that they had no permission to be there. Thus, the court ruled that there were no grounds for a civil lawsuit against the owner for injuries associated with a trespasser's unlawful entry on the premises.

Intentional Infliction of Emotional Distress

Sometimes called *extreme and outrageous conduct,* the tort of **intentional infliction of emotional distress** includes several types of outrageous conduct that cause severe emotional distress. Three conditions must be met to prove this tort:

1. The practitioner's conduct goes beyond behavior that is usually tolerated by society.
2. The conduct is calculated to cause mental distress.
3. The conduct actually causes the mental distress.

Rude and insulting behavior is not sufficient to recover under this tort; the behavior must be beyond all realms of decency. Depending on state law, patients' families who witness the conduct may also recover damages. A case that illustrates these points is *Angeles v. Brownsville Valley Regional Medical Center, Inc.* (1997).

After the mother delivered a stillborn fetus, she was told that, because of the fetus's weight and length, it had to be buried. The hospital's policy was that any stillborn fetus weighing more than 500 grams or more than 20 weeks' gestational age was to be buried.

When the mother contacted the pathologist four days later, he said that she could either designate a funeral home to recover the remains or give permission to the hospital to dispose of the remains in a respectful manner. The mother chose the latter option, believing that the hospital had a special place to bury babies.

Three months later, the parents learned that the fetus was still in the hospital morgue, primarily because no one knew what to do. The parents arranged for a funeral and burial, then filed this lawsuit.

Although the court did not condone the hospital's actions, it ruled that the actions were neither outrageous nor indecent. The actions were nonchalant and insensitive, but not atrocious or uncivilized. Thus, there were no grounds to sue the hospital for intentional infliction of emotional distress.

Unless the conduct goes outside the reasonable bounds of decency, courts are reluctant to allow plaintiff recovery for this tort. This tort can be easily avoided by treating patients and their families in the same civil, reasonable manner that one would want for oneself or loved ones.

■ EXERCISE 6–4

A private duty nurse was hired to care for an alcoholic patient in the patient's residence. While on duty, the patient and nurse argued and the patient threw a table lamp at the nurse, striking her on the head and upper torso. If she decided to sue the patient, what grounds would she assert in her case? Does the patient have grounds that he could assert in a court of law? If you were the judge, what would be your verdict?

QUASI-INTENTIONAL TORTS

The law also recognizes *quasi-intentional torts.* A tort becomes quasi-intentional when intent is lacking but there is a volitional action and direct causation. In other words, more than mere negligence is involved, but the intent that is necessary for an intentional tort is missing in quasi-intentional torts. As with intentional torts, quasi-intentional torts have no use to society and damages are not an issue. Table 6–4 outlines these torts.

Invasion of Privacy

The right to protection against unreasonable and unwarranted interferences with the individual's solitude is well recognized. The tort of *invasion of privacy* includes the protection of personality as well as the protection against interference with one's right to be left alone. This right to privacy concerns one's peace of mind in that he or she is allowed to be left alone without unwarranted publicity. Within a medical context, the law recognizes the patient's right against:

1. Appropriation or usage of the plaintiff's name or picture for defendant's sole advantage.
2. Intrusion by the defendant on the patient's seclusion or affairs.
3. Publication by the defendant of facts that place the patient in a false light.
4. Public disclosure of private facts about the patient by hospital staff or medical personnel.

Elements of invasion of privacy include:

1. An act that must intrude or pry into the seclusion of the patient.
2. Intrusion that is objectionable to the reasonable person.
3. An act or intrusion that intrudes or pries into private facts or publishes facts and pictures of a private nature.
4. Public disclosure of private information.

Information concerning the patient is confidential and may not be disclosed without authorization. Authorization may be either by patient waiver or pursuant to a valid re-

TABLE 6–4. QUASI-INTENTIONAL TORTS

Tort	Elements	Examples of Nursing Actions
Invasion of privacy	Act must intrude or pry into person's seclusion; intrusion must be objectionable to a reasonable person; intrusion must concern private facts or publish facts and pictures of a private nature; must be public disclosure of private information	Using a patients' pictures without their consent or in a manner that was not authorized by them Releasing confidential information to others without the person's consent Giving status reports about a patient to someone not authorized to receive such information
Defamation	Defamatory language about a living person that would adversely affect his/her reputation, published to a third person, damage to reputation	Making false chart entries about a patient's lifestyle or diagnoses Falsely accusing staff members in in front of visitors or other staff members

porting statute. Most hospitals and institutions have policies regarding who and under what circumstances information may be released. Liability could exist if nurses and hospital personnel fail to follow their published policies and procedures.

Nurses are to be cautioned about releasing information concerning current patients over the telephone. Remember, even family members may not be privileged to patient information. The patient may elect not to disclose information concerning diagnosis and treatments to family members. Short of a valid reporting statute, the nurse may not violate this privacy right.

Frequently, relatives and friends call to inquire about the patient's status, diagnosis, or prognosis. Before releasing any information, the patient must authorize such release, and the nurse should verify who the inquirer is, as most patients allow release of information only to family and close friends. For callers who are not allowable recipients of patient knowledge, an appropriate response is to ask the caller to contact the family or relatives directly.

Patients have a right to their names as well as to their pictures. Pictures or photos may not be used, even for medical journals or technical publications, without proper authorization (*Vessiliades v. Garfinckel's, Brooks Brothers*, 1985). In that case, the court held that a plastic surgeon had violated the privacy of a patient when he allowed, without her consent or prior knowledge, "before" and "after" pictures of her to be used for a department store presentation and by a television station.

A case that illustrates the court's reluctance to expand privacy rights is *Rothstein v. Montefiore Home* (1996). In this case, the deceased's wife had filed the original application for his admission to a nursing home. Included in the application packet were financial records and tax returns. The deceased died before the application could be processed and the application packet was returned to the deceased's daughter, not his widow.

According to the court, the daughter carefully examined the financial papers and, based on what she learned, filed a suit to contest her father's will in probate court. The will contest threatened the widow's position as beneficiary under the will, and the widow sued the nursing home for releasing the financial records to the daughter. The widow's case listed the cause of action as invasion of privacy.

In dismissing the invasion of privacy lawsuit, the court noted that such a lawsuit is meant to compensate a person for mental anguish when a private facet of a person's life is exposed to the public. The deceased, ruled the court, suffered no mental anguish. Additionally, the records were released in privacy to another member of the family, so no invasion of the widow's privacy occurred.

In limited circumstances, the newsworthiness of the event makes disclosure acceptable. The public's right to know can exceed the patient's right to privacy, as seen in the 1981 attempt on President Reagan's life or in the implantation of innovative life-support systems. Dr. Barney Clark (1982) would be an example of the latter, although his name might have been protected, as was done in the case of Baby K (1993).

Even though there may be a right to public knowledge, courts have not allowed the public disclosure to undermine a patient's dignity. Two landmark cases, *Barber v. Time, Inc.* (1942) and *Doe v. Roe* (1978), both stand for the need to protect the patient's privacy rights. One cannot divulge so much information about the patient that the patient's identity becomes readily obvious.

Valid reporting statutes may allow disclosure of limited patient data. Nurses must protect the patient's privacy over and above what is required by disclosure statutes (*Prince v.*

St. Francis-St. George Hospital, 1985). Chapter 7 discusses reporting statutes in more detail.

Defamation

Defamation, which is made up of the torts of slander and libel, is the tort of wrongful injury to another's reputation (his or her good name, respect, and esteem). It involves written or oral communication to someone other than the person defamed of matters concerning a living person's reputation. A claim of defamation may arise from inaccurate or inappropriate release of medical information or from untruthful statements about other staff members.

Five elements are necessary to prove the quasi-intentional tort of defamation:

1. Defamatory language that would adversely affect one's reputation
2. Defamatory language about or concerning a living person
3. Publication to a third party or to several persons but not necessarily the world at large
4. Damage to the person's reputation as seen by adverse, derogatory, or unpleasant opinion against the person defamed
5. Fault on the part of the defendant in writing or telling another the defamatory language

The tort may be harder to prove if the person affected is a public figure. The law recognizes that such public figures would have a greater possibility of publicly defending themselves than the private person and could more easily explain or counteract the potentially defamatory statement. For example, politicians could call a press conference or request that the local newspaper write their version. A private housewife or health care provider could not command such actions, and thus has greater protection for this quasi-intentional tort at law.

Generally, no actual damages need to exist for slander (oral communications), but must exist for libel (written defamation). Exceptions include slanderous statements that concern contagious or venereal diseases, crimes involving moral turpitude, or comments that prejudice persons in their chosen profession, trade, or business. Two older but still applicable cases illustrate this point. *Schessler v. Keck* (1954) concerned a case wherein a nurse told a second person that a particular caterer was currently being treated for syphilis, and the false statement destroyed the catering business. *Farrell v. Kramer* (1963) concerned a similar defamatory statement.

The nurse is to be cautioned against defamatory statements in chart references to patients. For example, charting that a patient is a prostitute or acts "crazy" may raise potential liability issues. When a person exhibits unusual behavior, chart exactly the behavior as perceived rather than conclusory statements.

■ EXERCISE 6—5

Imagine that you are required to design a one-hour continuing education offering for nurses to learn more about intentional torts. What content would you include in the presentation? How should you present the information to the audience? How should you evaluate the effectiveness of your continuing education offering?

DEFENSES

In some instances, a health care provider may commit an intentional tort and incur no legal liability. Called *defenses,* these specific instances and circumstances are the subject of the next chapter.

SUMMARY

Malpractice—negligence as it pertains to professionals—is the leading cause of lawsuits filed today in the medical arena. All six elements of malpractice must be proven in court for the injured party to prevail. There are guidelines to prevent or lessen the possibility of malpractice suits being filed against health care providers.

Intentional torts—those willingly performed with knowledge and intent—and quasi-intentional torts occur in a variety of ways in health care settings. To avoid committing such torts, the nurse must first comprehend their importance at law, and then understand how easily (and frequently) they can occur in clinical settings.

 GUIDELINES: INTENTIONAL TORTS AND QUASI-INTENTIONAL TORTS

1. Recognize that the patient has several rights at law for freedom from intentional torts and quasi-intentional torts and that the nurse must act to ensure these rights.
2. Know the elements of each of the intentional and quasi-intentional torts so that you will not violate the rights of patients for whom you care. Some torts are more common than others. The nurse should know that the tort of battery is the most common one seen within the health care arena and possibly the easiest one to commit. Stop and think before making unwarranted contacts with patients.
3. Know that there are limited circumstances in which the absolute rights of the patient may be transgressed. Understand the full impact of the law in these limited areas, and seek legal guidance before transgressing the patient's rights.
4. Treat all patients with the same competent, courteous care that you would want for yourself and your loved ones.
5. Be particularly selective when answering questions about patients over the telephone. Recognize that patients have the right to refuse, unless there exists a state reporting statute to the contrary, to allow disclosure of details about their illness and prognosis to others, including close family members.
6. Be cautious of the patient who is also a public figure. Public figures, whether voluntarily placed before the public eye or not, are owed the same privacy and reputation rights as the private patient.

AFTER COMPLETING THIS CHAPTER, YOU SHOULD BE ABLE TO

- Distinguish negligence from malpractice.
- List the six elements of malpractice and give examples of each element in professional nursing practice.
- Define the three tests currently used by courts in establishing cause-in-fact.
- Analyze the doctrine of res ipsa loquitor and give an example of when the doctrine would apply to professional nursing practice.
- Compare and contrast the locality rule to a national standard.
- List eight ways to avoid or lessen the potential of future malpractice cases.
- Define and differentiate between intentional and quasi-intentional torts.
- List the more commonly occurring intentional torts in health care settings and give an example of each.
- List the more commonly occurring quasi-intentional torts in health care settings and give an example of each.

APPLY YOUR LEGAL KNOWLEDGE

- What types of patients are more likely to bring nursing malpractice suits?
- When a patient injury occurs, is the nurse or another staff member always legally responsible?
- What are the more common types of nursing malpractice today?
- Why is the distinction between malpractice and negligence important?
- How do intentional torts differ from negligence and malpractice?
- If a teaching session were to be given on intentional torts seen in clinical settings, which torts would be included? Would you answer differently if time were limited and you could include additional materials?
- What can staff nurses do to protect patients from quasi-intentional torts? Does this differ from the nurse manager's role in preventing quasi-intentional torts?

YOU BE THE JUDGE

Dolores Lucas was admitted to St. Frances Cabrini Hospital complaining of back pain which had begun approximately six weeks prior to her admission. The pain was becoming steadily worse. She was admitted by a thoracic surgeon, who had performed heart surgery on her over three years before this admission. He referred the patient to a second surgeon, who determined that she should undergo a transabdominal hysterectomy and salpingo-oophorectomy. In preparation for the surgery, the patient was to be given a Fleet enema on the evening before surgery.

The enema was given by Ms. Roberts, a nurse at the facility. Ms. Roberts stated that she gave the enema without incident at about 7:30 P.M. The patient testified that, although she did not tell Ms. Roberts, she felt pain and burning when the enema was administered.

The next morning, the patient was taken to the operating room for her surgery. Shortly after beginning the procedure, the surgeon stated that he found retroperitoneal air present in the patient's pelvic area. He was unable to locate its origin. The anesthesiologist present during the surgery testified that there was no interior perforation. The hysterectomy was completed, and a third surgeon was consulted. He performed a loop sigmoid colostomy for proximal diversion of the fecal stream and closed the abdomen. He then did a rectal examination and found no obvious rectal perforation or any perforation of the colon.

Following her surgery, the patient remained in the hospital for three weeks. The colostomy was removed eight months later. The patient brought suit, alleging that Ms. Roberts was negligent in giving the preoperative enema. The lower court found for the plaintiff, and the hospital appealed.

Legal Questions

1. Was Ms. Roberts negligent in her care of this patient?
2. Does the fact that the patient said nothing during the administration of the enema affect the possible negligence?
3. Was there sufficient evidence to conclude that the doctrine of res ipsa liquitor might apply?
4. How would you decide this case?

REFERENCES

Annotations, 67 ALR 4th (1989). Applicability of Res Ipsa Loquitor in Cases of Multiple Medical Defendants—Modern Status, 544–601.

Anderson v. St. Francis-St. George Hospital, 614 N.E.2d 841 (Ohio, 1992).

Angeles v. Brownsville Valley Regional Medical Center, Inc., 960 S.W.2d 854 (Tex. App., 1997).

Arthur v. Lutheran General Hospital, Inc., 692 N.E.2d 1238 (Ill. App., 1998).

Baca v. Velez, 833 P.2d 1194 (N.M. App., 1992).

Barber v. Time, Inc., 348 Missouri 1199, 159 S.W.2d 291 (1942).

Blackman for Blackman v. Rifkin, 759 P.2d 54 (Colo. App, 1988), cert. denied (1988).

Bond v. Sacred Heart Medical Center, No. 86-2-03311 (February 1991).

Brown v. Southern Baptist Hospital, 715 So.2d 423 (La. App., 1998).

Crane v. Lakewood Hospital, 658 N.E.2d 1088 (Ohio App., 1995).

Creasy v. Rusk, 696 N.E.2d 442 (Ind. App., 1998).

Curtis v. MRI Imaging Services II, 956 P.2d 960 (Oregon, 1998).

Delaune v. Medical Center of Baton Rouge, Inc., 683 So.2d 859 (La. App., 1996).

Dent v. Memorial Hospital of Adel, 509 S.E.2d 908 (Georgia, 1998).

Depesa v. Westchester Square Medical Center, 657 N.Y.S.2d 419 (A.D. 1 Dept. 1997).

Dickerson v. Fatehi, 484 S.E.2d 880 (Virginia, 1997).

Doe v. Roe, 93 Misc.2d.201, 400 N.Y.S.2d. 958 (1978).

Donahue v. Port, Case #92-CIV-4477 (Pennsylvania, February 1994).

Estate of Chin v. St. Barnabas Medical Center et al., 711 A.2d 352 (N.J. Super., 1998).

Farrell v. Kramer, 193 A.2d 560 (Maine, 1963).

Fiesta, J. (1994). *20 Legal Pitfalls for Nurses to Avoid.* Albany, NY: Delmar Publishers, Inc.

Foflygen v. R. Zemel, 615 A.2d 1345 (Pennsylvania, 1992).

Fraijo v. Hartland Hospital, 99 Cal. Rptr.3d 331, 160 Calif. Rptr. 848 (1979).

Glassman v. St. Joseph Hospital, 631 N.E.2d 1186 (Illinois, 1994).

Harder v. F. C. Clinton, Inc., 948 P.2d 298 (Oklahoma, 1997).

Hardman v. Long Island Urological Associates, P.C., 678 N.Y.S.2d 365 (N.Y. App., 1998).

Hesler v. Osawatomie State Hospital, 971 P.2d 1169 (Kansas, 1999).

Jones v. Department of Health, 661 So.2d 1291 (Fla. App., 1995).

Kadyszewski v. Ellis Hospital Association, 595 N.Y.S.2d 841 (New York, 1993)

Keeton, W. P. (ed.) (1984). *Prosser and Keeton on the Law of Torts* (5th ed.). St Paul, MN: West Publishing Company.

Lane v. Tift County Hospital Authority, 492 S.E.2d 317 (Ga. App., 1997).

Loungbury v. Capel, 836 P.2d 188 (Utah, 1992).

Lunsford v. Board of Nurse Examiners, 648 S.W.2d 391 (Tex. Civ. App.–Austin, 1983).

Luby v. St. John's Episcopal Hospital, 631 N.Y.S.2d 773 (N.Y. App. Div., 1995).

McGraw v. St. Joseph's Hospital, 488 S.E.2d 389 (West Virginia, 1997).

Majca v. Beekil, Nos. 83677, 83886 (Illinois, 1998).

Manning v. Twin Falls Clinic and Hospital, 830 P.2d 1185 (Idaho, 1992)

Mohr v. Williams, 95 Minn. 261, 104 N.W. 12 (1905).

Moore v. Willis-Knighton Medical Center, 720 So.2d 425 (La. App., 1998).

Niece v. Elmview Group Home, 929 P.2d 420 (Washington, 1997).

Prince v. St. Francis-St. George Hospital, 484 N.E.2d 265 (App. Ohio, 1985).

Remmers v. DeBuono, 660 N.Y.S.2d 159 (N.Y. App., 1997).

Rothstein v. Montefiore Home, 689 N.E.2d 108 (Ohio App., 1996).

Saucier v. Biloxi Regional Medical Center, 708 So.2d 1351 (Mississippi, 1998).

Schessler v. Keck, 271 P.2d 588 (California, 1954).

Schloendorff v. Society of New York Hospitals, 211 N.Y. 125, 105 N.E. 92 (1914).

Silves v. King, 970 P.2d 790 (Wash. App., 1999).

Slease v. Hughbanks, 684 N.E.2d 496 (Ind. App., 1997).

Swift v. Northeastern Hospital of Philadelphia, 690 A.2d 719 (Pa. Super., 1997).

Van Horn v. Chambers, 970 S.W.2d 542 (Texas, 1998).

Vessiliades v. Garfinkel's, Brooks Brothers, 492 A.2d 580 (D.C. App., 1985).

Wingate v. Ridgeview Institute, Inc., 504 S.E.2d 714 (Ga. App., 1998).

Words and Phrases (1995). Assault. St. Paul, MN: West Publishing Co.

Ybarra v. Spangard, 154 P.2d 687 (California, 1944).

sevenseven

Nursing Liability: Defenses

■ PREVIEW

Health care providers are acutely aware of potential legal claims that may be filed against them. Much of this concern involves unknowns about the legal process and civil liability. But concern may also surface about possible defenses to lawsuits filed. This chapter explores possible legal defenses to nursing liability and how such defenses may lessen the individual practitioner's legal liability.

■ KEY CONCEPTS

defenses	abuse	assumption of the risk
consent	access	immunity
self-defense	qualified privilege	Good Samaritan laws
defense of others	release	statutes of limitations
necessity	exculpatory clause (contract)	products liability
truth	contributory (comparative)	collective liability
privilege	negligence	alternative liability
disclosure statutes	contributory negligence rule	

DEFENSES AGAINST LIABILITY

Several defenses are available to the health care practitioner in the event that a legal claim or lawsuit is filed. *Defenses* are "arguments in support of or arguments used for justification" (Boyer et al., 1991, p. 198). These defenses may be based on statutory law, common law, or the doctrine of precedent. These defenses may also be classified according to the cause of action filed against them.

DEFENSES AGAINST INTENTIONAL TORTS

Some of the defenses against intentional torts include: (1) consent; (2) self-defense; (3) defense of others; and (4) necessity (see Table 7–1).

108

TABLE 7–1. DEFENSES TO TORTS

Intentional Torts	Quasi-Intentional Torts	Nonintentional Torts
Consent	Consent	Release
Self-defense	Truth	Contributory negligence
Defense of others	Privilege	Comparative negligence
Necessity	Disclosure statutes	Assumption of the risk
Access laws	Immunity statutes	
Duty to disclose laws	Statutes of limitations	
Qualified privilege		

Consent

Consent may be either oral, implied by law, or apparent. There can be no suit for a battery if the patient approved of the touching. For example, Nurse Alicia is the medication nurse for an acute care nursing unit. She enters the patient's room with a syringe in one hand and an alcohol wipe in the other hand. As she enters the room she states, "Mr. Jones, I have your vitamin injection. In which arm would you prefer that I give it?" The patient extends his left arm and helps the nurse roll up his left sleeve with his right hand. *Apparent consent* has been given, because the reasonable person would infer from the patient's conduct that he both understood what was said to him and that he consented to the action of giving the injection.

Consent may also be *implied by law.* Many examples of implied consent occur in emergency settings. When the person is capable of neither giving nor denying consent, the law will adopt the granting of consent if the following four elements are met:

1. An immediate decision is made to prevent loss of life or limb.
2. The person is incapable of giving or denying consent.
3. There is no reason to believe that consent would not be given if the patient were capable of such.
4. A reasonable person in the same or similar circumstances would give consent.

A more thorough discussion on consent may be found in Chapter 8.

Self-Defense and Defense of Others

Self-defense and *defense of others* may be justifiable to protect oneself and others in the area from harm. For example, a patient suddenly becomes combative, and there is imminent danger to the nursing staff as well as to other patients and visitors. The nurses would be justified in forcibly restraining the patient, even though no order for restraints had been obtained. In such an example, defense of others could be extended to include the defense of the patient as well. The caveat is that one can use only reasonable force—that which is necessary to prevent injury to oneself or to defend others in the situation.

In *Mattocks v. Bell* (1963), a landmark case in this area, a male medical student was allowed to strike a 23-month-old child on the cheek to free his finger from the child's mouth. In finding that no battery or assault occurred, the court concluded that no unnecessary force was used nor was the force applied inappropriately. The court did say, however, that it was not condoning the striking of the child.

A more common example of self-defense and defense of others may be seen in the following example. A nurse is working in a medical–surgical unit of a large, urban, acute care institution. A male patient, newly postoperative from an appendectomy, approaches the nurse and demands "more pain medication now!" After being told that his next scheduled medication was not for over an hour, he grabs the nurse, saying, "I want my medicine now!" Since the nurse is alone and there is no one else available to assist her, she jabs her elbow into his sternum. Once freed, she returns to the central nurse's area and immediately calls security. Has the nurse acted prudently, using only "reasonable" force given the circumstances?

Many legal experts would agree with the nurse's action, given the specifics of this scenario. At court, a jury would be asked to determine if force was necessary and if the amount of force used was "reasonable." In the preceding scenario, because the patient was capable of using force and did so, added to the fact that he was angry, most experts would concur that force was appropriately used. The nurse struck only one blow, one that was sufficient for the patient to move away from the nurse and allow her to run for assistance. Again, striking a patient should not be one's first line of defense, but it may well be the most appropriate course of action given the circumstances. Remember to accurately document the incident and complete an unusual occurrence report; information on these issues is included in Chapter 9.

Necessity

Necessity, which is similar to self-defense, allows the nurse to interfere with the patient's property rights to avoid threatened injury. For example, suppose the suddenly combative patient approaches the staff with a knife or attempts to use a belt to strangle the nurse. This defense allows the nurse to take the knife or belt away from the patient. Thus, self-defense allows reasonable force against a person, while necessity allows the person's property to be confiscated. Two caveats to remember are:

1. A defense of necessity does not allow the nurse the right to search the patient's property.
2. The defense of necessity mandates that the patient's property must be the threatening factor.

DEFENSES AGAINST QUASI-INTENTIONAL TORTS

Consent

Consent may be a defense against the quasi-intentional torts of defamation and invasion of privacy as well as to the intentional torts. The nurse cannot be charged in a lawsuit with invasion of privacy if the patient allowed the nurse right of access to personal property. Consent does not need to be formal or well-thought-out. Allowing a nurse to remove a nightgown from a piece of luggage would also be consent to notice a stash of drugs packed alongside the nightgown.

■ EXERCISE 7–1

A patient who is suspected of being a drug substance abuser asks the nurse to "look in my shaving kit for my comb." While looking for the comb, the nurse sees a packet of a white, powdery substance. Thinking it might contain an illegal street drug, the nurse confiscated the packet. If the patient later brings suit for invasion of privacy for this occurrence, does the nurse have a valid defense? Would your answer change if, upon chemical analysis, no illegal drugs were found?

Truth

Truth is a valid defense against defamatory statements. Nurses should be aware that in using this defense, the entire statement must be true and not merely parts of the statement. Someone who states that "Many patients have perished for want of her skill" must be able to show that the entire statement is truthful or face a possible defamation suit.

Truth may be a defense against defamatory statements, but may also lead to other torts such as invasion of privacy. The nurse, in proving the truth of a defamatory statement, may unwillingly make public facts that concern the nature of the patient's hospitalization or the fact that the person was even a patient within a given setting. For example, for a nurse to prove that a specific patient was hospitalized for drug abuse, the nurse would need to divulge facts about the drug abuse that may invade the patient's privacy rights. As a practical matter, this usually does not occur, because the injured party or patient forfeits this privacy right when filing the lawsuit.

Privilege

Privilege, another defense against defamation, is a disclosure that might ordinarily be defamatory under different circumstances, but such disclosure may be allowable to protect or further public or private interests recognized by law. Examples of privilege include the mandate to report persons with certain diagnoses or diseases or those suspected of abusing others.

Disclosure Statutes

Both federal and state laws compel disclosure of health-related information to proper agencies for the protection of the public. The reporting laws that exist require health care providers to be familiar not only with the types of information that must be disclosed, but also with the governmental agency requiring the information. The giving of required information is protected, and there may be liability for disclosure of such privileged information to the wrong governmental agency.

Disclosure statutes mandate the reporting of certain types of health-related information to protect the public at large. A judge may also mandate that certain information be disclosed by issuing a subpoena. These statutes mandate that the health care providers or those standing in the place of health care providers voluntarily give the required information to the proper agency. The most common example of reporting statutes is vital statistics. All states require births and deaths to be reported, and a majority of states require an accounting of neonatal deaths and abortions.

Public health agencies may require a variety of disease states to be reported. Communicable and venereal diseases must be reported to protect the public. Additionally, some states require patients suffering from any type of seizure activity be reported to the state drivers' licensing agency. Cancer and other related diseases are to be reported in a handful of states.

If practitioners disclose only the limited information they must disclose, there is no liability for the disclosure under either a defamation or invasion of privacy law suit. These statutes, therefore, serve as a defense against both defamation and invasion of privacy.

Communicable disease reporting laws, informing public health officials of infectious cases, are among the oldest compulsory reporting statutes in most states. The statutes or regulations usually list the diseases to be reported and mandate practitioners to give local public health officials the patient's name, gender, age, address, and other identifying information as well as details of the patient's illness. In the cases of sexually transmitted diseases, other identifying information would include the names of all sexual partners within a reasonable time frame.

Because of the sensitivity of human immunodeficiency virus (HIV) and acquired immune deficiency syndrome (AIDS) issues, many states have enacted legislation regarding the confidentiality of HIV test results. This concept is more thoroughly explored in Chapter 9.

The National Childhood Vaccine Injury Act of 1986 mandates that all health care providers and institutions record each administration of any vaccine to a child and report any illness, disability, or death resulting from the administration of a vaccine to Health and Human Services. This act was passed following the national and international concern regarding the safety and efficacy of vaccines given to newborns and infants.

Child abuse is reportable to child welfare offices and/or other state-designated offices. Such statutes usually require that both suspected cases of child abuse and suspected neglect of a child be reported. *Abuse* incorporates physical, mental, and sexual assaults as well as physical, emotional, and medical neglect. Similar protection against abuse and neglect is currently being given adults in some states, particularly residents in nursing and convalescent homes.

Generally, the nurse reports any suspected cases through the administration of the institution. In most institutions, nurses report the suspected abuse to their immediate supervisor and the treating physician. All information concerning the notification is then documented in the patient's chart. Both civil and criminal liability may flow from the nonreport of such suspected cases, especially if further abuse or neglect occurs because of nondisclosure.

The landmark case of *Landeros v. Flood* (1976) held that a physician who fails to report suspected child abuse can be exposed for liability on the theory of medical malpractice. In that case, an 11 month old was brought to the emergency center with a leg fracture. The fracture was the type for which a reasonable and careful physician would have started an investigation of possible abuse. Instead, the child was treated and released to her parents. Shortly afterward, the child was admitted with severe and permanent injuries due to abuse. After being removed from her parents' care, this lawsuit was brought against the treating physician and health care institution.

In their findings, the court held that a hospital that, through its agents or employees, either knew of or should have suspected that a child requiring care was a victim of abuse, and failed to report the case, could be held liable for the subsequent injuries done to the child by her abusers. The decision makes it clear that liability for failure to report suspected child abuse is a greater risk than reporting suspected child abuse that, upon investigation, proves to be erroneous.

Nurses could easily have been part of the *Landeros* case. Reporting laws grant immunity from prosecution to those health care providers who do so in good faith and who report such violations to the correct governmental agency. This means that nurses who report a battered child to their supervisor and to the treating physician, following institution policy, have not violated the patient's or the parents' right to privacy.

In fact, nurses are more open to liability if they fail to report the abuse. If the parents fail to assert the child's rights against the nurse for nondisclosure of abuse, the state child welfare agency could sue the nurse in a civil suit for the injuries inflicted on the child after the failure to disclose (*Kempster v. Child Protection Services of the Department of Social Services,* 1987).

Health care providers are protected when they report suspected child abuse, even if the subsequent investigation shows the report to be groundless. In *Heinrich v. Conemaugh Valley Memorial Hospital* (1994), a Pennsylvania Superior Court found that the hospital was immune from suit when a child abuse report, which later proved groundless, was filed. Pensylvania's Child Protective Services Law mandates that suspected child abuse must be reported and that a plaintiff seeking to prove an injury resulted from a false report of abuse must show bad faith on the part of those reporting the suspected abuse. Courts presume good faith on the part of the health care providers unless shown to be incorrect.

A more recent case upholds this principle. In *Sager v. Rochester General Hospital* (1996), a 5-month-old child was taken to the emergency center with a fractured femur, an unusual injury for such a young child and one for which the parents had no explanation.

An orthopedist casted the leg and told the parents the child would be held for 24 hours for medical observation. The hospital social worker was notified of the child's admission, and after she consulted with her supervisor, she called the local protective services hotline. Child protective services posted a police officer at the child's hospital door to prevent the parents from removing the child. The child was subsequently placed in foster care and was then placed with a grandmother.

Criminal charges of abuse were never conclusively proven against the parents. The parents sued in civil court for intentional infliction of emotional distress, interference with the custodial relationship with their child, violation of their civil rights, and false imprisonment of their child.

The court dismissed the parents' causes of action. Hospital personnel, stated the court, must report evidence of apparent child abuse. They must hold the child pending completion of a child protective services investigation of possible abuse and the filing of legal procedures to remove the child into foster care. "When acting under a reasonable belief that their actions are warranted to prevent further imminent harm to an apparently abused child, hospital personnel are immune from liability in civil and criminal court for their actions" (*Sager v. Rochester General Hospital,* 1996, at 412).

Remember, though, that violations of the statutes, even in good faith, may not protect the nurse from liability. In *Perez v. Bay Area Hospital* (1992), a child was examined in the emergency room for genital irritation. Medication was prescribed, the child instructed in proper hygiene, and a culture obtained. The child was discharged, and the culture came back negative for sexually transmitted diseases.

Two days later, the Oregon Children Services Division (CSD) received a phone call from an unnamed nurse at the defendant hospital, stating that the child had tested positive for gonorrhea. Later that day, a CSD employee and a local police officer went to the child's school, told the school secretary that there was reason to believe the child had been infected with a sexually transmitted disease, and questioned the child. The child's mother was also questioned, in her home, by the CSD employee and the police officer. Later in the week, the mother was notified of the negative report by defendant hospital.

The mother subsequently filed this cause of action, asserting that the CSD employee was "negligent in disclosing information and identifying misinformation." The court granted summary judgment for the defendants on the grounds that the CSD employee's disclosures were protected by the Oregon abuse reporting statutes.

On appeal, the mother argued that the CSD employee should have contacted the hospital independently to verify the report, and that failure to do so constitutes negligence. The defendants countered that the Oregon law requires that the CDS immediately investigate reported abuse after receiving a report of suspected child abuse.

The trial court agreed with the plaintiffs and, had the case against the hospital been filed within the required statute of limitations, both the CDS employee and the defendant hospital would have been charged with negligence. Thus, very careful reporting of suspected abuse, according to the strict requirements of local and state law, is encouraged to prevent possible liability.

Access Laws

This group of statutory disclosure laws permits *access* to patient records and information without securing permission of the individual patient. The caveat is to know which given individuals or agencies may be allowed such access to patient information. Workers'

 ## GUIDELINES: DISCLOSURE STATUTES

1. Know both federal and individual state laws concerning the duty to report versus privileges to access laws.
2. Report only the information that is required to the proper governmental agency, and ensure that others who have a duty to disclose health-related information do so promptly.
3. Reporting must be done in good faith (as with abuse statutes), and civil and criminal liability may be incurred for failure to report under a statutory duty to disclose.
4. With access laws, follow hospital policy carefully, and ensure that those persons requesting access to medical records are allowed such access by law. Ask for proper identification as needed.
5. Remember, if you work in home health care or community settings, you may be the only person with the firsthand information that is needed to file reports to the appropriate governmental agency.
6. Breach of confidentiality is usually considered unprofessional conduct and grounds for disciplinary action by the state board of nurse examiners. Report only the information that is required; no freedom from liability exists for information that was not required or for information that is given to other than the proper governmental agency.

compensation statutes usually allow for access to medical records once a claim has been duly filed. If such a statute does not exist, the courts may rule that the filing of such a claim is a waiver under common law of the right of confidentiality in such health-related information.

Access laws seldom involve staff and midmanagement nurses. Usually, the medical records department and/or the administrative staff of the institution are apprised by the hospital attorney when charts may be accessed by law. Midmanagement nurses might become involved if access is sought to ongoing or current medical charts. This type of review of current records may be done in conjunction with the institution's Medicare and Medicaid reimbursement program. Before allowing access to medical records, nurses should take some precautions. First, they should receive written confirmation of such reviews from the hospital administration or the nursing service administration prior to the review. Then they should ascertain that the persons asking for access to the charts are the persons listed in the written confirmation, and ask for proof of identification as necessary. If any doubt persists concerning such a chart review, the nurses should contact their supervisors before allowing the charts to be seen. Finally, they should remain accessible to answer questions as needed. The reviewers may not clearly understand the nurse's system of charting, and nurses could be invaluable in interpreting the system to them.

Qualified Privilege

The defense of *qualified privilege* prevails when the person making the allegedly defamatory statements has a legal duty to do so, such as when a nurse manager reports, in good faith, on the professional performance of a staff nurse. Qualified privilege legally negates any inference of malice, because of the overriding public policy interest. When the quality of medical care is at issue, the reputation rights of health care professionals must concede to the greater social need.

Liability will not be imposed, even if the communications are false, as long as there is no malice and the communications are made in good faith to those persons who need to know such facts. The court, in the precedent-setting case of *Wynn v. Cole* (1979), found no liability on the part of a director of a health department who provided a prospective employer with information concerning a specific nurse's abilities. Such privileged communications exist for assessments provided by former employers to prospective employers. The caveat to be watchful is threefold:

1. The communications must be made through appropriate channels to persons needing the information.
2. Liability may be granted for untruthful communications released with malice.
3. The communications should be worded in objective and observable behavioral terms rather than judgmental descriptions.

Defamation may be *mitigated* (lessened or reduced) by such factors as retraction (one did all he or she could to rectify the previous statement) or by whether it was provoked or not. For example, the nurse may be provoked into a given statement by the anger and hostility aimed at the staff member by the patient or family. Although not an excuse for the defamation, such mitigating factors may serve to lessen the damages awarded the plaintiff.

■ EXERCISE 7–2

Interview nurse managers in hospital and community settings about privileges and qualified privileges. How do the nurse managers use these doctrines in their respective clinical settings? Does one manager use a particular privilege more than another privilege? Is there a trend in the use of privilege in the hospital versus community settings?

DEFENSES AGAINST NONINTENTIONAL TORTS

Defenses against negligent actions include (1) release; (2) contributory or comparative negligence; (3) assumption of the risk; (4) unavoidable accident; (5) defense of the fact; and (6) immunity statutes.

Release

A *release* may be signed, during the process of settling a claim, to prevent any and all future claims arising from the same incident. Once signed, the release bars (prohibits or prevents) future suits. In medical malpractice claims, a release is frequently a part of the out-of-court settlement. In effect, the plaintiff states that the settlement is the only compensation for the negligent action.

Releases are distinguished from *exculpatory clauses* or *exculpatory contracts*, which are signed before care is given and seldom serve as a successful defense. Usually, exculpatory contracts are signed to limit the amount of damages one receives in a suit or to prevent a future lawsuit based on the individual health care giver's actions. Such contracts usually fail on the grounds that they violate public policy. The court in *Cudnick v. William Beaumont Hospital* (1994) held that exculpatory agreements, which completely release a hospital from liability for an employee's negligence and which are signed by patients prior to receiving therapy, are against public policy and thus are invalid and unenforceable. The court further held that there are two exceptions to the rule invalidating exculpatory agreements for medical malpractice: (1) Experimental procedures are exempted because "they inherently require a deviation from generally accepted medical practices" (at 897); and (2) agreements releasing medical care providers from liability after treatment, pursuant to a lawsuit settlement agreement, are valid and enforceable.

Contributory and Comparative Negligence

Contributory and *comparative negligence* both serve as defenses and in essence hold injured parties accountable for their fault in the injury. Such fault by the plaintiff may occur for failure to follow prescribed treatments or if incorrect treatment is given based on the patient's false information to the physician.

Many states once used an all-or-nothing *contributory negligence rule:* Patients who had any part in the adverse consequences were barred from any compensation. Today, most jurisdictions use comparative negligence and reduce the money award by the injured party's responsibility for the ultimate harm done. For example, in a $500,000 reward, if the plaintiff is found to be 30% responsible for the negligence, then the plaintiff will be allowed a $350,000 award for damages. Some states further disallow compensation if the patient has 50% or greater responsibility in the ultimate harm done.

Legislatures and courts have adopted varying types of comparative negligence. Some jurisdictions apply the pure form of comparative negligence, wherein the plaintiff is allowed to recover the portion of the injury attributable to the defendant's negligence, regardless of which party was at greater fault. The majority of jurisdictions apply a modified comparative negligence rule, wherein the plaintiff whose negligence is found to exceed that of the defendant is barred from recovery.

The court in *Parkins v. United States* (1993) held that the patient has a duty to conform reasonably to prescriptions and treatments and to follow reasonable and proper instructions given by health care providers. Failure to so conform will prevent recovery in a court of law.

An exception to the preceding case law is *Harvey v. Mid-Coast Hospital* (1999). In that case, a 19 year old was treated for bipolar disease with Tegretol. He was found unconscious in his dorm room and was admitted through the emergency center to the intensive care unit. During the initial blood analysis at the time of admission, it was found that he had a toxic level of Tegretol in his blood.

While in the intensive care unit, he began having seizures and developed status epilepticus. The intensive care unit nurses did not notice the status epilepticus in time to avert neurological damage. The hospital's defense to a subsequently filed malpractice action was to assert a comparative negligence defense, alleging that the patient's self-inflicted overdose was the primary cause of the permanent neurological damage. In rejecting this defense, the court noted that in a professional malpractice suit the patient's own negligence could fall into one of four hypothetical categories:

1. A patient could refuse to follow advice or instructions.
2. A patient could delay seeking treatment or returning for follow-up.
3. A patient could furnish false, misleading, or incomplete information to a health care provider.
4. A patient's own self-injurious behavior could have caused the need for the medical treatment.

According to the court, the first three are situations in which the patient's own negligence can diminish or bar outright the patient's chances of success with a malpractice suit, because of comparative negligence. However, "when a patient's own negligent or intentional self-harm occurred before care was sought and only provided the occasion for needing care, the legal system does not apply the concept of contributory or comparative negligence" (*Harvey v. Mid-Coast Hospital*, 1999, at 37).

Assumption of the Risk

A defense similar to contributory and comparative negligence, *assumption of the risk* states that plaintiffs are partially responsible for consequences if they understood the risks involved when they proceeded with the action. A case example of this concept is *Lopez v. State of Louisiana Health Care Authority/University Medical Center* (1998). The patient was in his fourth day in the alcohol detoxification center of a state hospital. After breakfast, he and others lined up to be escorted outside for a smoke break. It was the eighteenth time since his admission that the patient had waited to be escorted for a smoke break.

The patient was leaning against a wall that had a door but no door handle. He stood right in front of the doorstop. All the other persons waiting for the smoke break were standing by the wall on the opposite side. A nurse opened the door from the other side and the patient was struck. He was immediately examined by the facility's physician and found to be unhurt, but sued the nurse and the facility for negligence.

The court ruled that the nurse, and thus the facility, was not negligent. If anything, the court said, it was the patient who was negligent. He knew that the door could and would open directly toward him. The patient was ambulatory and he elected to walk outside for a smoke break, demonstrating that he was not physically or mentally handicapped. There was an indication in his chart two hours before the incident that noted that the patient was "calm, steady, and aloof." The court concluded with the statement: "Health-care facilities do not have to protect patients from risks which patients who are aware of their surroundings and mentally capable should realistically anticipate and avoid on their own" (at 522).

Unavoidable Accident

This defense comes into play when nothing other than an accident could have caused the person's injury. For example, a staff member slips and falls in a patient's room. There is nothing on the floor that could have caused the accident and no one is a fault.

Defense of the Fact

This defense is used when there is no indication, direct or otherwise, that the health care provider's actions were the cause of the patient's injury or untoward outcome (e.g., the patient who receives an injection in the left arm and then begins to experience numbness and tingling in the right leg). There is no connection in the two events, and the defense to be pled is defense of the fact.

Immunity

Some states have enacted *immunity* statutes that serve to dismiss certain causes of action. The best example of a state immunity statute is the Good Samaritan statute. Because of the Good Samaritan laws, negligent actions against health care providers at scenes of accidents are rare.

Good Samaritan Laws

Legislation was at one time needed to encourage medical personnel to stop at the scene of an accident and to render appropriate medical care. In response to this need, all states have enacted *Good Samaritan laws*, which abrogate common law rescue doctrines in an effort to encourage health care providers to risk helping strangers in need of assistance, even when the health care providers have no duty to render such aid (*Jackson v. Mercy Health Center, Inc.*, 1993). While individual provisions of Good Samaritan laws vary greatly state to state, the laws have been instrumental in procuring necessary health care in emergency situations.

Good Samaritan laws are enacted to allow health care personnel and citizens trained in first aid to deliver needed medical care without unnecessary fear of incurring criminal and civil liability. The uniqueness of Good Samaritan laws is that they insulate a health care practitioner from his or her liability for rendering care at the scene of an accident.

Through legislative acts, society, for its own good, has given health care providers immunity from negligent acts or omissions when acting as a Good Samaritan at the scene of an emergency. State legislators have long recognized that persons who stop and render emergency care should be a protected class.

Dispute exists over which persons should be protected, the extent to which the protection extends, and the type of emergency that qualifies for Good Samaritan protection. Some states extend protection merely to licensed health care providers. Other states allow ordinary citizens to be covered under the legislation along with licensed health care providers.

At least one court has been willing to extend protection to individuals who volunteer to assist in emergencies. In *Boccasile v. Cajun Music Limited* (1997), a nurse volunteered her time to staff the first aid tent at an outdoor music festival where food was being sold and served to the public by festival promoters. A festival patron sampled the seafood gumbo, which contained a shellfish to which the man was allergic. The patron developed anaphylactic shock and died.

The first aid tent was staffed by the nurse and a physician, both unpaid volunteers. When it was reported that a patron was in distress, the physician quickly left the tent and went to his aid. The physician recognized the anaphylactic shock, instructed someone to call paramedics via the 911 distress line, and gave the man the only dosage of epinephrine that she had in her emergency bag.

As soon as someone else had come to relieve the nurse in the first aid tent, she too went to the patron's aid. She stayed with him while waiting for the paramedics to arrive. The patron quickly went into respiratory distress. The physician and the nurse began cardiopulmonary resuscitation but could not revive the man, and he died during transport to the hospital.

The Supreme Court of Rhode Island, using the Good Samaritan law, dismissed the wrongful death suit brought by the man's estate. Both health professionals were volunteers, the court concluded, rendering gratuitous services in an emergency situation, and there was no proof that either were guilty of "gross, willful or wanton negligence" (at 688).

The court was not persuaded that the nurse or physician was liable for ordinary negligence. Thus, even though the Good Samaritan law protected them, they did not need its application to be relieved from blame.

A newer trend is for states to mandate emergency assistance. Vermont was the first state to enact such a law requiring persons to assist others exposed to grave physical harm as long as the assistance could be given without endangering themselves. Reasonable assistance should be given, and violation of the statute is punishable by fines (*Vermont Statutes Annotated*, 1968).

The need for Good Samaritan laws becomes apparent because there is no legal duty to render assistance to a stranger in times of distress, unless so mandated by statute or unless the individual caused the stranger's distress. While one could argue that a moral or ethical duty should exist, no legal duty arises until the individual first initiates the giving of emergency care. Then the legal duty becomes one of reasonable or emergency care. Only when a person renders grossly negligent or willful and wanton negligent care is the health care provider not protected by the Good Samaritan immunity. As a practical matter, malpractice suits against Good Samaritans are relatively rare.

Before proceeding under a Good Samaritan law, nurses must recognize that the acts vary greatly among states. Consequently, they must be aware of exactly what is covered by an individual state act. Nurses should look for the following information when reviewing an individual state act:

1. Who is covered as part of the protected class? Some states cover all persons who give emergency care, some cover only physicians and nurses, and a few state acts cover only in-state physicians and nurses.
2. Where does the coverage extend? All state acts allow for aid at the scene of an accident, emergency, or disaster, with some states mandating that such accidents, emergencies, or disasters be roadside occurrences. Other states allow for emergency care wherever the need is, be it in a hospital, doctor's office, or outside a medically equipped place. Still other states specifically limit coverage under Good Samaritan laws to areas outside the workplace. The nurse must know what qualifies as the scene of an emergency before rendering aid under the Good Samaritan laws.

 GUIDELINES: GOOD SAMARITAN LAWS

1. Make your decision quickly as to whether you will stay and help. Remember, there is no common law duty to stop and render aid. Once you begin to provide care, you incur the legal duty to maintain a standard of reasonable emergency care.
2. Ask the injured person or family members for permission to help. Do not force your services once refused.
3. Care for the injured party where you can do so safely. This includes in the vehicle or at the exact site where the victim is found. Move the injured party only if you must do so without causing further harm and as needed to prevent further harm (e.g., off a major highway).
4. Apply the rules of first aid: Assess for and prevent bleeding, assess for the need to initiate cardiopulmonary resuscitation, cover the injured party with a blanket or coat, and so forth.
5. Continuously assess and reassess the person for additional injuries, and communicate findings of your assessment to the person or family members.
6. Have someone call or go for additional help while you stay with the injured party.
7. Stay with the person until equally or more qualified help arrives. Prevent unskilled persons from treating or moving the injured party.
8. Give as complete a description as possible of the care that you have rendered to the police and emergency medical personnel so that continuity of care exists. Give family members or police any personal items such as dentures, eyeglasses, and the like.
9. Do not accept any compensation (e.g., money or gifts) offered by the injured party or family members. Acceptance of compensation may change your care into a fee-for-service situation and cause you to lose your Good Samaritan protection.
10. Should you choose not to stop and render aid, stop at the nearest phone and report the accident to proper authorities so that the injured party may be aided.
11. Review legislative actions periodically for any changes in your state's Good Samaritan laws. Know the Good Samaritan laws in other states before giving assistance.

3. What is covered? Some states protect the individual during transportation to a medical facility. Another group of states protect against failure to provide for further assistance.

Most states require that the care be given in good faith and that it be gratuitous. Unfortunately, the acts may not define criteria to determine whether an emergency actually exists and what constitutes the scene of an emergency. Because of this, protection is uncertain in some states. To limit the nurse's liability and allow the nurse to participate in rendering needed care, the nurse should adhere to the guidelines on page 120.

■ EXERCISE 7–3

Explore your own state laws regarding Good Samaritan statutes. Are all health care providers included in the statutes? Are there other qualified persons who are covered? How do the statutes ensure that persons needing assistance will receive the needed help?

Recognizing that there may be no legal duty to stop and aid accident victims, is there an ethical duty to stop and render aid? Which ethical principles guide your answer to the question? Is there ever a time when you would be ethically bound not to stop and render care?

STATUTE OF LIMITATIONS

Statutes of limitations specify time limits for initiating claims. Unless specific exceptions apply, a suit must be filed within the time limit or the cause of action is barred (prohibited by law). Typically, individual states allow one to two years as the time frame for the filing of a malpractice suit. Therefore, injured parties must bring the suit within one to two years after they knew of the injury or had reason to believe that an injury was sustained. In the case of a minor, the statute of limitations may not begin to run (start) until the child reaches the age of majority, though there are a few states that restrict this tolling (stoppage) of statutes of limitations until children reach their majority (Aiken and Catalano, 1994). Review Chapter 2 for case examples of statutes of limitations.

PRODUCTS LIABILITY

Products liability refers to the liability of a manufacturer, processor, or nonmanufacturing seller for injury to a person or person's property by a given product. Under this type of action, the injured party may sue the maker of the product, or the seller of the product, or the intermediary distributors of the product, or all three entities. The landmark and leading case for imposing liability in this area of the law, irrespective of fault, is *Caprara v. Chrysler Corporation* (1981). In that case, the court declared that "the one in the best position to know of potential dangers and to have eliminated the same should respond to the injured party in damages" (at 124).

Theories of recovery for such products liability suits are based on either breach-of-warranty liability or strict liability. Under *breach-of-warranty liability*, the patient contends that the manufacturer or others in the chain of distribution breached either an expressed or implied warranty of fitness of the product. In a *strict liability action,* the plaintiff contends that the product is unreasonably dangerous due to a defect in its manufacture or design or due to inadequate labeling (*Corpus Juris Secundum,* 1984).

This area of law is really a mixture of tort and contract law. The expressed and implied warranties of fitness for a particular purpose and of merchantability are based in contract law. Tort law concerns the liability of a person in a civil action against the person or property of another and the violation of a duty owed the injured party. The warranties (from contract law) form the basis for finding liability without fault (from tort law) for injuries caused by the use of products.

The first hurdle for the plaintiff in products liability cases is to prove that there has been a sale of a product rather than the mere delivery of a service. The distinction is crucial because a products liability action does not exist if there is no sale of a product. Some courts have held there was no responsibility because there was service, not the sale of a product (*North Miami General Hospital v. Goldberg,* 1993), whereas other courts have suggested that the hospital owes a higher duty of care to the patient because the patient has no voice in the equipment or products used (Fiesta, 1994).

A second issue for products liability cases concerns defining products as opposed to services. A product has been defined as a "thing produced by labor" or "something produced by nature or the natural process" (Boyer et al., 1991, p. 492). For years, debate has centered around blood transfusions and whether they are products or services of a hospital. While some initial cases determined that blood transfusions were products for purposes of products liability cases, all jurisdictions, either by decisional law or by legislative statutes, have determined that blood transfusions by a hospital are a service incident to treatment and not a product sold by the hospital (Werthmann, 1984). More recent developments in this area concern whether a blood bank is a health care provider for purposes of statutes of limitations. In *Smith v. Paslode Corporation* (1993), the eighth circuit held that a blood bank was a health care provider in that the blood bank "provides health care services under the authority of a license or certification (at 3). This minority opinion illustrates the difficulty courts have with determining the status of blood banks and blood products.

Along the same line, a series of court decisions determined that radiation treatments were services and not products and that the dangers of the radiation treatment are not inherent in the radiation itself but result from (1) the professional medical decision to employ radiation therapy, (2) the manner in which it is administered, and (3) the amount given (*Dubin v. Michael Reese Hospital and Medical Center,* 1980).

A third issue concerns *unavoidably unsafe products.* To be considered unavoidably unsafe, a product must contain the following three criteria:

1. Its benefits must greatly outweigh its risks.
2. Its risks cannot be eliminated.
3. No safer product exists as an alternative.

If these three elements are proven, the manufacturer will be held liable for injuries only if there was failure to adequately warn of the risks. Prescription drugs usually are considered unavoidably unsafe, and case law concerns negligence for failure of inadequate warning rather than for product liability. One of the more interesting cases to date, *Detwiler v. Bristol-Meyers Squibb Company* (1995), found liability against a physician who implanted a silicone breast implant. While the majority of the decision concerned statutes of limitations, the court held that silicone implants failed to meet the standard of unavoidably unsafe.

Contrast the preceding holding with the holding in *King v. Collagen Corporation* (1993). In that case, the plaintiff was denied damages for injuries caused by the anti-wrinkle cream Zyderm because the corporation had submitted to and passed a rigorous premarket approval process required by the Food and Drug Administration. Thus, the corporation was allowed a safe harbor from state claims such as negligent design, failure to warn, and breach of warranty. This case may serve to reopen this entire line of legal thought.

As a general rule, proper warning to the physician will satisfy the drug manufacturer's duty to warn, since the patient can obtain the drug only through the physician. Exceptions to this requirement, when the patient must be directly warned (as through mass media newspaper communications), include situations in which (1) the drug may be given without an individual prescription (e.g., with mass inoculation for polio), and (2) Federal Food and Drug Administration regulations require package inserts (*Lukaszewicz v. Ortho Pharmaceutical Corporation*, 1981). Most state laws now require that pharmacists have this same duty to warn when a prescription is filled for an individual patient.

Nurses' duty to warn patients of unavoidably unsafe prescription medications has not been delineated in the majority of jurisdictions, but it would seem reasonable to anticipate that the nurse's duty to warn will be incorporated into patient discharge education. Advanced nurse practitioners and those nurses who, by legislative enactments, may prescribe medications are considered to have the same duty to warn as the physicians who prescribe medications.

COLLECTIVE AND ALTERNATIVE LIABILITY

Currently, two theories are emerging to aid plaintiffs who previously could not prove which manufacturer was at fault. *Collective liability* stems from cooperation by several manufacturers in a wrongful activity that by its nature requires the participation of more than one wrongdoer (concert of action). All the wrongdoers' actions result in an inadequate industry-wide standard of safety as to the manufacture of a product (enterprise liability). *Alternative liability* applies when two or more manufacturers commit separate wrongful or unreasonable acts, only one of which injures the plaintiff, but the plaintiff cannot identify the actual cause-in-fact defendant.

These theories rapidly emerged in light of the diethylstilbestrol (DES) lawsuits. Women injured by the drug directly and through their offspring attempted to sue manufacturers for failing to adequately test and label the drug and thus to warn of its risks. But it was virtually impossible to identify the manufacturer of the particular DES they took. This occurred because of (1) inadequate long-term record keeping by pharmacies, (2) the widespread practice of prescribing generic drugs, and (3) failure of the DES tablets to identify the manufacturer. Under these newer liability theories, injured women and their daughters gained compensation for the industry's failure to adequately test the drug on fetuses and to warn of its risks. (See, generally, *Abel v. Eli Lilly Company*, 1984, and *Collins v. Eli Lilly Company*, 1984).

CAVEATS IN PRODUCT LIABILITY LAWSUITS

Before deciding that a products liability action exists, several points need to be comprehended and remembered:

1. States often follow strict liability in medical or health-related causes of actions. Not to allow a strict liability cause of action would place an unfair burden on the plaintiff. Indeed, even with such a cause of action, compensation has been denied persons injured in health care settings.
2. The defendant must be a commercial supplier or be determined to be a commercial supplier for a products liability cause of action to exist in most jurisdictions.
3. The cause of action must be based on a sold product and not a service, or no action will exist under products liability.
4. There may also be a negligence cause of action. If the defendant passes all the hurdles and successfully defends against a products liability cause of action, the plaintiff may still be able to prove negligence.

■ EXERCISE 7–4

Think of all the equipment and products that you use daily in the care of clients and the pharmaceutical agents that you give to patients during the course of an average day or shift. What precautions or teachings do you take to further ensure the safe, competent care of clients?

SUMMARY

Defenses are available to health care providers to justify or partially explain why they acted as they did. Defenses explored in this chapter included those against intentional, quasi-intentional, and negligent torts; statutes of limitations; and product liability. Used correctly, these defenses can lessen the individual practitioner's potential liability.

AFTER COMPLETING THIS CHAPTER, YOU SHOULD BE ABLE TO

- Define the term *defenses* and give examples of defenses that may be used against intentional torts, quasi-intentional torts, and negligent torts.
- Analyze the concept of statute of limitations, including the importance this statute has in the health care field.
- Define and explain products liability defenses.

APPLY YOUR LEGAL KNOWLEDGE

- Which of the available defenses are more commonly used by professional nurses? Why?
- How do statutes of limitations protect professional nurse-defendants? Do they also protect the injured parties?
- Can products liability defenses prevent injured parties from showing negligence and liability against professional nurse practitioners?

YOU BE THE JUDGE

Mr. McGill filed a complaint alleging that the defendant, Dr. French, was negligent in diagnosing prostate cancer and not informing McGill or the referring physician, Dr. Woolfolk. Dr. French filed an answer denying the allegations and alleging contributory negligence on the part of the plaintiff.

McGill was a patient of Dr. Daniel Woolfolk, a physician specializing in internal medicine. Dr. Woolfolk treated McGill for respiratory problems. He then sent McGill to Dr. Barnett, for consultation on the patient's emphysema. Dr. Barnett noted a prostate enlargement and referred the patient to Dr. French, a board-certified urologist. Dr. French noted the enlarged prostate and scheduled the patient for a intravenous pyelogram, which showed mild prostate enlargement. Dr. French then tried unsuccessfully for several weeks to get in touch with McGill and share the test results with him.

Dr. French saw the patient approximately a year later, when the patient was admitted for urinary retention via the emergency center. During that hospitalization, Dr. French performed a prostatectomy on the patient. In the pathology report, prostatic cancer was diagnosed from the obtained specimen. Dr. French did not inform McGill of the results before his discharge, and the diagnosis was not included in the summary discharge note in the patient's chart.

McGill returned for a follow-up visit two weeks after being discharged from the hospital. At that time, Dr. French testified, he told the patient, for the first time, of the diagnosis of prostate cancer. Dr. French also testified that the patient was informed that the cancer was highly malignant and that it was necessary for him to carefully assess signs and symptoms of its advancement. Specifically, the patient was told to report any symptoms of back pain or bone pain. No treatment other than observation was made at that point, although Dr. French outlined a full treatment plan that he would undertake when the patient presented with symptoms.

The patient made another appointment for a month later, but came in early to see Dr. French. At that visit, he had denied any back or bone pain, and Dr. French testified that he had the same conversation with the patient that he had had the previous month. He also testified that he told Mr. McGill that early treatment was unnecessary, because the quality of his life would not change since he was currently asymptomatic. Another appointment was scheduled for three months later, and the patient was to schedule an earlier appointment if he became symptomatic.

The later appointment was not kept, and there is a disagreement regarding the sending by Dr. French's office of a reminder card when the appointment was missed. The office nurse testified that she first tried to call the patient when he missed the appointment, and then sent a postcard reminder.

Mr. and Mrs. McGill both testified that at no time were they told of the diagnosis of prostate cancer. Approximately nine months after the prostate surgery, Mr. McGill began experiencing stomach pain and saw Dr. Woolfolk. At that time, Dr. Woolfolk discovered that the patient had a cancer diagnosis, and the patient and his wife testified that this was the first time they were made aware of the diagnosis. Dr. Woolfolk testified that he became aware of the diagnosis by rereading the medical records completed after the patient's discharge following his prostate surgery.

During McGill's hospitalization for stomach problems, Dr. French was consulted, and he started the patient on therapy for the prostate cancer. Mrs. McGill testified that when she asked Dr. French why he had not told them earlier of the diagnosis of cancer, he replied, "Because it does not make any difference when you start therapy." The patient was discharged after seven days and given a follow-up appointment with Dr. French for a month later, which he failed to keep. Thereafter, the patient had no further contact with Dr. French.

During the same month he was to see Dr. French for the follow-up visit, the patient had a bilateral orchiectomy and was diagnosed with bone metastasis. He was later hospitalized for removal of two tumors from his colon and several courses of treatment for pneumonia. He began radiation treatment approximately eight months after his orchiectomy and died after six years of cancer therapy.

Legal Questions

1. Was Dr. French negligent in his care of the patient?
2. Was the patient's failure to keep his appointments and notify the physician of his continuing symptoms contributory or comparative negligence?
3. How would you resolve this case?

REFERENCES

Abel v. Eli Lilly Company, 343 N.W.2d 164 (Michigan, 1984).

Aiken, T. D., and Catalano, J. T. (1994). *Legal, Ethical, and Political Issues in Nursing.* Philadelphia: F. A. Davis Company.

Boccasile v. Cajun Music Limited, 694 A.2d 686 (Rhode Island, 1997).

Boyer, M., Ellis, K., Harris, D. R., and Soukhanov, A. H. (eds.). (1991). *The American Heritage Dictionary.* (2nd ed.). Boston: Houghton Mifflin Company.

Caprara v. Chrysler Corporation, 52 N.Y.2d 114 (New York, 1981).

Collins v. Eli Lilly Company, 342 N.W.2d 37 (Wisconsin, 1984).

Corpus Juris Secundum (1984). 72 Products Liability.

Cudnick v. William Beaumont Hospital, 525 N.W.2d 891 (Mich. Ct. App., 1994).

Detwiler v. Bristol-Meyers Squibb Company, 884 F. Supp. 117 (DSNY, 1995).

Dubin v. Michael Reese Hospital and Medical Center, 393 N.E.2d 588 (Ill. App. 1979), rev'd. 415 N.E.2d 350 (Illinois, 1980).

Fiesta, J. (1994). *20 Legal Pitfalls for Nurses.* Albany, NY: Delmar Publishers.

Harvey v. Mid-Coast Hospital, 36 F. Supp.2d 32 (D. Maine, 1999).

Heinrich v. Conemaugh Valley Memorial Hospital, 648 A.2d 53 (Pennsylvania, 1994).

Jackson v. Mercy Health Center, Inc., 884 P.2d 839 (Oklahoma, 1993).

Kempster v. Child Protection Services of the Department of Social Services, 515 N.Y.S.2d 807 (New York, 1987).

King v. Collagen Corporation, No. 92-1278, 1993 US App., LEXIS 432 (First Cir., January 15, 1993).

Landeros v. Flood, 551 P.2d 389, 17 Cal.3d 399 (California, 1976).

Lopez v. State of Louisiana Health Care Authority/University Medical Center, 721 So.2d 518 (La. App., 1998).

Lukaszewicz v. Ortho Pharmaceutical Corporation, 510 F. Supp. 961 (E.D. Wisc., 1981).

Mattocks v. Bell, 194 P.2d 307 (D.C. App., 1963).

National Childhood Vaccine Injury Act of 1986, 42 U.S.C., Section 300aa-25.

North Miami General Hospital v. Goldberg, No. 87-337 (Fla. App. Ct, February 23, 1993).

Parkins v. United States, 834 F. Supp. 569 (D. Conn., 1993).

Perez v. Bay Area Hospital, 829 P.2d 700 (Or. App., 1992).

Sager v. Rochester General Hospital, 647 N.Y.S.2d 408 (N.Y. Sup., 1996).

Smith v. Paslode Corporation, WL 392245 (8th Cir., 1993).

Vermont Statutes Annotated, Title 12, Sec. 519 (1968).

Werthmann, B. (1984). *Medical Malpractice Law: How Medicine Is Changing the Law.* Lexington, MA: Lexington Books.

Wynn v. Cole, 284 N.W.2d 144 (Mich. App., 1979).

eight

Informed Consent and Patient Self-Determination

■ PREVIEW

In the past, informed consent was a matter concerning the patient and the physician, a concept capable of being delegated to the nurse as the physician thought best. Too often, the consent was automatic and uninformed. Patients and their loved ones allowed the paternalistic health care system to do as it saw fit and asked far too few questions. Fortunately, this trend has changed, and nurses must understand the concept of informed consent to ensure that patient consent is truly valid and informed. Extensions of the concept of informed consent are patients' rights in research, genetic testing, and patient self-determination. This chapter explores the essential characteristics of consent, the power to consent, requirements for patients' consent in research, and patient self-determination through living wills and durable power of attorney for health care.

■ KEY CONCEPTS

consent	legal guardian or representative	durable power of attorney
informed consent	minor	for health care (DPAHC)
informed refusal	in loco parentis	medical durable power
expressed consent	court order	of attorney (MDPA)
implied consent	right of refusal	medical or physician directive
standards of disclosure	genetic testing	do-not-resuscitate directives
medical disclosure laws	patient self-determination	hospice center
therapeutic privilege	substituted judgment	assisted suicide
waiver	living will	
competency at law	natural death act	

ROLE OF CONSENT

Generally, the health care provider's right to treat a patient, barring true emergency conditions or unanticipated happenings, is based on a contractual relationship that arises through the mutual consent of parties to the relationship. *Consent* is the voluntary authorization by a patient or the patient's legal representative to do something to the patient. Consent is based on the mutual consent of all parties involved, and the key to true and valid consent is patient comprehension.

Consent becomes an important issue from a legal perspective in that patients may sue for a battery (unconsented touching) if they do not consent to the procedure or treatment and the health care provider goes ahead with the procedure or treatment. This means that patients may bring a lawsuit and be awarded damages even if they were helped by the procedure or treatment. For example, the therapy was performed correctly and the patient's health actually improved because of the therapy. The more current trend, however, is to argue consent under a negligence or malpractice cause of action.

Consent is an issue in its own realm. Consent does not always become a factor in a malpractice suit, although it may be a concurrent issue in a malpractice suit. Consent concerns the health care provider's right to treat a given individual, not the manner in which the treatment was delivered. Thus, one can deliver safe, competent care and still be sued for lack of consent.

The right to consent and the right to refuse consent are based on a long-recognized, common law right of persons to be free from harmful or offensive touching of their bodies. In a landmark case during the early part of this century, the court declared the reason for consent, and that case is still quoted today when referring to the consent doctrine. "Every human being of adult years has a right to determine what shall be done with his own body, and a surgeon who performs an operation without his patient's consent commits an assault for which he is liable in damages" (*Schloendorff v. Society of New York Hospitals*, 1914, p. 93).

Thus, two concepts are involved: (1) the prevention of a battery and (2) the person's right to control what is done to his or her body. Because of these rights, the health care provider has a duty to obtain consent prior to treating a patient. Consent, therefore, is not contingent on a request for information or clarification by the patient but must be actively sought by the health care practitioner.

CONSENT VERSUS INFORMED CONSENT

Consent, technically, is an easy yes or no: "Yes, I will allow the surgery" or "No, I want to try medications first, then maybe I will allow the surgery." Patients may not understand or may understand only vaguely what they are allowing.

The law concerning consent in health care situations is based on *informed consent*, which mandates to the physician or independent health care practitioner the separate legal duty to disclose needed material facts in terms that patients can reasonably understand so that they can make an informed choice. There should also be a description of the available alternatives to the proposed treatment and the risks and dangers involved in each alternative. Failure to disclose the needed facts in understandable terms does not negate the consent, but it does place potential liability on the practitioner for negligence. In other words, without any consent given, practitioner may be sued for a battery (an intentional tort). Without informed consent, practitioners open themselves to potential lawsuits for negligence.

The doctrine of informed consent has developed from negligence law as the courts began to realize that, although consent may have been given, not enough information was imparted to form the foundation of an informed decision. The right to informed consent did not become a judicial issue until 1957. In a landmark decision, the California courts found a doctor negligent for failing to explain the potential risks of a vascular procedure to a patient subsequently paralyzed by the procedure (*Salgo v. Leland Stanford, Jr. University Board of Trustees*, 1957).

Some courts have extended the right to informed consent to what might be called *informed refusal*. The practitioner may be liable for failure to inform the patient of the risks of not consenting to a therapy or diagnostic screening test. *Truman v. Thomas* (1980) was one of the first cases to recognize this important corollary to informed consent. In that case, the court awarded damages against a physician for failure to inform the patient of the potential risks of not consenting to a recommended Papanicolaou (Pap) smear.

INCLUSIONS IN INFORMED CONSENT

To be informed, patients must receive, in terms they can understand and comprehend, the following information:

1. A brief but complete explanation of the treatment or procedure to be performed (*Hecht v. Kaplin*, 1996).
2. The name and qualifications of the person to perform the procedure and, if others will assist, the names of qualifications of those assistants (*Lugenbuhl v. Dowling*, 1996 and *Grabowski v. Quigley*, 1996).
3. An explanation of any serious harm that may occur during the procedure, including death if that is a realistic outcome. Pain and discomforting side effects both during the procedure and following the procedure should also be discussed.
4. An explanation of alternative therapies to the procedure of treatment, including the risk of doing nothing at all (*Wecker v. Amend*, 1996).
5. An explanation that the patient can refuse the therapy or procedure without having alternative care or support discontinued (*Matter of Anna M. Gordy*, 1994).
6. The fact that patients can still refuse, even after the procedure or therapy has begun. For example, all of the radiation treatments need not be completed.

FORMS OF INFORMED CONSENT

Consent may be obtained in a variety of ways. Consent may be expressed or implied, written or oral, complete or partial.

Perhaps the easiest means of obtaining informed consent is when the consent is expressed. *Expressed consent* is consent given by direct words, written or oral. For example, after the nurse informs the patient that he or she is going to start an intravenous infusion, the patient says, "Okay, but could you put the needle in my left hand, since I am right handed?" As a rule, expressed consent is the type most often sought and received by health care providers.

Implied consent is consent that may be inferred by the patient's conduct or that which may legally be presumed in emergency situations. Implied consent has its foundation in the classic case of *O'Brien v. Cunard Steamship Company* (1899). In that case, a ship's female passenger joined a line of people receiving vaccinations. She neither questioned nor refused the injection. In fact, she willingly held out her arm for the vaccination. Later, she unsuccessfully brought suit for battery.

In the preceding example, rather than saying that he or she would allow an intravenous infusion to be started, suppose the patient merely extended the left arm and said nothing. The reasonable practitioner would infer from the conduct that the patient both understood the therapy and consented by action. Implied consent is frequently obtained by health care practitioners for minor procedures and routine care.

Implied consent may be presumed to exist in true emergency situations. For such consent, patients must not be able to make their wishes known, and a delay in providing care would result in the loss of life or limb. An important element in allowing emergency consent is that the health care provider has no reason to know or believe that consent would not be given were the patient able to deny consent. For example, the health care provider may not wait until the patient loses consciousness to order treatment that the patient had previously refused, such as a blood transfusion for a known Jehovah's Witness patient.

Consent may be *implied by law*, as in the instance in which the patient is a minor and the parent, or state standing in the place of a parent, consents to treatment. The law implies the minor's consent for the treatment.

Consent may be given *orally* or may be reduced to *writing*. Unless state law mandates written consent, the law views oral and written consent as equally valid. As a precaution, health care providers should recognize that oral consent is much more difficult to prove should consent or lack of consent become a legal issue. As a convenience and to prevent such court issues, most health care institutions require written consent.

Consent may be *partial* or *complete*. The patient may authorize the entire treatment or procedure or only part of the proposed therapy. For instance, if the patient authorizes a breast biopsy, but refuses to sign the consent form for a mastectomy based on the biopsy results, only a biopsy may be performed. The health care practitioner would then need to have a separate consent form signed before performing the mastectomy, should such surgery prove necessary.

STANDARDS OF INFORMED CONSENT

The various jurisdictions apply **standards of disclosure** for informed consent in one of three manners. These tests or standards of disclosure have evolved to ensure that patients are informed in their decisions and to allow a means of determining the adequacy of the disclosure.

The majority of states use a *medical community* standard, sometimes referred to as the *reasonable medical practitioner* standard. This standard evolved from the landmark *Karp v. Cooley* (1974) decision and is based on a model of medical paternalism. The standard requires that the medical or independent practitioner "disclose facts which a reasonable medical practitioner in a similar community and of the same school of medical thought would have disclosed regarding the proposed treatment" (*Karp v. Cooley*, 1974, at 411). This standard is fluid and changing, based on the prevailing medical thought and community, and is established at court through expert medical witness testimony. Generally, the patient must be told about inherent risks, but not necessarily unexpected risks that could occur after the treatment or procedure is initiated. Disclosure must include serious injuries that could occur, and courts favor more rather than less facts for full disclosure.

The last two tests involve the *reasonable (or prudent) patient standard.* One test, an *objective patient standard,* is based on disclosure of risks and benefits as determined by the needs of what a prudent person in the given patient's position would deem material. Thus, this standard is sometimes known as the *prudent patient standard* or *material risk standard.* Material facts are factors that may make a significant difference to the reasonable and prudent patient. It is imperative that the person has enough information on which to make a decision, including material risks (*Joswick v. Lenox Hill Hospital,* 1986, and *Arato v. Avedon,* 1993). The court in *Korman v. Mallin* (1993) stated that the "determination of materiality is a two-step process: (1) defining that existence and nature of the risk and the likelihood of occurrence; and (2) whether the probability of that type of harm is a risk which a reasonable patient would consider" (at 1149).

The second reasonable patient standard is based on a *subjective patient standard,* or the individual patient standard, which requires full disclosure that a particular patient, rather than a reasonable person, would have wanted to know. The fact finder must determine what risks were or were not material to the particular patient's decision with respect to the treatment accepted or refused. No expert testimony is required on the scope of disclosure, although such expert testimony may be required to establish risks and alternatives to therapy. Only a few states have adopted this standard.

Some states have attempted to bypass the three tests of disclosure by statutorily defining what must be disclosed to a patient prior to therapy or surgery. These *medical disclosure laws* mandate that certain risks and consequences be printed on the face of the consent form in language that the patient can be reasonably expected to understand.

Some states have adopted no one standard for disclosure but rely on individual case-by-case analysis, while others restrict informed consent to certain types of procedures such as operative or surgical procedures (*Jones v. Philadelphia College of Osteopathic Medicine,* 1993). A newer collaborative model for informed consent has been proposed by Piper (1994). This new standard proposes that the patient and physician define jointly what informed consent means to them. Such a standard would assign at least four responsibilities to patients: (1) to communicate their values and expectations of treatment to the physician; (2) to ask questions and seek clarification in patient–physician discussions; (3) to evaluate symptoms and report subjective impressions of how well treatment is satisfying their individual goals and values; and (4) to make reasonably good faith efforts to participate appropriately in treatment (Piper, 1994, p. 310).

Arguments for standards of full disclosure center on four key points:

1. Patients actually assume all the risks since it is their bodies and lives that are ultimately affected.
2. Informed consent mandates increased communications between the patient and the health care provider. With increased communications, one is less apt to violate the informed consent standards, and one is more likely to fully answer patients' questions.
3. Informed consent creates better health awareness by the consumer and ultimately encourages better health care practices.
4. Informed consent increases the quality of medical care because the health care provider is forced to explain all risks and benefits of the proposed procedure and to outline alternatives for the patient, thus selecting the best type and quality of care needed.

To bring a successful malpractice suit based on informed consent, the plaintiff must be able to prove, by a preponderance of the evidence, all of the following:

1. There was a duty on the part of the physician to know of a risk or alternative treatment.
2. There was a duty on the part of the physician to disclose the risk or alternative treatment.
3. There was a breach of the duty to disclose.
4. If the case is in a reasonable patient standard jurisdiction, a reasonable person in the plaintiff's position would not have consented to the treatment if he or she had known of the outstanding risk.
5. The undisclosed risk caused the harm or the harm would not have occurred if an alternative treatment plan was selected.
6. The plaintiff suffered damages.

■ EXERCISE 8–1

Explore your own state requirements for standards of informed consent. How did you go about discovering these standards? Do elective procedures and emergency situations use the same standard of informed consent?

EXCEPTIONS TO INFORMED CONSENT

The courts recognize the following four exceptions to the need for informed consent in circumstances in which consent is still required:

1. Emergency situations
2. Therapeutic privilege
3. Patient waiver
4. Prior patient knowledge

From a practitioner standpoint, consent is still needed to prevent charges of a battery, but the informed consent requirements are eased.

Emergencies give rise to implied consent. Some courts have recognized that if there is time to give information, a limited disclosure may be valid. If no time exists or the patient is incapable of understanding by virtue of the physical disability, then no information need be given.

Therapeutic privilege, which has its origins in the common law defense of necessity, allows primary health care providers to withhold information and any disclosures that they feel would be detrimental to the patient's health. The detrimental nature of the information must be more than fear that the information would lead to the patient's refusal. It must be a recognized and documented increased anxiety in the patient. Physicians, in using this exception, must be able to show that full disclosure of material facts would be likely to (1) hinder or complicate necessary treatment, (2) cause severe psychological harm, or (3) be so upsetting as to render a rational decision by the patient impossible (Rozovsky, 1990).

Therapeutic privilege is not favored by the courts and comes into play only when the patient is severely and emotionally disturbed, and the current medical status presents an imminent danger to the patient's life. Some courts have held that a relative must concur with the patient decision to consent and that the relative must be given full disclosure, whereas other courts have held that no relative need give concurrent consent. Once the risk to the patient has abated, the physician or independent practitioner must fully disclose the previously withheld information to the patient.

The patient may also agree to a *waiver* of the right to full disclosure and still consent to the procedure. The caveat to be avoided in this instance is that the health care provider cannot suggest such waiver. The waiver, to be valid, must be initiated by the patient.

Prior patient knowledge involves the patient to whom the risks and benefits were fully explained the first time the patient consented to the procedure. Liability does not exist for nondisclosure of risks that are public or common knowledge or that the patient had previously experienced.

Obtaining informed consent is a two-step process: communicating information to patients so that they are able to make informed decisions and documenting that decision. Communicating the plan of care is typically the role of the physician who performs the procedure or treatment. However, most nurses participate in the documentation phase.

ACCOUNTABILITY FOR OBTAINING INFORMED CONSENT

The physician or independent practitioner has the responsibility for obtaining informed consent (*Giese v. Stice*, 1997). Individual hospitals have no responsibility for obtaining informed consent unless (1) the physician or independent practitioner is an employee or agent of the hospital, or (2) the hospital knew or should have known of the lack of informed consent and took no action. Court cases and individual state statutes have repeatedly upheld this last principle.

The institution or hospital becomes responsible for informed consent only if those primarily responsible for ensuring that informed consent is obtained are employed by the hospital or institution or only if the hospital fails to take appropriate actions when informed consent is not obtained and the hospital is aware of that omission (*Lincoln v. Gupta*, 1985, and Cushing, 1991). In *Lincoln*, the court concluded that the patient should discuss risks of procedures with the physician, who "is the best person to inform the patient about the procedure and where to obtain proper services and facilities" (at 315).

While attorneys argue both sides of the accountability issue as it relates to the hospital or institution, most providers in the medical profession feel that to allow liability and thus to allow the hospital to monitor consent procedures and the actual disclosure of material facts upon which to base informed consent would destroy the professional relationship with the patient.

Nurses' Role in Obtaining Consent

Nurses who are not independent practitioners may become involved in the process of obtaining informed consent in one of several ways. Given that consent must be obtained for all procedures and treatments, not just medical procedures, one realizes the vast impact of this doctrine. This does not mean that nurses obtain written consent each time they give an injection or turn a patient. Most nursing interventions rely on oral expressed consent or implied consent that may be readily inferred through the patient's actions.

What the doctrine of informed consent means is that nurses must continually communicate with a patient, explaining procedures and obtaining the patient's permission. What it also means is that the patient's refusal to allow a certain procedure must be respected. Know the state laws on allowing the patient to refuse life-sustaining treatment. Even if the patient validly refuses life-sustaining treatment, the nurse could face charges for honoring or failing to honor this request. Each state has its own laws and applications of the laws. If the patient is unable to communicate, permission may be derived from the patient's admission to the hospital or obtained from the patient's legal representative.

A very real concern for nurses is in obtaining consent for the nursing aspects of medical procedures in which the primary procedure is performed by another practitioner. An example of such a concern is with postoperative care. Should the patient be taught about postoperative care before surgery, or should the nurse wait until after the surgery has been performed? Who is responsible for teaching postoperative care—the primary practitioner or the nursing staff? The answers from a legal perspective are far from clear. Possibly the best way to handle this dilemma is for the nurse to wait until after the patient has consented to the surgical procedure to give postoperative care information. This approach prevents interference with the physician–patient relationship and avoids potential conflicting explanations. Another approach is to have postoperative teaching materials and films developed to orient the patient to the entire procedure. This approach may be augmented by having a nurse available for questions or clarifications as needed. Many hospitals have implemented this latter approach with major procedures and operations such as heart catheterizations, vascular arteriography, and open heart surgery.

A third area of concern for the nurse is in obtaining informed consent for medical procedures provided completely by another practitioner. This obvious area of concern was perhaps the first one identified by most nurses. For years, nurses have been the health care providers obtaining the patient's consent for surgical or medical therapies performed by physicians. Some hospitals continue to permit nurses to obtain the patient's signature on the consent form. Other hospitals, to avoid this potential liability, prohibit nurses from obtaining signatures on consent forms.

It is important that nurses understand that physicians may legally delegate the responsibility of obtaining the patient's informed consent to the nurse. Physicians delegate this task at their own peril, for most medical practice acts hold that the physician is the responsible party for obtaining informed consent. Thus, any deficiencies in the informed consent as obtained by the nurse may be imputed back to the responsible physician. The nurse so delegated acts in the role of the physician or independent practitioner and must ensure that all material information is given to patients in language that they can understand. Therefore, the nurse may incur potential liability along with the delegating physician for the patient's informed consent (*Davis v. Hoffman*, 1997). Any additional information that the patient requests should be supplied by the physician, and the nurse is well advised to contact the physician immediately rather than attempt to talk a reluctant patient into the proposed procedure.

In *Davis*, the court ruled that the physician has the duty to obtain a patient's informed consent for surgery and that this duty does not apply to the hospital, even if the physician uses one of the hospital's operating rooms. The court also ruled that if a nurse assists in a procedure for which informed consent has not been given, the physician, but not the nurse, can be found liable for a civil battery. Since the nurse has no legal duty to obtain informed consent, reasoned the court, a nurse assisting in an unauthorized procedure lacks the legal intent to commit a battery. However, if the nurse takes on the task of explaining the operation to the patient, and the patient is harmed because the nurse's explanation of the operation is inadequate or incorrect, the patient can sue the nurse for negligence.

Some hospitals have begun to prohibit medical practitioners from delegating the accountability for obtaining informed consent to nurses. Once nurses become an integral part of the informed consent process, then the hospital also assumes liability under the doctrine of respondent superior.

Nurses also have an important role if patients subsequently wish to revoke their prior consent or if it becomes obvious that a patient's already signed, informed consent form does not meet the standards of informed consent. Most nurses have been faced with the problem of what to do when it becomes all too clear that the patient does not understand the procedure to be performed or believes that there are no major risks or adverse consequences inherent to the procedure. Remember, the nurse and the hospital may incur liability if there is reason to know that the standards of informed consent have not been met. In such instances, nurses should contact their immediate supervisor and the responsible physician. Both entities need to be informed of a patient's change of mind or lack of comprehension.

■ EXERCISE 8–2

A patient is admitted to your surgical center for a breast biopsy under local anesthesia. The surgeon has previously informed the patient of the procedure, risks, alternatives, desired outcomes, and possible complications. You give the surgery permit form to the patient for her signature. She readily states that she knows about the procedure and has no additional questions; she signs the form with no hesitation. Her husband, who is visiting with her, says he is worried that something may be said during the procedure to alarm her. What do you do at this point? Do you alert the surgeon that informed consent has not been obtained? Do you request that the surgeon revisit the patient and reinstruct her about the surgery? Since the patient has already signed the form, is there anything more that you should do?

CONSENT FORMS

Essentially two types of consent forms are presently in use. The *blanket consent form* that is required prior to admission is sufficient for care that is routine and customary. Routine and customary care may also be implied from the patient's voluntary admission into the hospital; therefore, this initial blanket consent form is needed only for insurance coverage and assignment of benefits.

Specific consent forms provide information, such as the name and description of the procedure to be performed, to be specifically named. Usually, the form also includes a section stating that (1) the person who signed the form was told about the medical condition, risks, alternatives, and benefits of the proposed procedure; and (2) any and all questions have been answered. With this type of form, the physician and hospital could show that no battery occurred because consent was given. However, the plaintiff may still be able to convince a court that informed consent was not given.

A second type of specific consent form attempts to prevent this latter possibility. This second specific type of form is a detailed consent form that lists the procedure, consequences, risks, and alternatives. It is this type of form that many states are now mandating through statutory medical disclosure panels.

Most of the latter forms have the following elements:

1. Signature of the competent patient or a legal representative
2. Name and full description of the proposed procedure
3. Description of risks and alternatives of the proposed procedure, including nontreatment
4. Description of probable consequences of the proposed procedure
5. Signatures of one or two witnesses according to state law

With such detailed forms, nurses should remember four things. First, witnesses are not required to make the consent valid. Witnesses merely attest to the competency of the patient signing the form and to the genuineness of the signature, not that the patient had all the information needed to make an informed choice (Switzer, 1995). Although nurses need not be witnesses for the consent form to make it valid, if they observe the signature and chart that such information was given at the time of the signing of the consent form, they would make excellent witnesses in an ensuing medical malpractice case.

A recent case illustrates the fact that nurses signing the informed consent form as witnesses do not make the hospital more liable in resulting malpractice lawsuits. In *Auler v. Van Natta* (1997), the patient had signed a consent form for a modified radical mastectomy and immediate reconstruction with a latissimus dorsi flap. When the patient later learned that a saline implant had been used, she sued the physician and the hospital.

Before going to trial, the hospital asked to be nonsuited in the case and the court agreed. The hospital, the court held, did not gratuitously take upon itself the duty to inform the patient and get her consent merely because a registered nurse signed her name on the informed consent form as a witness to the patient's signature.

Second, consent may be withdrawn at any time. There is nothing in the written form that precludes the patient's right to withdraw his or her consent at will. Third, consent forms, although strong evidence of informed consent, are not conclusive in and of themselves. Several challenges have surfaced, including:

1. Technical language that precluded reasonable patients from understanding what they actually signed.
2. The signature was not voluntary, but was coerced or forced.
3. Incompetency of the signer due to impairment by medications previously received.

Fourth, consent forms may be absent or the form may not address the performed procedure, and the nurse then has a duty to ensure that the physician and hospital administrative staff are knowledgeable of the deficiency. In a recent case from the Court of Appeals of Wisconsin, the physician performed an intraoperative tubal ligation during a cesarean section (*Mathais v. St. Catherine's Hospital, Inc*, 1997). When the surgeon asked for the instrument to do the tubal ligation, two nurses circulating in the delivery room looked for a signed consent form in the patient's chart and told the surgeon there was no consent form for a tubal ligation. The surgeon performed the tubal ligation despite the lack of a signed consent form. Three days later, one of the nurses who had been in the delivery room brought the patient a standard consent form for tubal ligation and asked her it sign it "just to close up our records."

The patient filed suit on the grounds of lack of informed consent. Nevertheless, the court held that the hospital and nurses faced no legal liability for the patient's civil lawsuit. To be able to rule in favor of the hospital, the court needed only to judge the nurses' actions at the time of the tubal ligation. The nurses in the delivery room checked the patient's chart to ascertain whether the appropriate signature was present on the informed consent form. One of the nurses informed the physician that there was no consent form for the procedure and observed the physician acknowledging hearing that fact.

At this point, the court said, the nurses had no legal duty to take further action. The court said that it may have been a clerical mistake that the form was absent or that there was some other valid reason that the surgeon continued with the operation. It is not necessarily true that the surgeon was performing an unauthorized procedure merely because there was no consent form on the chart. In any event, the nurses were not at fault. What happened was beyond the scope of their legal liability. The hospital also was not to blame, either as the nurses' employer or for having provided the operating room to this surgeon, who practiced independently.

Consent forms are considered to be valid until withdrawn by the patient or until the patient's condition or authorized treatments change significantly. Some hospitals use a 30-day guideline, but most hospitals prefer to have no set guidelines. Such guidelines could become cumbersome for the patient with a chronic, disabling diagnosis or for a patient who gave valid consent and then became incompetent to renew or sign new consent forms.

WHO MUST CONSENT?

Equally important to giving patients all material facts needed on which to base an informed choice is that the correct person(s) consent to the procedure or therapy. Informed consent becomes a moot point if the wrong signature is obtained.

Competent Adult

The basic rule is that if the patient is an adult according to state law, only that adult can give or refuse consent. Most states recognize 18 as the age at which one becomes an adult, although some actions might serve to classify the person as an adult prior to the legal age, for example, marriage. The adult giving or refusing consent must be competent to either sign or refuse to sign the necessary consent forms. *Competency at law* means that (1) the court has not declared the person to be incompetent, and (2) the person is generally able to understand the consequences of his or her actions. There is a strong legal presumption of continuing competency.

The actual determination of legal competency is not necessarily the function of the psychiatric medical staff. It is usually made based on the assessment of the person by a physician or other member of the health care profession. This assessment is often performed at the time informed consent is requested. Consultation with other health professionals is always a possibility and should be performed if there is (1) underlying mental retardation, (2) an obvious mental disorder, or (3) a disease that affects the patient's mental functioning.

Courts generally have held that there is a strong presumption of continued competency. Such cases involved persons whose minds sometimes wandered, who were disoriented at times, and, in one case, an individual who was confined to a mental institution. In each case, the court sought evidence to show that the person was capable of understanding the alternatives to the procedure as proposed and could fully appreciate the consequences of refusing consent to the procedure (*Matter of Roche*, 1996).

There are two exceptions to the legal adult's right to give or to refuse informed consent. The hospital must seek and abide by the decision of (1) a court-appointed guardian and (2) a person with a valid, written power of attorney. Such persons will present themselves to the hospital administration if they have previously been appointed and if the adult patient is incapable of giving or refusing consent.

Incompetent Adult

The *legal guardian or representative* is the person who is legally responsible for giving or refusing consent for the incompetent adult. Because the law is allowing someone other than the adult to make decisions for the adult, guardians and representatives have a narrower range of permissible choices than they would if deciding for themselves. Some states insist that the known choices of the patient be considered first. Any expressed wishes concerning therapy or refusal of therapy made while the patient was still fully competent should be evaluated and followed if at all possible.

To be appointed as a legal representative or guardian, the court must first declare the adult incompetent. The court will then appoint a guardian, either temporarily or permanently. If the court has reason to believe the adult is only temporarily incapacitated, then it will appoint a guardian until the adult is able to once again manage his or her affairs.

Guardians are usually selected from family members because the law feels that such persons will have the patient's best interests at heart and are in a position to best know the patient's desires. If the spouse of the incompetent adult is also elderly and ill, an adult child may be the appointed guardian.

Some persons are never adjudicated as incompetent by a court of law, and in selected states the family is asked to make decisions for the incompetent patient. For example, an automobile accident may render the patient incapable of making decisions and giving consent, and the physician will frequently ask the family about medical matters for the unconscious patient. The order of selection is usually (1) the spouse, (2) adult children or grandchildren, (3) parents, (4) grandparents or adult brothers and sisters, and (5) adult nieces and nephews.

The practitioner is cautioned to validate state laws and judicial decisions because *family consent* may not be valid consent in a handful of states. Lack of valid consent may lead to a court battle, especially if the practitioner acts on family consent and there was disagreement among family members as to the course of action to take.

Minors

Most states recognize a child under 18 as a *minor.* Parental or guardian consent is necessary for medical therapies unless:

1. The emergency doctrine applies.
2. The child is an emancipated or mature minor.
3. There is a court order to proceed with the therapy.
4. The law recognizes the minor as having the ability to consent to the therapy.

Some states also allow *in loco parentis* or the ability of a person or the state to stand in the place of the parents. Look to statutory law to see who may consent in the absence of a parent. If there is a family consent doctrine, it will be a grandparent, adult brother or sister, or adult aunt or uncle. A newer trend is allowing minor parents to consent for their children's medical and dental treatments.

As with adults, the law applies the doctrine of implied consent with medical emergencies, unless there is reason to believe that the parents would refuse such therapy. For example, if the patient were the child of Jehovah's Witness parents, medical personnel would have reason to believe that the parents might not consent to the giving of blood. The best course for the medical staff to follow if there is doubt about whether consent would be forthcoming is to seek a court order for the therapy unless there is a true emergency or life-threatening condition.

If the child's parents are married to each other or have joint custody, usually either parent can sign the consent form or make treatment decisions. Unless the divorce results in a sole custody arrangement or in total abrogation of parental rights, the parent with custody is generally considered the party to give or deny consent.

Such issues are state specific, and there are important exceptions to general rules. For example, a Georgia court has ruled that a do-not-resuscitate order could not be enforced without the signatures of both parents (Rutherford, 1994).

Emancipated minors are persons under the legal age who are no longer under their parents' control and regulation and who are managing their own financial affairs. Some states require parents to completely surrender the right of care and custody of the child to prevent runaways from coming under this classification. Such emancipated minors may validly consent to their own medical therapies. Examples of emancipated minors are married persons, underage parents, or those in the armed service of their country. Some states allow college students, living away from their parents, to fall in this category.

Mature minors may also consent to some medical care. This is a relatively new concept that is gaining legal recognition. Its origin is in family law and involves the right of the child to make a choice as to which parent will have custody of the child following a divorce. The concept of a mature minor was recognized as early as 1957 (*Madison v. Harrison*). The mature minor is a teenager, between the ages of 14 and 17, who is able to understand the nature and consequences of the proposed therapy, and who is making his or her own decisions on a daily basis and is independent.

The medical practitioner is encouraged to seek parental consent along with the consent of the mature minor in most circumstances. Such a practice aids in limiting potential liability and encourages family involvement.

Obtaining valid informed consent when minors declare themselves to be emancipated or sufficiently mature to consent in their own stead can be problematic. The best course of action when there is a question of valid consent is to temporarily postpone any elective procedure or treatment until it is determined if the minor can consent within state law. If a true emergency presents, then the practitioner may proceed under an emergency consent doctrine. The practitioner should carefully document in the medical record existence of valid informed consent or the need for emergency care.

The law also recognizes the right of minors to consent for some selected therapies without informing parents of the treatment. The reason for these exceptions is to encourage minors to seek needed treatment. Informing parents of the treatment might prevent minors from receiving the necessary therapy. Instances for which minors may give valid consent include:

1. The diagnosis and treatment of infectious, contagious, or communicable diseases.
2. The diagnosis and treatment of drug dependency, drug addiction, or any condition directly related to drug usage.
3. Obtaining birth control devices.
4. Treatment during a pregnancy as long as the care concerns the pregnancy.

Court orders may be obtained for the care of minors if the parents refuse to consent to needed procedures or treatment, although there is a trend toward nonintervention unless treatment is needed to save a life. For example, hospitals have often obtained court orders for blood transfusions when the parents have refused consent for the transfusion. In *In re Hamilton* (1983), the court ordered chemotherapy for a 12-year-old girl when the parents refused consent based on religious grounds. That court overruled the parents to improve the quality of the child's life during her dying.

 ## GUIDELINES: INFORMED CONSENT

Two criteria must be satisfied:

1. The consent is given by one who has the legal capacity for giving such consent
   a. Competent adult
   b. Legal guardian or representative for the incompetent adult
   c. Emancipated, married minor
   d. Mature minor
   e. Parent, state, or legal guardian of a child
   f. Minor for the diagnosis and treatment of specific disease states or conditions
   g. Court order
2. The person(s) giving consent must fully comprehend
   a. The procedure to be performed
   b. The risks involved
   c. Expected or desired outcomes
   d. Any complications or untoward side effects
   e. Alternative therapies, including no therapy at all

■ EXERCISE 8—3

Jimmy Chang, a 20-year-old college student, is admitted to your institution for additional chemotherapy. Jimmy was diagnosed with leukemia five years earlier and has had several courses of chemotherapy. He is currently in an acute active phase of the disease, though he had enjoyed a 14-month remission phase prior to this admission. His parents, who accompany him to the hospital, are divided as to the benefits of additional chemotherapy. His mother is adamant that she will sign the informed consent form for this course of therapy, and his father is equally adamant that he will refuse to sign the informed consent form because "Jimmy has suffered enough." You are his primary nurse and must assist in somehow resolving this impasse. What do you do about the informed consent form? Who signs and why?

Using the MORAL model, decide the best course of action for Jimmy from an ethical perspective rather than a legal perspective. Did you come to the same conclusion using both an ethical and a legal approach?

RIGHT TO REFUSE CONSENT

The right of consent involves the *right of refusal.* If persons have the right to consent, then they also have the right to refuse to give consent. The right to refuse continues even after primary consent is given. Patients or their guardians need only to notify the health care giver that they no longer wish to continue with the therapy. In some limited circumstances, the danger of stopping therapy poses too great a harm for the patient, and the law allows its continuance. For example, in the immediate postoperative period, the patient cannot refuse procedures that assure a safe transition from anesthesia. Likewise, the patient may not refuse immediate care for life-threatening arrhythmias following a myocardial infarction if that refusal would worsen the patient's condition. After the arrhythmias have abated, the patient may refuse further therapy.

The right for such refusal may be based on the common law right of freedom from bodily invasion or the constitutional rights of privacy and religious freedom. This right extends to the refusal to consent for lifesaving treatment in most states. In *Shine v. Vega* (1999), a young adult patient came into the emergency center for treatment for an acute asthmatic attack. She had a history of asthma, dating back to her early childhood.

The nurse began to monitor her, drawing and sending blood to the laboratory for blood gas analysis. When the results of the blood gas analysis came back, the nurse decided that the oxygen mask was not sufficient and convinced the physician to intubate her. The patient and her older sister both voiced adamant disapproval of the plan to intubate her, and they ran from the emergency center. They were chased through the hospital's corridors by security guards. The patient was caught, returned to the emergency center, strapped down in four-point restraints, and forcibly intubated. She recovered and was later discharged from the hospital.

Two years later, the patient died after refusing to go to the hospital for an asthma attack. The family filed a lawsuit, alleging that her death was attributable to fear of hospitals, doctors, and nurses stemming from the forced-intubation incident. The court agreed and upheld their right to sue for wrongful death.

The court, in its decision, noted that a medical emergency justifies nonconsensual treatment only when it is not possible or feasible to obtain informed consent from a person legally entitled to provide or withhold consent. Even in a life-threatening situation, care providers cannot substitute their own judgment for that of a mentally competent adult patient or family member. An earlier case had held that the patient's right to refuse treatment outweighed the physician's duty to treat (*Daniel Thor v. Superior Court of Solano County*, 1993).

The right of refusal is not without some potential consequences. The patient or guardian must be informed that the right of refusal may mean, and most often does mean, that the patient's physical condition continues to deteriorate and may hasten death. The right of refusal may also mean that third-party reimbursement may be denied, because most insurance policies have a clause that denies or limits reimbursement for refusing procedures that would aid in the diagnosis or reduction of the injury or illness.

Limitations on Refusal of Therapy

There are several instances in which the state may deny a patient's right of refusal. These state rights exist to prevent committing crimes and to protect the welfare of society as a whole. Limitations on refusal include:

1. Preservation of life if the patient does not have an incurable or terminal disease.
2. Protection of minor dependents.
3. Prevention of irrational self-destruction.
4. Maintenance of the ethical integrity of health professionals by allowing the hospital to treat the patient.
5. Protection of the public's health.

In cases filed to enforce the right to refuse care, the courts balance individual rights against societal rights (*Jefferson v. Griffin Spalding County Hospital Authority*, 1981; *Norwood Hospital v. Munoz*, 1991; *Daniel Thor v. Superior Court of Solano County*, 1993; and *Leach v. Akron General Medical Center*, 1984). In *Leach*, the court found that a patient has the right to refuse therapy based on a privacy right. In this case, the patient was incompetent and the issue was allowing the patient to forgo life-sustaining treatment.

LAW ENFORCEMENT

Medical personnel are often requested by the police and other law enforcement personnel to draw blood, remove stomach contents, remove bullets, and the like for the purpose of gathering evidence to be used against a suspect. The suspect will often refuse to give consent to the proposed treatments and procedures. As a health care provider, can you legally do as requested? Or will you open yourself to a potential lawsuit for battery?

The Supreme Court of the United States attempted for several years to answer these questions for the health care provider. In *Rochin v. California* (1950), the court ruled that the "removal of stomach contents shocks the conscience" and refused to permit the test results on the stomach contents from being introduced into evidence (at 757). Six years later, the court ruled that blood drawn from an unconscious person could be introduced into evidence, showing that the driver was legally intoxicated (*Breithaupt v. Adams*, 1957).

Finally, with the landmark *Schmerber v. California* decision in 1966, the court gave the health care provider some criteria for cooperating with law enforcement officials while staying relatively liability free. Five conditions must be present and documented:

1. The suspect must be under formal arrest.
2. There must be a likelihood that the blood drawn will produce evidence for criminal prosecution.
3. A delay in drawing the blood would lead to destruction of the evidence.
4. The test is reasonable and not medically contraindicated.
5. The test is performed in a reasonable manner (*Schmerber v. California*, 1966, at 763).

Remember, though, that state law may supersede the law enforcer's request; that is, in most states, the hospital or health care provider has no legal duty to perform the test as requested by the law enforcement official. State law may dictate who and under what circumstances blood may be involuntarily drawn.

Ruppel v. Ramsever (1999) illustrates these last points. In that case, the patient agreed to be brought in by paramedics to the hospital's emergency center after she hit a parked car. Once at the hospital, she refused care and demanded to leave. She was detained for 10 minutes by the hospital security guard while the police were called. They arrived, placed her under arrest for driving under the influence (DUI), and requested the physician and nurse to draw a blood sample for an alcohol level. The patient adamantly refused her consent to the drawing of blood.

The patient later filed a civil rights lawsuit against the hospital, which was dismissed by the court. Health care professionals, wrote the court, who are directed by law enforcement officers to collect samples of blood or urine for evidence, and who do so in good faith and with due care, cannot be sued for their actions. There is no requirement for health care professionals to second-guess whether the officer has probable cause.

INFORMED CONSENT IN HUMAN EXPERIMENTATION

Using vulnerable groups of people for research poses many potential problems because of the ease with which the subjects can be coerced. This is especially true of the mentally disabled, children, and prisoners. The major issue, other than coercion, seems to be that of informed consent.

Whenever research is involved, be it a drug study or a new procedure, the investigator(s) must disclose the research to the subject or the subject's representative and obtain informed consent. Federal guidelines have been developed that specify the procedures used to review research and the disclosures that must be made to ensure that valid, informed consent is obtained.

Since 1974, the Department of Health and Human Services (HHS) has required that an institutional review board (IRB) examine and approve the research study prior to any funding from HHS. This institutional review board determines whether subjects will be placed at risk and, if so, if the following criteria are met:

1. Risks to subjects are outweighed by the benefit to the subject and by the importance of the knowledge to be gained by doing the research.
2. The rights and welfare of the subject will be protected.

3. Legally effective consent will be secured prior to starting any data collection.

Specific requirements that the institutional review board must ensure before approving the research study are:

1. Risks to the subjects are minimized.
2. Risks to subjects are reasonable in relation to anticipated benefits, if any, to the subjects and to the importance of the knowledge that may reasonably be expected to result.
3. Selection of subjects is equitable.
4. Informed consent will be sought from each prospective subject or the subject's legally authorized representative.
5. Informed consent will be appropriately documented.
6. Where appropriate, the research plan makes adequate provision for monitoring the data collected to ensure the safety of the subjects.
7. Where appropriate, there are adequate provisions to protect the privacy of subjects and to maintain the confidentiality of data.
8. Where some or all of the subjects are likely to be vulnerable to coercion or undue influence, such as persons with acute or severe physical or mental illness or persons who are economically or educationally disadvantaged, appropriate additional safeguards have been included in the study to protect the rights and welfare of these subjects (45 CFR, Section 46.111).

The federal government has also mandated the basic elements of information that must be included to meet the standards of informed consent. These basic elements include the following:

1. A statement that the study involves research, an explanation of the purposes of the research and the expected duration of the subject's participation, a description of the procedures to be followed, and identification of any procedures that are experimental.
2. A description of any reasonably foreseeable risks or discomforts to the subject.
3. A description of any benefits to the subjects or others that may reasonably be expected from the research.
4. A disclosure of appropriate alternative procedures or courses of treatment, if any, that may be advantageous to the subject.
5. A statement describing the extent, if any, to which confidentiality of records identifying the subject will be maintained.
6. For research involving more than minimal research, an explanation as to any compensation and an explanation as to whether any medical treatments are available if injury occurs and, if so, what they consist of or where further information may be obtained.
7. An explanation of whom to contact for answers to pertinent questions about the research and research subjects' rights and whom to contact in the event of a research-related injury to the subject.
8. A statement that participation is voluntary, refusal to participate will involve no penalty or loss of benefits to which the subject is otherwise entitled, and the subject may discontinue participation at any time without penalty or loss of benefits to which the subject is otherwise entitled (45 CFR, Section 46.116).

The information given must be in language that is understandable by the subject or the subject's legal representative. No exculpatory wording may be included, for example, a statement that the researcher incurs no liability for the outcome to the subject. Subjects should also be advised of:

1. Any additional costs that they might incur because of the research.
2. Potential for any foreseeable risks.
3. Rights to withdraw at will, with no questions asked or additional incentives given.
4. Consequences, if any, of withdrawal before the study is completed.
5. A statement that any significant new findings will be disclosed.
6. The number of proposed subjects for the study.

Excluded from these strict requirements are studies that use existing data, documents, records, or pathological and diagnostic specimens, if these sources are publicly available or the information is recorded so that the subjects cannot be identified (45 CFR, Section 46.101[b], 1991).

Other studies that involve only minimal risks to subjects, such as moderate exercise by healthy adults, may be expedited through the review process (45 CFR, Section 46.110, 1991).

Concerns over the past abuses that have occurred in the area of research with children has led to the adoption of federal guidelines specifically designed to protect children when they are enrolled as research subjects.

Before proceeding under these specific guidelines, state and local laws must be reviewed for laws regulating research on human subjects. Proposals involving new investigational drugs or devices must meet Food and Drug Administration regulations (21 CFR, Parts 50, 56, 312, 314, and 812).

In 1998, Subpart D: Additional Protections for Children Involved as Subjects in Research was added to the code (45 CFR 46.401 et seq.). These sections were added to give further protection to children when they are subjects of research studies and to encourage researchers to involve children, where appropriate, in research. The sections present guidelines for involving children in research that:

1. Presents minimal risk.
2. Involves greater than minimal risk, but presents the prospect of direct benefit to the individual subjects.
3. Involves greater than minimum risk and no prospect of direct benefit to the individual subject, but is likely to yield generalizable knowledge about the subject's disorder or condition.
4. Is not otherwise approvable, which presents an opportunity to understand, prevent, or alleviate a serious problem affecting the health or welfare of children.

Since adopting these new guidelines, two federal agencies have now proposed further broadening the use of children as research subjects. The National Institutes of Health (NIH) and the Federal Drug Act (FDA) have recently taken action that is designed to increase the role of the child as research subject (45 CFR, Section 46.101[a][2] and National Institutes of Health, 1998). The goal of both these actions is to ensure that drugs that are being used and those proposed to be used in a pediatric population be properly labeled for pediatric indications and dosages. The NIH policy is that "children . . . must be included in all human subjects research. . . . unless there are scientific and ethical reasons not to include them (National Institutes of Health, 1998, p.1).

GUIDELINES: RIGHTS OF PATIENTS IN RESEARCH

1. Informed consent is the first hurdle to valid human experimentation. The nurse must ascertain that the patient or legal representative understands that a research study will be involved and that the patient or legal representative has a basic understanding of the research to be performed (nature of the study, expected results of the study, and the like).
2. The patient or legal representative must be given the choice to participate or not. This entails the giving of information in understandable terms and in sufficient quantity so that the patient or legal representative can make an informed choice of participation.
3. The patient or legal representative must know that he or she can choose to terminate participation at any point in the research study. This may be done without penalty, forfeiture of quality care and treatment, or loss of dignity.
4. The patient or legal representative should be aware of who is conducting the research study and how to contact this person(s) at any given time. All questions should be answered for the patient or legal representative as needed by the principal investigator.
5. The patient should be free from any arbitrary hurt or intrinsic risk of injury. Any physical or mental risks that the patient may be exposing himself or herself to should be explained as fully as possible when the initial informed consent is obtained. Likewise, medical care or treatment for such incurred risks should be made available to the patient by the researcher, and the patient or legal representative should be aware of these considerations at the time of the initial informed consent.
6. The patient always retains his or her right to privacy and confidentiality. If at all possible, the patient should never be capable of being identified through the research study, but a coding system should be devised and followed. If not possible, the patient should be known to as few persons as can be allowed by the research design.
7. The quality of research in which human subjects are involved is important. Institutional review boards should exist for all institutions in which human subjects are used for ongoing research studies. Institutional review boards should look first to the expected outcomes of the study and to that which is being studied in deciding if human persons may be used as subjects.
8. While the rights of the minor and of the mentally or developmentally disabled person are no greater than those of the competent adult subject in a research study, the need to protect these rights is greater. These persons are more likely not to understand the nature of the research or the fact that they can terminate their participation at will; they are also more easily coerced into becoming subjects for the proposed research study. The nurse must guard against such happenings and ascertain that valid legal representation exists for such underaged or disadvantaged persons.

GENETIC TESTING

Rapid scientific advances in the area of genetics, including scientists' ability to clone sheep and to create artificial human chromosomes, have created a number of issues for health care providers. Among these issues are the questions of informed consent for genetic testing, discrimination against persons with less than perfect genes, and the confidentiality of genetic testing. The first issue is addressed here and the confidentiality issue is addressed in Chapter 9.

Genetic testing is beginning to reveal whether symptomatic patients have a suspected genetic disorder and whether asymptomatic patients are predisposed to developing a genetic disease later in life or will pass the genetic disposition to their offspring. This ability to prevent some children from developing later illnesses has resulted in some states mandating that all newborns be screened for certain genetic disorders. For example, the test for phenylketonuria (PKU) has been mandated in all states except Maryland for a number of years. In Maryland, the test is voluntary.

The screening of newborns for other treatable conditions varies by state. For example, the screening for cystic fibrosis is mandatory in only five states (Arkansas, Minnesota, Nebraska, South Dakota, and West Virginia), with the remaining states allowing parents to refuse the test for causes such as religious grounds (Illinois Department of Public Health, 1996). The Institute of Medicine, a national health policy group, is recommending that genetic testing be performed only with the patients' or parents' informed consent (Andrews et al., 1994).

The issue of informed consent has the same requirements, be the informed consent for a surgical procedure, an invasive piece of monitoring, or evaluation of a genetic trait. Here, a simple blood test, with minimal risks to the patient, is needed for the testing to be done. Yet the implications are immense, because of the implications of the test to the person. All future life events may be affected by this simple test, including family planning, career choices, health insurance coverage, and the psychological well-being of the person and family.

The Institute of Medicine and the American Nurses Association recommend that the following elements also be included when informed consent is sought from either the patient or the parent. These elements include:

1. *Nature of the disorder.* The severity of the condition, whether it is treatable, and what the treatment entails should be addressed. Patients and parents may choose not to have the test performed if there is no treatment available.
2. *Efficacy of the test.* Patient and parent should be informed of the rate of false negatives and false positives with the test and whether further testing will be done based on a positive result. They should also be informed about the difference between probability of developing the condition or a certainty of developing the disease. Included in the discussion should be the ratio percentage of the probability of developing the condition, if such figures are known.
3. *Decisions that will follow if the test is positive.* For example, the pregnant patient who is positive for a genetic abnormality may be asked to decide whether to carry the fetus to term. Those attempting to conceive may be asked to decide about permanent sterility, rather than conceiving.
4. *Support services.* There are several agencies that offer support to patients or parents, and they should be informed of these potential services as part of the informed consent process.
5. *Disclosure and confidentiality issues.* The question of whether the patient wants to reveal positive tests results to other family members who may have inherited or may be at risk for the same genetic marker should be discussed. The patient or parent should also know that the insurance carriers and other health care providers may have access to the test result (Andrews et al., 1994, and Scanlon and Fibison, 1995).

To prevent the possibility of discrimination in insurance coverage, several states have already enacted laws concerning sickle cell trait (Alabama, Florida, and North Carolina) and hemoglobin C trait (North Carolina). The Health Insurance Portability and Accountability Act of 1996 provides protection from a national perspective. This act prevents using genetic information to determine insurance eligibility as well as preventing the limitation or denial of benefits using a preexisting exclusion clause. There are, however, no provisions to prevent plans from requiring genetic testing of those enrolled, excluding coverage for a particular condition, or charging higher premiums to those with genetic mutations. These additional provisions may be forthcoming as bills before both houses of the U.S. Congress address these issues.

Patient Education in Genetic Testing

The implications for patient education in this area of the law are immense. The nurse's knowledge of such issues is often limited because this is an area in which knowledge is literally exploding every day. Nurses will undoubtedly be asked many questions from frightened and concerned parents and patients, and they must first understand genetic testing, its limitations, and its potential for enhanced health care. Nurses must also understand and apply mental health interventions, since patients and parents are most vulnerable to self-doubt, guilt, hopelessness, and powerlessness at this time. Nurses can best meet the patients' and parents' needs by incorporating all members of the interdisciplinary health care team—specialists in genetics, social workers, mental health practitioners, religious counselors, and staff nurses.

The advocacy role of the nurse is extremely important during genetic testing and following positive test results. Nurses may need to assist the patients or parents in asserting their rights to all knowledge currently known about the condition/trait, in voicing their fears, and in facing some of the hard decisions that result from positive test results.

PATIENT SELF-DETERMINATION

Patient self-determination involves the right of individuals to decide what will or will not happen to their bodies. Usually, the right of self-determination is addressed in issues surrounding death and dying, but self-determination concerns all aspects of consent and its refusal.

THE ISSUE OF CONSENT

Before one can discuss the patient's right to die or to forgo life-sustaining procedures, one must address the issue of informed consent. Competent adults have long been recognized as having the right to refuse medical treatment, unless the state can show that its interests outweigh that right. Examples of such overriding state interests include:

1. Protecting third parties, especially minor children.
2. Preserving life, especially that of minors and incompetents.
3. Protecting society from the spread of disease.

Competent adults may decide which treatments they will receive and which medical procedures they will refuse. Usually, any decision to forgo medical treatment will need to survive a period in which the health care receiver is incompetent. Many states have attempted to help this classification of patient by statutory enactments.

Often, patients will express their desires in oral form. In some states, these oral wishes have been upheld by the judiciary. The courts examine documentation of these wishes and usually determine if the person knew of the terminal condition when expressing his or her wishes or whether the person was talking, in general terms, about future care when he or she became terminally ill. The courts have been reluctant to enforce generalities, and vague talk about potential happenings in the future usually have been held to have little weight by the court.

For years, legal experts have concluded that competent adults have the right to refuse medical treatment, even if the refusal is certain to cause death, a view that is consistent with the majority of states to decriminalize suicide. But it was not until 1984 that an appellate court directly confronted an issue in which a clearly competent patient refused necessary life-sustaining treatment. In *Bartling v. Superior Court* (1984), the California Court of Appeals' decision was eased because the patient died before the case was resolved. That tentativeness of the court was overcome by the next case to present itself, *Bouvia v. Superior Court* (1986).

The issue addressed in *Bartling* concerned the right of a competent adult patient, with a serious illness that was probably incurable but not necessarily terminal, over the objections of his physicians and the hospital, to have life-support equipment disconnected despite the fact that the withdrawal of such devices would hasten his death. Mr. Bartling, a severe emphysemic patient, entered the hospital for depression. While hospitalized, a tumor was noted on x-ray, and during the subsequent biopsy, his lung collapsed. Despite aggressive therapy, Mr. Bartling was trached and ventilator-dependent at the time this cause of action was heard. Though Mr. Bartling died during the course of the appeal, the appellate court did hold that the "right of a competent adult to refuse medical treatment is a constitutionally guaranteed right which must not be abridged" (at 192).

In *Bouvia v. Superior Court* (1986), the court addressed many of the same issues. Ms. Bouvia, a 28-year-old patient with severe cerebral palsy, sought removal of a nasogastric tube, inserted and maintained against her will for the purpose of involuntary forced feedings. Here, the court wrestled not only with the right of a competent adult to refuse medical therapy, but also with the facility's obligation to serve the autonomous interests of patients, as defined by those patients. In *Bouvia*, those autonomous decisions included medical support to prevent further pain and suffering during the dying process.

The legal history of the right of competent patients to forgo life-sustaining treatment is provided in a clear and accurate way through these two California opinions. The very strong unanimous court in *Bouvia* also demonstrates the consensus absent in 1984 that was beginning to solidify by 1986.

Incompetent patients present a totally different picture. The first court case to challenge the judiciary in this respect was *In re Quinlan* (1976). In a lengthy decision, the New Jersey Supreme Court held that although patients generally have the right to refuse therapy, guardians for the incompetent usually do not. "The only practical way to prevent destruction of the (privacy) right is to permit the guardian and family of Karen to render their very best judgment . . . as to whether she would exercise it in these circumstances" (at 664).

That court allowed the father of Karen Quinlan to authorize the withdrawal of life support systems for Karen. The decision was a difficult one to reach because Karen did not meet the Harvard criteria for brain death. While she was respirator-dependent at the time of the court case, she did have some brain activity on the electroencephalogram and some reflex movements. The decision was also difficult because it conflicted significantly with a precedent-setting New Jersey case that held that one should always save a life, even if the patient's objection to lifesaving procedures was based on religious beliefs (*John F. Kennedy Memorial Hospital v. Heston*, 1971).

The decision reached by the court in *Quinlan* was to allow Karen's father the right to remove Karen from life-support systems. It should be clear, however, that the father made the final decision. The court system gave him the right to make the ultimate decision, but did not influence that decision.

The next significant decision in this area of the law was *Superintendent of Belchertown State School v. Saikewicz* (1977). Here, the Massachusetts Supreme Court deviated from the Quinlan case in two significant ways:

1. This court used the doctrine of **substituted judgment** (subjective determination of how persons, were they capable of making their opinions and wishes known, would have chosen to exercise their right to refuse therapy) to decide what Joseph Saikewicz would have wanted to be done with his right to refuse therapy.
2. No ethics committee was suggested by the court. Unlike Quinlan, the Saikewicz opinion met with general disfavor because the court totally rejected the notion that these types of decisions should be made by families and physicians with the aid of ethics committees. Indeed, the *Saikewicz* court held that the decision to discontinue therapy "must reside with the judicial process and the judicial process alone" (p. 475).

Eichner v. Dillon (1980), the third case to further define allowing patients the right to forgo life-sustaining procedures, restricted the termination of extraordinary life-support treatments to the patient who was terminally ill or in a "vegetative coma characterized as permanent or irreversible with an extremely remote possibility of recovery" (p. 468). *Eichner* also combined the substituted judgment doctrine as followed in *Saikewicz* with the *best interest* (personal preferences made while the now incompetent patient was rational and capable of stating what he or she would want in the event of a catastrophic happening) test as derived from *Quinlan*. Although not a perfect solution, the decision did seem to soften the negative impact of *Saikewicz*.

The final decision concerning the incompetent patient's right to die seems to have been settled in 1990. In *Cruzan v. Director, Missouri Department of Health* (1990), the court made explicit that right-to-die issues will be decided on a state-to-state basis and that there will be little, if any, U.S. constitutional limits on what states may do. Following the *Cruzan* decision, cases have allowed more latitude to family members, and courts have struggled to find instances in which patients had made some expression, however fleeting, about their desires for sustaining life with artificial or life-support measures.

Two recent cases exemplify those points. In *In re Fiori* (1995), a Pennsylvania court held that a hospital may terminate life-support treatment for a patient in a persistent vegetative state without a court order if the hospital obtained the consent of close family members and the consent of two physicians. The court limited this holding to patients in a persistent vegetative state with no cognitive powers, no chance of recovery, and who never clearly expressed a preference for termination. In a previous case, *Grace Plaza of Great Neck, Inc. v. Elbaum* (1993), the court had held that where doubt exists as to an incompetent's desired course of treatment, a judicial determination is necessary before life support can be terminated. The court further stated that proof of a patient's desires, such as through a living will or prior statement, will serve to limit a provider's autonomy in denying termination of treatment.

LIVING WILLS

Living wills, started in the 1960s, gained popularity following these cases. *Living wills* are directives from competent individuals to medical personnel and family members regarding the treatment they wish to receive when they can no longer make the decision for themselves (Figure 8–1). The living will is not necessary if the patient is competent and capable of making his or her wishes known. It becomes important when the previously competent person becomes seriously ill and incompetent.

Usually, the language of a living will is broad and vague. It gives little direction to the health care provider concerning the circumstances and actual time the declarant wishes the living will to be honored. There is typically no legal enforcement of the living will, and medical practitioners may choose to abide by the patient's wishes or to ignore them as they see fit. There is also no protection for the practitioner against criminal or civil liability, and many physicians have been afraid to proceed under a living will's direction for fear that family members or the state will file charges of wrongful death.

NATURAL DEATH ACTS

To protect practitioners from potential civil and criminal lawsuits and to ensure that patients' wishes are followed when they are no longer able to make their wishes known, a special type of living will, known as the *natural death act*, was enacted into law. These natural death acts are legally recognized living wills in that they serve the same function as living wills but with statutory enforcement, and virtually all states have enacted some form of natural death legislation. Recognizing that the physician may be unwilling to follow the directive, several of these laws require a reasonable effort on the part of the physician to transfer the patient to a physician who will abide by these wishes.

Statutory provisions for natural death acts vary from state to state. Generally, persons over 18 years may sign a natural death act. Such persons must be of sound mind and capable of understanding the purpose of the document that they sign. The natural death act document is usually a declaration that withholds or withdraws life-sustaining treatment from the patient should he or she ever be in a terminal state. The natural death act must be in written form, signed by the patient, and witnessed by two persons, each of whom is 18 years or older.

Some states also specify that the witnesses to the natural death act not be:

1. Related to the patient by blood or marriage.
2. Entitled to any portion of the estate of the patient by will or intestacy.
3. Directly financially responsible for the patient's medical care.
4. The attending physician, his or her employee, or employee of the facility in which the declarant is a patient.

LIVING WILL DECLARATION

To My Family, Doctors, and All Those Concerned with My Care

I, _____, being of sound mind, make this statement as a directive to be followed if for any reason I become unable to participate in decisions regarding my medical care.

I direct that life-sustaining procedures should be withheld or withdrawn if I have an illness, disease or injury, or experience extreme mental deterioration, such that there is no reasonable expectation of recovering or regaining a meaningful quality of life.

These life-sustaining procedures that may be withheld or withdrawn include, but are not limited to:

SURGERY   ANTIBIOTICS   CARDIAC RESUSCITATION
RESPIRATORY SUPPORT   ARTIFICIALLY ADMINISTERED FEEDING AND FLUIDS

I further direct that treatment be limited to comfort measures only, even if they shorten my life.

You may delete any provision above by drawing a line through it and adding your initials.

Other personal instructions:

These directions express my legal right to refuse treatment. Therefore, I expect my family, doctors, and all those concerned with my care to regard themselves as legally and morally bound to act in accord with my wishes, and in so doing to be free from any liability for having followed my directions.

Signed _____ Date_____

Witness _____ Witness _____

PROXY DESIGNATION CLAUSE

If you wish, you may use this section to designate someone to make treatment decisions if you are unable to do so. Your Living Will Declaration will be in effect even if you have not designated a proxy.

I authorize the following person to implement my Living Will Declaration by accepting, refusing and/or making decisions about treatment and hospitalization:

Name _____

Address _____

If the person I have named above is unable to act on my behalf, I authorize the following person to do so:

Name _____

Address _____

I have discussed my wishes with these persons and trust their judgment on my behalf.

Signed _____ Date_____

Witness _____ Witness _____

FIGURE 8-1. EXAMPLE OF A LIVING WILL (Courtesy of the Society for the Right to Die, 250 West 57th St., New York, NY 10107.)

5. The person who, at the request of the patient, signed the declaration because the patient was unable to sign.

Other states incorporate some of these restrictions.

The form of the natural death act also varies state to state. Some states provide no suggestion as to the contents of the document, whereas other states have a mandatory form that must be filled in by the declarant. Still other states suggest a form but provide that additional directions may be added if they are not inconsistent with the statutory requirements. For states that have no set form, private organizations have suggested formats for these special living wills.

Once signed and witnessed, most natural death acts are effective until revoked, although some states require that they must be reexecuted every five years. In some states, the patient who is pregnant may not benefit from the provisions of the natural death act during the course of the pregnancy. It may be advisable for the declarant to review, re-date, and re-sign the natural death act every year or so. This assures family members and health care providers that the directions contained in the natural death act reflect the current wishes of the patient.

The natural death act may be revoked by physical destruction or defacement, by a written revocation, or by an oral statement indicating that it is the person's wish to revoke the previously executed natural death act. Some states have less restrictions on revocation; for example, the revocation may take place without regard to the mental condition of the patient, and the revocation is ineffective until the attending physician is notified of the revocation.

Once a valid natural death act exists, it is effective only when the person becomes qualified, that is, the person is diagnosed to have a terminal condition and the removal or withholding of life-support systems would merely prolong the patient's process of dying. Most states require that two physicians certify in writing that any procedures and treatments will not prevent the ultimate death of the patient but will serve only to postpone death in a patient with no chance of recovery. Medications and procedures used merely to prevent the patient's suffering and to provide comfort are excluded from this definition.

Today, many states also allow an oral invocation of a natural death act and/or another person to invoke a natural death act for the patient. States were exploring a variety of options to ensure that natural death acts met the needs of patients when the durable power of attorney for health care become more prominent.

DURABLE POWER OF ATTORNEY FOR HEALTH CARE

The *durable power of attorney for health care (DPAHC)* or the *medical durable power of attorney (MDPA)* allows competent patients to appoint a surrogate or proxy to make health care decisions for them in the event that they are incompetent to do so. These legislative enactments were the next logical step following limitations with living wills and natural death acts. No longer did the family or health care provider need to guess if this was the time that the patient would have wanted the living will to be followed, as there was a person, given the authority of the patient to either accept of refuse care, to speak for the patient.

Power of attorney is a common law concept that allows one person (an agent) to speak for another (the principal), and is a concept of the agency relationship. At common law, the power of attorney terminates upon the death or incapacity of the principal. To prevent this occurrence when the patient most wants the power of attorney to be effective, legislatures adopted the Uniform Durable Power of Attorney Act. This act sanctions the right of an individual to grant a durable power of attorney—one that would be valid even if the principal was incapacitated and legally incompetent.

Under most of the DPAHC statutes, individuals may designate an agent to make medical decisions for them when they are unable to make such decisions. The power includes the right to ask questions, select and remove physicians from the patient's care, assess risks and complications, and select treatments and procedures from a variety of therapeutic options. The power also includes the right to refuse care and/or life-sustaining procedures. Health care providers are protected from liability if they abide, in good faith, on the agent's decisions.

Agents further have the authority to enforce the patient's treatment plans by filing lawsuits or legal actions against health care providers or family members. Agents have the right to forgo treatment, change treatment plans, or consent to additional treatment. In short, they have the full authority to act as the principal would have acted. Thus, the DPAHC is the best form of substituted judgment currently available for an otherwise incompetent patient.

Most patients are cautioned to appoint persons as agents who understand what the patient would want and are capable of making those hard decisions. Friends, relatives, or spouses may be appointed as agents. Most states allow the patient or potential patient to appoint subsequent agents. In the event the first named person cannot serve or is unwilling to serve in this capacity, then a second or third person has the principal's authority. Without this latter provision, patients' wishes might still not be honored.

MEDICAL OR PHYSICIAN DIRECTIVES

Some states allow for a directive that lists a variety of treatments and lets patients decide what they would want, depending on the patient's condition at the time. For example, the patient can select life-sustaining therapy if the condition is not terminal to disallowing life-sustaining therapy if the condition is terminal and irreversible. Generally known as a *medical or physician directive,* this document has legal worth comparable to the living will.

UNIFORM RIGHTS OF THE TERMINALLY ILL ACT

The act, adopted in 1989, is narrow in scope and limited to treatment that is merely life prolonging and to patients whose terminal condition is incurable and irreversible, whose death will occur soon, and who are unable to participate in treatment decisions. The act's sole purpose is to provide alternative ways in which a terminally ill patient's desires regarding the use of life-sustaining procedures can be legally implemented. To date, 12 states have adopted the act.

This act was passed because no two states have living will or natural death act provisions that are identical. Perhaps the act was passed because the political nature of the right to die had driven the legislature to enact virtually meaningless statutes to avoid political fallout.

Many of the provisions of the act look identical to some state natural death act provisions. For example, the qualified patient must be diagnosed as terminal and life-sustaining procedures would only prolong the dying of the patient. Physicians who are unwilling to comply with patients' requests not to begin or continue life-support procedures should take all necessary steps to transfer the patient to a physician who will comply with the provisions of the declaration. Patients diagnosed as being in a persistent vegetative state are not qualified patients.

PATIENT SELF-DETERMINATION ACT OF 1990

In November 1991, the Patient Self-Determination Act of 1990 was enacted into law as part of the Omnibus Budget Reconciliation Act of 1990. This act was in direct response to the Nancy Cruzan case in Missouri, and it mandates that patients must be queried about the existence of advanced directives and that such advanced directives be made available to them, if they so wish.

In 1983, Nancy Cruzan was involved in a one-car automobile accident. She was discovered lying face down in a ditch without cardiac or respiratory functioning, and life support was started. She eventually was diagnosed as being in a persistent vegetative coma, and her parents requested the removal of artificial hydration and nutritional support. The trial court allowed such removal because Cruzan "expressed thoughts at age 25 in a somewhat serious conversation with a friend that if sick or injured she would not wish to continue her life unless she could live at least halfway normal" (*Cruzan v. Director, Missouri Department of Public Health*, 1990, at 2843). The Supreme Court of Missouri reversed that decision, stating that such statements were unreliable for the purpose of determining her intent and further held that the family was not entitled to direct the termination of her treatment in the absence of a living will or "clear and convincing, inherently reliable evidence absent here" (at 2844).

The U.S. Supreme Court held that states had the authority to impose legal requirements on decisions to discontinue therapy for incompetent patients. The case was then remanded back to trial level in Missouri and, on retrial, the court concluded that the friend's statement of Nancy Cruzan's desires was sufficient to allow the removal of the feeding tube. Ms. Cruzan died on December 16, 1990.

Justice Scalia, in his separate concurrence, praised states for beginning to grapple with the issue of terminating medical treatment through legislation. Almost every state recognizes some form of advanced directive, from living wills to durable powers of attorney for health care. The problem, though, is that few people prepare advance directives. Thus, the Patient Self-Determination Act was passed to ensure that persons did know about such advanced directives and that they would be assisted in making such directives, if they so desired.

There were three basic purposes for the Patient Self-Determination Act as outlined in 1991:

1. Patients who are informed of their rights are more likely to take advantage of them.
2. If patients are more actively involved in decisions about their medical care, then that care will be more responsive to their needs.
3. Patients may choose care that is less costly (Rouse, 1991, p. 21).

The act merely lets people know about existing rights and does not create any new rights for patients, nor does it change state law. Perhaps the act has served as incentive for more states to pass durable powers of attorney for health care statutes, but it does not mandate such passage. The act does not require that patients execute advanced directives. It merely provides for patient education about such directives and provides assistance for those patients wishing to execute such directives. The legislation specifically states that providers may not discriminate against a patient in any way based on the absence or presence of an advanced directive.

Nor does the act legislate communication or conversation. Yet one of the purposes of the act is to encourage communication and conversation about existing directives, at a time when the patient is competent to understand and to execute advanced directives.

To make the Patient Self-Determination Act a reality, health care providers must themselves understand the act, its purposes, and how to answer patients' and families' questions. Quality care could be enhanced as health care providers often struggle to determine appropriate courses of care complicated by lack of knowledge about patients' preferences for treatment. Patient education about advanced directives should ideally take place outside the acute care setting, and nurses may become involved in consumer education programs. Nurses can also become involved in assessing the patients' readiness to prepare an advanced directive in the acute care setting.

The most challenging aspect of the process of preparing an advanced directive is assisting patients to identify their preferences for treatment. Some individuals have clear opinions, while other patients are more comfortable trusting future choices to family members without articulating specific wishes. It is also important for health care providers and patients to remember that preferences change over time and that the willingness to undergo aggressive treatment is in large part dependent on perception of the likely outcome of that treatment.

An expression of patient wishes for or against treatment choices is important. If these preferences are known, then the standard one applies in life-threatening situations is that of substituted judgment, which holds that the decision is the one the patient would have made if competent to make such a decision. If the preferences are not known, then the standard becomes one of best interests in light of everything that is known about the patient. Often, it is helpful to the patient's family and friends to articulate this latter standard, because they may be experiencing denial, guilt, or attachment.

Early in this inception, Lynn (1991) listed three types of patients for which advanced directives are most important. These individuals include:

1. Patients for whom a legally designated surrogate does not exist or could be controversial, such as an acquired immune deficiency syndrome (AIDS) patient who chooses to designate a long-term mate rather than a parent or sibling.
2. Patients with unusual or highly specific preferences.
3. Patients and families for whom the existence of a a document will reduce anxiety.

The Patient Self-Determination Act offers nurses an opportunity for greater participation in decision making. Nurses may enter discussions with patients about their hopes and fears that can be the basis for planning future care. Although one may not always understand the treatment preferences expressed by patients and family members, one can respect the courage required to confront the issues.

DO-NOT-RESUSCITATE DIRECTIVES

Some health care organizations have initiated ***do-not-resuscitate directives*** that patients may execute upon admission to health care institutions. Per the patient's request, the physician will then follow hospital policy in attaching such orders to the patient record. Most institutions require that there is documentation that the patient's decision was made after consultation with the physician regarding the patient's diagnoses and prognosis. The order should then be reevaluated according to institution policy.

Three states (New York, Georgia, and West Virginia) are among the minority of states that address do-not-resuscitate orders in acute care and long-term care facilities. New York's law is one of the most comprehensive in the nation. This law establishes the hierarchy of surrogates who may request a do-not-resuscitate status for incompetent patients and has also mandated that all health care facilities inquire of patients, as they are admitted, their desires concerning resuscitation. The act was promulgated by worry about the overuse of cardiopulmonary resuscitation. Frequently, the issue concerning do-not-resuscitate turns on whether the patient was fully informed when a physician ordered a no-code for the patient. *Payne v. Marion General Hospital* (1990) represents the first case in this area of the law.

There are two recent cases that address the issue of consequences when health care providers go against patient wishes in this area. In *Wendland v. Sparks* (1998), the patient had been hospitalized for two months for fibrotic lung disease and multiple myeloma. She was in remission and was fairly stable, given her underlying disease state.

Neither the family nor the patient had ever requested a do-not-resuscitate order. The patient had been resuscitated three times during the hospital stay and had never requested that she have a do-not-resuscitate order. In fact, shortly after one of the successful resuscitations, the patient's husband told the attending physician that he wished his wife placed on a ventilator if that became necessary to save her life.

The patient sustained a cardiopulmonary arrest at 4:40 A.M. One nurse brought the crash cart, while another went to get her physician, who was close by. When the physician arrived, she checked her pulse, listened for a heartbeat, listened for respiratory effort, and looked at the pupils. Stating, "I just cannot do it to her," she ordered the nurses to cease their efforts at resuscitation and the patient was pronounced dead by the physician.

The nurses testified that, if they had not been ordered otherwise by the physician, they would have performed a full code resuscitation on the patient. The court ruled that the physician's judgment was faulty and that the family had the right to sue the physician for wrongful death. Even though this patient had no practical chance of surviving her preexisting medical condition and faced the very real prospect of a diminished quality of life, she had a right to life. The loss of even a small chance of survival and rehabilitation is worth something and cannot be taken away arbitrarily. The court, though finding fault with the physician, did not fault the nurses for following her instruction.

In *Allore v. Flower Hospital* (1997), the patient had signed a living will. He had signed the living will in June upon admission to the hospital. He survived that hospitalization and was discharged. He was later admitted again and discharged, then admitted in August for the third and last time.

He went into respiratory distress during the night. The nurse was unaware of the living will, and there was no copy of the document in his current chart. When he coded, the nurse attempted to reach the physician, but he could not be reached. The nurse then called the cardiologist on call, who had no way of knowing of the patient's living will. They successfully resuscitated the patient.

The Court of Appeals ruled that the nurse had acted correctly by obtaining blood gases, by calling the cardiologist on call, and by sending the patient to the intensive care unit, where he was intubated and placed on a ventilator. He died later that day. The nurse, said the court, had followed the accepted nursing standards for life-saving measures for a patient in respiratory distress and could not be faulted for her care.

MATURE MINORS AND THE RIGHT TO DIE

In 1989, the Illinois Supreme Court became the first court in the United States to rule that a minor patient should be permitted to refuse medical treatment necessary to save her life. *In re E. G.* involved a 17-year-old leukemia patient whose doctors recommended a course of treatment that included a series of blood transfusions. She objected to these blood transfusions, based on her religious convictions, and the court upheld this right of refusal. They stated:

> Although the age of majority in Illinois is 18, that age is not an impenetrable barrier that magically precludes a minor from possessing and exercising certain rights normally associated with adulthood. . . . If the evidence is clear and convincing that the minor is mature enough to appreciate the consequences of her actions . . . then the mature minor doctrine affords her the common law right to consent to or refuse medical treatment (*In re E. G.*, 1989, at 327–328).

To a great extent, the court in reaching that momentous decision carefully weight the fact that E. G. was a very mature teenager, and that her religious convictions were based on deeply held, family-shared values. The psychologist testified at court that she had the maturity of a 22 year old.

In the years following that decision, there have been at least three other cases involving this area of the law (*O. G. v. Baum*, 1990; *In the Matter of Long island Jewish Medical Center*, 1990; and *Belcher v. Charleston Area Medical Center*, 1992). Taken together, they reflect the problems posed by such requests and that their resolution is not quickly decided. In these later cases, the patients were younger and much less mature than E. G. and ultimately the decisions regarding maturity have been very subjective.

In the Matter of Long Island Jewish Medical Center (1990) illustrates this point. Philip Malcolm, weeks shy of his eighteenth birthday, refused to consent to a blood transfusion based on religious convictions. At first glance, the facts of this case are very similar to *In re E. G.* The judge noted, however, that Philip and his family had only recently joined the Jehovah's Witnesses, some three years before this request. He did understand the basic tenets of the religion, but was not sufficiently mature to make this decision on his own. The court stated:

> He has never been away from home and has never dated a girl. He consults his parents before making decisions and when asked whether he considered himself an adult or a child, he responded, "Child." There was no evidence that Philip had been urged by his parents to make his own decision regarding blood transfusions (at 244).

The stakes are extraordinarily high in these cases, and legal authorities are starting to believe that these issues must be addressed soon. This is especially true in light of the various standards adopted by states concerning mature minors and their right in deciding issues that concern their welfare. Much of the argument has centered around an agreed definition of maturity, especially in the medical realm. Many courts still rely on the parents and their decision-making capacity. Would courts truly uphold minors' rights if they were totally different than their parents wishes?

There are two possible answers to this dilemma. One would be to lower the age of medical competency, identifying an age at which minors could either give consent or refuse to give consent. Current research indicates that between the ages of 12 and 14, adolescents undergo a major shift in cognitive functioning that enables them to reason abstractly, as well as to consider cause-and-effect relationships (Irwin and Millstein, 1992). Thus, there is reason to advocate a standard treating 14 year olds as competent in health care decision making.

Unfortunately, such an age-based standard creates several problems. It is no less arbitrary than the current standard of 18 as the age of majority. The same research that establishes the adolescent onset of cognitive functioning also recognizes that these abilities are acquired gradually, and that they reflect both a biological and an environmental component. Moreover, it is likely that some minors younger than the age of competency will seek to consent to their own health care treatment, reinforcing the same process now in place through the courts.

A second alternative is to adopt a uniform best interest approach, denying all adolescents autonomy until they reach the age of maturity. This standard has the advantage of not having to discern the adolescent's competency or maturity, but also has the disadvantage of taking decision making away from competent minors. Neither of these two approaches is likely to prevail, and the courts will continue to debate such issues.

■ EXERCISE 8—4

Find out what your hospital does about advanced directives. How is the patient made aware of these options and who assists the patient desiring to complete such a directive? If patients come to your institution with advanced directives, how are staff alerted to their existence? Are any provisions taken to ensure the validity of advanced directives prior to a patient's death? Give suggestions you might have for a more effective usage of such documents.

HOSPICE CARE

Some terminally ill patients prevent the need for natural death acts and living wills by entering hospice centers. A *hospice center* allows patients to receive the nursing and medical care that is required and to be kept comfortable, without the fear that they will be resuscitated or placed on life-support systems when death occurs. Some states are also beginning home hospice care to allow patients to receive the benefits of hospice centers in their own homes.

Congress recognized the need for such terminal care apart from the hospital setting and authorized Medicare reimbursement for hospice care (P.L. 97-248, 1982). Medicare reimbursement is limited to a six-month time interval, and this does not indicate that

GUIDELINES: ADVANCED DIRECTIVES

1. Nurses should review the state statutes and provisions for durable powers of attorney for health care, natural death acts, and living wills. Realize that the requirements may vary greatly state to state, and have the in-hospital attorney hold classes for nurses so that the nursing staff is fully aware of any statutory requirements and the means by which these advanced directives are enforced.

2. Review the hospital policy and procedure manual for any hospital guidelines in this area. If no policies exist, suggest to the committee or persons responsible for such policies the need for guidance in this area.

3. Should the patient or family tell you that a signed advanced directive exists, you should make that known to the physician and hospital administration immediately. Document the existence of the declaration in the patient's medical record, and ask for a copy of the declaration for the medical record.

4. Should the patient revoke the declaration or tell the nurse that he or she desires to revoke the declaration, the nurse is obligated to document such in the record and to immediately notify the attending physician and hospital administration. This is true even if the competency of the patient is questionable because some statutes allow for revocation even if the declarant is not of sound mind.

5. It is advisable that the nurse not be a witness to the living will or natural death act because many natural death acts forbid a witness from being employed by the attending physician or facility in which the patient is hospitalized. Usually, a friend or someone unrelated to the patient serves as the witness for this declaration.

6. Should the patient have a copy of the living will or natural death act in his or her medical record, read it carefully to ascertain the scope of its provisions. It is much easier to clarify the declaration while the patient is still competent than to try directives in the document. Document in the medical record any clarification that the patient gives to you, and ensure that the attending physician also understands the scope of the patient's declaration.

7. In most states, the nurse or another person may write and sign advanced directives as proxy of the competent patient. Here, the nurse must be sure that the patient is of sound mind, because competency is an important issue in the execution of such a directive. Document in the record what occurred and the circumstances that made it necessary for a second person to sign for the patient (partial paralysis or whatever the medical reason for the competent patient to be unable to sign).

8. Assist the family members in this time of crisis by being available and by answering as many of their questions as possible. Tell the family members of any existing ethics committee or other persons available to talk with them. Remember that they need time to internalize what is happening, especially if they are called on to concur with the patient's directive or to insist on the implementation of the patient's directive.

Congress meant that patients with a longer life expectancy should seek or accept more aggressive care.

The problem encountered with hospice centers is that the usual patients seeking such care are competent—the very same patients who could refuse heroic care if they were in a formal hospital setting. Problems encountered with allowing a patient to die are usually confined to incompetent, hospitalized patients.

ASSISTED SUICIDE

Although suicide as a crime has been abrogated in all states, most states still prohibit **assisted suicide.** Some states treat assisted suicide harshly, whereas other states prohibit only causing suicide, not assisting it. While other states have tried unsuccessfully through legislation to pass assisted suicide statutes, only Oregon has such a statute. The Oregon Death with Dignity Act was first passed by the voters in November 1994, then reviewed judicially, and on November 4, 1997, it was reasserted by a 60 to 40% margin when the voters opposed repeal of the act. In the full first year of its enactment, eight people (average age 71) had died in accordance with the act's provisions (*Brown University Long-Term Quality Advisor,* 1998). Table 8–1 recounts case law and major legislative decisions that have led to assisted suicide as it currently exists in the United States.

The act allows physicians who choose to participate to write lethal drug prescriptions for competent, terminally ill adults who are residents of the state. Other provisions that must be met before the prescription is written include:

1. Both the attending physician and a consulting physician must certify that the patient has no more than six months to live.
2. The patient must make both an oral and a written request for the prescription, followed by a second oral request 15 days or more after the first requests.
3. The attending physician must refer the patient for counseling if a psychological illness or depression is suspected.
4. The doctor must wait at least 48 hours after the third request before prescribing the medication.

Michigan is another state that has dealt with this issue in great degree. Because of Dr. Jack Kevorkian's "death machine," assisted suicide has taken on new meaning. Michigan originally filed murder charges against Kevorkian, but they were dismissed. Michigan then passed a statute "prohibiting one who has knowledge that a person intends to commit suicide from intentionally providing the physical means or participating in the phys-

TABLE 8–1.   RIGHTS OF THE TERMINALLY ILL: CASE LAW AND MAJOR LEGISLATIVE DECISIONS

Year	Case/Legislation	Description
1976	*In re Quinlan*	Right to remove person in prolonged vegetative state from ventilator
1990	*Cruzan v. Director, Missouri Department of Health*	Right given to states to decide whether families can remove artificial feeding tubes from persons in prolonged vegetative states
1991	Patient Self-Determination Act	Requires health care facilities receiving Medicare funds to provide information to patients at the time of admission about advanced directives
1994	Oregon Death with Dignity Act	Allows competent terminally ill adult patients to obtain prescriptions for lethal drugs
1996	Ninth Circuit Court Decision	Court decision stating that the Washington State ban on the right of terminally ill adult patients to request assistance in committing suicide from a qualified professional was unconstitutional
1997	*Vacco v. Quill* and *Compassion in Dying v. Glucksberg*	Supreme Court rules that states can ban physician-assisted suicide; states may also legalize and regulate physician-assisted suicide

ical act by which the person attempts or commits suicide," but the prohibition does not apply to "withholding or withdrawing by a licensed health care professional" (Kamisar, 1993, p. 37). This law has been challenged, and Dr. Kevorkian is now under legal constraint.

The question of whether mentally competent, terminally ill patients have a constitutional right to seek a physician's aid in ending their lives was answered by the U.S. Supreme Court in 1997. Both Washington and New York state courts had held that their states' attempt to ban physician-assisted suicide violated the constitutional due process rights of terminally ill patients who seek to hasten their deaths by using physician-prescribed medications. At the core of the matter is whether states may distinguish between patients who choose to refuse or withdraw medical treatment (allowing to die) and those who choose to extend this right to include medication-assisted suicide (assisting to die).

The U.S. Supreme Court, in one of the most important decisions of the 1990s, rejected the challenge to the constitutional right of the person to die, and, in essence, said that courts could ban physician-assisted suicides (*Compassion in Dying v. Glucksberg*, 1997, and *Vacco v. Quill*, 1997). Although finding no constitutional right to die, the court explicitly left open the door for states to legalize and regulate physician-assisted suicide, if the state chose to do so. This decision by the Supreme Court came just months before the Oregon voters passed the Death with Dignity Act for the second time. There is now a Model State Act to Authorize and Regulate Physician-Assisted Suicide being developed (Baron et al., 1996). To prevent potential managed care abuses with physician-assisted suicide, the model act requires that four conditions be met before one can receive assistance. These requirements, all having the effect of limiting managed care abuses, include:

1. The patient must be competent, defined as "based on the patient's ability to understand his or her condition and prognosis, the benefits and burdens of alternative therapy, and the consequences of suicide."
2. The patient must be fully informed.
3. The choice must be voluntary, one that is made independently, free from coercion or undue influences.
4. The choice must be enduring, in that the request must be stated to the responsible physician on at least two occasions that are at least two weeks apart, without self-contradiction during that interval (Baron et al., 1996, p. 20).

The nurse's role in this area is still developing. The American Nurses Association opposes the movement and opposes nurses' participation either in assisted suicide or active euthanasia because they violate the ethical traditions embodied in the *Code for Nurses* (ANA, 1994a and 1994b). In Michigan, the Michigan Nurses Association has come out in support of the legalization of assisted suicide for "competent persons whose suffering cannot be relieved or satisfactorily reduced with alternative strategies" (Michigan Nurses Association, 1994). The Oregon Nurses Association has requested specific standards within which nurses can operate without fear of disciplinary action, since physician are the only health care providers whose role is directly addressed in the act (Woolfrey, 1998).

If nurses are asked directly by patients to assist with their suicide, the nurse must refuse. But, before closing the door to open communications, look beyond the request to what the patients may be saying. They may be expressing a need for greater pain control or for someone to talk to about the fears of a terrible death. At this time, nurses must be clear that they cannot assist patients in this aspect, but may be able to assist with procuring medications for more effective pain control or by supplying needed forms to assist patients with advanced directives. Another avenue may be to ensure that patients speak with a chaplain or representative of their faith or with a social worker. Ensure that the patients know that someone cares and assist them in ways that nursing can intervene.

In recognition of the universal need for humane end-of-life care, the American Association of Colleges of Nursing, supported by a Robert Wood Johnson Foundation grant, convened a roundtable of nurse experts and other health care providers to begin communications surrounding this area. This roundtable was in accord with the 1997 International Council of Nurses mandate that nurses have a unique and primary responsibility for ensuring that individuals at the end of life experience a peaceful death.

This group of experts in health care ethics and palliative care developed the End-of-Life Competency Statements.* While developed as terminal objectives for undergraduate nursing students, they apply to all nursing professionals. These competencies are:

1. Recognize dynamic changes in population demographics, health care economics, and service delivery that necessitate improved professional preparation for end-of-life care.
2. Promote the provision of comfort care to the dying as an active, desirable, and important skill, and an integral component of nursing care.
3. Communicate effectively and compassionately with the patient, family, and health care team members about end-of-life issues.
4. Recognize one's own attitudes, feelings, values, and expectations about death and the individual, cultural, and spiritual diversity existing in these beliefs and customs.
5. Demonstrate respect for the patient's views and wishes during end-of-life care.
6. Collaborate with interdisciplinary team members while implementing the nursing role in end-of-life care.
7. Use scientifically based standardized tools to assess symptoms (such as pain, dyspnea, constipation, anxiety, fatigue, nausea/vomiting, and altered cognition) experienced by patients at the end of life.
8. Use data from symptom assessment to plan and intervene in symptom management using state-of-the-art tradition and complementary approaches.
9. Evaluate the impact of traditional, complementary, and technological therapies on patient-centered outcomes.
10. Assess and treat multiple dimensions, including physical, psychological, social, and spiritual needs, to improve quality at the end of life.
11. Assist the patient, family, colleagues, and oneself to cope with suffering, grief, loss, and bereavement in end-of-life care.
12. Apply legal and ethical principles in the analysis of complex issues in end-of-life care, recognizing the influence of personal values, professional codes, and patient preferences.
13. Identify barriers and facilitators to patients' and caregivers' effective use of resources.

---

*Source: From American Association of Colleges of Nursing, *Peaceful Death: Recommended Competencies and Curricular Guidelines for End-of-Life Nursing Care* (1999). Washington, DC, used with permission.

14. Demonstrate skill at implementing a plan for improved end-of-life care within a dynamic and complex health care delivery system.
15. Apply knowledge gained from palliative care research to end-of-life education and care (American Association of Colleges of Nursing, 1999).

SUMMARY

This chapter has detailed informed consent from a variety of aspects: from the competent person's consent for minor surgery to the incompetent person's right to die without life-sustaining procedures and devices. The American public places great value and respect in one's right to determine what will happen to the person. Nurses must understand and use measures that ensure one's right to control his or her own destiny.

AFTER COMPLETING THIS CHAPTER, YOU SHOULD BE ABLE TO

- Define informed consent, comparing and contrasting it with consent.
- Describe means of obtaining informed consent, including expressed, implied, oral, written, complete, and partial.
- Compare and contrast three standards of informed consent.
- Describe four exceptions to informed consent.
- Describe who has responsibility for obtaining informed consent.
- Describe types of consent forms in use in health care settings.
- Analyze whose signature must be obtained to ensure informed consent.
- Describe one's right to refuse consent for medical care.
- Describe the patient's right to either consent to or deny consent for research.
- Discuss the various issues that arise with informed consent and genetic testing.
- Describe advanced directives, including living wills, natural death acts, and durable power of attorney for health care and do-not-resuscitate directives.
- Discuss legal issues surrounding assisted suicide.
- Enumerate end-of-life competencies as developed by the American Association of Colleges of Nursing.

APPLY YOUR LEGAL KNOWLEDGE

- How does the distinction between consent and informed consent have implications for professional health care providers?
- What should the nurse do when told by a patient that he or she has an advanced directive?
- How does the nurse decide if a patient's consent is truly voluntary and informed?
- What type of role should nurses have securing informed consent? In assisting with research studies? In assisting with genetic testing?
- How do you incorporate end-of-life competencies in your daily nursing practice?

YOU BE THE JUDGE

Charlotte Butler sought treatment for relief of chronic pain she began to experience in her left chest and rib cage area after undergoing surgery, radiation, and chemotherapy treatments for breast cancer. She was referred by her oncologist to Dr. Kim, a member of the Fulton Anesthesia Associates and an anesthesiologist working as an independent contractor at South Fulton Medical Center, Inc. Dr. Kim administered epidural steroid injections to Butler on January 20, 1988, and February 17, 1989. In September 1989, when the steroid injection failed to give long-term relief, Dr. Kim gave Butler a thoracic sympathetic (neurolytic) block, which, unlike the two previous steroid injections, was an injection of the nerve-destroying agent phenol. In January 1990, Dr. Kim performed a second neurolytic block on Butler, following this procedure almost immediately, in February 1990, with a third neurolytic block.

In August 1990, Butler called Dr. Kim requesting additional treatment for her pain. Although the informed consent form filled out by the hospital nursing staff and signed by Butler identified this last procedure as an "epidural steroid injection," Dr. Kim actually administered a fourth neurolytic block using the agent phenol. This last injection was administered too close to Butler's spinal column, with the phenol penetrating the spinal column, and rendering Butler a ventilator-dependent C1 quadriplegic.

Butler settled her claim against Dr. Kim and subsequently filed this action against South Fulton Medical Center, Inc., alleging the hospital was negligent in two ways:

1. The hospital's nursing staff did not fulfill their duties and obligations with regard to the obtaining of consent forms from Butler.
2. The hospital failed to adequately supervise Dr. Kim in that it allowed him to perform sympathetic neurolytic blocks without the requisite credentials.

The trial court granted South Fulton Medical Center, Inc.'s motion for summary judgment as to Butler's claim that it had negligently hired and supervised Dr. Kim. They dismissed her cause of action against the hospital nursing staff for failing to identify the correct procedure on the informed consent form. It was significant that Butler noted in her deposition that she never read any of the consent forms before she signed them. Also significant was that Dr. Kim never told her anything specific about any of the procedures he performed in his effort to relieve her chronic pain and that Butler candidly admitted that she did not know the difference in the various procedures that were performed, but that she was relying on Dr. Kim to select the procedure that was "right for her."

Legal Questions

1. Was the court correct in dismissing the informed consent cause of action from the nursing staff of South Fulton Medical Center, Inc.?
2. Did Butler give informed consent for any or all of the procedures that were performed on her?
3. What were the nurses' informed consent responsibilities with regard to this patient?
4. Did the nurses have a responsibility to ensure that Butler knew about the procedure before they let her sign the informed consent form?
5. How would you decide this case?

REFERENCES

Allore v. Flower Hospital, 699 N.E.2d 560 (Ohio App., 1997).

American Association of Colleges of Nursing (1999). *Peaceful Death: Recommended Competencies and Curricular Guidelines for End-of-Life Nursing Care.* Washington, DC: Author.

American Nurses Association (1994a). *Position Statement on Assisted Suicide.* Washington, DC: Author.

American Nurses Association (1994b). *Position Statement on Active Euthanasia.* Washington, DC: Author.

Andrews, L. B., Fullarton, J. E., et al. (eds.). (1994). *Assessing Genetic Risks: Implications for Health and Social Policy.* Washington, DC: National Academy Press.

Arato v. Avedon, 858 P.2d 598 (California, 1993).

Auler v. Van Natta, 686 N.E.2d 172 (Ind. App., 1997).

Baron, C. H., et al. (1996). A model state act to authorize and regulate physician-assisted suicide. *Harvard Journal on Legislation* 33, 1–34.

Bartling v. Superior Court, 163 Cal. App.3d 186, 209 Cal. Rptr. 220 (Cal. App. Ct., 2d Dis., 1984).

Belcher v. Charleston Area Medical Center, 422 S.E.2d 827 (South Carolina, 1992).

Breithaupt v. Adams, 352 U.S. 432 (1957).

Bouvia v. Superior Court, 179 Cal. App.3d 1127, 225 Cal. Rptr. 297 (Cal. App. Ct, 2d. Dis., 1986).

Cushing, M. M. (1991). Demystifying informed consent. *American Journal of Nursing* 91 (11), 17–19.

Compassion in Dying v. Glucksberg, 117 S. Ct. 2258 (1997).

Cruzan v. Director, Missouri Department of Health, 497 U.S. 261, 110 S. Ct. 2841, 111 L.E.D. 2d 224 (1990).

Daniel Thor v. Superior Court of Solano County, 855 P.2d 375, 21 Cal. Rptr. 2d 357 (Cal., 1993).

Davis v. Hoffman, 972 F. Supp. 308 (E.D. Pa., 1997).

Eichner v. Dillon, 73 App. Div. 2d 431, 426 N.Y.S.2d 517 (2d. Dept., 1980).

Eight Die in Oregon Under Assisted-Suicide Law. (1998). *The Brown University Long-Term Quality Advisor* 10(10), 6.

45 CFR, Sec. 46.111, 46.101(b), 46.110, and 46.116 (1991).

45 CFR, Sec. 46.401 et seq. (1998).

45 CFR, Sec. 46.101(a)(2) (1997).

Giese v. Stice, 567 N.W.2d 156 (Nebraska, 1997).

Grabowski v. Quigley, 684 A.2d 610 (Pa. Super., 1996).

Grace Plaza of Great Neck, Inc. v. Elbaum, 82 N.Y.2d 10 (New York, 1993).

Hecht v. Kaplan, 645 N.Y.S.2d 51 (N.Y. App., 1996).

Illinois Department of Public Health (1996). *Newborn Screening: An Overview of Newborn Screening Programs in the United States, Canada, Puerto Rico, and the Virgin Islands.* Springfield, IL: Author.

In re E. G., 4549 N.E.2d 322 (Illinois, 1989).

In re Fiori, 652 A.2d 1350 (Pennsylvania, 1995).

In re Hamilton, 657 S.W.2d 425 (Tenn. App., 1983).

In re Quinlan, 70 N.J. 10, 335 A.2d 647 (1976).

In the Matter of Long Island Jewish Medical Center, 557 N.Y.S.2d 239 (New York, 1990).

Irwin, C., and Millstein, S. G. (1992). Risk taking behaviors and biopsychosocial development during adolescence. pp. 75–102. In E. J. Susman et al. (eds.). *Emotion, Cognition, Health, and Development in Children and Adolescents.* Hillsdale, IL: Erlbaum.

Jefferson v. Griffin Spalding County Hospital Authority, 247 Ga. 86, 274 S.E.2d 457 (1981).

John F. Kennedy Memorial Hospital v. Heston, 58 N.J. 576 (1971).

Jones v. Philadelphia College of Osteopathic Medicine, 813 F. Supp. 1125 (Pennsylvania, 1993).

Joswick v. Lenox Hill Hospital, 510 N.Y.S.2d 803 (New York, 1986).

Kamisar, Y. (1993). Active versus passive euthanasia: Why keep the distinction? *Trial* 29 (3), 32–37.

Karp v. Cooley, 493 F.2d 408 (5th Cir., 1974).

Korman v. Mallin, 858 P.2d 1145 (Alaska, 1993).

Leach v. Akron General Medical Center, 13 Ohio App.3d 393, 469 N.E.2d 1047 (Ohio, 1984).

Lincoln v. Gupta, 370 N.W.2d 312 (Michigan, 1985).

Lugenbuhl v. Dowling, 676 So.2d 602 (La. App., 1996).

Lynn, J. (1991). Why I don't have a living will. *Law Medicine and Healthcare* 19, 101–104.

Madison v. Harrison, #68651 (Massachusetts, 1957).

Mathias v. St. Catherine's Hospital, Inc., 569 N.W.2d 330 (Wis. App., 1997).

Matter of Anna M. Gordy, 658 A.2d 613 (Delaware, 1994).

Matter of Roche, 687 A.2d 349 (N.J. Super. Ch., 1996).

Michigan Nurses Association (1994). *MNA Human Rights/Ethics Committee Position Statement on Assisted Voluntary Self-Termination.* Okemos, MI: Author.

National Institutes of Health (1998). *NIH Policy and Guidelines on the Inclusion of Children as Participants in Research Involving Human Subjects.* Rockville, MD: Author.

Norwood Hospital v. Munoz, 564 N.E.2d 1017 (Massachusetts, 1991).

O'Brien v. Cunard Steamship Company, 154 Mass. 272, 28 N.E. 226 (1899).

O. G. v. Baum, 790 S.W.2d 839 (Tex. App.–Houston [1st District], 1990).

Payne v. Marion General Hospital, 549 N.E.2d 1043 (Ind. App. 2d Dis., 1990).

Piper, A., Jr. (1994). Truce on the battlefield: A proposal for a different approach to medical informed consent. *The Journal of Law, Medicine, and Ethics* 22(4), 301–313.

Public Law 97-248 (1982).

Rochin v. California, 342 U.S. 165 (1950).

Rouse, F. (1991). Patients, providers, and the Patient Self-Determination Act. *Hastings Center Report* 21(1), S2–S3.

Rozovsky, F. A. (1990). *Consent to Treatment: A Practical Guide* (2nd ed.). Boston: Little, Brown and Company.

Ruppel v. Ramsever, 33 F. Supp.2d 720 (C.D. Ill., 1999).

Rutherford, M. (1994). Small patients, big legal risks. *RN* 57(9), 51–57.

Salgo v. Leland Stanford, Jr. University Board of Trustees, 317 P.2d 170 (Cal. Dis. Ct. App., 1957).

Scanlon, C. & Fibison, W. (1995). *Managing Genetic Information: Implications for Nursing Practice.* Washington, DC: American Nurses Association.

Schmerber v. California, 384 U.S. 757 (1966).

Schloendorff v. Society of New York Hospitals, 211 N.Y. 125, 105 N.E. 92 (1914).

Shine v. Vega, 709 N.E.2d 58 (Massachusetts, 1999).

Superintendent of Belchertown State School v. Saikewicz, 373 Mass. 728, 370 N.E.2d 417 (1977).

Switzer, K. H. (1995). Informed consent for inserting a CVC. *American Journal of Nursing* 95(6), 66–67.

The Patient Self-Determination Act, Sections 4206 and 4751 of the *Omnibus Reconciliation Act of 1990,* Public Law 101-508, November 1990.

Truman v. Thomas, 27 Cal.3d 285, 611 P.2d 902 (1980).

21 CFR, Parts 50, 56, 312, 314, and 812.

Vacco v. Quill, 117 S. Ct. 2293 (1997).

Wecker v. Amend, 918 P.2d 658 (Kan. App., 1996).

Wendland v. Sparks, 574 N.W.2d 327 (Iowa, 1998).

Woolfrey, J. (1998). What happens now? Oregon and physician-assisted suicide. *Hastings Center Report* 28(3), 9–17.

nine

Documentation and Confidentiality

■ PREVIEW

A major responsibility of all health care providers is that they keep accurate and complete medical records. Much of what is collected and recorded remains very sensitive information. Understanding the need for clear and concise records and knowing which portions of the record may be discovered and introduced during trials should enable the nurse to be a proficient recorder of patient care. The newest area of confidentiality is with computer documents, electronic mail, and Internet access. This chapter presents guides for documentation—both the patient record and incident reports—and issues of confidentiality.

■ KEY CONCEPTS

medical records

standards for record keeping

effective documentation

computerized charting

charting by exception

alteration of records

retention of records

omnia praesumuntur contra
   spoliatorem

patient access to medical records

incident, variance, situational, or
   unusual occurrence report forms

patient's right to privacy

confidentiality of medical records

common law duty to disclose

MEDICAL RECORDS

Medical records and a medical records library are mandated by federal governmental and nongovernmental agencies. Additionally, agencies such as the Joint Commission for the Accreditation of Healthcare Organizations (JCAHO) and state and local rules and regulations further define this complex area.

From a nursing perspective, the most important purpose of documentation is communication. The *purposes of medical records,* as identified by JCAHO, are to:

1. Assist in planning patient care and in continuing the evaluation of the patient's condition and ongoing treatment.

2. Document the course of the patient's medical evaluation, treatment, and change in condition.
3. Document communication between the practitioner responsible for the patient and any other health professional who contributes to the patient's care.
4. Assist in protecting the legal interest of the patient, the hospital, and the practitioner responsible for the patient.
5. Provide data for use in continuing education and in research (1999).

Thus, such records not only record what has transpired but also serve as a vital communication link among members of the health care team as well as further educational and research programs.

To accomplish the primary purposes of record keeping, the JCAHO *Accreditation Manual for Hospitals* (1999) also specifies **standards for record keeping.** These standards attempt to ensure:

1. Patient identification.
2. Medical support for the selected diagnoses.
3. Justification of the medical therapies used.
4. Accurate documentation of that which has transpired.
5. Preservation of the record for a reasonable time period.

Although the *Accreditation Manual for Hospitals* previously specified only inpatient care, the latest edition dictates that the same high standards apply to emergency care patients, patients seen through the hospital's ambulatory clinics (outpatients), and patients seen in conjunction with a hospital-based home health care program (JCAHO, 1999).

CONTENTS OF THE RECORD

Basic information that should be recorded for any patient includes:

1. Personal data such as name, date of birth, gender, marital status, occupation, and person(s) to be contacted for emergencies.
2. Financial data such as health insurance carrier with assignment of rights, patient employer, and person responsible for payment of the final bill.
3. Medical data.

These last data entries form the bulk of the record and include, but are not limited to, a history of signs and symptoms, diagnoses, treatments, medical tests, laboratory results, consultation reports, anesthesia and operating room records, signed informed consent forms, progress notes, respiratory therapy records, and nurses' notes. In some states and in some instances, marital status may not be recorded. For example, some states prohibit inclusion of the parents' marital status on birth certificates to prevent the stigma of illegitimacy.

The accreditation standards also specify that documentation of nursing care be reflective of the individual patient status. Thus, nurses' notes should address patient needs, problems, limitations, and patient responses to nursing interventions. Individualized, goal-directed nursing care is provided to patients through the use of the nursing process. Each patient's nursing needs are assessed by a registered nurse at the time of admission or within the period established by the nursing department/service policy. Patient education and patient/family knowledge of self-care are given specific consideration in the nursing plan. The plan of care is documented and reflects current standards of nursing practice (JCAHO, 1999).

The observations charted should lead to nursing diagnoses. Pertinent patient quotes about symptoms and feelings should be included in the medical record. It is advisable to use some form of nursing process in charting so that no pertinent information is overlooked or forgotten.

Documentation must show continuity of care, interventions that were used, and patient responses to the therapies implemented. Nurses' notes are to be concise, clear, timely, and complete. Even if the patient condition does not change, that absence of change should be recorded at least once per shift. The complete patient assessment performed by the nurse caring for a selected patient should be reflected, in its entirety, in the patient's medical record.

EFFECTIVE DOCUMENTATION

The American legal system has helped nurses recognize what must be included in charting and, through case law, has given tips on how to chart entries correctly. These tips for *effective documentation* are enumerated in the following paragraphs.

Make an Entry for Every Observation

If no mention has been made of a change in a patient's condition, the jury can infer that no observation of the patient was conducted. In *Houlton v. Memorial Hospital* (1997), a patient was admitted through the emergency center for numbness below the waist and tingling in her leg. The diagnostic tests performed in the emergency center disclosed a low fever and an elevated white blood cell count. The patient had no loss of lower body motor function or loss of bowel or bladder control.

The patient's physician listed two different medical diagnoses to rule out: an epidural abscess from osteomyelitis or a malignant spinal tumor. According to the medical evidence the court said it considered before making its decision, an epidural abscess would tend to cause sensation and lower body motor function to decline gradually and progressively, whereas a spinal tumor would tend to cause a sudden loss of motor function and loss of bowel and bladder control from an acute infarct affecting the blood supply to the spinal cord.

On the afternoon following admission, the neurologist's provisional diagnosis was a spinal tumor, as there had been no loss or even the onset of decline in lower body motor function. However, later that afternoon, the patient started having trouble moving her legs. She got out of bed and walked to the bathroom unassisted, but had to ring for help to arise from the commode. She said her legs "were numb and did not seem to work." Two aides got her into a wheelchair, then helped her back to bed, but did not tell the charge nurse, and no one notified the physician. The nurses' notes stated that the patient had not experienced any significant change in her condition during the shift.

The night nurse knew that the patient was having difficulty moving her legs, but did not believe that this was a significant change in her condition, did not chart it, and did not notify the physician. In the morning, the day nurse found the patient completely paralyzed below the waist and called the physician. The neurosurgeon erroneously concluded the paralysis was a sudden onset, and he believed this was consistent with a spinal tumor.

The patient, in fact, had a spinal abscess from osteomyelitis. The court ruled that she could have benefited from surgery, but a correct medical diagnosis was not made in time to do the surgery. The cause, ruled the court, was the negligent nursing assessment and documentation, for which the jury returned a substantial verdict against the hospital.

The lesson from this case is that even routine checks of patients must be recorded, because failure to record such data leads to the inference that the patient had not been checked. Here, the nurses attempted to show that they had assessed the patient, but it was clear from the notes that this patient was not adequately assessed.

A similar finding occurred in *Webb v. Tulane Medical Center Hospital* (1997). In this case, a 23-year-old man had been diagnosed with sickle cell anemia when he was less than a year old. He had suffered poor health throughout his short life, with continued bouts of pneumonia and repeated sickle cell crises. He was admitted to the acute care setting for intravenous antibiotics and pain medications, and discharged on oral antibiotics after seven days. He was told to report for a follow-up visit in the hospital's sickle cell clinic six days after discharge.

On the morning of his clinic visit, he came in, stating that he had chest and abdominal pain. He was not immediately seen by the physician, but was admitted to the acute care setting through the emergency center with a diagnosis of multiple pulmonary infarcts. The patient continued to deteriorate. His chest pain continued, he developed a low-grade fever, and antibiotics had little effect on his overall condition.

At midnight, the physician ordered and the nurses started two units of packed cells to transfuse over a total of approximately eight hours, and they were completed about eight o'clock in the morning. By noon, the patient's temperature was 103.8°F, and he was having more severe chest and abdominal pain. The physician was notified, blood gases were drawn, and the patient was coded about 10 minutes later.

A visiting friend had called for help. The patient was revived after a lengthy code but remained comatose in the intensive care unit until his death seven days later.

At trial, the patient's mother prevailed against the hospital. The Court of Appeals agreed with the trial judge's belief that there was evidence of nursing negligence. The court agreed that, once the blood was begun, the patient should have been observed frequently and carefully monitored for potential complications. Failure to do so, said the court, is a breach of the legal standard of care for nursing practice.

The court also believed that, although the blood transfusion had been completed for over four hours, his continued high fever, chest pains, labored breathing, and abdominal pain warranted close monitoring by the nurses. Failure of nursing to provide such close monitoring was also a breach of the nursing standard of care. The courts found a serious problem with the fact that there were no nursing notes charted after 10:00 A.M. that any nurse had checked on the patient. Thus, the court concluded, that no care had been given for the two to three hours just prior to this patient's arrest.

Ultimately, the nurses were found not to be liable for the patient's death because an autopsy revealed that the cause of death had been a cardiopulmonary infarct acutely precipitated by aspiration of vomitus, a very sudden event that could have happened even with the closest of monitoring and the best nursing care possible. The court believed that this was the end stage of a tragic progression of the sickle cell disease.

Follow Up as Needed

Merely charting changes in patient status may not be adequate. The landmark decision of *Darling v. Charleston Community Memorial Hospital* (1965) showed that follow-up measures must be taken. James Darling, an 18-year-old high school football player, had broken his leg during a Saturday afternoon game and had the leg casted at the local hospital. Following the casting, he was admitted for observation. The nursing staff continued to assess Darling's casted leg, noting repeatedly in the patient record his deteriorating condition, the foul odor being emitted from the casted extremity, and the patient's ever-increasing pain. The nurses did share their observations with the primary physician, but took no further action when the primary physician failed to take corrective action.

The court concluded that the follow-up and evaluation of the patient's responses were equally important to the initial assessment and that the nurses had a further duty to the patient, and that merely assessing and charting Darling's condition were insufficient. That court also inferred that proper documentation, no matter how accurate and timely it is, can never be a substitute for quality nursing care. Rather, the nursing staff should have reported their observations and lack of subsequent medical interventions to the nursing supervisor. The supervisor should have consulted the medical chief for the service.

Complete records, however, may help to protect the staff from legal liability. In a classic Kentucky case, periodic observations plus accurate charting coupled with timely physician contact and medical management allowed a jury to conclude that there was no liability against either the nursing staff or the physician (*Engle v. Clarke*, 1961). This principle has since been indirectly upheld in *Pellerin v. Humedicenters, Inc.* (1997). In that case, the court noted that failing to chart the site and mode of an injection does not affect how the injection was actually administered, but it does tend to indicate that the nurse did not follow accepted policy and procedure in carrying out her job responsibilities.

Read Nurses' Notes Before Giving Care

Few nurses have been encouraged to read the nurses' notes prior to caring and/or charting on a patient. By taking the time to read the entry prior to the current one, it is possible to determine whether there has been a change in the patient's condition. Even physicians have a duty to read nurses' notes, the court concluded in a 1988 case. There, a patient's leg incision failed to heal properly following heart bypass surgery. After the patient mentioned her discomfort and continuing discharge from the leg incision, the nurse made an entry in the record. The patient subsequently continued to experience problems with her leg, and a year after the initial surgery, x-rays revealed that hemoclips had been left in her leg.

Though the defendants prevailed because no medical expert witness was called to testify, if there had been expert testimony both the physician and the hospital would have had difficulty explaining why no one, particularly the surgeon, paid attention to the patient's complaint or the nurse's notes. The court concluded that the nurse's notes literally and figuratively stand out "like a red flag" (*Regan Report on Nursing Law*, 1988, at 1).

Always Make an Entry, Even if It Is Late

Record entries must be timely, charted as close to the happening as possible. Time dulls even the best memories, and a nurse may have to strain to recall what actually transpired. Too often, valuable information is then omitted for lack of recall. If one must chart after the fact, it is more important that all pertinent data are included rather than preserving the chronological order of the chart. To show timeliness, remember to include the complete date and time of charting in the entry. The usage of military or 24-hour time has aided in accuracy of timed entries.

There is no rule against charting out of time sequence, and a late entry is far superior to no entry at all. However, the longer the time interval between the actual patient care and the charting of that care, the more likely it is that the court becomes suspicious that the additional entry is merely to prevent liability.

If a late entry is made, never try to squeeze the information into a small space or along the margins of the chart. Such crowding in data often is perceived in a courtroom as an attempt to cover up information. The nurse may want to add a note stating why the entry is late or somehow to explain why the charting had not been done earlier. Such a note could be as simple as "first day back from three scheduled days off" or "patient chart unavailable at 03:00."

Likewise, never leave several blank lines for a colleague to enter notes. The colleague should make his or her entry as a late entry.

Remember, too, that after a certain time period, most states hold that the chart must be "complete." This usually occurs 30 to 60 days after the patient's discharge from an acute care setting or an ambulatory surgical setting. After that time period, no further changes may be made.

Make the Chart Entry After the Event

Never chart in advance of a happening, treatment, or medication. The patient may not tolerate the procedure as had been intended, or taken the medication, or the nurse may have been unable to complete what he or she had intended to do. For example, another patient on the unit may have arrested or needed assistance immediately and the already charted procedure was never completed, or the patient may be in a full code and the vital signs as recorded show an acceptable heart rate, respiratory rate, and blood pressure. Although it seems a small issue, if it can be shown that the nurse charted in advance, an attorney may be able to lessen the nurse's credibility in the eyes of a jury.

Accurate nurses' notes form the basis of the patient medical record. Too often, this charting reflects the expected as opposed to the actual. In *Genao v. State* (1998), a nurse documented a sedated psychiatric patient's condition three times without ever seeing the patient. When the patient was finally "seen," she was found after being raped by another patient.

Use Clear and Objective Language

For years, nurses have been taught to use somewhat vague terminology in charting rather than drawing conclusions. Entries were used as "appears to be asleep" or "seems to be resting comfortably" or, even more vague, "had a good night." These types of entries were thought to protect the nurse against drawing conclusions or being accused of making medical diagnoses. Today's attorney looks at such vague verbiage and is inclined to ask questions that cast doubt on the nurse's observational powers or that serve to imply that what the nurse actually saw was quite different from what was charted. Thus, the nurse should chart, using objective, definite terms so that there is no doubt about the certainty of the entry.

A case that speaks directly to the clarity of the entry is *Shahine v. Louisiana State University Medical Center* (1996). The patient sued the surgeon and the hospital over persistent numbness in her right hand, which she first noticed after her total right hip replacement. Her suit alleged that the numbness was an ulnar nerve injury from improper positioning or from the surgeon's pressing against her arm or hand during the surgery.

The Court of Appeals exonerated all defendants from liability. The reason for this favorable result was the effort the circulating nurse made to document in precise detail how the patient had been positioned, stabilized, and padded before surgery, and specifically her documentation of the steps taken to extend the patient's arms out of harm's way and to pad her arms and hands to avoid pressure- or positioning-related injuries.

The court found it was critical that the nurse wrote a detailed factual statement describing to the smallest detail how the patient had been positioned, and that she refrained from unsubstantiated judgmental assertions such as stating that the patient was positioned properly or in a manner designed to avoid injury.

Mental capacity can also be established by the factual charting of nurses. In *Mitsinicos v. New Rochelle Nursing Home, Inc.* (1999), a nursing home resident had filed a lawsuit against the nursing home. The court had to decide if the resident had sufficient mental capacity to file a lawsuit or whether a guardian was necessary. To resolve the issue, the court read nursing documentation to conclude that the resident's intermittent confusion did not render him legally incompetent.

When charting is not specific, the court may find against the hospital and staff. In *Griffin v. Methodist Hospital* (1997), the court stated that to defend against malpractice, it is not good enough to generalize about the standard of care's having been met. An expert witness must be able to find in the chart what specific examinations and treatments were performed. Saying after the fact that a patient was monitored appropriately is useless without nursing notes of the specific actions that constituted monitoring of the patient's condition.

Time of occurrences have always caused some confusion, especially when trying to discover if a code has been called in a timely manner or if the appropriate treatment has been timely initiated. At least one court case has addressed time confusion as being detrimental to the defense of a filed lawsuit. In *Landry v. Clement* (1998), the issue was at what time a physician was notified of late decelerations on a fetal heart monitor strip. The nurses' notes said that the physician phoned at 4:30 P.M. and was notified of the late decelerations. But the fetal heart monitor strip clock noted that the deceleration occurred at 5:30 P.M. At trial, a nurse testified that the fetal heart monitor clock was fast by one full hour and that the actual time of the deceleration was 4:30 P.M. Although the court did not say that the time discrepancies directly affected the quality of the patient's care, the legal record was seriously compromised by the fact that the fetal heart monitor clock was set one hour ahead of the real-time clock.

Be Realistic and Factual

Nurses should also chart a realistic picture of the patient, particularly patients who refuse to comply with therapeutic regimes or are difficult to care for because of abusive and threatening language. These patients may well have a less than satisfactory outcome, especially if they were noncompliant. Charting what the patient said, instances of non-compliance, and threats against nursing personnel help to prevent such a case from coming to court. Prospective attorneys will be hesitant to represent clients who caused or contributed to their unsatisfactory outcome.

Noted observations should be factual and should describe objectively the patient's symptoms, appearance, and behaviors. Avoid any language of blame or negligence in charting. If needed, use quotation marks to include actual patient statements. Never use conclusory statements without giving supportive objective data, such as "patient states he was trying to climb over the bedrail and that is why he fell."

Chart Only Your Own Observations

It is advisable that nurses refrain from charting for other nurses, unless absolutely necessary. For example, the physician insists on giving a particular injection and the nurse notes that medication received by the patient, as well as the person who administered the medication. Because patient records may be used in a variety of courts, the nurse doing the charting will be unable to remember particulars about the patient, diagnoses, and nursing care. Yet the nurse will be called to testify because his or her name appeared on the chart. For the same reason, chart only what is observed or assessed.

Some institutions still require that professional nurses chart for nonlicensed personnel or "cosign" charts for these personnel. Charting for others or cosigning notes makes the charting nurse potentially liable for care, observations, or omissions as charted. Always read and investigate what has been charted before cosigning. Nurses should further investigate ways of changing such policies.

Chart Patient's Refusal for Care

If the patient refuses care or ordered treatment, ensure that the refusal is documented timely. Remember, too, that patient education about the consequences of that refusal must be included in the medical record. In a case that illustrates this principle, the patient refused a mammogram after a lump had been discovered in her breast. The court noted that the standard of care requires that a physician recommend a mammogram, and if the patient refuses, the physician should explicitly chart that refusal. The physician should also insist that the patient return for a follow-up examination no later than one month and that refusal should also be charted, if the patient indicates that she needs no further care (*May v. Jones*, 1996).

Clearly Chart All Patient Education

Nurses inevitably combine patient education with a variety of other physical tasks, such as teaching the patient proper foot care while bathing the diabetic patient, instructing about meal plans while assisting with the feeding of a newly diagnosed congestive heart failure patient, or demonstrating how to correctly change a toddler's dressing while showing the parents how to observe for signs of wound infection. Some of this patient education is carefully documented, especially if the patient is to be discharged later that day or early the next morning. All patient education must be documented in the patient record, with an evaluation of the teaching also documented.

To document patient comprehension, ask pertinent questions about material that was just taught. Another strategy is to have the patient perform a demonstration of the task or select appropriate foods from the daily menu selection to verify that learning has occurred. Finally, listen carefully to the patient's questions for appropriateness and content mastery. When documenting, reference that teaching has been done, rather than "discussed with the client how he would select low-sodium foods." Include all teaching that is done for reinforcement of needed knowledge and revalidation that the patient is retaining the information. If printed materials are sent home with the patient, retain a copy of the information sheet for the medical record.

Correct Charting Errors

The legal system has also given guidance in the area of how to rectify charting errors. There is adequate case law to support the contention that if there are errors in part of the record, the jury could find that errors might just as easily exist elsewhere as well, and thus the entire record could be found to be erroneous. Recognizing that anyone could make an error or misspell a word, the error in question should have a single line drawn through it with the correct entry placed above the error or next to the erroneous entry. Also include the time and date of the correction and to initial or sign the correction to show by whom, when, and why a new notation was made. The nurse may explain the correction with an entry such as "Entry made on wrong chart" or "Spelling error." To avoid charting on another patient's chart, each page of the patient's medical record should be stamped with the patient's name, medical record number, and other institution identifiers.

If the reason for the striking of a portion of charting is self-evident, no additional note need be made and the nurse should just initial the cross-out. For example, if a misspelled word is crossed out and the correctly spelled word is the next entry, it is obvious why the correction was made. Frequently, this is seen when right is crossed out and left inserted or vice versa. It is obvious that the wrong extremity was first charted and then the correct extremity was identified.

Many institutions discourage the usage of "error" (such as "spelling error" or "error in charting) when correcting a chart entry. There is some concern that using the word error may be interpreted as though the entire entry is in error, and nurses are urged to avoid using the word error on the chart.

Nurses should never, under any circumstance, totally obliterate the entry, tape a new entry over the erroneous entry, or use a more imaginative way to prevent the reading of the error in their charting. Correction fluid was not invented to obliterate a medical record entry and should not be used for this purpose. Such obliterations or erasures serve only to raise suspicion in the minds of others and questions of what was hidden arise. Innocent though the entry may have been, it is hard to defend a lawsuit with altered records. In *Ahrens v. Katz* (1984), white-outs of part of the nursing notes in the original chart were discovered and the records x-rayed so that the injured party's counsel could determine what the nurse had originally written.

For the same reason, charts should never be destroyed or recopied, for the question is always asked about what it was that the nurse was trying to hide. Additionally, records should not be altered if the nurse knows that a lawsuit is pending. The attorney for the patient already has a copy of the record, and additions or changes will not be on his or her copy. Thus, the attorney for the patient will introduce that a new version of the chart has been made.

Physicians do not have the right to demand that nurses alter records, nor may physicians alter nurses notes. In *Henry v. St. John's Hospital* (1987), a patient in active labor was administered 6 cc of Marcaine intramuscularly in each hip by the resident, and the nurse recorded the drug, dosage, and person administering the medication in the nursing notes. After the neonate was born with fetal distress, the resident went back and amended the dosage to a lesser amount. The court found against the resident and defendant hospital.

Attorneys for injured patients examine charts for evidence that later materials have been included or that there has been a total substitution of a part of the record. Examples of such alterations include:

1. Writing crowded around existing entries.
2. Changes in slant, pressure, uniformity, or other differences in handwriting.
3. Use of different pens or typewriters to write a single entry.
4. Additions of different dates written in the same ink, while original entries were written in a separate but consistent ink.
5. Differences between pages as to folds, stains, offsets, holes, tears, and type of paper used.
6. Use of forms not in use at the purported time of entry.
7. Use of later years (1996 for 1995), especially if corrected (Nygaard and Deubner, 1988).

A different color of ink was the clue that the record had been altered in *Rotan v. Greenbaum* (1959). The plaintiff died from an allergic reaction to penicillin, which had been ordered during treatment for mumps. The record indicated that the penicillin was given "for mumps and pharyngitis." However, the words "and pharyngitis" were written in a different color of ink, clearly because penicillin would be an appropriate treatment for pharyngitis but not an appropriate therapy for mumps.

Above all, the record must be readable and charted in ink. One of the primary purposes of charting is to communicate with other health care workers about the patient's condition, response to therapies, and progress. If nurses cannot write clearly and their writing cannot be read, then they should print the entry. There is no communication if the primary entry maker is unable to read the entry.

Writing should be legible and only standard, institution-approved abbreviations used. If nurses have difficulty remembering an abbreviation or frequently confuse the abbreviation among several meanings, they should not use it. It is far better to spell out an entry than to be unable to explain the abbreviation to the jury. Counsel for the injured party frequently review the records with the author during deposition, insisting that each illegible word and comment be explained.

Nurses' notes should be organized and written as neatly as possible. Although writing sloppy notes has no bearing on the quality of care delivered, opposing attorneys will make the observation if the nurse is disorganized and sloppy in charting, then he or she is most likely disorganized and sloppy in the delivery of nursing care. Many jurors will accept these statements as true and find against the health care provider and for the injured patient.

Since documentation is done to communicate to other health care deliverers the status of the patient, never invent new abbreviations that have meaning to only one or two persons or to one nursing unit in the hospital. Such self-coined abbreviations hinder rather than assist the communication process. A second and equally valid reason not to coin new abbreviations is that the nurse is likely not to remember what the abbreviation meant when asked by opposing counsel. It is difficult to show quality, competent care when the primary nurse is unable to ascertain what happened to the patient.

Perhaps the best reason not to use self-coined abbreviations is how they appear to the patient or what they signify. In a 1990 case, the family had been concerned about the quality of health care delivery during the elderly patient's hospital stay. The family brought suit, especially after they discovered the "PBBB" notation in the physician's progress note stood for "pine box by bedside." The case settled before going to court (Mangels, 1990).

Never Alter a Record at Someone Else's Request

Never alter a record at someone else's request, even if the request seems harmless. Seasoned malpractice or personal injury attorneys will be able to see that the record has been altered, alerting them that something irregular has happened. At trial, the attorney may well use this irregularity to bolster the case. This brings into question both your credibility and behavior for the judge and jury. Deliberately altering a medical record could also be grounds for disciplinary action by the state board of nursing.

Identify Yourself After Every Entry

At the conclusion of all entries, nurses identify themselves by full name and title. This is true whether or not the nurse has been previously identified. Some institutions allow the nurse to use initials at the conclusion of a page entry if the nurse has signed the bottom portion of the page where all personnel charting are identified by name and status.

Use Standardized Checklists or Flow Sheets

To prevent routine care from being omitted from the chart and to ensure that frequent observations are both performed and charted, many hospitals have adopted graphic sheets or flow sheets. Even checking that patients have received take-home instruction sheets is significant in preventing subsequent liability (*Roberts v. Sisters of St. Francis*, 1990). These simple checklist approaches to charting are legally valid and prevent the need for long chart entries. This method also seems to prevent some of the shorthand charting that left large gaps in the chart.

Leave No Room for Liability

One last point to remember is that the nurse should chart on all lines in sequence and should ensure that additional entries cannot be squeezed in later. Blank spaces allow others to enter information over the previous nurse's signature, in which case the previous nurse may then be legally liable for the entry.

GUIDELINES: CHARTING (WHAT SHOULD THE RECORD CONTAIN?)

1. All the information that is necessary to communicate the patient's progress:
   a. Initial assessment data
   b. Description of actual and/or potential problems
   c. Record of all procedures, treatments, medications, and care
   d. Record of health teaching
   e. Description of patient reactions to treatments, procedures, medications, and teaching
   f. Record of actions taken and persons contacted
2. Information presented in a form that communicates the patient's progress:
   a. Notes made at the time of or immediately following the event recorded, with correct time and date
   b. Notes written and properly signed by the person doing or observing the event being recorded
   c. Notes made in chronological order
   d. Notes free of omissions, personal opinions, generalizations, and ambiguous abbreviations
   e. Notes that are concise, precise, spelled correctly, accurate, and unambiguous
   f. Notes that are legible and neat
   g. Notes that have no unused spaces or blank lines
3. Information that is recorded from a legal perspective:
   a. Record the obvious: Record what you actually saw, did, or communicated to another.
   b. Do not allow inaccuracies to be charted: Record what actually happened, even if you wish you had done something differently.
   c. Do not obliterate an entry: Draw a single line through an error, mark it "mistaken entry," and sign it using your first initial, last name, and correct title.
   d. Do not destroy parts of the record: Follow the same advice as for obliteration of an entry.
   e. Describe events and behaviors: Do not use labels or medical terms you are unsure of in charting.
   f. Document all communications to others and any intermediary steps taken; if you question an order, document that you recontacted the physician and clarified the order.
   g. Record all routine assessments and nursing care; help develop a flow sheet for more accurate records if needed.

■ EXERCISE 9–1

For your last two patients (or any two patients), compare the nursing notes against the guidelines presented in this chapter. Can they be written more completely to adhere to the guidelines? If the answer is yes, do so. Has this exercise changed your opinion of the importance of nursing documentation? Explain your answer.

COMPUTERIZED CHARTING

Many institutions have now adopted, either in part or in whole, *computerized charting*. The use of computers increases accurate recording of facts and allows for prompt charting, particularly when bedside computers are used. Nursing information systems (NIS) allow for accuracy at all stages of the nursing process, from assessment to evaluation. In fact, some systems prompt the nurse if a portion of the nursing process is omitted. Perhaps one of the more important reasons for computers in hospitals is the improved patient care that results with computers. Necessary test and laboratory results are instantly available, medication errors are reduced, and problems with charting, such as illegible writing, misspellings, unapproved abbreviations, and time needed for writing entries, are eliminated by computers.

Issues of concern with using computers for hospital records usually focus on privacy and confidentiality rights of the patient. With a properly designed and implemented computer program, there can be more security than in current, more traditional charting procedures. Security is enhanced because:

1. There are fewer points of access into the system.
2. Each person's access can be restricted to a limited scope of information, with only those portions of the records that are relevant for one's functioning being accessible. The person can be "locked out" if violations occur.
3. The information sought through individual access codes can be monitored, making misuse easier to detect.
4. Passwords are changed on a regular basis.
5. Access to the system is terminated when the employee resigns employment status.
6. Confidentiality statements are signed by users to acknowledge their awareness of legal and institution requirements for usage.

The desire for privacy and confidentiality is well founded. In 1991, then President Bush announced that work had begun on a uniform national health insurance billing system. Every individual with health insurance would receive a computer-encoded health care "smart card" that could be used to electronically access a central database containing the person's insurance information and medical records. Although not yet a reality, work continues on such a system within the Health and Human Services Department of the federal government.

An early Supreme Court case addressed medical information privacy. *Whalen v. Roe* (1977) determined that a New York State database of lawful users of abusable medications was allowable, because the prohibitions on public disclosure of the information in the database were adequate to prevent any constitutional harms to the persons listed in the database. The court considered all provisions that were in place to protect the database. The stringent physician and administrative procedures protecting the patient's interest in privacy also played a part in the court's ultimate ruling. Interestingly, the court did not address whether compilation of the information was itself a violation of privacy, nor did they question whether there were adequate security measures present.

There are some privacy measures in effect, primarily because the U.S. Constitution contains certain privacy rights. The Privacy Act of 1974 prevents the federal government from collecting private information for one purpose and then using it for another purpose (5 U.S.C., Section 552a, 1974). The Computer Fraud and Abuse Act of 1986 defines a federal fraud offense as an offense for the alteration, damage, or destruction of information contained in a federal interest computer. The act made it a crime to traffic in computer passwords, and declared that tampering with computerized medical records warrants punishment without a showing of monetary loss or any showing of incorrect or harmful treatment (42 U.S.C., Section 290dd-3, 1988).

An issue that still remains concerns the machines themselves. Computer-based records can be altered, destroyed, or rendered inaccessible by computer viruses or other acts of sabotage. Technology changes can render a record storage system obsolete long before the need for the records stored in them has ended. Thus, hospitals may need to find new ways of storing records so that they remain retrievable.

CHARTING BY EXCEPTION

This abbreviated system of charting radically differs from the more traditional methods of charting. *Charting by exception* requires documentation of only significant or abnormal findings, and previously entered standardized or expected results are not entered into the chart. The charting by exception format uses preprinted guidelines, such as nursing diagnosis-based standardized care plans and protocols, flow sheets, and graphic records to show the progress or lack of progress of the patient. Bedside charting is increased, so that there is immediate access to patient data by health care workers. Charting by exception streamlines documentation by combining three essential elements:

1. Standards of nursing care
2. Flow sheets
3. Bedside access to chart forms

Institutions can personalize charting by exception to fit their own needs. For example, they can use only the preprinted guidelines, or allow for individualization of patient care within the preprinted guidelines. To be successfully used, though, the institution must establish standards that are uniformly used by all health care personnel and establish what are normal findings and expected outcomes so that all significant data are considered when assessing patient outcomes.

Charting by exception is not without some legal perils. Charting by exception may fail to provide enough information to alert practitioners to potential problems. For example, in *Lama v. Borras* (1994), the patient underwent surgery for a herniated disk. Two days later, there was an entry noting that the surgical dressing was "very bloody," and pain at the site of the incision was noted on the following day. By the fourth day postoperatively, the surgical dressing was again "soiled," and severe incisional pain was noted on the fifth day postoperatively. On the sixth day after surgery, the physician diagnosed diskitis and began antibiotic therapy.

Review of the patient's chart failed to show what happened during the time that the patient's dressing became bloody and he experienced increasing pain. Vital signs and medications are charted, but important details such as the status of the incision and duration and intensity of pain were not charted. Lacking, too, are possible nursing and medical interventions that accompanied the changing surgical drainage and pain or any communications that occurred between the nursing and medical staffs.

The jury in this case concluded that more complete charting could have answered questions that charting by exception failed to answer. The jury also concluded that the infection might have been diagnosed sooner if more traditional charting methods had been followed. "Intermittent charting failed to provide the sort of continuous danger signals that would be the most likely to spur early intervention by a physician" was the final holding of this court (at 278). The court further found that this type of charting failed to meet the regulations of the Puerto Rico Department of Health, which requires that qualitative nurses' notes be recorded for each patient by each nursing shift.

Charting by exception may make it impossible to show the attentiveness of the nursing staff to patients, particularly patients in whom complications develop. Charting by exception may not assist nurses in being able to defend themselves, because even they cannot recreate what was done and not done for an individual patient. Remember that it may be two years before the nurse knows that a lawsuit is filed.

ALTERATION OF RECORDS

Essentially two types of *alterations of records* may be necessary to ensure a truthful, accurate record. The first concerns *minor errors,* such as those that occur in spelling, notations of laboratory data, incorrect phraseology, and the like. These types of errors are usually corrected by the person making the entry at the time of the entry or shortly after the entry was made. The error should be marked through with a single line and the correct information entered, timed, dated, and signed. Incorrect entries should never be erased or obliterated, because such actions raise suspicion in the jurors' minds.

The second type of alteration concerns *substantive errors,* such as incorrect test data, omitted progress notes, incorrect orders, and the like. Only administrative staff or the primary physician should correct such substantive errors, and all persons misled by the error should be contacted and advised of the correct information. Correction for these types of errors include the addition of new materials with the explanation of why they were necessitated, who made the addition, the date, and the time.

An addendum to the record by a physician or other health care provider should not be seen as proof of an error. Occasionally, an addendum may be written based on new information that was just received. However, because a patient's record should reflect as closely as possible concurrent treatment and observation, adding information at a later date is unusual. The further away in time the charting occurs, the more suspicious a reviewer can be about the provider's purpose.

Patients may wish to correct or modify an entry in the medical record. Usually, the patient is permitted to add to the original chart a letter of explanation regarding the modification or addition. Staff agreeing with the letter of modification or addition may also add their own letters of support. This approach preserves the original document while clarifying the source and nature of the change.

RETENTION OF RECORDS

Health care facilities have a responsibility to maintain and protect patient records (*Fox v. Cohen,* 1980). This obligation, **retention of records,** is codified in state statutes that impose a clear duty on facilities not to lose or destroy records within certain time frames. The time frame usually coincides with state statutes of limitations for medical negligent causes of action.

Record retention varies according to state law, with the majority of states preserving the record for the period of time in which suits may be filed (state statutes of limitations) or for five years, whichever time interval is the longest. As a practical matter, most institutions save records for longer periods of time.

The impact of lost medical records can be devastating to meeting the burden of proof. If records are lost, are incomplete, or have disappeared, there is a tendency by the court to presume negligence, and juries have no difficulty finding for the injured party. Known as *omnia praesumuntur contra spoliatorem* (all things are presumed against a despoiler), courts have allowed such disappearances and lack of records to suggest a presumption of guilt. In *May v. Moore* (1982), the Alabama Supreme Court held that even testimony about a physician's lost records (and this physician had a record of losing charts when there was a bad outcome) was admissible and was sufficient to create an inference of negligent treatment.

A more recent case has defined the four elements that are required before the plaintiff can prevail in a lawsuit when spoilage is a factor. In *Proske v. St. Barnabas Medical Center* (1998), the patient sued her physician for failure to diagnose her breast cancer more quickly. The patient's hospital records contained all her mammography reports, and the earlier reports contained indeterminable findings or concluded there were calcifications present that appeared benign. The court was unable to decide either for or against the plaintiff because all of her mammography films had disappeared. The plaintiff then added allegations against the hospital where the films had been taken. These additional allegations were for spoilage of the evidence.

The Superior Court of New Jersey ruled in favor of the hospital on the patient's allegations of spoilage. The films, they said, were innocently misplaced while being removed for storage at a remote location by an outside medical records services vendor. There was no proof of actual intent to tamper with or to destroy the evidence. The court would have ruled for the plaintiff if there had been evidence of deliberate tampering with the evidence.

The court ruled that a patient can sue a health care provider for spoilage of the evidence when:

1. The provider, who may or may not be a defendant or potential defendant, knows malpractice litigation is pending or probable.
2. The provider intentionally tampers with or destroys evidence to try to disrupt the patient's legal case.
3. The patient's malpractice case is compromised.
4. The patient suffers a monetary loss.

Because the patient could not prove these four elements, the court ruled for the defendant.

Destruction of medical records may be performed to protect confidentiality, and destruction should be complete. Should a patient request the destruction of his or her medical record prior to the retention interval lapsing, many courts favor sealing the record over total destruction. Sealing preserves the record while preventing its discovery.

OWNERSHIP OF THE RECORD

Because the chart is the business record of the institution, the hospital is the rightful owner of the entire record. Correspondingly, the individual physician owns the chart records of patients seen in the physician's office. Courts have recognized this right of hospital ownership by declaring that since hospital records are essential to proper administration, hospital records become the property of the hospital.

This ownership right of hospitals to their business records does not preclude the patients' property rights in the same records. The patient generally has the right to all the information contained within the record and to a copy of the original record. The hospital may charge the patient a reasonable fee for the copy of the record. Some exceptions are made for certain psychiatric records, and state law may forbid the patient access to some psychiatric records.

A recent case defined patients' and providers' rights and responsibilities as they pertain to the medical record (*Cornelio v. Stamford Hospital*, 1998). According to the court, the law allows a patient, a patient's physician, or a patient's legal representative to examine any and all materials contained in the patient's medical record. This includes original pathology specimens, pathology slides, x-ray films, lab specimens, physicians' notes, reports, correspondence, bills, insurance forms, and the like. The patient does not have to first file a lawsuit against the health care provider to be entitled to access the materials contained in the patient's medical record. A patient or patient's representative seeking access to a patient's health care record does not have to have a subpoena or even a reason for desiring access to the chart.

Copy expenses for materials that can be copied are the patient's or patient's representative's responsibility. Patients may have the right to copies of the medical records they need in order to pursue disability or industrial insurance claims at a reduced cost or at no cost. Providers must consult their own attorneys to make themselves aware of how their state laws cover this special circumstance. Using an outside photocopy vendor, rather than making copies of the patient's chart in-house, is not a violation of a patient's right to medical confidentiality.

Certain materials cannot be copied, but the patent still had rights of access to examine them, as in the case of pathology slides. The originals stay in the custody of the health care provider. Once pathology specimens or smear slides are obtained by the health care provider, they are no longer part of the patient's personal property, but remain with the health care provider. Even though the patient may have a copy of medical records, health care providers are still required by law to keep the original records and pathology materials.

The court noted that the right to access and the right to copy materials that can be copied are two separate or independent rights. The patient has the right to come to the health care facility and view the original, not be placated with copies. When the patient or representative comes to view the chart, the person can be seated in a designated area and closely supervised while in possession of the chart. The hospital should make available x-ray viewers and microscopes for examination of the originals.

ACCESS TO MEDICAL RECORDS

Besides a legal right to the record, there are some practical reasons for allowing the *patient access to medical records.* Allowing patients access to their medical records helps to dispel feelings that the physician was lying about the severity of the illnesses or that the physician was unsympathetic to their illnesses. Allowing access helps reassure patients that their care was based on actual medical findings.

Most states require that the record be completed prior to the patient's right of access, and statutes have been enacted to establish procedures for such patient access. For example, the policy may provide that access be between the hours of 9 A.M. and 5 P.M. Monday through Friday and only when a hospital representative is present to answer questions. It is also generally recognized that the competent patient can authorize this right of access to others. These others include insurance carriers, legal representation, and outside professionals acting on behalf of the patient.

One of the problems concerning access of patients to their medical records arises when patients are incompetent, minors, or die prior to exercising their right. In such instances, others may be able to authorize access to a patient record. As a general rule, a guardian of an incompetent patient stands in the place of the patient and can authorize access. If there is no court-appointed guardian, hospitals may rely on the authorization of the next of kin or the person responsible for authorization and payment of the medical treatment. Access may be refused if family confidences or information about other than the patient would be needlessly disclosed through access to a mentally incompetent patient's medical record. *McDonald v. Clinger* (1982) denied access of a patient record to a spouse with a showing that such disclosure would cause a danger to the patient, spouse, or other person.

Access to charts of minors also presents a recurring problem, especially in the event of treatment for sexually transmitted diseases, pregnancy, or substance abuse. As a rule, if minors are authorized under state law to consent to their own care, then parents will not have a right of access to the record. Additionally, payment of care may help to decide access questions. If minors, even mature minors, rely on their parents for payment of care, then the parents may have right of access to the record or of disclosure from the primary health care provider.

In the event of a patient's death, the next of kin or the executor of the estate may authorize access to the record. If the spouse has predeceased the patient, it would be advisable to obtain the authorization of all adult children rather than rely on the authorization of only one of the adult children.

Access may be gained to a patient record by law. Examples of *access by law* include subpoenas of records of a party if the party's mental or physical condition is relevant to the lawsuit, subpoenas of records for suspected billing fraud by the health care provider, and when there is a statutory duty of disclosure.

In *Florida Department of Health and Rehabilitative Services v. V. M. R., Inc* (1991), a warrant was issued allowing the Florida Department of Health and Rehabilitative Services to enter a women's medical center and inspect the clinic's premises and records. The clinic and two patients moved to quash the warrant, claiming that the medical records could not be released without written authorization from patients. The court agreed and noted that, although there may be an exception to the privacy provisions in limited circumstances, no such exception had been accorded this agency. Additionally, the court found that the agency's right to examine records did not extend to such personal information as a patient's name, address, and medical history. The impact of such decisions respects the state's authority to regulate, but the power does not allow a governmental agency to make public private medical records.

A second major area of concern with access problems is the patient's right to privacy and confidentiality. Such privacy rights encourage candor by the patient and optimize proper medical treatment and diagnosis. Privacy rights also allow nurses to be truthful and open in their assessments and recording of patient care. For example, in *Head v. Colloton* (1983), the Iowa Supreme Court held that the records of a potential donor for a bone marrow transplant were hospital records and, as such, were exempt from release as public records under the state's freedom of information law.

In general, health care providers involved in the direct care of the patient have access to the record, and records should be housed where they will be the most accessible for patient care providers. This encourages prompt recording as well as quality patient care. Administrators and hospital staff members have access for auditing, billing, quality assurance purposes, and defending potential claims.

Exceptions to the preceding statement include substance abuse treatment or substance abuse treatment records. In *Lugar v. Baton Rouge General Medical Center* (1997), a man who had previously been treated for alcohol abuse applied for life insurance from the same company with whom he was working as an insurance agent. He indicated that he had never received alcohol treatment or been arrested for alcohol abuse.

In doing the background check, the company knew the man had been treated at a certain hospital, but did not know for what he had been treated. The insurance company asked the man to sign a release for medical records. The hospital released his confidential medical records to the insurance company. The records showed that he had sought treatment and had been admitted for a long history of alcohol abuse. He lost his job with the insurance company and brought suit against the hospital for breach of medical confidentiality.

Under state and federal law, a general release for medical records does not authorize the provider to divulge the fact of substance abuse treatment or substance abuse treatment records. That requires a written release, signed by the patient, that specifically applies to such information and records. Unfortunately, the man had signed such a release when he signed the insurance company's legal release form.

Researchers may also have access to medical records. Staff members and qualified students generally may review charts for research purposes without prior patient consent. An internal or external review panel to protect the rights of human subjects is required prior to allowing researchers access to medical records if the institution receives federal funding.

INCIDENT REPORTS

Incident, variance, situational, or unusual occurrence report forms were originally designed to be part of the overall risk management or quality assurance effort of any health-oriented institution. JCAHO standards dictate the establishment of an incident reporting system (1999), with the main function of incident reports being the review and evaluation of patient care. If one uses the definition of an incident to be an unfavorable deviation of expectations involving patient care that may be the result of medical management, it is easy to see that incident reports were devised to augment and improve the quality of patient care. Other obvious uses of such forms are to enhance the hospital's in-service educational offerings, to alert hospital administrative staff to potential problem areas, to minimize injuries from the incident, and to decrease the likelihood of similar incidents in the future.

Incident reports may serve to aid the hospital attorney in planning defense strategy and in deciding whether a case should be litigated or settled out of court. The hospital's liability carrier frequently asks for such reports when investigating claims. Because of their confidential status in most states, nurses traditionally have been instructed to be candid in their remarks on incident reports so that the quality of care can be upgraded.

The root of the confidential nature of incident reports lies in a hospital or business record privileged communication doctrine. Although not a common law right, hospitals have long declined to divulge such reports, arguing that disclosure would make the incident report virtually useless.

In today's legal atmosphere, more and more justices are ruling that plaintiffs, through their attorneys, do have a right to discover incident reports. Declaring that plaintiffs still must show the need for their right to incident reports, several cases have allowed such discovery.

Nurses must exercise caution in completing such reports and should always fill out the forms as though they are discoverable. No language that admits liability should be included, and there should be no mention of the incident report form's having been completed in the patient's chart. Indicating that there is an incident report *incorporates by reference* the incident report into the chart and makes it as discoverable as the original patient chart. The ideal incident report is a checkoff list, with a limited area for a brief, written description of the occurrence.

 ## GUIDELINES: INCIDENT REPORTS

1. The incident report should be initiated by the one who directly observes the incident or by the first person to arrive at the site of the incident.
2. Incorporate the patient's account of the happening into the incident report and state his or her comments as direct quotes. If the patient is unable to give an account, describe exactly what you witnessed or discovered. For example, "the patient fell out of bed" is appropriate if you actually saw the fall. Statements such as "Patient found on floor at foot of bed" or "Patient states, 'I was trying to get up and lost my balance'" are more appropriate if you were the first person to discover the patient on the floor.
3. Write only the facts. Do not infer assumptions or draw conclusions. Do not add what you would like to have done after the fact. Above all, never imply liability. A question such as, "How could this incident have been prevented?" should be left unanswered or answered in the negative.
4. Have other witnesses assist you in preparing the report and have them cosign the final report.
5. If appropriate, have the patient or injured party seen by a physician and document any actions taken and treatment given.
6. Avoid writing in the medical record that an incident report was completed or else it will become incorporated by reference into the total patient chart. Document what happened and the actions taken if the incident report involved a hospitalized patient.
7. Forward the report to nursing service, the hospital attorney, the quality assurance committee, and anyone else so designated by hospital policy.
8. Ensure that only one copy of the report exists. If other departments or committees would like to see the report, the original may be forwarded to them in succession.
9. Should your hospital require multiple copies of incident reports, initiate action to reduce the number of copies to one.

It is also advisable to abandon multiple copies of the form because such copies tend to deny a privileged communication. For an incident report to be considered privileged under the attorney–client privilege, it ideally will be completed and forwarded directly to the hospital attorney or the in-house representative.

■ **EXERCISE 9–2**

Acquire a copy of your facility's incident or variance report form. Does the form adhere to guidelines suggested in this chapter? If it does, explain how it adheres to these guidelines. If not, explain areas that are in conflict with the materials presented. Now design a form that could be substituted for the form you are currently using.

FAXING OF MEDICAL RECORDS

Using fax machines to send health information is another way to ensure that material is received promptly and accurately. Difficulty arises in assuring the *patient's right to privacy.* The JCAHO requires that facilities have safeguards in place that protect the security and confidentiality of computerized and paper-based records (1999). Thus, medical information should be faxed only if urgently needed and must be accompanied by a signed release form. A cover sheet indicating the confidentiality of the material and to whom it is to be given should accompany all medical faxes. Additionally, fax machines should be located in an area with restricted access.

CONFIDENTIALITY OF MEDICAL RECORDS

The primary reason for *confidentiality of medical records* is to promote candor by patients and health care providers to optimize medical and nursing treatment. The second reason for confidentiality is that violation of that right opens the health care provider to a potential lawsuit. Confidentiality respects patient privacy issues. In *Claim of Gilbert* (1998), the court upheld the firing of an AIDS program coordinator at a community health center for violating her employer's confidentiality policy. The program coordinator had divulged information about a prospective client to a colleague who was not a coworker.

Health Insurance Portability and Accountability Act of 1996

In August 1996, President Clinton signed the Health Insurance Portability and Accountability Act (HIPAA) into law (Public Law 104-191). This act mandates the development of a centralized electronic database containing all health records for every patient in the United States as a means of administrative simplification. Despite the requirement that standards for the electronic exchange of individually identifiable health information be developed, the provision does not mandate a federal policy protecting those records until February 21, 2000. Although this data bank would help further medical research and potentially cut millions of dollars in health care costs, it creates serious privacy concerns when vast amounts of personal information are collected and stored in a data bank.

The act is sweeping legislation that provides for:

1. The portability of health care coverage.
2. An antifraud and abuse program.
3. The streamlining of the transfer of patient information between insurers and providers.
4. Tax incentives toward the acquisition of health insurance and accelerated benefits.
5. The establishment of the federal government as a national health care regulator.

Title II of the act mandates the creation of a central electronic database for the transmission of health care information among health care providers, insurers, government, and health plans. The current law does not require consent from patients to have their medical records included in the data bank.

Presently, federal law does not protect patient confidentiality in medical records. Protection is given through limited federal law and a patchwork of state laws, varying in degrees of protection. Under this act, it will become the responsibility of the secretary of the Department of Health and Human Services to promulgate comprehensive standards to facilitate the transmission of medical data, administrative records, and financial records.

Although the advantages of the HIPAA are enormous, confidentiality concerns prevail as medical information will be on computer networks that can easily be accessed, copied, and distributed. Safeguards can be implemented, including coding, encryption, and voice activation, but many fear that these safeguards will easily be eliminated with the "click of a hacker's mouse" (Sweeney, 1997). At the same time, the amount of information kept by health care providers on their patients is ever increasing, due to requirements made by managed care organizations and employers offering self-funded health insurance programs for their employees.

On September 11, 1997, Secretary Shalala submitted to Congress her recommendations, entitled *Confidentiality of Individually Identified Health Information*. These recommendations include the following:

1. Hospitals, insurers, doctors, and other organizations with health information must protect against deliberate or inadvertent misuse or disclosure. The information must be secured against improper use by employees and outsiders.
2. Health care providers and insurers must give patients a written explanation of how they will use, keep, and disclose medical records. Patients could get copies of those records and propose corrections. Providers and payors would have to maintain a history of disclosures.
3. Criminal penalties, including fines and imprisonment, for obtaining health information under false pretenses and for knowingly disclosing or using medical information in violation of the federal privacy law.
4. Any individual whose rights under the law have been violated, whether negligently or knowingly, should be permitted to bring an action for actual damages and equitable relief. For knowing violations, attorney's fees and punitive damages should also be available.

Regardless of the final provisions that are ultimately implemented, the HIPAA provides only floor protection. State laws can still provide greater protections, and it is anticipated that states will pass a variety of other laws to further protect the patient's rights to privacy and confidentiality.

Electronic Mail and the Internet

The age of information presents some unique challenges. The increasing use of electronic mail (e-mail) via the Internet is an area of potential liability for health care providers. Communicating patient care in a paper world is fraught with potential for wrongful disclosures. Although there are safety measures that can be used with e-mail, such as encryption or an electronic "lock and key" system, it is not perfect. Messages are "locked" by the sender, making the message unreadable except by the intended recipient, who has a "key" or electronic password to decrypt the message. Thus, there is some measure of privacy. The danger lies in the possibility of an unauthorized decrypt of the message, much like the "hacker" in computer systems.

Similar issues arise with Internet messages, because there is no greater security when Internet communication is in transit over phone lines than there is with an ordinary phone call. Messages can be intercepted and read as they pass through routers. Although federal laws give some protection in the area, privacy issues for messages sent via Internet remain a hotly debated topic.

REPORTING AND ACCESS LAWS

The law compels disclosure of medical information in contexts other than discovery or testimony. Reporting laws require that information be given to governmental agencies, both federal and state. Examples include vital statistics, child abuse, elder abuse, public health, and wounds.

Some statutes do not mandate reporting but allow access to medical records without the patient's permission. Examples of such access laws include workers' compensation, state public records laws, and federal freedom of information act.

COMMON LAW DUTY TO DISCLOSE

The *common law duty to disclose* recognizes a duty to disclose medical information in limited circumstances. Persons who could have avoided injury if information were disclosed have filed successful lawsuits against those with a duty to disclose.

Contagious Diseases

With contagious diseases, there is a duty to warn others at risk of exposure unless forbidden by statute. This includes family members and health care providers, as well as others at risk. In most states, there is no duty to warn all members of the public individually, but states vary on this requirement. For example, the State Supreme Court in South Carolina has held that a hospital could be held liable for the death of a patient from meningitis. The child's friend had been diagnosed and treated for meningitis at Oconee Memorial Hospital, and the hospital failed to notify persons who had had contact with the child during the contagious period (*Phillips v. Oconee Memorial Hospital,* 1986).

Threats to an Identified Person

Some courts have ruled that there is a duty to warn identified persons when a patient has made a credible threat against them. The first decision to affect this duty was *Tarasoff v. Board of Regents of the University of California* (1976). In that case, a nonhospitalized psychiatric patient told his psychiatrist that he would kill his former girlfriend. The threat to kill was made more than once, and there was no doubt in the psychiatrist's mind that the patient could make good his threat. After Tarasoff was killed, her parents brought this lawsuit for wrongful death, and the court concluded that the psychiatrist or his employer did have a duty to either warn the potential victim or to warn others who could have advised the victim of her potential danger. In a later decision, *Thompson v. County of Alameda* (1980), the same court clarified the scope of this duty to warn by ruling that only threats to readily identifiable persons created a duty to warn, and there is no corresponding duty to the public at large.

Courts have slowly applied the duty to warn principle, and most courts are now holding that there is a duty to warn identifiable individuals. For example, in *State v. Bright* (1996), the court ruled that it is not a breach of medical confidentiality for a health care professional to warn a potential victim of a patient's dangerous propensities. "Courts around the United States are not just overlooking the traditional definition of medical confidentiality to protect potential victims, but are imposing an affirmative duty on psychiatrists, psychologists, therapists, and other mental health workers, in inpatient and outpatient settings, to warn identifiable victims when patients make threats toward them" (at 1057).

In *Bright*, an armed forces veteran was receiving outpatient therapy for chronic alcohol abuse. Over the past 20 years, he had been considered bipolar. It was known to his therapist that he had killed his brother some years before but was found not guilty by reason of insanity. During the course of the therapy, the patient repeatedly voiced an intention to kill his ex-wife. The ex-wife had left the state and was living in hiding because of the patient's harassment, intimidation, and threatening conduct.

Finally, the patient stated that he was leaving town that evening to find his ex-wife and kill her. The therapist called the local police and the police in the county where the ex-wife lived. Working together, the two police agencies apprehended the man, one and one-half miles from the intended victim's residence. The patient had with him a newly purchased hunting knife and a roll of duct tape in his trunk. He was charged with making terrorist threats and attempted murder. The court had nothing but praise for the therapist's actions.

There is a beginning trend to extend this duty to warn to the general public. For example, in *Kathleen K. v. Robert B.* (1984), the court allowed a woman to sue her sexual partner for deliberate and/or negligent failure to warn her that he had genital herpes. A more recent case, *Reisner v. Regents of the University of California* (1995), held that a man who discovered in 1990 that he had contracted the acquired immune deficiency syndrome (AIDS) virus from his girlfriend may sue a physician for failing to inform her she had received contaminated blood in 1985.

A further trend in the duty to warn concerns genetic diseases. The court in *Safer v. Pack* (1996) held that the physician has a duty to warn individuals, including the patient's immediate family members, who are at risk of avoidable harm from a genetically transmitted condition. This holding was based on the premise that a genetically transmissible condition is sufficiently similar to a contagious disease.

Robert Batkin, the father of plaintiff Donna Safer, was diagnosed in 1956 with multiple polyposis and colorectal cancer. Despite Dr. Pack's efforts to excise the cancer, Mr. Batkin died of metastatic disease in 1964. In 1990, Safer, then 36 years old, was diagnosed with a cancerous blockage of the colon and multiple polyposis. After undergoing a colectomy with ileorectal anastomosis, it was discovered that the cancer extended beyond her bowel. The finding of the additional metastases led to removal of her left ovary and a regimen of chemotherapy.

In 1991, Ms. Safer obtained her father's medical records. They revealed that he had suffered from multiple polyposis, which she claimed is a hereditary disease leading to colorectal cancer. She filed a complaint alleging that Dr. Pack had been professionally negligent by failing to warn her of the risk posed to her health. Safer further contended that the medical standards prevailing at the time required Dr. Pack to inform her of the risk so that she could benefit from early diagnosis and treatment.

The lower court found for Dr. Pack, and Safer appealed. The superior court said:

> We see no impediment, legal or otherwise, to recognizing a physician's duty to warn those known to be at risk of avoidable harm from a genetically transmissible condition. In terms of foreseeability especially, there is no essential difference between the type of genetic threat at issue here and the menace of infection, contagion, or a threat of physical harm. . . . The individual or group at risk is easily identified, and substantial future harm may be averted or minimized by a timely and effective warning (*Safer v. Pack,* 1996, at 1192).

The superior court then decided that a physician must reasonably attempt to inform those likely to be affected or to make the information available. This duty, the court held, extends beyond the patient to members of the immediate family, who may be adversely affected by the failure to warn. The court did note in their discussion that there may be some confidentiality issues if the father in this case had specifically asked that his family not be informed of his genetically transmissible disease. This latter issue will undoubtedly be adressed by courts in the future.

Some states have passed statutes concerning the duty of a health care provider to warn about potential risks to patients during invasive procedures. New Hampshire has passed a law that health care workers infected with hepatitis B or human immunodeficiency virus (HIV), must disclose this fact to patients before performing invasive, exposure-prone procedures. The law also requires them to notify previous patients for whom they had performed invasive, exposure-prone procedures (1994). A Pennsylvania court, in *Scoles v. Mercy Health Corporation* (1995), was permitted to require an HIV-positive surgeon to prove that he had disclosed his HIV status to prospective patients before performing surgery. The court noted that the nature, severity, and duration of harm overshadowed the physician's claim that the disclosure was in violation of the Americans with Disabilities Act and the Rehabilitation Act of 1973.

LIMITATIONS TO DISCLOSURE

Several statutory and common law limitations on disclosure have evolved that assist in preserving confidentiality and impose sanctions for some violations of confidentiality.

Substance Abuse Confidentiality

Special federal rules deal with confidentiality of information concerning patients treated or referred for treatment for substance abuse. These rules apply to any facility receiving federal funding, including Medicare and Medicaid reimbursement. These rules prevent disclosure, and even acknowledgment of the patients' presence in the facility.

Information may be released with the patient's consent, if the consent is written and contains all of the following elements:

1. The name of the person or program to make the disclosure
2. The name or title of the person or organization to receive the disclosure
3. The name of the patient
4. The purpose of the disclosure
5. How much and what kind of information is to be disclosed
6. The patient's signature
7. Date of signature
8. A statement that the consent may be revoked
9. The date when the consent will automatically expire

A court order, including a subpoena, does not permit release of information unless these eight elements have all been met (42 CFR, 1988).

Child abuse reports may be made under state law without patient consent or court order, but release of records to child abuse agencies must have consent or an order. Staff members must be oriented to these rules. In *Heng v. Foster* (1978), a nurse successfully challenged her dismissal for failure to report a fellow staff member's theft of patient files by establishing the reasonableness of her belief that the federal regulations prohibited the report.

HIV/AIDS Confidentiality

Special characteristics of HIV and AIDS and of the AIDS epidemic present new and unique challenges to health care providers trying to maintain patient confidentiality while meeting their obligations to disclose medical information. First, widespread fear of AIDS and ignorance about its transmission have made concerns of privacy and confidentiality even more important and urgent. If information about a person's AIDS infection or HIV positivity reaches employers, insurers, schools, or friends, it may have disastrous effects. Confidentiality is at the heart of HIV and AIDS testing, for most individuals will not submit to HIV testing and counseling unless there is assurance of confidentiality.

Second, the fact that the transmission of AIDS and HIV is not through close proximity or casual contact limits the need for disclosure of information about infection. This argument can be expounded both as a need not to warn as the rate of infection is somewhere around .0001 per exposure, to an affirmative duty to warn, particularly in the transmission to unborn children.

Third, the fact that AIDS at present is incurable (though medications now exist to give the patient a longer quality life) makes prevention all the more essential. One can use this statement to argue either for strict confidentiality to allow persons to be tested and counseled or for limited confidentiality to protect persons who may be exposed.

States have adopted a variety of legislative and administrative approaches to confidentiality and disclosure of information regarding AIDS and HIV. All 50 states require reporting of AIDS cases, without the patients' consent, to the Centers for Disease Control and Prevention or to the state health department for epidemiological purposes. Twenty-six states require the reporting by name of all people diagnosed with HIV. Two other states, Texas and Connecticut, require the reporting of HIV infection only in children who are less than 13 years of age. Most states allow disclosure to medical personnel who are involved in the patient's treatment, though not necessarily to all caregivers. For example, California permits disclosure only to those providing direct care, and Kentucky permits disclosure only to the patient's treating or personal physician.

The majority of states have adopted statutes maintaining the strict confidentiality of AIDS-related information, including California, Florida, and Massachusetts. Other states have passed statutes permitting disclosure of AIDS testing to certain persons or under certain circumstances, such as Texas (disclosure to spouse permitted), Georgia (disclosure to spouse, sexual partner, or child permitted under limited circumstances), and New York (disclosure permitted if infected person refuses to do so after counseling and warning that the physician will disclose the information if the infected person does not do so).

There is also some limited movement toward mandatory testing for HIV/AIDS. In July 1996, the American Medical Association endorsed the mandatory testing of all pregnant women and newborns. In February 1997, New York became the first state to mandate the screening of all newborns for HIV and the disclosure of the test results to the newborns' mothers. Supporters of the bill argued that early identification and treatment of HIV is saving lives. Research has shown that providing zidovudine prenatally and to newborns significantly reduces the incidence of perinatal transmission (Centers for Disease Control and Prevention, 1994).

A number of states permit the state health department to engage in contact tracing or partner notification. Some states notify all sexual and needle-sharing contacts while others have chosen a more limited means of notifying contacts, such as the contact of all individuals who have received infected blood products. Health care providers are urged to investigate their state statutes in this regard.

Because standards of care are constantly evolving in patients with AIDS, the issues of liability often depend on when the care of the patient actually occurred. For example, in *Doe v. Johnson* (1991), the issue centered on a blood transfusion the patient received in 1985 and whether there was a duty to inform patients about the possibility of contracting AIDS from the blood supply. Since this was not a standard of care at the time of the blood transfusion, the court said that the jury should decide if the blood transfusion was a reasonable treatment alternative at the time the patient underwent surgery.

Almost uniformly, courts have upheld privacy rights when disclosure of test results have been made without the patient's consent (*Doe v. High-Tech Institute, Inc.*, 1998; *Biddle v. Warren General Hospital*, 1998; *Jane Doe v. Marselle*, 1996; and *In re Sealed Case*, 1995).

■ EXERCISE 9–3

You have been appointed to a panel to establish a national standard for nursing documentation. Hopefully, this will assist in preventing future litigation that centers around documentation. What types of uniform charting forms should be developed and why?

Can one form or one set of forms be developed for national usage? List the pros and cons of a national standard for documentation.

Are there ethical principles involved in documentation, especially confidentiality and truthfulness in documentation? From an ethical perspective, would a national standard for documentation more completely protect the ethical principles involved in documentation? Why or why not?

SUMMARY

Medical records ensure that communications concerning individual patients will be available to health care providers, including patients' diagnoses, treatments, procedures, interventions, and response to those treatments, procedures, and interventions. Communications also exist for research, quality assurance, third-party payors, and legal defense. This chapter has outlined the reasons for written communication, explained how to document effectively, and stated general rules concerning when patient data may be disclosed to others.

AFTER COMPLETING THIS CHAPTER, YOU SHOULD BE ABLE TO

- List and explain the five purposes of medical records.
- Define and describe basic information to be included in the medical record.
- List and give examples of 10 guidelines for accurate documentation.
- Analyze the concepts of:
  a. Alteration of records
  b. Retention of records
  c. Ownership of the medical record
  d. Access to medical records
  e. Computerized charting
- Describe four important aspects of incident reports.
- Compare and contrast charting by exception to traditional charting.
- Define confidentiality and relate that concept to:
  a. Substance abuse conferences
  b. AID/HIV conferences
  c. Access laws
  d. Child/elder abuse conferences
  e. Electronic mail and Internet service

APPLY YOUR LEGAL KNOWLEDGE

- How can a staff member ensure confidentiality in clinical settings?
- What makes charting effective, and how can professional nurses ensure that their charting is effective?

- After learning the purposes and guidelines for documentation, how might one design a better chart?
- What safeguards can be used to ensure confidentiality when sending medical information by fax or by electronic mail?

YOU BE THE JUDGE

While being treated at the Albany Memorial Hospital Emergency Center, Ms. Fosby reached for a blanket and felt a sharp pinprick, which she discovered was caused by a needle embedded in her right index finger. She removed the needle and gave it to the nurse, who informed Fosby that she would get a copy of the incident report and that would tell her how the needle had been previously used. Later, the hospital refused to give Fosby the incident report and advised her that she should consider the needle infectious and be tested for HIV at three-, six-, and twelve-month intervals. Fosby followed this advice and, fortunately, tested negative for the HIV antibodies.

Claiming that the hospital's refusal to provide her with information regarding the prior use of the needle and its advice to undergo HIV testing led her to believe that she was at grave risk for developing AIDS, the plaintiff and her husband commenced this "AIDS phobia" cause of action. At trial level, the court allowed a motion for summary judgment in favor of the defendants upon their showing by two expert medical witnesses that the needle was unused, as there was no blood or other hemoglobin present, and thus there was zero probability that HIV could have been transmitted via the needle to Fosby.

Fosby appealed, maintaining that she had a viable cause of action because the records contained sufficient evidence to show that she had a rational basis for contracting AIDS, particularly in light of the hospital's refusal to share the incident report with her and their insistence that she be tested for HIV.

Legal Questions

1. Does this plaintiff have a valid case against the defendant hospital as she asserts in her cause of action?
2. Was there negligence on the part of the hospital?
3. Does the hospital's refusal to share the incident report with the plaintiff have any bearing on the outcome of this case?
4. How would you decide this case?

REFERENCES

Ahrens v. Katz, 595 F. Supp. 1108, (N.D. Ga., 1984).

Biddle v. Warren General Hospital, No. 96-T-5582 (Ohio App., 1998).

California Health and Safety Code, Section 199.21

Centers for Disease Control and Prevention (1994). Recommendations of the U.S. Public Health Service Task Force on the use of zidovudine to reduce the perinatal transmission of human immunodeficiency virus. *MMWR* 43 (RR-11), 1.

Claim of Gilbert, 679 N.Y.S.2d 452 (N.Y. App., 1998).

Computer Fraud and Abuse Act of 1986, 42 U.S.C. Section 290dd-3 (1988).

Cornelio v. Stamford Hospital, 717 A.2d 140 (Connecticut, 1998).

Darling v. Charleston Community Memorial Hospital, 33 Ill.2d 326, 211 N.E.2d 253 (1965), cert. den'd. 383 U.S. 946 (1965).

Doe v. High-Tech Institute, Inc., No. 97CA0385, 1998 WL 379926 (Colo. Ct. App., 1998).

Doe v. Johnson, 476 N.W.2d 28 (Iowa, 1991).

Engle v. Clarke, 346 S.W.2d 13 (Kentucky, 1961).

Florida Department of Health and Rehabilitative Services v. V. M. R., Inc, No. 90-2779, 1991 Fla. App. LEXIS 6122 (July 2, 1991).

Florida Statutes Annotated, Sec 14A, Sec. 381609 (2)(f).

Fox v. Cohen, 406 N.E.2d 178 (Ill. App. Ct., 1980).

42 *CFR,* 1988.

Genao v. State, 679 N.Y.S.2d 539 (New York, 1998).

Griffin v. Methodist Hospital, 948 S.W.2d 72 (Tex. App., 1997).

Head v. Colloton, 331 N.W.2d 870 (Iowa, 1983).

Health Insurance Portability and Accountability Act of 1996, Public Law 104-191 (1996).

Heng v. Foster, 63 Ill. App.3d 30, 379 N.E.2d 688, 19 Ill. Dec. 816 (1st Dis., 1978).

Henry v. St. John's Hospital, 512 N.E.2d 1044 (Illinois, 1987).

Houlton v. Memorial Hospital, 679 N.E.2d 1202 (Illinois, 1997).

In re Sealed Case, 67 F.3d 965 (D.C. Cir., 1995).

Jane Doe v. Marselle, 675 A.2d 835 (Connecticut, 1996).

Joint Commission for the Accreditation of Healthcare Organizations (1999). *Accreditation Manual for Hospitals.* Oakbrook Terrace, IL: Author.

Kathleen K. v. Robert B., 198 Cal. Rptr. 273 (Cal. App., 1984).

Lama v. Borras, 16 F.3d 473 (1st Cir. [PR], 1994).

Landry v. Clement, 711 So.2d 829 (La. App., 1998).

Lugar v. Baton Rouge General Medical Center, 696 So.2d 652 (La. App., 1997).

Massachusetts General Legislative Chapter 111, Section 70f.

Mangels, L. (1990). Chart notes from a malpractice insurer's hell. *Medical Economics,* November 12.

May v. Moore, 424 So.2d 596 (Alabama, 1982).

May v. Jones, 675 So.2d 276 (La. App., 1996).

McDonald v. Clinger, 84 A.D.2d 482, 446 N.Y.S.2d 801 (4th Dept., 1982).

McKinley's *New York Public Health Law,* Section 2782(4)(a) and (b).

Mitsinicos v. New Rochelle Nursing Home, Inc., 685 N.Y.S.2d 758 (N.Y. App., 1999).

Nygaard, D. A., and Deubner, S. J. (1988). Altered or lost medical records. *Trial* 24(6), 6–55.

New Hampshire Rev., Stat. Ann. Section 141-F, 9-b, 1994.

Pellerin v. Humedicenters, Inc., 969 So.2d 590 (La. App., 1997).

Phillips v. Oconee Memorial Hospital, 290 S.C. 192, 348 S.E.2d 836 (South Carolina, 1986).

Privacy Act of 1974, 5 U.S.C. Section 552a (1974).

Proske v. St. Barnabas Medical Center, 712 A.2d 1207 (N.J. Super., 1998).

Regan Report on Nursing Law (1988), 29(6), 1.

Reisner v. Regents of the University of California, 37 Cal. Rptr. 518 (California, 1995).

Roberts v. Sisters of St. Francis, 566 N.E.2d 662 (Illinois, 1990).

Rotan v. Greenbaum, 273 F.2d 830 (D.C.Cir., 1959).

Safer v. Pack, 677 A.2d 1188 (N.J. Super. Ct App. Div., 1996)

Scoles v. Mercy Health Corporation, No. 92-6712 (E.D. Pa., 1995).

Shahine v. Louisiana State University Medical Center, 680 So.2d 1352 (La. App., 1996).

State v. Bright, 683 A.2d 1055 (Del. Super., 1996).

Sweeney, L. (1997). Weaving technology and policy together to maintain confidentiality. *Journal of Law, Medicine, and Ethics* 25(1), 98–110.

Tarasoff v. Board of Regents of the University of California, 17 Cal.3d 425, 551 P.2d 334 (1976).

Thompson v. County of Alameda, 27 Cal.3d 741, 614 P.2d 728 (1980).

Vernon's *Annotated Texas Revised Civil Statutes,* Article 4419b-1, Section 9.03.

Webb v. Tulane Medical Center Hospital, 700 So.2d 1141 (La. App., 1997).

Whalen v. Roe, 429 U.S. 589 (1997).

ten

Professional Liability Insurance

■ PREVIEW

With the advent of the malpractice crisis of the 1970s, health care providers rapidly became acutely aware of the vast scope of potential lawsuits that could be filed against them, either individually or collectively. This malpractice scare served to alert health care providers of their unique vulnerability. Lawsuits could be filed by any health care consumer at almost any time. Physicians quickly acquired and increased their liability coverage. Nurses, like their physician counterparts, should not be without professional liability insurance. This chapter explores issues that nurses should consider and investigate when choosing a policy that will give them the best protection should a subsequent lawsuit be filed against them.

■ KEY CONCEPTS

insurance policy (insuring agreement)	claims-made policies	reservation of rights
policyholder	employer-sponsored coverage	defense costs
professional liability	declarations	covered injuries
occurrence-based policies	limits of liability	supplementary payments
policy period	deductibles	coverage conditions
	exclusions	indemnity

INSURANCE POLICIES

An *insurance policy,* sometimes called an *insuring agreement,* is a formal contract between the insurance carrier and an individual or corporation. For a stated premium (fee per year), the insurance policy will provide the insured party or *policyholder* with a specific dollar amount of protection when certain injuries are caused by the person(s) insured by the policy. The conditions of the coverage and the extent of coverage are detailed in the policy itself.

Regardless of the policy chosen, there are some common elements of all *professional liability* policies. The policies provide payment for a lawyer to represent the insured nurse in the event of a claim or lawsuit. Most insurance carriers insist that the nurse use a lawyer whom the insurance company has on retainer, because this assures both the nurse and the insurance carrier that the selected lawyer will be versed in medical malpractice issues. All policies specify the limits of legal liability. Insurance carriers will pay settlements or jury awards but will not cover the cost of any moral obligations that nurses might feel they owe the injured party.

TYPES OF POLICIES

There are essentially two ways of classifying types of insurance policies. The first way is as either occurrence-based or claims-made insurance coverage. *Occurrence-based policies* cover the nurse for any injuries arising out of incidents that occurred during the time that the policy was in effect, known as the *policy period.* This holds true even if the subsequent lawsuit is filed after the policy has expired and the policy was not renewed by the policyholder. *Claims-made policies* provide coverage only if an injury occurs and the claim is reported to the insurance company during the active policy period or during an uninterrupted extension of that policy period. The uninterrupted extension, or *policy tail*, allows the claims-made policy to be enforced for a specific period of time following the policy period.

The occurrence-based policy is preferable for most nurses because lawsuits may not be filed immediately, particularly in cases involving children and neonates. Claims-made coverage is adequate if the policy is continuously renewed and kept active or if a policy tail is purchased for extended coverage. If there is doubt regarding coverage needed, consult the insurance agent or an attorney.

A second way of classifying types of insurance policies is individual, group, or employer-sponsored coverage. *Individual coverage* is the broadest type of coverage and is specific to the individual policyholder. This type of policy covers the *named policyholder* on a 24-hour basis, as long as actions fall within the scope of professional nursing practice, including both paid services and voluntary services. This type of policy is tailored to meet the needs of the individual nurse. *Group coverage* involves insuring a group of similarly licensed professionals and may be advantageous in some private clinics or businesses. Group coverage is frequently obtained by professional practitioners where all of the insured individuals practice during office hours and have essentially the same job descriptions. *Employer-sponsored coverage,* which is obtained by institutions, is perhaps the narrowest of coverage for individual nurses since they must first show that they are practicing within the scope of their employment as well as within the scope of professional nursing practice. Those covered are called the *insureds,* or they may be legally referred to as "former insureds for acts committed while insured." Employer-sponsored coverage is favored by the institution as the coverage is written specifically for the business and its major concerns.

■ EXERCISE 10–1

Using your own professional clinical area, list arguments for purchasing either occurrence-based or claims-made insurance policies. Determine which coverage would be best for you as an individual policyholder. What type of coverage is most often written within your state? Is this type of coverage adequate for your potential needs?

DECLARATIONS

The first part of the policy is known as the *declarations.* Included under this section are the policyholder's name, address, covered professional occupation (such as general staff nurse, advanced family nurse practitioner, or emergency center staff nurse), and the covered time period. This sections also lists the company's limits of liability coverage and state requirements for information that may modify the policy.

LIMITS AND DEDUCTIBLES

The insurance policy should have a section marked *limits of liability.* This section usually has language about two separate dollar figures. For example, it could read $500,000 each claim, $1,000,000 aggregate, or $1,000,000 each claim, $3,000,000 aggregate. These dollar figures indicate what the insurance company will pay during a given policy period. The insurance company will pay up to the lower limits for any one claim or lawsuit and up to the upper limits of the policy during the entire policy period.

All claims arising from the same incident or occurrence are considered a *single claim* for purposes of the insurance coverage. For example, if a professional nurse inadvertently gave patient A the medications that were ordered for patient B, both patients could file suit for injuries caused by this single medication error. Most insurance companies would consider these two separate lawsuits as a single claim (arising from the same incident) and would pay up to the lower limits of the policy. The upper limit figure or aggregate figure is the total amount that the insurance carrier will pay for all claims made in a calendar year or policy period.

Deductibles include any amounts that the insurance carrier deducts from the total amount available to pay for plaintiff damages. Some policies deduct the amount paid for the nurse's legal defense from the total limits of liability.

ADDITIONAL CLAUSES IN INSURANCE POLICIES

Exclusions are items not covered in the insurance policy. In professional liability policies, such exclusions frequently describe circumstances or activities that will prevent coverage of the insured party. Exclusions also include the absence of appropriate licensure or certification. These exclusions may be covered in the policy under the general title *reservation of rights,* so entitled because the company reserves the right to deny coverage once the facts are known. When and if it is determined that a restricted activity has been involved, then the insured nurse must reimburse the insurance company for incurred expenses of legal defense. Other insurance companies insist that the insured nurse pay all expenses out of pocket until it is shown that an excluded activity has not been involved.

Some of the more common examples of excluded activities involving inappropriate behavior include:

1. Criminal actions.
2. Incidents occurring while the insured was under the influence of either drugs or alcohol.

3. Physical assault, sexual abuse, molestation, habitual neglect, licentious and immoral behavior toward patients whether intentional, negligent, inadvertent, or committed with the belief that the other party was consenting.
4. Actions that result in punitive damages to the plaintiff. This last provision is included because coverage of punitive damages would defeat the purpose of punishing the wrongdoer.
5. Actions that violate state nursing practice acts.

More recent additions to the preceding list include exclusion for the transmission of AIDS/HIV from the health care provider to a patient and exclusions for expanded roles in nursing. Sometimes, this last exclusion is worded as "exclusions for liability incurred in the position of proprietor, superintendent, or executive officer of a clinic, laboratory, or business enterprise."

Exclusions also include any claims or suits resulting from the practice of a profession that does not appear on the certificate's declarations. Nurses should alert their insurance company when there is a change in professional status to ensure that the nurse is fully covered during the policy period.

Terms in the *coverage* section indicate when the insured is actually covered and for what activities. Policies that have fairly broad coverage sections will include language similar to the following: ". . . professional services by the individual insured, or by any persons for whose acts or omissions such insured is legally responsible . . ." will be covered in this policy. Such verbiage indicates that insureds are covered both for their own actions and for actions performed by nurses under their direct and indirect supervision. This coverage is vital for nurses who hold supervisory positions, such as nursing supervisors, charge nurses, and nursing faculty.

Defense costs are included in most policies. These include all reasonable and necessary costs incurred in the investigation, defense, and negotiation of any covered claim or suit. Most companies pay these in addition to the limits of liability. Additionally, if the nurse is required to appear before the state board of nursing or a governmental regulatory agency, the company will pay attorney fees and other costs resulting from investigation or defense of the proceeding, up to $1,000 per policy period. This latter amount is in addition to the coverage limits.

Covered injuries outlines the types of injuries and provisions that the insurance company will honor. Usually, insurance companies include personal (bodily) injury, mental anguish, property damage, personal injury to a patient such as invasion of privacy, libel, and slander, and economic damages as covered injuries. The lawsuit must specifically note that the suit is for monetary damages. In other words, the insurance company will cover the cost of litigation and awards if money damages are involved. The insurance company will not cover the cost of litigation if the action sought is a specific performance as in the instance of a lawsuit brought to prevent a nurse practitioner from performing medical acts. *Sermchief v. Gonzales* (1983) is a good example of such a specific performance lawsuit. See Chapter 12 for details of this case.

Supplementary payments include provisions for additional payments to the insured party. Some policies may supplement lost earnings or reasonable expenses incurred by the insured as well as the cost of appeal bonds and costs of litigation charged against the insured. These latter provisions may also be termed *defense costs*.

Conditions or **coverage conditions** outline the insured nurse's duties to the insurance carrier in the event a claim or lawsuit is filed, provisions for cancellation of the policy, prohibition of assignment of the policy, and subrogation of rights. Many insurance policies will cover policyholders only if they give written notice to the insurance carrier immediately upon the filing of a claim or lawsuit and forward to the insurance carrier every demand, notice, summons, or other process received.

Also in this section are the nurse's right to select counsel and the right to request a settlement. Most policies allow the insurance carrier to settle without the policyholder's consent and deny the policyholder the right to retain counsel apart from the insurance company. As explained under general provisions, most insurance companies prefer to retain attorneys known to have expertise in medical matters, rather than allow the insured the right to obtain attorneys unknown to them.

GUIDELINES: PROFESSIONAL LIABILITY INSURANCE POLICIES

1. Read the policy carefully before purchasing it and ask for explanations as needed. Make sure that the policy will augment an employer-sponsored policy or will adequately protect your interests if you are independently employed.
2. Make sure that the per-claim and aggregate coverage limits are adequate for your specific nursing needs. As a double check, scan your geographic area for the tendency of nurses to be named in lawsuits and the average dollar damages being awarded plaintiffs in lawsuits that name nurses as defendants.
3. Check on any information that relates to malpractice claims in your area. Resources to be explored include the local law library, insurance carriers, health claims arbitration boards, and hospital attorneys.
4. Look to see that the policy gives you optimal coverage. Ideally, it should be occurrence-based coverage and include protection for both your direct professional actions as well as the professional actions of those you supervise. If your area allows only the purchase of claims-made coverage, investigate the availability and cost of a policy tail. Investigate other options that are covered by the policy. Does this policy cover appeal bonds or supplementary benefits? Can you select your own counsel or request a settlement out of court?
5. Understand the exclusions of the policy. Will you still be covered if you accept a job as an independent practitioner? If the exclusions also exclude your job description, as in the instance of advanced practice nurses, investigate additional insurance policies.
6. Be aware that there are areas of nursing practice in which the risk of lawsuits is higher. These areas include, but are not restricted to, critical care areas, home health care, emergency centers, the operating room, and maternal and child health areas. Thus, the need for individual coverage is most acute.
7. Above all, remember that you are a member of a profession with the potential to have lawsuits constantly filed against its members. Do not consider practicing professional nursing without the valuable protection provided by liability insurance.

■ EXERCISE 10–2

Using the sample policy found in Figure 10–1, find the various provisions that were just discussed, including:

1. Limits of liability.
2. Declarations.
3. Deductibles.
4. Exclusions.
5. Reservation of rights.
6. Covered injuries.
7. Defense costs.
8. Coverage conditions and supplementary payments.

Did you have difficulty finding some sections? Would this be a policy that you would consider purchasing for your own liability coverage? Why or why not?

INDIVIDUAL VERSUS EMPLOYER LIABILITY COVERAGE

Should a nurse have individual professional liability coverage or should the nurse rely on the employer's insurance policy in the event of a malpractice action? Many nurses have been assured by hospital administrative staff and by competent lawyers that they can depend on the hospital's insurance policy to cover them in the event of a subsequent legal action. However, the actual truth is that nurses who relied on hospital policies most often were not adequately protected monetarily, nor were they adequately represented by legal counsel in the lawsuit.

There are several reasons for this situation. First, many institutional liability insurance policies have limited coverage and cover employees only while they are performing work as hospital employees. Thus, private-duty nurses and off-duty employees are automatically excluded from coverage. Nurses who volunteer their professional services likewise are not covered. School nurses and community or home health care nurses may not be covered at all in most medical insurance policies, though the newer trend is to protect these nurses in the performance of their employment.

Second, the hospital's policy is designed to meet the needs of the large institution, and hospital attorneys may not be able to protect the individual nurse's best interests. For example, the hospital may elect to settle out of court rather than pursue a particular case, even though the nurse's best interests can be served only through a court hearing. Also, should the hospital wish to bring an indemnity claim against the nurse for the incident that triggered the lawsuit, the hospital policy will not cover the nurse nor will it pay for his or her representation. **Indemnity** claims are those brought by the employer for monetary contributions from the nurse or nurses whose actions or failure to act caused the original patient injury.

A recent case illustrates the concept of indemnification. In *Patient's Compensation Fund v. Lutheran Hospital* (1999), the fund paid a $10,000,000 settlement to a patient and then attempted to recover from the nurse and her individual policy. The patient was admitted to the facility for treatment of ureteral stenosis, for which morphine sulfate and belladonna suppositories were prescribed postoperatively. The morning following the sur-

In consideration of payment of the premium, in reliance upon the statements in the declarations and subject to all of the terms of this policy, agrees with the named insured as follows:

COVERAGE AGREEMENTS

The company will pay on behalf of the insured all sums that the insured shall become legally obligated to pay as damages because of:

COVERAGE—INDIVIDUAL PROFESSIONAL LIABILITY

Injury arising out of the rendering of or failure to render, during the policy period, professional services by the individual insured, or by any person for whose acts or omissions such insured is legally responsible, except as a member of a partnership, performed in the practice of the individual insured's profession described in the declarations including service by the individual insured as a member of a formal accreditation or similar professional board or committee of a hospital or professional society.

EXCLUSION

This insurance does not apply to:
1. Liability of the insured as a proprietor, superintendent, or executive officer of any hospital, sanitarium, clinic with bed and board facilities, laboratory or business enterprise other than as stated in the above declarations;
2. Liability of the insured as a nurse-anesthetist or as a nurse midwife.

LIMITS OF LIABILITY

Individual Professional Liability
The limit of liability stated in the declarations as applicable to each claim is the limit of the company's liability for all damages because of each claim or suit covered hereby. All claims arising from the same rendering of or failure to render the same professional services shall be considered a single claim for the purposes of this insurance. The limit of liability stated in the declarations as aggregate is, subject to the above provision respecting each claim, the total limit of the company's liability under this coverage for all damages. Such limits of liability shall apply separately to each insured.

SUPPLEMENTARY PAYMENTS

The company will pay, in addition to the applicable limit of liability:
1. All expenses incurred by the company, all costs taxed against the insured in any suit defended by the company, and all interest on the entire amount of the judgment therein which accrues after entry of the judgment and before the company has paid or tendered or deposited in court that part of the judgment that does not exceed the limit of the company's liability thereon.
2. Such premiums on appeal bonds required in any such suit, premiums on bonds to release attachments in any such suit for an amount not in excess of the applicable limit of liability of this policy, and the cost of bail bonds required of the insured because of accident or traffic law violations arising out of the use of any vehicle to which this policy applies, not to exceed $250 per bail bond, but the company shall have no obligation to apply for or furnish such bonds.
3. Reasonable expenses incurred by the insured at the company's request in assisting the company in the investigation or defense of any claim or suit, including actual loss of earnings not to exceed $25 per day.

DEFINITIONS

"Insured" means any person or organization qualifying as the policy holder in the person's insured provision of this policy. The insurance afforded applies separately to each insured against whom claim is made or suit is brought, except with respect to the limits of the company's liability.

"Damages" means all damages, including damages for death, which are payable because of injury to which the insurance applies. "Named insured" means the person or organization named in the declarations of this policy.

CONDITIONS

Insured's duties in the event of occurrence, claim or suit

1. Upon the insured's becoming aware of any alleged injury to which this insurance applies, written notice containing particulars sufficient to identify the insured and also reasonably obtainable information with respect to the time, place, and circumstances thereof, and the names and addresses of the injured and of available witnesses, shall be given by or for the insured to the company or any of its authorized agents as soon as practicable.
2. If claim is made or suit is brought against the insured, the insured shall immediately forward to the company every demand, notice, summons, or other process received by him or his representative.
3. The insured shall cooperate with the company and, upon the company's request, assist in making settlements, in the conduct of suits and in enforcing any right of contribution or indemnity against any person or organization who may be liable to the insured because of injury or damage with respect to which insurance is afforded under this policy; and the insured shall attend hearings and trials and assist in securing and giving evidence and obtaining the attendance of witnesses. The insured shall not, except at his own cost, voluntarily make any payment, assume any obligation, or incur any expense.

SUBROGATION

In the event of any payment under this policy, the company shall be subrogated to all of the insured's rights of recovery therefore against any person or organization, and the insured shall execute and deliver instruments and papers and do whatever else is necessary to secure such rights. The insured shall do nothing after loss to prejudice such rights.

ASSIGNMENT

The interest hereunder of any insured is not assignable.

CHANGES

Notice to any agent or knowledge possessed by any agent or by any other person shall not effect a waiver or change in any part of this policy or stop the company from asserting any right under the terms of this policy; nor shall the terms of this policy be waived or changed, except by endorsement issued to form a part of this policy, signed by a duly authorized representative of this company.

FIGURE 10–1. SAMPLE PROFESSIONAL LIABILITY INSURANCE POLICY

gery, the patient sustained a cardiac arrest and was resuscitated, though he sustained permanent brain injury due to hypoxia.

Only one of the nurses named in the suit had professional liability insurance, though all the nurses who cared for the patient in the early postoperative period were named in the lawsuit. The nurses prevailed on a technicality in that they were not valid "health care providers" as defined in the Patient Compensation Fund. However, this case serves to illustrate that insurance companies and other health care agencies can and do file lawsuits for expenses incurred on behalf of nurses and other health care providers.

Finally, most hospital insurance policies do not have supplementary payments for the nurse-defendant. This means if nurses incur additional expenses in investigating the claim or lose days of work defending the claim, then they must cover the expenses out of pocket.

Employer-based coverage, though, is a good starting point for prudent nurses. They should ask to either see and read the hospital policy or ask about specific provisions in the employer-sponsored coverage and then acquire their own individual coverage to augment the employer's policy. Nurses should also take into consideration the following factors:

1. The type of nursing that they normally do (staff versus charge versus supervision)
2. The dollar amount of the average awards in their particular geographic area
3. The unit or type of nursing in which they normally work (critical care versus general medical–surgical nursing)
4. The propensity for lawsuits against nurses in that same geographic area

The hospital attorney can provide nurses with information regarding trends in malpractice in their locality. Then nurses should find a policy that provides the necessary coverage. They can extend coverage as their job status changes or as they expand practice roles.

■ **EXERCISE 10–3**

Consult with your risk manager or institution legal counsel. What types of provisions are made in the institution policy for individual nurses? What type of coverage would be advisable for nurses working in the institution to purchase?

REASONS TO PURCHASE INDIVIDUAL LIABILITY INSURANCE

Nurses need liability insurance for several reasons:

1. Perhaps the most convincing reason is that defending against a lawsuit, no matter what the merit of the case, is costly. There are attorney fees, court costs, and costs of discovery, not to mention the actual award (or settlement) if the nurse is found negligent. Few nurses can sustain such financial strain without insurance coverage.
2. Professional liability insurance is relatively inexpensive. Many nurses can purchase adequate coverage for between $50 and $150 a year.
3. A popular reason for insurance coverage is the assurance of adequate protection should a lawsuit be filed. Malpractice is not synonymous with incompetence or guilt;

even the most conscientious nurses could be sued for performing their actions below the acceptable standard of care if an untoward happening occurs and they are in the direct line of causation. For example, even though nurses are covered during patient transfers from one facility to a second facility, events happen that place nurses at risk. What if, during the transfer, the nurse temporarily leaves the side of the patient to speak with the pilot or driver? Is this abandonment of the patient and, thus, not within the scope of the nurse's authority? One's mental health is well worth the cost of the insurance policy.

4. Having one's own professional liability insurance does not automatically trigger an employee indemnity lawsuit. But should the institution choose to sue the nurse for reimbursement, he or she is protected.

5. The fact that professionals assume accountability for their own actions or omissions is an additional reason for acquiring such liability coverage. Inherent in accountability is responsibility (and ability to pay) should the plaintiff be negligently injured by the professional's actions or omissions.

6. Malpractice insurance premiums are currently a tax-deductible business expense.

ARGUMENTS FOR HAVING PROFESSIONAL LIABILITY INSURANCE

There is no valid reason for nurses to be without professional liability insurance. A favorite argument of many in-hospital attorneys is to remind nurses that they are more lawsuit prone if they have an individual insurance policy. However, in today's society the nurse is, in essence, the conduit either to the hospital's potential liability or to the physician's potential liability through the doctrine of respondeat superior or through a dual servant role. The nurse's expanding role, with its autonomy and advocacy components, has led to heightened legal accountability and increased potential for being named in lawsuits.

In selected states, tort reform acts have limited the amount of economic liability against individual defendants, particularly physicians and health care corporations. Thus, nurses may find themselves named in more, not fewer, lawsuits as attorneys seek means to find additional sources of revenue for injured clients.

It is immaterial to the patient bringing the lawsuit whether or not the nurse has insurance. Typically, when injured parties file lawsuits, they have no idea of whether or not the nurse is insured. But it should matter greatly to nurses, since the cost of defense could very well financially destroy them. In most states, the judgment remains open until satisfied or dropped. That means that a nurse may be paying on a prior judgment for several years after the judgment; in states that allow garnishment of wages for adjudicated debts, one's wages may be garnished for several years after the initial judgment.

■ EXERCISE 10–4

Poll nurses with whom you work about the advantages of professional liability insurance. Do those you interviewed have individual policies? List the reasons they gave for having or not having individual policies. Which reasons are listed most frequently? Were the reasons valid as opposed to mere guesses by the nurses you interviewed? List arguments that you could use to educate these nurses about the value and necessity of having individual professional liability insurance coverage.

Using ethical principles, list reasons why nurses should have professional liability insurance. Does having such coverage make nurses more autonomous in their practice? Do any of the ethical principles negate having such coverage?

SUMMARY

Individual malpractice insurance may not prevent potential liability, but does assist the nurse if a lawsuit is filed or the nurse is a named party in a lawsuit. Policies, though difficult to understand at first glance, are really not that difficult once the reader understands the various terms and phrases.

AFTER COMPLETING THIS CHAPTER, YOU SHOULD BE ABLE TO

- List elements common to all professional liability insurance policies.
- Differentiate types of professional liability insurance policies available commercially to professional nurses.
- Identify issues to be considered when deciding between individual coverage, group coverage, and employer-sponsored coverage.
- List and refute reasons given against having individual coverage.

APPLY YOUR LEGAL KNOWLEDGE

- What do the terms and language in insurance policies mean to the policyholder?
- Are there insurance policies that are more desirable for nurses who work in different clinical areas in acute care settings? Do these policies differ for nurses working in home care settings or in ambulatory settings?
- Are there times when it would be advisable to have no individual professional liability coverage?

REFERENCES

Patient's Compensation Fund v. Lutheran Hospital, 588 N.W.2d 8880 (Wisconsin, 1999).
Sermchief v. Gonzales, 600 S.W.2d 683 (Mo. en banc, 1983).

IV IMPACT OF THE LAW ON THE PROFESSIONAL PRACTICE OF NURSING

eleven

Nurse Practice Acts, Licensure, and the Scope of Practice

■ PREVIEW

Throughout the years, an elaborate system of licensure and credentials for health care providers has evolved to ensure that only qualified persons deliver health care. Both licenses and credentials have as their primary purpose the protection of the public at large. Through proper issuance of licenses and credentials, qualified health care providers are distinguished from unqualified persons. The first group is given a license to practice, whereas the latter group is prohibited from harming society in a health care role. This chapter outlines the relationship between state nurse practice acts, entry into professional practice, and the scope of practice issues. The chapter also discusses the multistate licensure issue and alternative (complementary) therapies.

■ KEY CONCEPTS

credentials
professional licensure
  mandatory licensure
  permissive licensure
  institutional licensure
nurse practice acts
grandfather clause
reciprocity
endorsement

licensure by examination
licensure by waiver
temporary license
disciplinary action
diversion programs
articulation with medical practice
  acts
standing orders
joint statements

scope of practice
continuing education
National Practitioner Data Bank
  (NPDB)
certification
alternative or complementary
  therapies
multistate licensure
mutual recognition compact

CREDENTIALS

Credentials are proof of qualifications, usually in written form, stating that an individual or organizations has met specific standards. Two types of credentials are used in health care: licensure and certification.

PROFESSIONAL LICENSURE

Professional licensure is the legal process by which an authorized authority grants permission to a qualified individual or entity to perform designated skills and services in a jurisdiction in which such practice would be illegal without a license. Licenses are issued by governmental agencies and are enforced by the police power of the state. For nurses, the authorized authority is the *state board of nursing* or the *state board of nursing examiners.* The qualified individual is the candidate for licensure, and this candidate is a graduate nurse who has successfully completed all requirements for licensure or a nurse with licensure in another state. The designated skills and services are professional nursing actions.

Licensure is enacted through state legislative action. Licensure statutes measure minimum competency of the person licensed and are intended to protect health care consumers. Licensure laws, an example of a state's exercise of its police power, exist to protect the public against unqualified practitioners.

Individual state legislative bodies enact into law their specific licensing procedures, stating which professions must be licensed to practice within the state. In most states, physicians and dentists were the first professionals to be licensed, with nurses generally the next licensed professional. Part of the statutory law in all jurisdictions of the United States is the state nurse practice act. Each state, the District of Columbia, and territories of the United States have individual nurse practice acts, bringing the total number to 61.

State Boards of Nursing

Individual legislators do not directly enforce statutory law. The means of ensuring enforcement of nurse practice acts is through the state board of nursing or the state board of nurse examiners. This board is created by language in the selected nurse practice act, and is ultimately accountable to the legislators for professional nursing within a given jurisdiction. A board of nursing has no greater authority than that which the statute, enacted by the legislature, grants to it. Therefore, the board of nursing is limited by the language of the given nurse practice act.

State boards of nursing are mandated in the state nurse practice acts. The specific act sets the number of members of the board, qualifications for membership, and the term of appointment. States vary in the numbers of persons on the board, and currently there are 7 to 17 members on the state boards of nursing. The individual nurse practice act may allow for legal or expert members, or for election (North Carolina) rather than appointment of the members. In all but 6 states there is one board of nursing for both professional and practical nursing. The remaining six states have two separate boards.

Boards of nursing have an executive director who is responsible for administering the work of the board and seeing that the nurse practice act provisions as well as rules and regulations of the board are followed. The American Nurses Association (ANA) recommends that boards of nursing:

1. Govern their own operation and administration.
2. Approve or deny approvals to schools of nursing.
3. Examine and license applicants.
4. Review licenses, grant temporary licenses, and provide for inactive status for those already licensed.
5. Regulate specialty practice.
6. Discipline those who violate provisions of the licensure law (ANA, 1990).

The board is given the authority to set standards by promulgating rules and regulations and has as a charge the enforcement of such rules and regulations. Most state boards of nursing have published standards of professional conduct and guidelines for unprofessional conduct, with enforcement assured by the board's ability to revoke, stipulate, or suspend a previously granted license or to deny licensure.

The board's authority arises from various sources of law. Its authority may be:

1. Legislative, through the promulgation of rules and regulations.
2. Quasijudicial, through hearings.
3. Administrative, through licensure control.

State legislatures may also require that licensure be either mandatory or permissive.

Mandatory Licensure

Mandatory licensure requires that all persons who are compensated as a member of a licensed profession obtain licensure prior to practicing actions of the profession. Mandatory licensure regulates the practice of the profession and requires compliance with the statue if an individual engages in activities defined within the scope of that profession (Aiken and Catalano, 1994). Thus, both the title of registered nurse and the professional actions are protected.

A case that illustrates the power of the board of nursing to regulate nursing practice is *People v. Stults* (1997). In that case, a nonlicensed medical assistant obtained a position in a medical clinic that had previously been held by a registered nurse with a pediatric specialty.

The medical assistant had worked in pediatric clinics for nearly two decades after completing a college-level medical assistant program with an emphasis in pediatric care. She knew the pediatric nurse who had the position and was contacted by the physician and asked to take the position when the pediatric nurse resigned.

The physician assumed that the medical assistant was a registered nurse. Three years later, a new office manager asked for the medical assistant's license, which was conspicuously absent from the clinic's files. She had no license and was reported to the state board of nursing.

It could not be proven in court beyond a reasonable doubt that the medical assistant had ever claimed or pretended to be a registered nurse. To uphold her conviction for unlicensed nursing practice, however, the court did not need proof that she had misrepresented that she had a nursing license.

In the clinic, the medical assistant had performed tasks that required a nursing license within the state of Illinois. Falsely claiming or leading others to believe one is a licensed nurse is illegal but is not the only way to violate the nursing practice act and the law. The medical assistant was performing nursing functions illegally without a registered nurse or practical nurse license, said the court. Giving injections and immunizations to pediatric clients and performing physical assessments cannot be done by a nonlicensed person, ruled the court. She had also been doing phone triage of patients, giving specific medical advice to mothers about their sick children, and offering general advice to patients, such as how to manage feeding problems and when to switch babies from formula to solid foods. The ultimate holding of the court was that a nonlicensed person cannot counsel patients about their health care concerns.

Direct physician supervision of a nursing function being carried out by a nonlicensed person does not take nonlicensed nursing practice out of the scope of the nursing practice act or make it legal, the court ruled. Thus, the appellate court upheld her conviction.

Several exceptions to mandatory licensure within a jurisdiction that requires mandatory licensure are:

1. Performance of nursing actions by unlicensed practitioners in emergency conditions.
2. Practice by nursing students incidental to their current course of study, including students who are licensed and those who are not licensed.
3. Nursing actions by employees of the federal government, provided the nurse holds a valid and current license in another state or territory.
4. Practice by graduate nurses for a specific length of time during which licensure is being processed, provided the nurse has been issued a temporary permit to practice nursing within the state.
5. Nursing care given to patients by qualified nurses during transportation of the patient through a given state.
6. Unpaid persons caring for family members or friends.
7. Nurses working for the Red Cross during a disaster.
8. Caregivers who conduct religious services and rites and who do not report to be registered nurses.

Nurses in the armed services or nurses employed by federal agencies must hold a current state license, but not necessarily from the state in which they are currently employed or assigned.

Permissive Licensure

Permissive licensure (Texas) regulates only the use of the title and does not protect nursing actions. Thus, nurses cannot use the title registered nurse (RN) unless duly licensed, but they can perform many or all of the same nursing actions as long as they do not call themselves an RN. For example, in a state with permissive licensure, a licensed practical or vocational nurse (LPN or LVN), working under the supervision or through direct orders of a physician, could perform most of the same actions that an RN performs as only the title is protected, not the nursing actions.

Permissive licensure correlates best with the initial registration acts of the early 1900s. The term *registered nurse* was defined as a person who had graduated from an acceptable school of nursing and had passed an examination, rather than a person engaged in a specific type of practice. These first registration acts provided for permissive licensure.

The state board of nursing may have as its concern only the professional practice of nursing or may incorporate both professional and practical licensed nurses (RNs as well as LPNs or LVNs), and 44 states now have joint boards. If the charge of the state board of nursing is merely professional licensure, then a separate board of nursing for the practical nurse will also exist within the same jurisdiction. Whether one or two separate boards exists, the restriction of mandatory or permissive licensure may vary within the given state. For example, professional nurses may have mandatory licensure, while practical nurses may have permissive licensure, or both may have mandatory or permissive licensure.

Institutional Licensure

Institutional licensure is the process by which a state government regulates health institutions. Institutional licensure is the alternative to individual licensure. Most government agencies issue licenses to health care facilities, granting permission for the facility to operate, and the issuing body holds the facility responsible for maintaining sanitation, fire safety, staffing, and equipment. Institutional licensure of individuals gives these facilities the added right to decide who is qualified to perform what tasks and duties, and awards licenses as the facility deems appropriate.

Institutional licensure grants the institution authority to directly regulate staff members' practice as well as requirements for administration, equipment specifications, fire safety, footage regulations, and minimal nursing staff requirements. Usually, the process is implemented, not controlled, by individual state monitoring agencies or national organizations, such as the Joint Commission on Accreditation of Healthcare Organizations (JCAHO). Theoretically, institutional licensure gives nonprofessionals the regulation of a given profession without standard criteria for such regulation.

There is a growing impatience by consumers with the seeming indifference of the health care community to individual consumer needs. Many of these consumers feel that the current licensing laws are at fault. The licensing laws have been characterized as more protective of professional jurisdiction than public safety, costly to apply, and too rigid to accommodate the changing needs of the health care delivery system and society at large. Licensing laws are often silent on the more critical issues of competency and quality (Joel, 1995).

Advocates of institutional licensure insist that these issues will be eliminated and rectified by the renewed interest in institutional licensure. Reasons cited include allowing nurses more flexibility in their practice and the opportunity to more effectively expand the practice of nursing. Proponents also claim that institutional licensure will allow professionals to be more responsive to changing needs, that such licensure will allow providers to take on and relinquish activities as the situation and their abilities demand, and that it will be more cost-effective, thus saving consumers money.

Perhaps the crucial differences between institutional and individual licensure are more philosophical than practical. Individual licenses reinforce the responsibility of the professional to the individual client rather than to the employer. In an environment that often sacrifices quality in an attempt to lower costs, this would seem a most fundamental argument against institutional licensure. Would nurses feel they could speak against an employer who is also a regulator? And would nursing become lost on a board that has as its charge all regulated areas of practice (Joel, 1995)?

■ EXERCISE 11–1

Make a list of the pros and cons of institutional versus state licensure for nursing. Now repeat that list from the perspective of a consumer rather than that of a professional. How does institutional licensure undermine professional nursing?

NURSE PRACTICE ACTS

Nurse practice acts, which originated to protect the public at large, define the practice of nursing, give guidance within the scope of practice issues, and set standards for the nursing profession. The state nurse practice act is the single most important piece of legislation for the nurse because the practice act affects all facets of nursing practice. The nurse practice act is the law, and state boards of nursing cannot grant exceptions or waive its provisions. For example, if licensure can be granted only to individuals who graduate from an approved school of nursing, then the board must refuse licensure to a candidate who did not graduate from an approved school of nursing even if the candidate can show evidence of competency and equivalency.

By the early twentieth century, the minimum requirements for nursing practice were beginning to take shape. *Nurse registration acts,* permissive precursors to nurse practice acts, were emerging, and in 1901 the state nurses associations adopted proposals supporting commitment to passage of state laws to control the practice of nursing. North Carolina was the first state to pass a permissive nurse practice act in 1903. By 1923, every state had passed some type of nurse registration act and New York State, in 1938, was the first to enact a mandatory nurse practice act, establishing two levels of nursing practice: licensed RNs and LPNs. Other states followed suit, and by 1952 all states, the District of Columbia, and the U.S. territories had enacted nurse practice acts.

The early acts mainly regulated registration and fee structures. With the advent of mandatory acts, only licensed professionals could practice nursing. Some states enacted definitions of professional nursing, whereas other states had no formal definition of professional nursing. In 1955, the ANA approved a model definition for nursing practice and continued through the years to broaden the definition, amending the definition in 1970 to incorporate nursing diagnosis and further allowing for an expanded scope in 1979. To provide for some consistency in individual state nurse practice acts, the ANA published a model act for state legislators in 1980 and again in 1990. This latest model nurse practice act incorporates the advanced nurse practitioner as well as the registered nurse (ANA, 1990).

Individual nurse practice acts continue to be worded differently, with varying concepts of professional nursing. All nurse practice acts are worded in fairly general terms, and there is no laundry list of specific actions to ensure that the nurse stays within the given act. Rather, the acts' general provisions should give guidance as to acceptable actions. For example, one reason that specific actions are not listed is that, as statutory law, the nurse practice acts are slow in changing to conform with modern practice and technological advances. If actions were specifically enumerated, one would be required to follow the nurse practice act exactly, even though current practices might have changed.

An example may assist with understanding this last statement. Imagine that the state nurse practice act has no provision for nursing diagnosis, yet the JCAHO standards re-

1955 MODEL ACT: PRACTICE OF NURSING

The practice of professional nursing means the performance for compensation of any act in the observation, care, and counsel of the ill, injured, or infirm, or in the maintenance of health or prevention of illness of others, or in the supervision and teaching of other personnel, or the administration of medications and treatments as prescribed by a licensed physician or dentist; requiring substantial specialized judgment and skill and based on knowledge and application of the principles of biological, physical, and social science. The foregoing shall not be deemed to include acts of diagnosis or prescription of therapeutic or corrective measures.

Source: American Nurses Association approves a definition of nursing practice (1955). *American Journal of Nursing* 55(12), 1474. Reprinted with permission.

quire that nursing diagnoses be written for each patient within hospitals that have JCAHO accreditation. If enumerated actions in the nurse practice act specifically omitted nursing diagnoses as part of the professional practice of nursing within the state, the professional nurse would run the risk daily of violating the act or of working in a nonaccredited institution.

Further, suppose that the institution's policies and procedures mandate that nursing diagnoses are part of the assessment due each patient, just as the patient's progress, response to nursing interventions, and nursing care needs are part of the nursing protocol. Now the dilemma would concern the nurse practice act and one's livelihood. Does the individual nurse violate the nurse practice act or ignore the hospital's policy and procedure manual and refrain from making a nursing diagnosis? Such a scenario could happen if nurse practice acts were checklists for approved nursing actions.

1976 MODEL PRACTICE ACT: PRACTICE OF NURSING

The practice of nursing means the performance for compensation of professional services requiring substantial specialized knowledge of the biological, physical, behavioral, psychological, and sociological sciences and of nursing theory as the basis for assessment, diagnosis, planning, intervention, and evaluation in the promotion and maintenance of health; the casefinding and management of illness, injury, or infirmity; the restoration of optimal function; or the achievement of a dignified death. Nursing practice includes but is not limited to administration, teaching, counseling, supervision, delegation, and evaluation of practice and execution of the medical regimen, including the administration of medications and treatments prescribed by any person authorized by state law to prescribe. Each registered nurse is directly accountable and responsible to the consumer for the quality of nursing care rendered.

Source: American Nurses Association (1980). *The Nursing Practice Act: Suggested State Legislation.* Kansas City, MO: Author. Reprinted with permission.

1990 MODEL PRACTICE ACT: DEFINITION OF NURSING

The "practice of nursing" means the performance of services for compensation in the provision of diagnosis and treatment of human responses to health or illness;

"Professional nursing practice" encompasses the full scope of nursing practice and includes all its specialties and consists of application of nursing theory to the development, implementation, and evaluation of plans of nursing care for individuals, families, and communities. Professional nursing practice requires substantial knowledge of nursing theory and related scientific, behavioral, and humanistic disciplines. Professional nursing practice includes, but is not limited to:

(1) assessment, diagnosis, planning, intervention, and evaluation of human responses to health or illness;
(2) the provision of direct nursing care to individuals to restore optimum function or to achieve a dignified death;
(3) the procurement, coordination, and management of essential client resources;
(4) the provision of health counseling and education;
(5) the establishment of standards of practice for nursing care in all settings, including the development of nursing policies, procedures, and protocols for a specific setting;
(6) the direction of nursing practice, including delegation to those practicing technical nursing;
(7) the supervision of those who assist in the practice of nursing;
(8) collaboration with other independently licensed health care professionals in case finding and the clinical management and execution of intervention as identified to be appropriate in a plan of care; and
(9) the administration of medication and treatments as prescribed by those professionals qualified to prescribe under the provision of (cite state statute[s]).

"Technical nursing practice" includes the skilled application of nursing principles in the delivery of direct care to individuals and families within organized nursing services. Technical nursing practice requires the study of nursing within the context of the applied sciences. Technical nursing practice includes, but is not limited to:

(1) participation in the development, evaluation, and modification of a plan of care;
(2) the provision of direct care to individuals to restore optimum function or to achieve a dignified death;
(3) patient teaching;
(4) the supervision of those who assist in the practice of nursing;
(5) the administration of medication and treatments as prescribed by those professionals qualified to prescribe under the provisions of (cite state statute[s]).

Source: American Nurses Association (1990). *Suggested State Legislation: Nursing Practice Act, Nursing Disciplinary Diversion Act, Prescriptive Authority Act.* Washington, DC: Author. Reprinted with permission.

Thus, nurse practice acts are not checklists. The practice acts contain general statements of appropriate professional nursing actions. Nurses must incorporate the nurse practice act with their educational background, previous work experience, institutional policies, and technological advancements. If the main purpose of nurse practice acts is to protect the public from unsafe practitioners, then the ultimate goal of nurse practice acts must be to provide competent, quality nursing care by currently qualified practitioners.

■ **EXERCISE 11–2**

Read your state's nurse practice act, emphasizing the general provisions defining nursing actions. Does the act give sufficient guidance for nurses to know if an action is either within the act or outside its scope?

ELEMENTS OF NURSE PRACTICE ACTS

Definition of Professional Nursing

All state nurse practice acts define nursing. As previously stated, some state definitions include nursing diagnoses and speak of collaboration with other professionals. Some nurse practice acts allow for individual treatment, while others specify nursing interventions and therapies. Basically, there are three approaches to statutory definitions of professional nursing:

1. The *traditional approach* is based on the ANA's original model definition. This approach does not include diagnosis, treatment, or prescription. Most states currently following this model definition have not addressed expanded practice or advanced practice issues. Some states use a more restrictive definition and then allow for some limited expanded roles for nursing by having broad delegatory language in the state medical practice act.
2. The *transitional approach* may also allow some expanded roles beyond those described in the nurse practice act through the use of standing orders and through supervision by a responsible physician. Some states with transitional approaches add an additional action for nurses, for example, the legal permission to diagnose and evaluate patients but not to treat them.
3. The *administrative approach* is seen in the majority of states. This approach uses a broader definition of nursing and allows additional acts as may be authorized by appropriate state agencies. Advanced nurse practitioners and expanded nursing roles are incorporated, relying on the authority granted to the state board of nursing to promulgate rules for such advanced roles. These rules and regulations are then administered and enforced through the state board of nursing. This approach may also allow for overlap between physician and professional nursing roles and functions. For example, this approach allows both physicians and nurses to diagnose and treat patients, within the respective realms of their disciplines.

Requirements for Licensure

Requirements usually center on personal characteristics and educational requirements to ensure that the candidate is at least minimally competent to practice professional nursing. These criteria include academic and clinical performance, a passing score on the licensing examination, and personal qualities.

Academic and clinical performance are validated by transcripts from approved schools of nursing. The state board may use its own criteria for approval or may rely on national accreditation agencies such as the National League for Nursing (NLN) and the American Association of Colleges of Nursing (ACCN), through their respective accrediting arms.

All states administer licensing examinations and use a standardized, nationally normed test. With the advent of computers and the availability of computer-generated examinations, states now allow candidates for licensure to schedule times to take the national examination. Provisions are made for handicapped candidates in accordance with the Americans with Disabilities Act. With the increasing numbers of nurses seeking reciprocity (recognition of licensure from one state to another state) from other state boards, states have adopted to continue the practice of national norms for successful passage of the examinations.

Personal qualifications and attributes screened include citizenship or visa permits, physical and mental health fitness, minimal age requirements, fluency in English requirements, and good moral character references.

Payment of fees is another area to meet licensure requirements. These fees include processing and administration fees for the licensure examination, interim work permit fees, and temporary licensure fees.

Exemptions

Most states allow exemptions from state licensure in very few circumstances. Some of the valid exemptions have previously been enumerated, such as exemptions for professional students in current course work and for graduate nurses during the application process.

Another form of exemption is the *grandfather clause.* This term applies to certain persons working within the profession for a given period of time or prior to a deadline date. These individuals may be granted the privilege of applying for a license without having to meet all the requirements for licensure or without having to take the licensing examination. Such a grandfather clause was used to allow World War II nurses, or those with on-the-job training and expertise, licensure even though they had not graduated from an approved school of nursing or passed the licensure examination.

The grandfather clause is also projected to be used if the ANA proposal for professional entry into practice for baccalaureate nurses is fully implemented. In 1964, the ANA proposed that the entry level for professional nursing should be the baccalaureate of science in nursing degree (BSN) and that this would be implemented by 1985. Associate degree nurses (ADNs) would be technical nurses and those previously licensed will be allowed the right to retain the title RN in the proposed new licensing schema. But new graduates will need an earned baccalaureate degree to use the title RN (Hood, 1985).

In 1984, the ANA revised the timetable for implementation, and to date little success has been attained in this direction. By 1988, 30 state nurses associations had addressed the issue and 28 had adopted resolutions advocating the BSN as the professional entry requirement. The ANA House of Delegates in 1995 reaffirmed this commitment to the BSN as entry level into professional nursing and voted to assist states in implementing strategies that would make such a goal a reality (ANA, 1995).

Today, only two states have succeeded in changing the entry requirements (North Dakota and Maine), and other states are at varying degrees of attempting to achieve this goal (George and Young, 1990). Maine continues to allow both the BSN and the ADN nurse to function within the state without requiring that nurses earn a BSN within a reasonable time period. North Dakota remains the only state to have fully implemented this provision. The only schools of nursing in North Dakota offer a BSN degree or higher, and ADN nurses coming into the state are granted provisional licensure, with an eight-year provision for completion of the BSN degree. If they have not completed the BSN within that time frame, they are not allowed to renew their licenses as registered nurses (North Dakota Century Code, 1997).

Licensure Across Jurisdictions

Because each state has its own nurse practice act and because most states have mandatory licensure, provisions are included within state nurse practice acts for licensing nurses with valid licenses in other jurisdictions. There are essentially four means of granting licensure across jurisdictions:

1. *Reciprocity* is an agreement by two or more states granting recognition to licensure by other state boards of nursing. For reciprocity, the licensing requirements of the involved states must be equivalent. Such a provision allows licensed nurses to be granted additional licensure merely by application and by payment of required fees. The concept of reciprocity also allows states with similar disciplinary actions to revoke a license in a state based solely on revocation in a sister state (*Schoenhair v. Pennsylvania*, 1983).
2. Under *endorsement,* a similar concept, a state may grant licensure to an already licensed nurse from another state if the two states' qualifications and licensure requirements are comparable. Usually, the state granting endorsement requires that a similar licensure examination exists in both states. This means of granting licensure is distinguished from reciprocity in that no prior agreement existed between the two involved states, and individual nurses must petition for licensure by endorsement. Their cases are decided on an individual basis.
3. *Licensure by examination* is required when the petitioned state does not grant licensure by reciprocity or by endorsement. Essentially, licensure by examination means that the individual must meet all of the state requirements and successfully complete a licensing examination before licensure is granted.
4. *Licensure by waiver* is similar to licensure by examination. If the petitioning candidate meets or exceeds some of the requirements for licensure, that portion previously demonstrated may be waived for the candidate, while other requirements must be demonstrated by the candidate. States may choose to waive educational requirements, experience requirements, or examination requirements while requiring that deficiencies be met.

As with any new graduate within the state, a given state may grant a *temporary license* to out-of-state nurses. Temporary licenses allow nurses to practice while permanent licensure is pending or may allow them to practice for a limited period of time. For example, the state may grant temporary licensure for a semester or two while the nurse completes graduation requirements for an advanced nursing degree.

Foreign nursing school graduates desiring to practice nursing in the United States must meet the requirements of the state or territory in which they reside and must pass the licensing examination. Each state nurse practice act specifies requirements for foreign nursing school graduates. All states require that graduates of a foreign school apply for an occupational visa and have successfully completed a VisaScreen, verifying proficiency in English, and that they have either earned a certificate from the Commission on Graduates of Foreign Nursing Schools or passed the National Council Licensure Examination for Registered Nurses (NCLEX-RN).

The Committee on Graduates of Foreign Nursing Schools (CGFNS), sponsored independently by the ANA and NLN, administers an examination to foreign-educated nurses that addresses their command of the English language as well as knowledge of nursing concepts and skills and serves as a guide for their ability to successfully pass the licensing examination. Following successful passage of the CGFNS examination, foreign nurses are allowed to obtain an occupational visa in the United States. The committee also has a Credentials Evaluation Service (CES) to evaluate transcripts and credentials from foreign countries.

In 1998, legislation was passed in the House of Representatives in Washington, D.C., which would have allowed additional foreign nurses to practice in the United States in hospitals with a documented nursing shortage. Called the Health Professional Shortage Area Nursing Relief Act (1998), the bill was designed to provide an expedited means of allowing foreign nurses to practice in areas of critical need in the United States. Opposed by President Clinton and reluctantly supported by the ANA, the bill was defeated before it reached the U.S. Senate.

Disciplinary Action and Due Process Requirements

To give credence to the state board of nursing's ability to enforce licensure requirements, the board also has the authority for *disciplinary action.* There are various actions that may be taken, depending on the severity of the violation. Allowable disciplinary actions include:

1. Private reprimand or warning.
2. Public reprimand.
3. Probation.
4. Suspension of licensure.
5. Refusal to renew licensure.
6. Revocation of licensure.

Not all of the preceding measures have the same significance. For minor violations, the individual nurse may receive a warning or reprimand. Continued violations may be cause for probation or temporary suspension of licensure. Major violations are dealt with through licensure revocation or refusal to reissue licensure. Some of the possible violations for which disciplinary actions may be instigated include, but are not limited to:

1. *Conviction* of a felony or crime involving *moral turpitude* (an action that is done contrary to justice, honesty, modesty, or good moral principles).

2. Use of *fraud* or *deceit* in obtaining licensure.
3. *Violation* of the provisions of the nurse practice act.
4. *Aiding* or *abetting* any unlicensed person with the unauthorized practice of nursing.
5. *Revocation, suspension,* or *denial of licensure* to practice nursing in another jurisdiction.
6. *Habitual use* of, or *addiction* to, alcohol or drugs.
7. *Unprofessional conduct* that is likely to deceive, defraud, or injure the public or patients.
8. *Lack of fitness* by reason of physical or mental health that could result in injury to the public or individual patients.

During licensure suspension or probation, the board of nursing has the authority to impose conditions such as:

1. Obtaining substance abuse rehabilitation and counseling.
2. Obtaining special counseling.
3. Requiring supervision for specific techniques or procedures to validate competency.
4. Requiring satisfactory completion of educational programs.

Disciplinary actions may arise in one of several ways, depending on applicable state law. Generally, a written complaint is filed with the state board of nursing by an individual, a health care agency, or a professional organization. This single complaint triggers action on part of the board. The complaint may be initiated directly by the state board of nursing in some states. The complaint is screened, and an investigation is initiated, if appropriate. A board hearing is then scheduled, and the nurse is entitled to a clear statement of the charges, the right to question and produce witnesses, the right to an attorney, and the right to a fair determination based on the evidence presented. The board may also request that the nurse provide a written response to the board regarding the allegations. This process is outlined in Table 11–1.

During the investigation phase, the board will contact any and all witnesses for information and statements about the complaint. They usually subpoena patient records and obtain copies of the health care institution's policies and procedures. The board may also retain an independent nurse consultant to review nursing notes and actions taken by the nurse being investigated for appropriateness. In cases in which diversion of drugs is suspected, the Drug Enforcement Agency (DEA) may also become involved. The DEA, if involved, usually conducts its own investigation and may use undercover agents to monitor the nurse at work. The DEA's evidence will later be used by the board at the hearing.

Because state boards of nursing are agencies of state administrative law, the nurse is constitutionally allowed due process rights. This means that the practicing nurse has the right to adequate notice of the alleged misconduct, an opportunity to present information concerning the alleged misconduct, and the right to appeal the board's action. Some states impose stricter rights; for example, not only do nurses have the right to be heard, they also have the right to call witnesses and to be represented by legal counsel. Some states also schedule a conference with their attorney and the nurse before commencing the formal hearing.

During the hearing, both sides are allowed to present witnesses and to be represented by legal counsel. At the conclusion of the hearing, the board of nursing decides if the evidence presented merits disciplinary action or not, and the board of nursing will specify any disciplinary action at this time.

TABLE 11–1. PROCESS FOR DISCIPLINARY HEARINGS

Filing of the sworn complaint
   Individual complaint
   Health care agency complaint
   Professional organization complaint
Review of the complaint
   Notice of hearing to the involved nurse
   Hearing before the board of nursing
   Evidence presented by board and nurse
   Witnesses called by board and nurse
   Decision by the board of nursing
Disciplinary action
   If found not guilty of misconduct, no action by board of nursing
   If found guilty of misconduct, the board of nursing may:
      Issue a reprimand, public or private
      Place the nurse on probation
      Deny the renewal of licensure
      Suspend the nurse's license
      Revoke the nurse's license
      Allow the nurse to enter a diversion program
Court review
   Review the board decision and concur with its finding
   Order a new trial
   Appeal to a higher court

Following the announcement of the disciplinary action to be taken (as warranted), the nurse may file a lawsuit to appeal the board's decision. Depending on the jurisdiction, the nurse may file the case in the lowest court of the state or in a special court that handles appeals from state agencies. The appropriate court reviews only the state board of nursing's original decision against the nurse, not the nurse's alleged misconduct. The court's charge is to determine if the board acted properly. Whether the nurse or the state board of nursing prevails, the losing side may further appeal the decision through the court process to the highest court in the given state.

Among the more common reasons for the state board of nursing to investigate a nurse are:

1. Negligent or substandard care provided a patient (*Leahy v. North Carolina Board of Nursing,* 1997, and *Mississippi Board of Nursing v. Hanson,* 1997).
2. Incompetence, a charge applied to the nurse who is not qualified to provide care to a specific patient.
3. Abusive behavior, either physical or oral (*Hill v. Pennsylvania Department of Health, Division of Nursing Care Facilities,* 1998).
4. Substance abuse (*Regester v. Indiana State Board of Nursing,* 1998).
5. Physical or mental impairment.
6. Fraud, usually committed in the application process.

Failure by the state board of nursing to comply with the constitutional rights of due process or of state law may result in the reversal of the board's decision by the judiciary.

The court in *Colorado State Board of Nursing v. Hohn* (1954), the landmark case in this area of the law, ordered the nurse's license reinstated, because the hearing was held with less than the full board present and state law mandated a full board hearing.

Typically, state nurse practice acts require that a quorum of the board be present for a disciplinary hearing and for disciplinary decisions. For example, the court in *Stevens v. Blake* (1984) held that a majority of the board of nursing must be in accord for final disciplinary decisions. The court further held that it is not necessary that a majority be present physically for each step involved in the process.

Adequate notice of an alleged misconduct means more than just 10 to 20 days' notice that a hearing will be held by the state board of nursing. Adequate notice encompasses knowledge or reason to have the knowledge that the particular conduct is prohibited by the state nurse practice act. This means that the wording of nurse practice acts may not be too vague or overly broad. This is usually avoided by a standard of conduct that is widely recognized as unprofessional. For example, the court in *Leahy v. North Carolina Board of Nursing* (1997) upheld a one-year revocation of a nurse's license for what the board ruled were two significant lapses in professional judgment. The nurse appealed the ruling by filing this lawsuit. In both the instances that ultimately caused the registered nurse in question to lose her license, she did not respond to reports from the LPNs under her supervision that there was grave concern for the condition of the patients the LPNs were monitoring. One patient's respirations had dropped from 20 to 8 per minute, and another patient had blood in his urine.

In the first instance, the LPN first notified the RN, then reported the patient's condition to a supervisor. The supervisor immediately assessed the patient, notified the physician, and administered the Narcan as ordered. In the second instance, the RN told the LPN not to call the urologist, even though another RN had requested that the physician be notified. The charges filed against the nurse were failing to set her priorities appropriately in determining which patients presented the greatest danger and most needed care, failing to recognize her patients' conditions, failing to supervise appropriately the care given patients by LPNs, and failure to make patient information available to other health care providers, namely the supervisor and the physician.

At the hearing, the board of nursing did not have an expert witness testify to the standards of care owed by this nurse. Instead, the board served as expert witnesses in determining the standard of care owed these patients and in determining the accountability of the nurse. At trial, the Supreme Court of North Carolina agreed with the board that no expert witnesses were necessary because the licensing board may use its own experience and specialized knowledge to evaluate a situation presented before it for a ruling. Thus, the nurse's challenge to revocation of her license failed.

A 1994 case in Iowa, *Burns v. Matzen*, decided a provision in an Iowa law requiring licensing boards to revoke the licenses of habitually intoxicated health professionals had been upheld by the Supreme Court of that state. The board of nursing placed a registered nurse on probation in accordance with the statute after finding that the nurse was habitually intoxicated. The nurse challenged the decision and the statute. The nurse argued that the law was unconstitutionally vague because licensees could not sufficiently discern what conduct would constitute habitual intoxication and therefore could not avoid violating the statute. The court upheld the statute, ruling that a "person of ordinary intelligence should easily understand what type of conduct is to be avoided" (at 4). The court concluded that the licensing board could determine whether a nurse violated the statute on a case-by-case basis without developing a specific definition. The nurse's probationary status was upheld.

In *Mississippi Board of Nursing v. Hanson* (1997), the Supreme Court of Mississippi also found for the board of nursing, despite an appellate court ruling that held in favor of the nurse. In this case, the nurse was charged with reckless disregard for the health and safety of her patient. She had removed an infant from an incubator, holding the infant around the neck with one of her hands. She carried the infant around the unit by his neck, jesting as she held the naked infant and allowing his unsupported body to dangle. During a one-year period, the nurse endangered babies by holding them under their armpits, removing babies from incubators and carrying them to distant parts of the unit, thus compromising the maintenance of a stable body temperature and unnecessarily exposing them to risk of infection. During the same time frame, she also was noted to stimulate neonatal intensive care patients' hearts by rapidly flipping the levers on their incubators to jostle them as they lay in the incubator, increasing the risk of intraventricular hemorrhage.

The court did not discount the credibility of the nurses witnessing these events, even though two of the nurses waited 30 days before coming forth to discuss the incidents with their charge nurse. Nor did the court fault their credibility merely because each told a slightly different version of the events. The court was unimpressed with the nurse's expert witness, who stated that none of the babies could be proven to have been harmed by her conduct.

The court ruled that the board of nursing was capable of making a fair decision, despite the fact that the nurse alleged they were prejudiced based on a federal civil rights lawsuit she had previously filed against the board collectively and each member individually. The legal system, held the court, presumes that administrative bodies are fair and honest. The court ruled that it would not allow the board's deliberations and decision to be drowned out with unsupported allegations of bias and upheld the permanent revocation of the nurse's license.

Fraudulent conduct may be the basis for disciplinary action. In *Thompson v. Olsten Kimberly Qualitycare, Inc.* (1997), a home health nurse was fired for alleged double billing of patients, for signing documents as an RN when she was really an LPN, for absenteeism, and for being verbally abusive toward coworkers. The grounds for her termination were reported to the state board of nursing, and she sued for defamation.

A person licensed as a professional health care provider must report to the board of nursing personal knowledge of any conduct of a licensed professional nurse believed to be grounds for disciplinary action. This includes conduct that appears incompetent, unprofessional, unethical, fraudulent, or indicative that the nurse is mentally or physically unable to engage safely in the profession of nursing. Any person, facility, or corporation making such a report to the board in good faith is immune from civil liability or criminal prosecution over such a report. The nurse was entitled to her day in court to attempt to prove that her employer was not acting in good faith, however, and the case was remanded to the trial court for decision on this one issue.

In *Regester v. Indiana State Board of Nursing* (1998), the nurse had been writing prescriptions and forging the names of physicians she worked with on the prescription. This was done without their knowledge, and for medications that the nurse admitted she was using habitually. She was charged with practicing medicine without a license or authority and voluntarily submitted to a treatment program. Her case was reviewed by the board of nursing. Because of her fraudulent actions in obtaining prescription drugs and the fact that she was addicted to these same drugs, the board of nursing suspended her license indefinitely.

The hearing before the board was held within the prescribed time frame, and the board stipulated that she could reapply for her license in six months. They were to review her progress at the time of her reapplication for licensure. The nurse brought this case, alleging that the suspension of her license was an arbitrary opinion by the board, rather than a decision based on facts. The court, finding for the board of nursing, could find no evidence that this was an arbitrary opinion or a decision made purely as an opinion. The fact that the board stipulated that she could apply for relicensure in six months supported the thoroughness of the decision-making process in this court's determination.

In 1983, the Texas Court of Appeals upheld the suspension of a nurse's license for "unprofessional and dishonorable conduct . . . likely to injure the public" (*Lunsford v. Board of Nurse Examiners,* 1983, at 391) when the nurse failed to adequately assess a potential cardiac patient. The nurse argued that she had acted according to a direct physician order and could not have allowed admission for the patient to the hospital whether or not she had completed the patient assessment. The board, and subsequently the court, ruled that her failure to assess and implement appropriate nursing actions was within the adequate notice provision of the state nurse practice act and was within the specific rule promulgated by the Texas Board of Nurse Examiners. Other cases uphold this type of judicial finding, including *Scott v. State of Nebraska, ex rel. Board of Nursing for the State of Nebraska* (1976) and *Ex parte Smith* (1983).

The message for individual nurses seems to be twofold:

1. Nurses must carefully monitor the rules and regulations as they are published by the state board because, as practitioners, they will be held accountable for such rules and regulations.
2. Nurses must remain knowledgeable about standards of their specific communities because unprofessional conduct is frequently established by expert opinion of nurses as that which falls below the standard of care necessary for the protection of the public interest.

Penalties for Practicing Without a License

Most nurse practice acts allow for a fine or imprisonment for practicing without a license. Fines or confinement represent charges that may be pursued against the illegal practitioner. Generally, fines range from $50 to $500, and the term of confinement does not exceed 60 days.

Civil suits may also be filed against the nonlicensed practitioner. Such suits may be filed prior to, concurrent with, or after criminal charges. The civil suits are brought by those harmed by the nonlicensed practitioner and usually concern standards of care.

DIVERSION PROGRAMS

The nursing profession, through diversion programs, is showing a commitment to the rehabilitation of nurses who are psychologically unable to function or addicted to either drugs or alcohol. Rather than disciplining these nurses through the traditional discipli-

GUIDELINES: STEPS IN DISCIPLINARY PROCEEDINGS FOR NURSING MISCONDUCT

1. A sworn complaint is filed with the state board of nursing by an individual, a health care agency, or a professional organization, or the complaint may be originated by the board of nursing itself.
2. If there is sufficient evidence, the state board of nursing will hold a formal review of the matter, during which both sides may be represented by legal counsel and witnesses are called. Sometimes, a less formal meeting with the nurse and the state's attorney will occur before the formal board hearing.
3. Depending on the outcome of the hearing, the board may take disciplinary action.
4. The nurse may appeal the board's decision in state court. The court reviews the actions of the board, not the original act of misconduct by the nurse, and either upholds the board's action or grants a new trial.
5. Whichever side loses at trial level may decide to further appeal the court decision to the next highest court in the state. That court may also uphold the lower court's decision or reverse the decision, and the court may also reinstate the nurse's license if the nurse filed the appeal.

nary process, these nurses are diverted to rehabilitation programs. Diversion programs also allow the state board of nursing to protect the public while complying with the Americans with Disabilities Act of 1990 (ADA). See Chapter 20 for a more complete discussion.

A case that supports this compliance with the ADA is *Scott v. Beverly Enterprises-Kansas, Inc.* (1997). The nurse failed to mention in his interview for a charge nurse position in a nursing home that his license was restricted. He was not allowed access to narcotics or other mind-altering medications. The restriction had been imposed following a long history of trouble with narcotics addiction. When he finally produced and tendered his license to his employer as required by law, shortly after being employed, he was immediately fired. He sued for disability discrimination.

He claimed that he was a successfully rehabilitated drug abuser, having been "clean" and sober for 30 days before he reported to work at this job. The nurse's suit alleged that he was a "qualified individual with a disability," protected from employment discrimination by the ADA. The District Court for Kansas dismissed his lawsuit.

First, the court noted, a nurse with a restricted license who cannot have access to narcotics is not a "qualified individual with a disability" with respect to a nursing position for which the job description requires the ability to administer and/or account for narcotics and other mind-altering drugs on a daily basis. Second, this nurse was not a "successfully rehabilitated drug user," merely because he had been clean and sober for a 30-day period. He was still a current drug user, based on the court's 20/20 hindsight after he was fired. Unfortunately, for employers who must make difficult decisions, and for employees who have successfully overcome addictions, the courts have not clearly defined just how long persons with past problems must be in remission before they get protection from the antidiscrimination laws.

Voluntary alternatives to traditional disciplinary actions, *diversion programs* (sometimes referred to as *peer assistance programs*) entail attendance at group sessions such as Alcoholics Anonymous, Narcotics Anonymous, or counseling sessions; voluntary submission of urine samples for substance abuse; and special provisions by employers. Facilities that allow diversion program nurses to work within their units must comply with specific guidelines, generally the filing of quarterly reports with the board of nursing; working on general nursing units rather than emergency centers, intensive care units, and postanesthesia care units; working no overtime while in the program; and working daytime hours as opposed to night shifts. Some programs also forbid the recovering employee from assuming charge positions and from administering narcotics to patients.

Nurses may petition the board for reinstatement of full licensure after 12 to 24 months and must show compliance with the provisions of the program and the ability to perform in the workplace. The advantage of the program is that recovering nurses are allowed to fully be rehabilitative and productive in their chosen career as opposed to being denied licensure to work in the nursing profession. If nurses fail to comply with the provision of the program, the board of nursing institutes more traditional disciplinary provisions.

■ EXERCISE 11–3

Investigate the existence of a diversion or peer assistance program for substance abuse and/or mental illness within your state. If so, find out how it is administered and its success rate. How does the program assist these nurses? If there is no program, what does the state board of nursing do for nurses who have substance abuse or mental illness issues? Are the members of the board of nursing working to implement such a diversion program?

What are the ethical responsibilities of nurses who know that a coworker or peer has a substance abuse problem? Does the mere knowledge of such information increase one's ethical responsibilities to patients who may be cared for by the affected nurse? What are the ethical issues involved from the perspective of the entire profession?

ARTICULATION WITH MEDICAL PRACTICE ACTS

Medical practice acts are to physicians what nurse practice acts are to nurses: state laws that allow the individual to practice in a given discipline. Most medical practice acts define medicine as acts of diagnosis, prescription, treatment, and surgery. Some states' acts include only the first three elements.

Incorporated into the language or the intent of medical practice acts is *broad delegatory language,* enabling the physician to delegate to qualified and skilled persons the legal ability to perform certain actions and skills. This broad delegatory language, coupled with standing orders and protocols, has increased the functions of nurses while causing an overlap between nurse practice acts and medical practice acts—*articulation with medical practice acts.* For example, nurses in intensive care units and coronary care units may actually perform some medical acts because of valid standing orders and protocols. When the electrocardiogram rhythm strip shows ventricular fibrillation (a medical diagnosis), the nurse may inject lidocaine or perform electric cardioversion (a medical treatment).

Not all jurisdictions recognize and implement *standing orders* in the same manner. Some states allow standing orders to take precedent if the patient fits a particular classification (because the patient is in the coronary care unit, the coronary care standing orders are immediately valid), while other states mandate that the patient be seen by the physician and the standing orders be signed by a physician before they may be implemented. However a particular state approaches standing orders and protocols, they are a means of expanding the scope of nursing practice.

Another way of incorporating medical practice acts with nurse practice acts is by passing laws that make some functions common to both professions. For example, some state laws allow both nurses and physicians to diagnose and treat patients as long as the nursing diagnosis does not alter the patient's medical regimen. Other states allow nurses to evaluate and diagnose patients but not to treat them. The more modern nurse practice acts are beginning to allow for the treatment and diagnosis of patients by professional nurses.

A third approach to increase nursing's role is by *joint statements* between the disciplines of medicine and nursing. Joint statements are part of an evolving process and, in fact, are stopgap measures until states are able to develop and implement broader definitions of nursing practice. Joint statements thus serve as the basis for expanded nursing practice. There would be no need for joint statements if nurse practice acts were amended at the same time the joint statements were written.

SCOPE OF PRACTICE ISSUES

In recent years, the courts have attempted to settle scope of practice issues and the articulation of medical practice acts with nurse practice acts. As a general rule, negligence issues have caused scope of practice issues to be considered second, rather than first.

Scope of practice issues speak to the actions or duties of a given profession. The phrase "scope of practice" legally refers to permissible boundaries of practice for the health professional, and the scope of practice is defined by statute, rule, or a combination of statute and rule. For example, in a state that statutorily allows nurses to diagnose and treat patients, individual, licensed nurses may diagnose and treat the patients that they encounter. In a state that expressly forbids diagnosis and treatment as a nursing function, nurses would be practicing medicine without a license if they undertook to diagnose and treat the patient. In a state in which both nurses and physicians may diagnose and treat patients, the scope of practice issues overlap, and reasonable and customary practice become key issues.

From a legal perspective, scope of practice issues usually arise in one of two instances: (1) Some negligent act was associated with the scope of practice issue, or (2) the standard of care owed the patient is increased because of the medical or nursing action.

A landmark case that illustrates the first instance is *Cooper v. National Motor Bearing Company* (1955). One of the first cases that mandated nurses to be patients' advocates, this case concerned an occupational health nurse who failed to recognize the patient's signs and symptoms as being indicative of cancer, and who further failed to refer the patient to his physician for treatment. The court ruled that occupational health nurses should be able to diagnose sufficiently well to know whether to treat the patient or to refer the patient. Thus, diagnosis—outside the scope of nursing practice at that time—was called for in a limited scope. Note that the court failed to question or decide the greater issue of when such diagnoses were outside nursing's scope of practice.

Standards of care issues frequently arise with nurses in expanded roles, such as nurse anesthetists and nurse midwives. In these types of cases, the court usually applies a medical standard of care, reasoning that a greater duty is owed the patient because the nurse is performing actions that physicians typically perform. *Whitney v. Day* (1980) held that nurse anesthetists are professionals with expertise in an area of medicine and as such are held to those higher standards. *Mohr v. Jenkins* (1980) reached a similar conclusion.

One possibility for preventing scope of practice issue differences concerns the hospital or institutional policy and procedure manuals. Since nursing and technology are both fluid and dynamic, up-to-date policies and procedures may ensure that the nurse practices within nursing's scope of practice. Policies and procedures accomplish this goal because they tend to be much more narrow than nurse practice acts and give clarity to actions that the nurse may or may not perform. For example, the nurse practice act may have a standard that reads "makes judgments and decisions about the nursing care for the client or patient by using assessment data to formulate and implement a plan of goals and objectives." The hospital policy and procedure manual has a procedure that states, in laundry list fashion, how the patient assessment will be done, when it is to be performed, and specific guidelines for documentation of the patient assessment. The nurses' assessment data may be inclusive of broad hemodynamic measurements, and the hospital policy and procedure manual should also have a procedure for the performance of hemodynamic measurements and monitoring, arterial lines, thermodilution pulmonary artery catheter lines, and central lines.

Policies and procedures specify the allowable scope of practice within the given setting. They may be more narrow than the scope of practice stated within the nurse practice act, but they may not extend the nurse practice act scope of practice. The professional nurse must choose the nurse practice act over the hospital policy if there is a discrepancy. Professional standards and the nurse practice act mandate quality care for all patients. Professional standards and the state board of nursing's rules and regulations were the central themes reinforced in *Lunsford v. Board of Nurse Examiners* (1983).

To be of maximum value to nurses, the policies and procedures must be current. Ideally, they should be developed jointly by medical and nursing committees and updated periodically. The policies and procedures should be reflective of community standards. The committee developing them must be aware of the nursing role within the given community, and policies and procedures written so as to allow nurses to meet and exceed the public standard.

Institutional policies and procedures mandate that nurses remain current in their practice, either through continuing education classes, in-service education classes, or reading current journal articles. Institutional policies and procedures also help nurses prevent potential liability if they can show how individual nursing actions were within the policies and procedures and thus within the allowable scope of practice.

Other means for preventing scope of practice differences include:

1. Listing accepted procedures in the nurse practice act.
2. Requesting the attorney general's opinions for clarification on allowed or prohibited procedures.

3. Reviewing recent judicial decisions for definition of roles.
4. Requesting joint statements from professional organizations clarifying roles and practices.
5. Reviewing rules and regulations of the state board of nursing concerning the permitted scope of practice.

Scope of practice issues also concern an individual nurse's right to refuse patient assignments. The ANA *Code for Nurses* (1985) upholds the right of individual nurses to refuse assignments for ethical reasons. In 1996, the JCAHO acknowledged that right by adding a standard to both its hospital and home care accreditation manuals. The standard requires employers to establish policies and mechanisms to address staff requests not to participate in aspects of care that conflict with their cultural values or religious beliefs. The new standard requires each facility to:

1. Specify aspects of patient care that might conflict with staff members' values and beliefs.
2. Have a written policy on how requests to be excused from care are handled and make that policy available to all staff members for review.
3. Develop a process for deciding whether staff requests not to participate in care are legitimate and should be granted.
4. Ensure the safe delivery of care in instances in which a staff member's request to be excused is granted.

Courts have generally upheld the nurse's right to refuse an assignment based on religious beliefs. For example, nurses can refuse to care for and be a party to abortion, if abortion is against their religious tenets. Discrimination in employment on the basis of

GUIDELINES: REFUSAL OF CARE BASED ON RELIGIOUS AND MORAL PRINCIPLES

1. If you have such beliefs, inform your supervisor or nurse manager and request that you not be assigned to such cases. Beliefs normally do not occur in a relatively short time period but are deeply held and should be conveyed to management when you are hired.
2. If you are currently caring for a client and conditions suddenly warrant an aspect of care that you object to, alert your supervisor or nurse manager so that the patient can be reassigned or other alternative arrangements made.
3. Once you have accepted assignment for a patient's care, you are legally responsible for that care until the patient has been reassigned. If an emergency occurs, you must provide for the care as required, regardless of any personal objections you may have.
4. In a nonemergency situation, follow the institution's policy and procedures for refusing assignments. Whether a written policy exists or the institution is in the process of writing such a policy, be clear that your refusal is based on religious or moral grounds.
5. If there is a dispute about the appropriateness of your refusal, work with the nursing team, risk manager, or other appropriate persons to resolve the issue to everyone's satisfaction.

religion is one of the protected rights under Title VII of the Civil Rights Act of 1964. One of the early cases in this area of the law was *Kenney v. Ambulatory Center of Miami* (1981), in which an operating room supervisor was demoted after she objected on religious grounds to assisting in an abortion case. The court ruled that the center had a legal duty to accommodate Kenney's religious beliefs and ordered that she be reinstated to her former position.

A newer case in this area of the law illustrates that nurses may only refuse to assist with procedures that are against religious tenets. In *Larson v. Albany Medical Center* (1998), the nurse refused to participate in an elective abortion because of her religious beliefs. Instead of a simple refusal, the nurse used the request from her supervisor to assist in the abortion as an opportunity to launch into an argument about abortions. This action, said the court, was not protected by the religious beliefs of the nurse and was insubordinate behavior, and the nurse could be disciplined by the institution.

States today typically have *conscience clauses* that provide for more explicit protection. Forty-four states now have such clauses that allow for refusal of care based on moral or ethical beliefs, not just religious beliefs. There is also a Federal Conscience Clause (42 U.S.C. 3009.7), which applies to facilities that receive specific types of governmental funding, such as grants under the Public Health Service Act and Community Health Centers Act. As with the state clause, the federal clause protects only nurses who refuse to assist with abortions and sterilizations because of religious or moral beliefs.

 GUIDELINES: NURSE PRACTICE ACTS

1. Obtain a current copy of your state's nurse practice act. This may be done by writing or contacting the state board of nursing or the local or state office of the state nurses association. Additionally, copies may be available at a bookstore specializing in medical and nursing literature or at the local medical library.
2. Read the act carefully for the following elements, ensuring that you understand what each element means to you as a professional nurse:
   a. Definition of professional nursing
   b. Requirements for licensure
   c. Exemptions
   d. Grounds for disciplinary actions
   e. Criteria for out-of-state licensure
   f. Creation of the state board of nursing
   g. Penalties for practicing without a license
3. Know the state board of nursing rules and regulations regarding professional standards of care and dishonorable conduct. As you read the rules and regulations, know what each enumerated rule and regulation means, and apply each to your individual nursing practice.
4. Know who to contact and what to do if the nurse practice act is violated by licensed or unlicensed practitioners. Remember, you have an obligation to uphold the state nurse practice act and to see that others likewise uphold the act.

UPDATING NURSE PRACTICE ACTS

There are several ways to update individual nurse practice acts. Updating may call for a *simple revision* of the original act or a complete rewriting of the act. Because nurse practice acts are legislative enactments, any changes must be channeled through the state legislative body.

Amendments add to the nurse practice act or its regulation, usually giving nurses the needed legal permission to perform actions and functions that have become part of the community standard. Amendments have the same force of law as does the original act, and many state nurses acts are amended annually by state legislatures.

Redefinitions involve a rewriting of the definition of nursing and as such automatically change the force of the entire act, for example, rewriting the definition of nursing to include diagnosis and treatment or to clarify diagnosis to mean nursing diagnosis. The act is thus clarified for the practicing profession, the scope is broadened, and there has been no repeal or piecemeal amendment to the original act.

Application of sunset laws also aids in keeping nurse practice acts current. Such laws call for a review of the act at a fixed time, such as six to ten years after the enactment of the original act. The purpose of sunset laws is to force a periodic review by legislative bodies and thus prevent an act from becoming hopelessly outdated. The practice act affected automatically expires at the designated date. Most acts are updated during the legislative year immediately preceding application of the sunset law.

The dynamic process of nursing may also necessitate some needed action before the nurse practice act is actually revised or amended by the appropriate legislative body. Professional organizations, such as the state nurses association and the state board of nursing, may lobby for needed changes in the nurse practice act and thus force redefinition or amendment of the act. Or the state board of nursing may enact new rules and regulations to ensure that the nurse practice act meets the prevailing community standards. Thus, practicing professional nurses must do more than just know the original nurse practice act. They must remain current on newly adopted rules and regulations of the state board of nursing and understand the lobbying efforts of the professional organizations, because both may have great impact on an individual nurse's scope of practice.

CONTINUING EDUCATION FOR PRACTICING NURSES

Many nurse practice acts speak to **continuing education** for professional nurses. Whether mandatory or voluntary, the concept of continuing education centers around a means of ensuring that nurses remain current in their practice. With expanded and ever-increasing scope of practice issues and increased accountability for technical nursing skills and functions, nurses must maintain current and competent practice standards. Although state boards of nursing and professional nursing organizations continue to argue for and against mandatory continuing education, there is no argument that nurses must remain competent to practice in all practice settings.

Today, much of the debate has turned toward developing mechanisms to ensure continuing competency, rather than accrual of continuing education hours. Such validation of continuing competency would more greatly ensure that nurses are competent to care for specialty patients, to perform management roles, or to function as quality nursing educators. Merely attending a continuing education session or completing a short quiz about the content of a journal article does not ensure that the nurse remains competent, nor that any learning actually occurred. In fact, many continuing education programs are designed to explore broader topics such as alternative therapies or newer roles in nursing—issues that the nurse may not be able to readily incorporate into practice arenas. Continuing competency, it is hoped, will be able to better ensure that nurses are lifelong learners and that they remain competent, whatever their role or field in nursing. They will still attend sessions that explore new paths for nurses or revisit the history of nursing, and state boards of nursing will have a better benchmark upon which to renew licenses.

REPORTING PROFESSIONAL VIOLATIONS OF THE NURSE PRACTICE ACT

An important concept for professional nurses concerns the difficulty of knowing how and when to report a coworker for violations of the state nurse practice act. Reporting may be for unprofessional conduct, extended scope of practice, or substance abuse. Looking the other way may be easier, but all nurse practice acts require the reporting of violations of the act. Failure to report violators is usually grounds for additional disciplinary action. For example, most nurse practice acts also hold the nonreporting nurse to be in violation of the nurse practice act. Nurses who report in good faith are protected from defamation lawsuits, since they are required to report violations of the nurse practice act.

Unprofessional conduct includes, but is not limited to, failing to report to the board or the appropriate authority in the organization in which the nurse is working, within a reasonable time of the occurrence, any violation or attempted violation of the nurse practice act or duly promulgated rules, regulations, or orders.

The most obvious means of reporting violations is within the organizational structure. Most nurses have a direct chain of command to hospital or institutional administrations, and the staff nurse should report violations of the act to the immediate supervisor, usually a nurse-manager or charge nurse. Reports should be factual and documented in writing. Reports should include as complete a description of the violation as possible, listing other witnesses and giving patient names, as appropriate. The report should be complete so that administrative staff can investigate and gather additional evidence.

Administrative personnel have a duty to act on reported violations. They may insist that the violator receive counseling, further education classes, or supervised demonstrations to ensure quality nursing actions. The administrative personnel may not allow the violator merely to terminate employment, thus allowing the violator to change places of employment without ever seeking help or changing actions. In such a case, the hospital administrator has a duty to report the violator to the state board of nursing.

Individual staff nurses may also incur the same duty. Suppose an individual nurse reports a nurse for substance abuse or substandard nursing care to the appropriate supervisor. Later, the reporting nurse learns that the reported nurse has quit her job and is now working for another hospital within the same city (or state). Upon questioning the supervisor, the reporting nurse learns that no action was taken by the hospital administration. The nurse was merely questioned and voluntarily resigned. To date, the second hospital has not asked for a reference concerning the nurse. If there was sufficient evidence to report the nurse to your supervisor in the first place, then there is sufficient evidence to file that same report with the state board of nursing. An affirmative duty to report the nurse to the state board of nursing exists in such a case.

Reporting a violator of the nurse practice act may be done by writing to the state board of nursing, describing the substance abuse or substandard care, and including all pertinent documentation. Sign the letter, because anonymous complaints are summarily disregarded by most boards of nursing and administrators, and the nurse has not fulfilled the affirmative duty to safeguard nursing practice by an anonymous letter. Most state boards of nursing will preserve confidentiality. This last step usually proves unnecessary. Once the nurse is reported through the proper hospital channels, administrative staff will aid the nurse with necessary counseling, education, or rehabilitation.

NATIONAL PRACTITIONER DATA BANK

The *National Practitioner Data Bank (NPDB)* was created by the Health Care Quality Improvement Act of 1986 and became operational on September 1, 1990. Although primarily aimed at affecting the practice of medicine, the NPDB also affects the professional practice of nursing. The NDPB records three types of data:

1. Information relating to medical malpractice payments on behalf of health care practitioners.
2. Information relating to adverse actions taken against clinical privileges of physicians, osteopaths, and dentists.
3. Information concerning actions by professional societies that adversely affect membership.

The information is then available to health care facilities needing the information to verify credentialing of potential practitioners. Failure to report results in fines and penalties if mandatory reporting is identified.

The NDPB affects nursing from the perspective of advanced nursing practice because nurse practitioners, nurse midwives, clinical nurse specialists, and nurse anesthetists are subject to credentialing procedures similar to those named in the act as well as the quality of care at facilities that also employ nurses. Although far from a perfect system, it is the beginning of a nationwide effort to track and identify professionals found liable of malpractice or who have had professional memberships or professional privileges revoked.

CERTIFICATION

Certification is a form of credentialing that has both legal and professional implications. Certification indicates a level of competence above minimum criteria for licensure and verifies that an individual has met certain standards of preparation and performance.

Certification of individuals awards the person so certified with the right to use the title conferred by the certificate. Certification affirms the special qualifications that the individual has achieved in a defined area of clinical practice.

Many specialty nursing organizations offer certification to professional nurses. Some organizations mandate advanced degrees in nursing as prerequisites for certification, whereas others do not add this prerequisite. The ANA offers a wide variety of certifications as do other professional organizations. For example, the Emergency Nurses Organization, the American Association of Critical-Care Nurses, and the Association of Operating Room Nurses offer specialty certification in those areas of clinical practice.

■ EXERCISE 11—4

Interview personnel within your facility to see what certificates are required to hold various nursing positions within the facility. Is there a pay differential for certification? How are staff nurses (e.g., critical care nurses or emergency center nurses) urged to attain certification?

ALTERNATIVE THERAPIES

Alternative or complementary therapies, modalities not normally used by health care providers to treat illnesses such as therapeutic touch, biofeedback, guided imagery, acupuncture, and massage therapy, are becoming more popular in the United States as patients are beginning to understand and value their effectiveness. In 1992, the National Institutes of Health established the Office of Alternative Medicine to promote the unbiased study of nonconventional therapies. Even medical and nursing schools are beginning to offer such course work, usually as elective courses rather than required courses for a given degree program.

Athough the popularity for alternative therapies is increasing, few studies have been done to validate the efficacy of such therapies, and no uniform standards of practice exist to provide guidance to nurses and physicians who regularly use such therapies. Some states explicitly outlaw certain alternative therapies, whereas others require licensure or certain standards of education before performing certain alternative therapies. In Utah, for example, acupuncturists must meet a minimum level of training for licensure. In New York, nutritional therapists are permitted to practice under the Alternative Medical Practice Act (*Gonzales v. New York State Department of Health,* 1996).

Nurses must know their state law before performing such therapies. For example, in a state that does not recognize a certain therapy, the nurse who practices the therapy could be charged with practicing a therapy that is not legally authorized (Elder et al., 1997). If the state requires licensure in order to perform a specific therapy, such as massage, and the nurse does not have a license, the charge against the nurse will be practicing without a license. Sometimes, the practice is permitted, but institution policy forbids its usage. Thus, nurses must know and follow state law and individual institution policy.

Before considering the use of alternative therapies, remember a few basic issues. Patients should be fully informed about the alternative therapy before its use, including information about the value and projected outcomes. In some states, certain therapies are still considered experimental, so that signed informed consent similar to that used for any research subject is required. After using the therapy, ensure that it is fully documented in the patient record. Finally, answer fully any questions about alternative therapies.

The landmark case concerning alternative therapies in nursing is *Tuma v. Board of Nursing of the State of Idaho* (1979). In that case, Ms. Tuma, a nursing instructor who was in the hospital for the sole purpose of supervising nursing students, was asked by a patient about other therapies for cancer, including natural products such as laetrile and chaparral. At the patient's urging, Tuma agreed to return to the hospital later in the evening so that she could explain the alternative therapies to the patient's family.

The patient's daughter-in-law told the physician about the meeting, and he ordered the chemotherapy discontinued because he felt that the patient no longer wanted the chemotherapy treatments. After talking with Tuma, the family resumed the chemotherapy treatments, and the patient died shortly thereafter.

The physician reported the incident to the director of nursing, and the hospital subsequently filed a complaint with the state board of nursing, alleging that Tuma had interfered with the physician–patient relationship. The board suspended her license for six months, and Tuma appealed. The Supreme Court of Idaho held that Tuma's actions did not fall within the board's legislative language of "unprofessional conduct" and reinstated her license.

Hopefully, given the climate of informed patients and patient empowerment, such a case would never be filed today. But the case does give some direction. Ensure that patients are referred to the physician for questions they might have about their conventional therapy and the alternative therapy. Remember, if the patient or a family member asks about alternative practitioners, some states, such as California, prevent physicians from referring patients to alternative practitioners. If they do, they can be charged with "aiding and abetting the unlicensed practice of medicine" (Gates, 1997).

MULTISTATE LICENSURE AND MUTUAL RECOGNITION COMPACTS

Advances in the health care delivery system have resulted in a variety of changes. One of the changes with which all health care providers are struggling is the increasing use of new telecommunication technologies. The new technologies are raising questions related to the regulation of health care.

Historically, regulation of health professionals has been a state-based function whereby each state or territory regulates the health care workforce within its geographic boundaries. Thus, all health care professionals practicing within a state or territory are required to be licensed by the jurisdiction in which they practice. However, with soaring technologies, including telehealth consultation, telephone triage, and air transport nursing, to name but a few, practice is no longer limited by geographic boundaries.

The ANA (1998) described telehealth as the removal of time and distance barriers for the delivery of health care services and related health care activities. Communication technologies provide a means for health care professionals to practice across state lines. In many instances, this may mean providing services in states in which the professional does not hold a current license. Some telehealth employers and nurses may not consider the provision of telehealth services as "practicing," or may consider it unnecessary to obtain licenses in all jurisdictions in which patients who receive their services reside. Yet this provision of service in various states has posed a potential problem of widespread unlicensed practice and presents challenges for boards of nursing in states where patients receive services from nurses located in different states.

Many suggestions have been offered to address the regulatory problem raised by telehealth, such as institutional licensure, federal licensure, and the Ontario model. The Pew Health Professional Commission Report (1995) called for sweeping changes in the regulation of health professionals. The question that remains, however, is whether such changes are truly needed.

Over the past 10 to 15 years, the health care delivery system has been restructured significantly, including such changes as the transition from independent hospitals and facilities to integrated multistate delivery systems. During recent years, the pace of hospital system mergers and acquisitions have been such that few facilities remain unaffiliated with larger, integrated delivery systems. In fact, the number of multistate health care systems had grown exponentially, with some systems marketing their services throughout the entire country. Additionally, managed care has focused attention on revised mechanisms for payment of health care services. Fee for service is increasingly being replaced by capitation, resulting in shifts in the allocation of financial resources within many institutions. Finally, a well-documented movement away from acute care to home care and assisted living settings has altered the health care delivery system.

A second major factor is the explosion in technological advances. Telenursing, the compliment to telehealth or telemedicine, is but one piece of this technological explosion. The National Council of State Boards of Nursing (NCSBN) defines telenursing as "the practice of nursing over distance using telecommunciations technology" (1998a, at 256). Rather than the model used in medicine in which the physician is in direct consultation with other physicians, telenursing is the nurse in direct consultation with the patient(s). Some would argue that this is not a direct practice of nursing because there is no direct hands-on care and that telephone triage nurses typically use physician-approved protocols for reference. Nurse practice acts, in all states and territories, define nursing much more broadly than merely "hands-on" care; therefore, the consensus has been that a nurse utilizing the knowledge, skill, assessment, judgment, and decision making inherent in nursing education and licensure is indeed practicing nursing.

The third major driving force in this equation is the demand by consumers to be involved in decisions about their care. With the acceptance of the World Wide Web, people have unprecedented access to information about the diagnoses and treatments of illnesses, often without appropriate safeguards to determine the accuracy or efficacy of the information or mechanisms to determine whether the information is appropriate to their needs. The implications of this newfound consumerism are profound for the following reasons:

1. Consumers will demand care when and where they want it.
2. Consumers will demand to be included in all decisions about their own health care.
3. Consumers are increasingly comfortable using technology to access health care information.
4. Society will expect increased emphasis on health and healthy behaviors.

Any one of these three driving forces, taken individually, may have allowed nursing and health care delivery systems to maintain the status quo. Taken collectively, the question of whether current licensure, defined as the granting of legal authority to engage in certain practices, and nursing regulation, defined as the system of laws and rules that govern the practice of nursing, will be able to ensure public protection within a radically different structure arises.

A regulatory issue that must be addressed, given these new expectations, is how licensure should be addressed in the future. Currently, states do not have the ability to grant a nurse authority to practice in other states, although mechanisms are in place to allow nurses to request authority from other states. A second issue, as yet undecided by case law, is whether care occurs at the location of the patient, the location of the health care provider, or both. Many argue that since nursing interventions and consultation are generated by the provider, care must occur at the location of the provider. Others argue that it is unrealistic to expect consumers to figure out where the person providing electronic care is based, and thus care is defined by the location of the recipient of the care.

Because of such issues, in 1994, the NCSBN board of directors authorized the beginning of formal mechanisms to evaluate and analyze nursing regulation. After recognizing that the essential dilemma is that licensure remains state-based and state lines no longer bind nursing practice, identification of options and alternatives was initiated, with the goal being a state-based license, nationally recognized, and locally enforced.

A number of potential regulatory models were identified and evaluated against these criteria. Among these models were:

1. *Fast endorsement*—a speedy system for each state to approve each individual licensure application.
2. *Reciprocity*—a system in which states enter into agreement to accept each others' licensees without individual review.
3. *Corporate credentialing (institutional licensure)*—a conceptual idea that involves issuance of a credential by an employer. There is currently no legal authority in existence for such a model.
4. *The Ontario model*—a system that focuses on authorizing certain professionals to perform certain acts.
5. *Mutual recognition*—a system used primarily in Australia and the European Union, which facilitates states recognizing credentials as authorized by other states. Mutual recognition is sometimes referred to as the *driver's license model*.
6. **Multistate licensure,** a conceptual idea for issuing a "special license" to authorize multistate practice.

After extensive deliberation about developing a new multistate license, it was recognized by the NCSBN that the implementation issues were essentially the same as the implementation issues for mutual recognition, a regulatory system in which states enter into agreement to mutually recognize licenses of other states. The study group formed by the NCSBN determined that the regulatory system with the greatest potential of meeting the stated goal as an adaptation of mutual recognition. The advantages of the model as determined by the NCSBN are:

1. Authority is granted to practice in any state that has signed a **mutual recognition compact.**
2. Dual jurisdiction for discipline is established.
3. Uniform standards are not required.
4. The model can be phased in over time, so that not all states will be affected at the same time.

5. A central licensee information system, which does not currently exist, is a required component of the infrastructure.

The mechanism to implement the mutual recognition model of nurse licensure is the interstate compact. Not a new concept, interstate compacts were in existence in the early 1900s. Essentially, an interstate compact is an agreement between two or more states, entered into for the purpose of addressing a problem that transcends state lines. The compact must be initiated and voted on by the state legislative bodies to be enforceable. Like any other contract, modification of the compact is possible only by the unanimous consent of all party states. In addition, because the compact is law, it is subject to the traditional principles of statutory interpretation. An interstate compact gains its forcefulness because of its dual contract nature.

The mutual recognition model for the regulation of nursing that has been adopted by two states, Utah and Arkansas, specifically addresses four areas:

1. Jurisdiction
2. Discipline
3. Information sharing
4. Administration of the compact

The interstate compact was drafted in such a way that it is compatible with existing state laws. Although the compact supersedes state provisions that are in direct conflict, all provisions that are not addressed by the compact, or even in direct conflict, will continue to be in full force and operation. The compact was drafted to address only those issues essential to facilitate practice across state lines without unduly overriding state law.

Jursidiction

The compact calls for a nurse to be licensed in the state of residence or "home state." The nurse must meet that state's licensure requirements and abide by the nurse practice act and other applicable laws, as is currently required. A rather substantial consideration in using residence rather than primary practice site as the link for licensure was that simply defining practice site posed administrative difficulties. Additionally, using the primary practice site would mean that nursing practice would be defined in the compact, rather than in the state nurse practice act.

Other states (that have signed on the compact) where the nurse practices but does not live are called *remote states*. These remote states grant the nurse the privilege to practice in their state as a provision of the interstate compact. This is not an additional license. The nurse practicing in the remote state is expected to practice within the scope of practice and according to the standards of the remote state.

Discipline

Both the state of residence and remote state boards of nursing must be able to take disciplinary action in order to protect the citizens regardless of where the nurse or the citizen is located. Both the state of residence and the remote state may take action to limit or stop the practice of an incompetent or unethical nurse in their state. The state of residence acts against the license per se, using probation, suspension, or revocation as its mechanisms of action, and the remote state acts against the practice privilege granted by the compact by limiting or stopping the practice with a cease and desist order. Both processes include due process of law and the effects of both processes are essentially the same.

Under the compact, nurses have the authority to practice on an expanded scale, in greater numbers of states. Likewise, in the compact, the states' boards of nursing authority to discipline matches the nurses' ability to practice. The broadening of authority also necessitates the broadening of information sharing to allow state boards of nursing to discipline, if discipline is required.

Information Sharing

An essential component of the interstate compact is the ability for state boards of nursing to have timely licensure and discipline information on each nurse. The compact provides for reporting and maintenance of licensure and discipline information. The NCSBN has committed to improving the Disciplinary Data Bank system and to developing information for endorsement. The states that joined the interstate compact are expected to underwrite the expenses for creating this information system. When operational, the system will be a closed, secure system, primarily for use by the state boards of nursing, but with levels of limited access to comply with providing public information to employers and consumers as exists under the current regulatory system.

Administration of the Interstate Compact

The interstate compact provides for the ability to administer the compact through the formation of compact administrators. The compact defines these administrators as the head of the nurse licensing authority in each participating state. The compact also gives these administrators the authority to write rules and regulations to implement the compact.

The act specifies what will be regulated, and the state rules and regulations specify how the act will work. The compact is written in such a way as to define the legal framework with the allowance for detail to be addressed in the rules. Thus, the compact is often referred to as an overlay to the state nurse practice act.

Eight states introduced the mutual recognition interstate compact during the 1999 legislative session. The status of those eight states as of July 1999 includes:

1. Arkansas, where the act has been adopted and signed by the governor.
2. Iowa, where the compact is still in process.
3. Maryland, where the act has been adopted and awaits the governor's signature.
4. Nebraska, where the compact is still in the legislature.
5. North Carolina, where the compact has passed one state house and has been introduced into the other house.
6. Texas, where the compact has passed one house and has been introduced in the other house.
7. Wisconsin, where the compact is still in the legislature.
8. Utah, the first state to pass the compact, has now adopted and amended the compact.

Additional states are considering introducing the compact into the 2000 legislative year, and some states have declared that they will not introduce the compact in any legislative session. With the passage of the compact language in both Arkansas and Utah, it is likely that nurses from these two states may begin to practice in either state, using a single license from their state of residence, as early as July 1, 2000. Additionally, the eight states as listed have also agreed to begin a five-year evaluation of the compact, starting in the year 2000.

Many nurses have expressed major concerns over the mutual recognition model and the concept of multistate licensure, claiming that such a system is unnecessary and will undermine the professional delivery of competent nursing practice. Though positive in its initial description, there are many unanswered questions that continue to surface about the model, which must be addressed before the model is fully implemented. Among these concerns are the following issues:

1. *Standards within a state will be weakened.* California is the sole state that allows licensure for individuals who successfully pass the registered nurse and licensed vocational nurse examinations, but who have not graduated from formal nursing education programs. Under the language of the compact, these nurses who today cannot receive reciprocity licensure would be allowed to practice on the license they received in their state of residence. North Dakota, the only state requiring the baccalaureate degree for nursing licensure, would be unable to enforce this requirement on out-of-state nurses who practice in North Dakota.

   Many states have provisions in their statutes addressing continuing competency. Some require continuing education hours, whereas others require hours of practice. These provisions, just like the initial requirements for licensure discussed above, would not be enforced on out-of-state nurses. Thus, support of the model may inadvertently lead to policy decisions that the nursing profession does not support and that may not be in the best interest of consumers.

2. *Consumer protection is not improved with the model.* The developers of the mutual recognition model claim that it is needed to improve public protection by regulating telehealth and telenursing. The NCSBN cited the increased use of tecnhology to provide care to patients remote from the physical location of the nurse as the reason for development of the model and desire for rapid implementation across the country. When examined, however, the model offers no improved consumer protection sufficient to warrant such a major change in nursing licensure.

   Standards of practice and regulation have arisen from the individual states. Generally, these standards that improve consumer protection and advance the ability of nurses to provide care to the public start in one state and are adopted by other states as their value is understood, and adoption becomes politically possible. Thus, these standards are tested on a state-to-state basis. Nurses who are residents and licensees of a state working with their regulatory agency can exert the necessary pressure on their state legislature to make changes. One only has to look at the many consumer protections advocated by state nursing associations and ultimately adopted by their respective state legislatures through the state nurse practice act to see how this concept is applied in practice. It is unclear how this process can continue to be implemented when some nurses are exempted from the standards. Exerting the necessary political force on an agency of the federal government or some new regional entity would be much more difficult than dealing with one's state legislative body, with whom nurses in many states already have a relationship.

3. *State boards of nursing will be weakened.* The economic effect on state boards of nursing is enormous since the boards receive their revenues through licensure fees. These fees underwrite the board's ability to meet in a central location at given times during a calendar year; conduct site visits and approve schools of nursing for initial licensure and, in some states, advanced practice licensure; conduct investigations supporting the need for disciplinary hearings; support peer assistance or diversity programs for nurses with substance abuse issues; and conduct board hearings, among other activities. With the expected loss of revenue to a given state, state boards of nursing may be financially unable to continue to protect the public and regulate those who come under its auspices.

4. *Uncertainty about the centralized data base (NURSYS).* Throughout the discussions about the mutual recognition model, questions have addressed this centralized computer database. Now, after two years, there is still only limited information from the NCSBN about the centralized database, other than that it will be secure and that confidentaility will be maintained. The early language used about "significant investigatory information" has recently been defined, yet nurses and nursing organizations have pressed for this information since 1997. In 1998, due to pressure brought by the ANA House of Delegates, a beginning clarification on the issue was published:

> Current significant investigative information means: 1) investigate information that a licensing board, after a preliminary inquiry that includes notification and an opportunity for the nurse to respond if required by state law, had reason to believe is not groundless and, if proved true, would indicate more than a minor infarction; or 2) investigative information that indicates that the nurse represents an immediate threat to public health and safety regardless of whether the nurse had been notified and had an opportunity to respond [NCSBN, 1998, Article (d)(1)[d)(2)].

This new clarification represents a vast improvement over the initial language and addresses part of the concerns of nurses and consumers. It does not, however, address how security will be implemented and assured.

5. *Ability of state nursing associations to achieve optimal standards, working conditions, and compensation for nurses may be compromised.* This concern mainly arises in states where collective bargaining is authorized. Some states have statutes that preclude licensure in a new state solely for the purpose of participating in labor disputes or acting as a "strikebreaker." If nurses can practice in a state without being licensed in that state, the effect and enforcement of these statutes would be nullified. Although strikes by nurses are rare, they are usually precipitated by quality concerns and professional practice issues, not by pure economic issues. It would be unfortunate if nurses coming into a state to provide care during a strike offer lower-quality competency than those nurses they replace.

6. *Lack of clarity about dual disciplinary actions.* Under the compact, nurses can be disciplined for actions both in their home state and a remote state where care was delivered. Nurses are expected to know the standards of each state in which practice occurs and apply them to each patient interaction. When an incident occurs in which action by a board of nursing is necessary, the standards of two states may apply. In the event the board of nursing in the remote state decided to take action, those standards may be different than the standards of the state in which the nurse is licensed. Thus, a nurse may receive a sanction in one state for acting in a manner that is totally consistent with the nurse's own state laws and rules.

The compact, as currently written, requires each nurse to practice consistent with the laws and rules of the state in which the patient is located. While this concept is clear, what remains unclear is how each state that is a party to the compact will handle the same incident. For example, what remains wholly unclear is whether nurses, disciplined in one state, will have to defend themselves in all other states that are party to the compact. Or would nurses merely defend themselves in the state in which the patient resided and the state in which they have initial licensure?

7. *Exclusion of advanced practice nurses.* Some nursing groups have raised concerns that, because advanced practice nurses have been excluded from the language of the compact, the profession will be automatically divided into "basic nursing" as provided by registered nurses and licensed practical or vocational nurses, and "advanced practice nursing" as provided by nurse practitioners, nurse midwives, nurse anesthetists, and clinical nurse specialists. Such a split would reject the concept of nursing as a continuum of practice, contends the ANA (1997).

8. *Any major change in nursing licensure should be made by the profession and the consumers it serves.* An argument may also be made for the importance of the profession to be the driving force in any and all legislation that affects the profession. In many states, there exists a successful partnership between the board of nursing and professional nursing organizations. This partnership relies on each partner to act in concert with its mission whereby the public is protected and the profession is promoted, and to work collaboratively toward sound policy. Many of the individual state boards of nursing have questioned this mutual recognition model within their own organization and have been met with some of the same lack of answers and willingness to discuss the issues as have professional organizations. This leads many to believe that all avenues should be explored and evaluated before going forward with this present model.

There are other models that address concerns related to licensure that do not involve such a drastic change from the current state-based system. While evaluating these other models, some basic questions must also be answered, such as the provision of anonymous telehealth care, the affordability of such a model, and whether the license is tied to the location of the provider or the recipient. Once some of these basic issues are addressed and resolved, nursing can implement a system that is usable by nursing and acceptable to the consumers to whom care is committed.

SUMMARY

Credentials, proof of the qualifications of individuals, include both licensure and certification. The first licensure laws for nurses were, in reality, permissive registration acts. Today, all states and territories have nurse practice acts and administrative boards of nursing that regulate registered and practical nursing practice. Professional nursing organizations and licensing boards offer certification for nurses in advanced clinical practice roles and in advanced nursing practice.

Issues are arising that greatly impact the future of professional nursing, including alternative therapies and multistate licensure. These issues must be addressed by nursing so that the profession continues to be committed to consumers served by the profession.

AFTER COMPLETING THIS CHAPTER, YOU SHOULD BE ABLE TO

- Define licensure, including mandatory, permissive, and institutional licensure.
- Describe the process for creating state boards of nursing and their authority, including limitations on their authority.
- Describe the process of how state nursing acts define the professional scope of practice.
- Describe entry into practice in relationship to state nurse practice acts.
- Describe the legal ramifications of alternative therapies.
- Compare and contrast multistate licensure and mutual recognition compacts within the context of the current state-based licensure system.

APPLY YOUR LEGAL KNOWLEDGE

- How do nurse practice acts provide for consumer protection and for nursing advancement?
- Does the state board of nursing have the authority to change the practice of professional nursing?
- What are the main differences between licensure and credentialing? Is that difference crucial to consumer protection?
- How does multistate licensure both strengthen and weaken professional nursing?
- Are mutual recognition compacts needed in the professional practice of nursing?

YOU BE THE JUDGE

Barbara Hilder and Virginia L. White were employed by North Arundel Nursing and Convalescent Center, Inc. (the nursing home). The nursing home terminated their employment on the day after an emergency situation arose involving a chronically ill 69-year-old patient. The patient lived at the nursing home, on the unit known as Station Two Back. On October 6, 1994, Robin Anderson, LPN, was assigned to Station Two Back and was the nurse assigned to the patient. White, also an LPN and a nursing supervisor, was responsible that day for Station Two Back and for two other nursing units. Hilder, a registered nurse, was the Assistant Director of Nursing. Hilder had been employed by the nursing home since November 1989, and White had been employed there since August 1992.

At about 12:30 on October 6, a page was broadcast into the multipurpose room where White, Hilder, and Activities Director Sandra Osborne, Assessment Nurse Melinda Miller, and Food Services Supervisor Lorraine Hill were working on resident care plans. White answered the page, using the telephone in the multipurpose room and, after hanging up, asked those in the room if they had ever heard the patient complain of heart problems, specifically his "heart hurting." Miller responded that she had not and that such a complaint warranted further investigation. Hilder then asked White to help her retrieve supplies from Hilder's car for a bridal shower that was to be held in the nursing home later that day. According to Osborne, White replied, "We'll get the food out of the car, and then dial 911 when we get back." Hilder and White left the multipurpose room, laughing, and exited the building.

Concerned for the well-being of the patient, Miller went to check on him. When she arrived, she found him to have an elevated pulse, diaphoretic, and stating repeatedly, "My heart hurts." After consulting with the Director of Nursing Marcy Eley, Miller called 911, and the patient was transferred to North Arundel Hospital.

During the hearing, Hilder and White both denied that a page had ever come into the multipurpose room regarding the patient's condition. They stated that the first time the patient's status was brought to their attention was in the hallway as they were about to exit the building. There Anderson, the charge nurse, approached them to give them an update on the patient's condition. Hilder and White both testified that Anderson did not ask them for assistance or convey to them that the patient was in distress. They said that Anderson only wanted to tell them that she had medicated the patient for agitation in accordance with the physician's orders. Hilder testified that when she asked Anderson what the patient's vital signs were, Anderson said she had not taken them. Hilder told her to return and take the vital signs. Hilder and White then left the buiding and returned in about five minutes to discover that 911 had been called.

Anderson testified that when she approached Hilder and White she told them she thought the patient should be sent to the acute care hospital via 911 because he was complaining of chest pains. Although she did not use the word "emergency," Anderson testified that she conveyed to both nurses her opinion that it was indeed an emergency and the patient should be evaluated at an acute care facility. Anderson testified that Hilder and White told her to return to the patient's room and take his vital signs. Anderson said that White appeared to be confused when Anderson spoke to her in the hall and that it occurred to her later that White may not have been the one who responded to the page.

Both White and Hilder were terminated by the nursing home on October 7, 1994, following a brief fact-finding investigation.

Legal Questions

1. Did the agency err in dismissing the two employees?
2. Was there sufficient evidence to show that they were negligent in the care of this patient? Was it willful negligence?
3. What type of action should the board of nursing take against their licenses?
4. How would you decide this case?

REFERENCES

Aiken, T. D., and Catalano, J. T. (1994). *Legal, Ethical and Political Issues in Nursing.* Philadelphia: F. A. Davis Company.

American Nurses Association (1985). *Code for Nurses with Interpretive Statements.* Kansas City, MO: Author.

American Nurses Association (1998). *Competencies for Telehealth Technologies in Nursing.* Washington, DC: Author.

American Nurses Association approves a definition of nursing practice. (1955). *American Journal of Nursing* 55(12), 1474.

American Nurses Association (1980). *The Nursing Practice Act: Suggested State Legislation.* Kansas City, MO: Author.

American Nurses Association (1997). *Policy Series Backgrounder: Multistate Regulation of Nurses.* (No. 98-BAC-05). Washington, DC: Author.

American Nurses Association (1990). *Suggested State Legislation: Nursing Practice Act.* Washington, DC: Author.

American Nurses Association (1995). *Report of the House of Delegates: 1995.* Washington, DC: Author.

Burns v. Matzen, #93-100 (Iowa, 1994). In *Hospital Law Manual* 2(11), 4.

Colorado State Board of Nursing v. Hohn, 129 Colo. 195, 268 P.2d 401 (Colorado, 1954).

Cooper v. National Motor Bearing Company, 136 Cal. App.2d 229, 288 P.2d 581 (1955).

Elder, N. C., Gillcrist, A., and Minz, R. (1997). Use of alternative healthcare by family practice patients. *Archives of Family medicine,* 6(2), 181.

Ex parte Smith, 435 So.2d 108 (Alabama, 1983).

Federal Conscience Clause, 42 *U.S.C.* 3009.7.

Gates, R. P. (1997). Legal issues in alternative medicine. *Alternative and Complementary Therapies,* 4 (4), 143.

George, S., and Young, W. B. (1990). Baccalaureate entry into practice. *Nursing Outlook,* 29(8), 41–45.

Gonzales v. New York State Department of Health, 648 N.Y.S.2d 827 (N.Y. App., 1996).

Health Professional Shortage Area Nursing Relief Act, H.R. 2759 (1998).

Hill v. Pennsylvania Department of Health, Division of Nursing Care Facilities, 711 A.2d 1068 (Pa. Cmmwlth., 1998).

Hood, G. (1985). At issue: Titling and licensure. *American Journal of Nursing,* 85(5), 92–94.

Joel, L. A. (1995). Your license to practice: Variations on a theme. *American Journal of Nursing,* 95(11), 7.

Joint Commission for the Accreditation of Healthcare Organizations (1996). *1996 Accreditation Manual for Hospitals: Volume 1, Standards.* Oakbrook Terrace, IL: Author.

Kenney v. Ambulatory Center of Miami, 400 So.2d 1262 (Fla. App., 1981).

Larson v. Albany Medical Center, 676 N.Y.S.2d 293 (N.Y. App., 1998).

Leahy v. North Carolina Board of Nursing, 488 S.E.2d 245 (North Carolina, 1997).

Lunsford v. Board of Nurse Examiners, 648 S.W.2d 391 (Tex. Civ. App.–Austin, 1983).

Mississippi Board of Nursing v. Hanson, 703 So.2d 239 (Mississippi, 1997).

Mohr v. Jenkins, 393 So.2d 245 (La. Ct. App., 1980).

National Council of State Boards of Nursing (1998a). Boards of nursing approve proposed language for an interstate compact for a mutual recognition model for nursing regulation. *Multistate Regulation Task Force: Communique* 9(1), 256.

National Council of State Boards of Nursing (1998b). *Nurse Legislative Compact,* Article II, Sections (d)(1) and (d)(2).

North Dakota Century Code (1997). Chapter 43-12-1-09-3.

People v. Stults, 683 N.E.2d 521 (Ill. App., 1997).

Pew Health Professional Commission Report (1995). *Reforming Health Care Workforce Regulation: Policy Considerations for the 21st Century.* Author.

Regester v. Indiana State Board of Nursing, 703 N.E.2d 147 (Indiana, 1998).

Scott v. Beverly Enterprises-Kansas, Inc., 968 F. Supp. 1430 (D. Kan., 1997).

Scott v. State of Nebraska, ex rel. Board of Nursing for the State of Nebraska, 244 N.W.2d 683 (Nebraska, 1976).

Schoenhair v. Pennsylvania, 459 A.2d 877 (Pennsylvania, 1983).

Stevens v. Blake, 456 So.2d 795 (Ala. Civ. App., 1984).

Thompson v. Olsten Kimberly Qualitycare, Inc., 980 F. Supp. 1035 (D. Minn., 1997).

Tuma v. Board of Nursing of the State of Idaho, 100 Idaho 74, 593 P.2d 711 (Idaho, 1979).

Whitney v. Day, 100 Mich. App. 707, 300 N.W.2d 380 (Ct. App. Mich., 1980).

twelve

Advanced Nursing Practice Roles

■ PREVIEW

During the past few decades, several dynamic factors have helped to shape and support the trend away from traditional, hospital-based roles in nursing. Now the focus on advanced practice roles in nursing is even more critical, as the nation wrestles with health care reform and primary health care. The Health Security effort of 1993 emphasized security, savings, simplicity, choice, quality, and responsibility—all components of nursing's advanced practice roles in an environment where a legal system realizes the full potential of advanced practice nursing.

Nurses today require an advanced practice arena that will support advanced education and advanced skills. Increasingly larger numbers of nurses are becoming dissatisfied with traditional staff nursing roles and returning to educational institutions for higher degrees in nursing. The roles of the nurse anesthetist, nurse midwife, advanced nurse practitioner, and clinical nurse specialist continue to evolve and to expand, improving the quality of health care in a nation that is cost-conscious, yet demanding of access and quality care.

■ KEY CONCEPTS

advanced practice roles	prescriptive authority	reimbursement
scope of practice	admitting privileges	direct access
standards of care	antitrust issues	

HISTORICAL OVERVIEW OF ADVANCED NURSING PRACTICE ROLES

Early in America's history, women were fulfilling the role of autonomous nursing practitioners and midwives (Reverby, 1987). During the late 1800s, physicians usurped the autonomous health care deliverer status that prevails today. This was accomplished through state medical practice acts and the strong organizational structure of the American Medical Association (Stevens, 1971). The modern *advanced practice roles* originated in the late 1960s and early 1970s when the shortage of primary physicians led to new initiatives to meet America's health care needs.

Today, advanced nursing practice encompasses four distinct practice roles. The hallmark of these four roles is that nurses have the ability to combine the caring role of the nurse with the more traditional curing role of the physician. Advanced practice nurses are committed to providing basic health care to all people, ensuring health promotion and maintenance, increasing the quality of care, and ensuring the development of better informed consumers (Inglis and Kjervik, 1993).

Interestingly, roles that nurses performed became their occupational titles. While the public is now requiring a specialized body of knowledge rather than a title distinction, advanced practice nurses are still known by these occupational titles.

Nurse Anesthetist

Perhaps the oldest of the expanded roles in nursing is that of the *nurse anesthetist.* In 1878, Sister Mary Bernard was administering anesthesia at St. Vincent's Hospital in Erie, Pennsylvania. Agatha C. Hodgins served as a nurse anesthetist in Cleveland, Ohio, at the turn of the century and was as well known for her ability to administer anesthesia as she was for teaching doctors and nurses her techniques (Mannino, 1982).

The two world wars, as well as the Korean and Vietnam wars, increased the need for nurses proficient in administering anesthesia. Both at home and at the war front, nurses were needed to expand the numbers of medical personnel giving anesthesia. The physician shortage of the early 1960s continued to support the need for this expanded nursing role, and schools of nurse anesthesia quickly opened. Nurse anesthetists are registered nurses who have completed a formal program of clinical education in planning anesthesia care, administering anesthetic agents, and monitoring the anesthetized patient. Nurse anesthesia was the first expanded role in nursing to seek recognition via certification and education. Most state boards of nursing require that the nurse anesthetist be master's prepared, and all states require current certification through the American Association of Nurse Anesthetists.

Nurse anesthetists currently provide anesthesia for a variety of procedures, including dental, surgical, and obstetrical procedures, in acute care settings, outpatient facilities, and physician and dental offices. Nurse anesthetists administer approximately 70% of all anesthetics given the patients yearly, and they are the sole providers of anesthetics in 85% of rural hospitals (American Association of Nurse Anesthetists, 1998). Today, an increasing number of nurse anesthetists are responsible for pain management in preoperative and postoperative patients in a variety of clinical settings, including long-term care facilities and home care agencies. Practice agreements for the nurse anesthetist range from hospital employee to a member of a professional anesthesiology group to a member of a independent group of nurse anesthetists.

The first legal challenges to this role arose in the mid-1930s. In what has become a landmark decision, the California Supreme Court in 1936 held that the giving of anesthesia by nurses was not "diagnosing nor prescribing by nurses within the meaning of the California Medical Practice Act" (*Chalmers-Francis v. Nelson*, 1936, at 402). Thus, nurses could administer anesthesia within the scope of nursing practice.

Nurse Midwifery

The practice of *nurse midwifery* also has its origins in the late 1800s and early 1900s. At that time, midwifery was becoming a regulated, legally recognized profession through state legislative enactments. Prior to such state enactments, the art of midwifery was a lay art, practiced by women who learned about childbirth either by their own experiences or through others trained in the art. After the state enactments, the art of midwifery became more common among nurses. The first nurse midwifery educational program was opened in 1952 by the Maternity Association of New York City.

The practice of nurse midwifery still has some legal uncertainties. Authorization of nurse midwifery may be found in nurse practice acts, medical practice acts, rules and regulations specific to nurse midwives, allied health laws, public health laws, or a combination of any of these. Some states, depending on the jurisdiction, also regulate nurse midwifery through state agencies.

The practice of nurse midwifery involves the independent management of essentially normal prenatal, intrapartum, postpartum, and gynecological care of women, as well as the care of the normal newborns. Usually, there is a complex system for medical consultation and collaboration, and in some states all care is given with the understanding that a referral physician is always available. Some states allow the full range of practice, whereas other states allow more restrictive practices.

Working in acute care settings, freestanding clinics, health departments, ambulatory care facilities, and physician offices, certified nurse midwives offer holistic, continuous care; education of women through the childbearing period and years; and primary care for women's health needs. Certified nurse midwives offer an alternative childbearing experience to the low-risk patient, typically through active participation of the woman and her family through pregnancy and childbirth. All states require the certified nurse midwife to be master's prepared, and all require current certification.

As with nurse anesthesia, the earliest cases in nurse midwifery addressed the issue of whether the practice constituted the practice of medicine. The case of *People v. Arendt* (1894) held that the midwife in question was guilty of practicing medicine without a license. Since that time, nurse midwives have worked to develop a clear definition of the status of the role of nurse midwife.

Advanced Nurse Practitioners

Known in some states as nurse practitioners, the role is clarified as advanced nurse practitioners for states that refer to all registered nurses (RNs) as nurse practitioners. This role began in 1965 when Drs. Loretta Ford and Henry Silver began a program at the University of Colorado that placed nurses in new practice settings and increased their traditional patient care responsibilities. Goals of the advanced nurse practitioner movement were to prepare nurses with master's and doctorate degrees for independent expert practice, teaching, and clinical research. The advanced nurse practitioner has a client caseload much as a practicing physician carries a client caseload. Long-term goals included increased access to quality health care as well as expanded use of nursing skills in health assessment and maintenance. This increased access to quality health care was mainly seen in rural areas and was used by patients for whom minimal health care was available.

Today, advanced nurse practitioners typically are master's prepared nurses who have specialized in one or more practice specialties, including gerontology, women's health, family, pediatric, adult health, acute care, mental health, oncology, or emergency care nursing. Most provide primary care to low-risk patients and many serve as the primary health care provider. Practitioners work in acute care settings, ambulatory settings, occupational settings, college and university student health settings, long-term care facilities, assisted living facilities, public health departments, nursing service centers, physician offices, or their own offices. Some states require a master's degree to practice in the state, and 46 states require certification, either through the American Nurses Association or other certifying agency. There are in excess of 50,000 nurse practitioners in the health care delivery system today (Flanaghan, 1998).

Advanced nurse practitioners may work independently, in a peer relationship with physicians, or dependently under the physicians' standing or direct orders. Depending on the state nurse practice act, the nurse may independently diagnose, treat, and prescribe for a given patient or may be limited to managing the care of the patient as a delegated role. The advanced nurse practitioner may also be limited by the state nurse practice act to diagnose and treat, but not prescribe for the patient.

Legal challenges for this role have included scope-of-practice issues, much like the challenges to nurse anesthetists and nurse midwives. One case upheld the suspension of a nurse's license for treating patients without a physician's supervision (*Hernicz v. State of Florida, Department of Professional Regulation,* 1980). Other cases have upheld the right of the nurse to practice as an advanced nurse practitioner (*Sermchief v. Gonzales,* 1983, and *Bellegie v. Board of Nurse Examiners,* 1985).

Idaho was the first state to enact specific legislation defining and promoting the independent role of the advanced nurse practitioner in 1971. Currently, advanced nurse practitioners are authorized by their individual state boards of nursing through certification, licensure, official recognition, registration, or approval. Educational requirements vary depending on state requirements, with most states requiring advanced nursing degrees, demonstrated nursing skills, or additional nursing course work. The trend is toward requiring a master's degree for all advanced nurse practitioners.

Clinical Nurse Specialist

Although the major development of the *clinical nurse specialist* role occurred during the 1960s and 1970s as changes in nursing science and practice were rapidly developing, the first program was started by Rutgers University in 1954. The concept of a master's level nurse prepared as a specialist in a clinical area was a departure from the the traditional functional preparation in teaching, administration, and supervision. Clinical nurse specialists were developed for the purpose of improving the quality of nursing care provided to patients and their families during the 1960s when significant advances in technology paralleled advances in specialty medicine, primarily cardiovascular and pulmonary surgical specialties.

This role evolved in response to needs expressed by both patients and nurses. Traditionally, as nurses advanced in nursing, they moved away from the bedside and entered either administrative or educational roles. Nurses with advanced nursing knowledge and skills who tried to stay within staff positions usually failed due to the economics of the hospital because it was more cost efficient to have staff nurses and licensed practical nurses give direct patient care.

Several schools of nursing began to offer curricula that would allow nurses to obtain an advanced nursing degree and to specialize in clinical nursing so that they could continue to work directly with patients, family members, and staff. The specialization also allowed the nurse to be proficient in teaching, research methodology, and consultation. This allowed the clinical nurse specialist not only to be directly involved with patient care but to be indirectly involved with increasing the quality of nursing care throughout the institution.

Early clinical nurse specialists were described by a variety of titles, including nurse clinician, clinical associate, liaison nurse, and clinical supervisor. An early analysis of the core functions of the clinical nurse specialist identified them as:

1. The assessment of nursing needs of patients and the development of nursing care plans based on the knowledge of nursing, medical, biological, and social sciences and generally directing the provision of nursing care in the patient unit.
2. Consulting with others as needed and making appropriate use of available administrative and organizational channels in support and maintenance of nursing performance.
3. Setting and evaluating standards of clinical nursing practice in the unit.
4. Teaching to improve a clinical competence of the nursing staff on the unit and teaching patients.
5. Introducing nursing practice innovations and refining nursing procedures and techniques and investigating specific nursing practice problems (Georgopoulos and Christman, 1970).

In 1974, at the American Nurses Association (ANA) Congress for Nursing Practice, the role was defined as requiring a master's degree in nursing. Ideally, the clinical nurse specialist is a practitioner holding a master's degree with a concentration in specific areas of clinical nursing. The function of the clinical nurse specialist is unique with respect to the particular use of clinical judgment and skills regarding client care, service as an advocate when the client is unable to cope with a particular situation, and influence for change as necessary in the nursing care and in the health care delivery system (ANA, 1976). The clinical nurse specialist can also be certified through a variety of certification opportunities.

Traditionally, subroles of the clinical nurse specialist are divided into two broad categories: (1) direct care functions, which include expert practitioner, role model, and patient advocate; and (2) indirect care functions, which include change agent, consultant or resource person, clinical teacher, researcher, liaison person, and innovator. Today, the clinical nurse specialist's roles include those of case manager, coach, systems coordinator, and gatekeeper. In these newer subroles, the clinical nurse specialist is able to contribute to improved quality and cost-effective services during the transition of health care delivery from the acute care setting to community to integrated, seamless health care. The involvement of the clinical nurse specialist in these roles is predictable given the clinical nurse specialist's history as change agent. All of the roles may be independent, collaborative, or supervised, depending on the state nurse practice act.

The roles of the advanced nurse practitioner and the clinical nursing specialist are beginning to blend, so that it is often difficult to distinguish the two roles. Like nurse practitioners, clinical nurse specialists work in a variety of practice settings, including acute care settings, mental health settings, long-term care facilities, home health settings, public health departments, college and university student health settings, hospice settings, physicians' offices, and their own offices. Clinical nurse specialists may have independent prescriptive authority, provide primary or secondary care, and have admitting privileges. A trend is toward using a more general title to include both clinical nurse specialists and nurse practitioners as their roles are so similar in practice settings today. In 1996, there were 7,082 nurses with the credentials of both the clinical nurse specialist and the nurse practitioner compared to 1,909 in 1992 (Moses,1992).

■ EXERCISE 12–1

Investigate the use of advanced practice nurses within your area. Do such roles exist? How do these nurses function in the community and hospital health care delivery systems? Is the state nurse association and/or other professional organizations working to expand the role of these nurses?

LEGAL LIABILITY OF EXPANDED NURSING ROLES

In some ways, professionals practicing in expanded nursing roles have dual legal liabilities:

1. They are licensed to practice by the state board of nursing and are accountable for its rules and regulations.
2. They have acquired advanced standing under the delegatory language of the state medical practice act or have acquired advanced standing under the state nurse practice act, public health laws, or other state laws, and are accountable for this independent or interdependent role.

Several questions arise from a legal perspective regarding the potential liability of the practitioner in an expanded role. Most of the questions come under the overall classification of standards of care and scope of practice.

SCOPE OF PRACTICE

A major legal issue is the permissible *scope of practice,* which refers to the permissible boundaries of practice for a health professional, as defined by statute, rule, or a combination of statute and rule, and which defines the actions and duties of nurses in these roles. Physicians were the first professionals in virtually all states to define their scope of practice, and by the 1800s had defined medicine to include curing, diagnosing, treating, and prescribing. Physicians also ensured against interference in their practice by incorporating provisions that made it illegal for anyone not licensed as a physician to perform acts included in their definition.

Nurses gained legal control of their profession in the early 1900s. By 1930, all states had passed nurse practice acts. *Autonomous practice* was defined as supervision of patients, observation of symptoms and reactions of patients, and accurate recording of patient information. The remainder of the nursing scope of practice was defined as *complementary* (interdependent) or dependent to the physician. With the advent of advanced nursing practice, it became apparent that such a definition of scope of practice would prevent independent practice, and several courses of action were undertaken to remedy the situation.

One means of increasing the scope of practice was by amending or totally altering state nurse practice acts. States began to accomplish this by promulgating rules and regulations to expand the scope of practice. In 1971, Idaho became the first state to broaden its definition of nursing to statutorily include diagnosis and treatment as part of the scope of practice of the advanced nurse practitioner. Although the intent of the statute was clear, the statute also required that acts of diagnosis and treatment be authorized by rules and regulations jointly developed by the boards of nursing and medicine, and that all institutions employing advanced nurse practitioners develop policies and guidelines for their practice. This latter requirement resulted in constraints in their practice.

Currently, all states and the District of Columbia have enacted legislation regarding the advanced nurse practitioner's scope of practice. The majority of states' statutes require that the advanced nurse practitioner have a sponsoring or supervising physician, greatly diminishing their scope of practice, though the trend seems to be moving toward a more collaborative, nonsupervisory role. Twenty-five states and the District of Columbia have removed statutory requirements for either physician supervision or mandated collaboration, thus allowing full independent practice by nurse practitioners (Flanaghan, 1998).

A second means of expanding the legal scope of practice is by court decisions concerning the nature of the advanced nurse practitioner's role. Two significant decisions have been made in this area, and they remain the landmark cases today. *Sermchief v. Gonzales*, a 1983 Missouri Supreme Court decision, held that the Missouri legislature, when it enacted the nurse practice act, had intended to avoid statutory constraints on the evolution of new nursing roles and thereby gave advanced nurse practitioners practice authority through the broad wording of professional nursing. In actuality, the court found that professional nursing in that jurisdiction had the right to practice within the limits of their education and experience.

In *Sermchief*, a group of advanced nurse practitioners were routinely providing gynecological care, including routine Pap smears, pregnancy testing, and birth control measures, pursuant to protocols jointly developed by nursing and supervising physicians. The Missouri Nurse Practice Act did not require direct physician supervision, but defined professional nursing in more general terms, according to specialized education, judgment, and skill. A group of physicians, predominantly those whose practice had declined because of the advent of the advanced nurse practitioners' practice, brought suit claiming that the nurses, rather than practicing nursing, were instead engaged in the illegal practice of medicine. In a lengthy decision, the court held that the advanced nurse practitioners were indeed practicing within the scope of their education and skills and within the scope of nursing as the Missouri legislature had intended.

Sermchief was a significant decision for nursing. A second significant decision was *Bellegie v. Board of Nurse Examiners* (1985). In that case, the Texas Medical Association and the Texas Hospital Association challenged the authority of the Texas Board of Nurse Examiners to promulgate rules and regulations regarding advanced nursing practice within the state. In finding for the Board of Nurse Examiners, the court held that the Board's regulatory authority was not limited to regulating titles, but extended to regulating the activities and education of nursing within their jurisdiction.

These two decisions clearly began the establishment of nursing's legal status as a full-fledged, independent profession. If nursing is to continue to expand as a truly autonomous professional role, then nurses must work at state and national levels to promote the most effective use of the advanced practice nurses.

At the federal level, scope-of-practice issues are tied to reimbursement issues. One of the most significant pieces of legislation for advanced practice nursing was the passage of Medicare reform in 1997 (Public Law 105-33). That piece of legislation included Medicare reimbursement for both nurse practitioners and clinical nurse specialists, regardless of geographic setting. Effective January 1, 1998, services are reimbursable by Medicare, if the same services were eligible for reimbursement if provided by a physician and the services are within the scope of practice of the nurse practitioner and the clinical nurse specialist. The true significance of the decision was to disavow the payment for services only if they were in "rural settings," narrowly defined to mean a nonmetropolitan statistical area county. Also significant is that the nurse practitioner or clinical nurse specialist may function in a variety of clinical settings, including nursing homes, which had previously been a restricted area for reimbursement. Finally, the legislation was significant in that the "collaborative" practice deferred to collaborative as defined by state nurse practice acts, rather than the more restrictive language of the federal government (Rules and Regulations, 1998).

A positive outcome is that this piece of legislation also gave nursing educational requirements not set by state law. Effective January 1, 2003, both certification and an earned master's degree will be required for all nurse practitioners and clinical nurse specialists to be eligible for direct reimbursement for serving Medicare patients.

One limitation in the legislation is the reimbursement for nurse practitioners and clinical nurse specialists at 85% of the physician reimbursement for the same service. While this is basically the same payment provision that existed under the current insurance codes for reimbursement in states that allowed such reimbursement, it continues to devalue the service of the nurse who is providing identical services as their physician counterparts (Public Law 105-33, 1997).

Interestingly, the passage of the Medicare Reimbursement Reform Bill as part of the Balanced Budget Act of 1997 addressed (though not necessarily satisfactorily) the three main issues that advanced practice nurses have continually included in their lobbying efforts:

1. Elimination of restrictions that allow nurses to practice only in certain geographic settings (for example, rural and undeserved areas)
2. Elimination of requirements that make nurses dependent on physician supervision or collaboration
3. Establishment of requirements that same services should result in same payments by insurers and third-party payors, regardless of the specialty or profession of the provider.

At the state level, nurses must continue to work to ensure that the sole authority for advanced nursing practice is placed within the board of nursing, and that the board has the authority to promulgate rules regarding the practice of advanced practice nurses, passage of statutory definitions of advanced nursing practice, and granting of clinical and admitting privileges to advanced nurse practitioners (Safriet, 1992).

Malpractice Issues

Areas in which advanced practice nurses have incurred liability include:

1. Conduct exceeding the scope of expertise that causes harm (*Gugino v. Harvard Community Health Plan et al.*, 1983).

2. Conduct exceeding physician-delegated authority that results in harm (*Tatro v. State of Texas*, 1983).
3. Independent practice in a state where advanced nurse practitioners must have a sponsoring physician (*Hernicz v. State of Florida, Department of Professional Regulation*, 1980).
4. Failure to refer when the advanced nurse practitioner's skills are exceeded (*Lane v. Otis*, 1982, and *Azzolino v. Dingfelder*, 1994). The failure to refer is the most prevailing cause of action, and advanced practice nurses must refer patients in a timely manner when they see that their expertise will soon be exceeded.
5. Negligence in the delivery of health care (*Goodliffe v Parish Anesthesia Associates*, 1995).
6. Failure to adequately diagnose (*Topp v. Logan*, 1990; *Adams v. Kreuger*, 1993; and *Jenkins v. Payne*, 1996).

Lawsuits involving advanced nurse practitioners raise inevitable questions about whether the nurse involved was performing an activity that was:

1. Generic to nursing and thus within the nursing scope of practice.
2. A medical activity that is permitted by law as germane to the advanced practice nurse's scope of practice.
3. A medical activity not within the scope of practice of the advanced practice nurse.
4. A nursing activity that overlaps with a medical activity.

Additional questions center on the elements of malpractice such as the duty owed the patient, breach of that duty as owed, foreseeability, causation, and damages.

If the activity involved in the lawsuit was purely nursing function, then nurses will serve as expert witnesses in determining the standard of care owed the patient. If the activity was a medical function not allowed within the nurse scope of practice, the expert witness will testify to medical standards of care. As the next section illustrates, the courts and nursing are still struggling with standards of care when the activity involved is a nursing function that overlaps with a medical function as opposed to an activity allowable within the scope of the advanced practice nurse.

STANDARDS OF CARE

The question that arises frequently in negligence cases is what legal *standard of care*, or duty of care, is to be applied to nurses in expanded roles. Nurses who perform functions and actions traditionally recognized as medical should be familiar with court decisions concerning standards of professional care. Earlier cases mainly held that nurses in expanded roles are held to the medical standard of care (*Hendry v. United States*, 1969, and *Harris v. State through Huey P. Long Hospital*, 1979). *Whitney v. Day, M.D. and Hurley Hospital* (1981) held that nurse anesthetists are professionals who have expertise in an area akin to the practice of medicine. Because their responsibilities lie in an area of medical expertise, the standard of care is to be based on the skill and care normally expected of those with like education and expertise. A 1925 case (*Olson v. Bolstad*) disallowed any liability on the part of the physician involved and found that the nurse midwife was solely negligent. While that court also set the medical standard as the standard of care for the midwife, it specifically stated that the physician incurred no liability in relying on the midwife to perform her duties properly.

Fein v. Permanente Medical Group (1985) was one of the first cases to disagree with this line of holdings. In *Fein*, the court set the standard of care for the advanced nurse practitioner. In that case, a patient was misdiagnosed by an advanced nurse practitioner and, subsequently, by a physician as having muscle spasms rather than a myocardial infarction. After examining the patient and obtaining a history, the nurse diagnosed muscle spasms and gave the patient a prescription for Valium. The court labored to find that the advanced nurse practitioner was held to the standard of a nurse practitioner performing diagnosis and treatment, not to the standard of a physician performing diagnosis and treatment. Specifically, the court held that "the examination or diagnosis cannot be said—as a matter of law—to be a function reserved to physicians rather than to registered nurses or nurse practitioners" (at 140). Therefore, a physician working with advanced practice nurses or an advanced nurse practitioner functioning in a similar setting would be qualified to establish the standard of care.

Another case regarding professional standards of care was *Paris v. Kreitz* (1985), which concerned the standard of care of a physician's assistant. The court addressed the liability of the physician's assistant and concluded that "the argument that physicians' assistants are subject to the same standard of care as physicians is without merit" (at 244). Citing the standard jury instruction, which states that a health care provider is subject to the standard of practice among members of the same health care profession with similar training and experiences and situated in the same or similar communities, the court concluded that it was clear that a physician's assistant was not subject to the same standards as a medical doctor. Had the defendant been an advanced nurse practitioner, the conclusion of the court would have been the same: The advanced nurse practitioner is not subject to the same standards as medical doctors.

Court cases continue to uphold standards of care when applied to advanced practice nurses. In *Ray v. Anesthesia Associates of Mobile* (1995), a nurse anesthetist was liable for the failure to correctly place an endotracheal tube, resulting in the death of the patient. In *Goodliffe v. Parish Anesthesia Associates* (1995), the nurse anesthetist was liable for the faulty endotracheal tube placement that resulted in the patient's dislocated jaw. In *Jenkins v. Payne* (1996), a nurse practitioner was liable for not recognizing the symptoms of breast cancer, resulting in the patient's death from metastasis.

Recent court cases may also herald new areas of liability for advanced practice nurses include *Cohen v. State Board of Medicine* (1996) and *Ruggiero v. State Department of Health*, (1996). Though both of these cases involved physicians' licenses, they address issues that could equally affect advanced practice nurses. In *Cohen*, a physician had prescribed controlled substances susceptible to abuse, including narcotics, barbiturates, and benzodiazepines, without seeing the patient and without determining the medical necessity and appropriateness of the medications. One patient, an admitted addict, received prescriptions for Dilaudid for himself, his wife, and his son and daughter. The wife came into the office but was never examined. His children were never seen in the office. Another patient received a prescription for Esgic over the telephone one day and was admitted for detoxification and chemical dependency treatment the next day. The physician's license was revoked for a five year period.

In *Ruggiero*, the physician's license was revoked for failure to maintain proper patient records and improper infection control practices. Records consisted of a journal in which the physician noted patients he had seen that day. At a later date, he relied on his memory to write entries about the patients into their medical records. Food and medications were improperly stored together in the same refrigerator, the sink designed for handwashing was filthy, and used instruments were left on open trays without disinfectant.

A final question about advanced nursing practice and standards of care is who may serve as an expert witness in establishing the prevailing standard of care of specific professions. The rule that a medical expert witness must be from the same medical specialty as the physician involved in the case has been eroded (*Samii v. Baystate Medical Center,* 1979). In one California case, an obstetrical nurse practitioner was permitted to establish the prevailing standard of care in a case that concerned an obstetrician. That was because the services provided were the same as those that could be provided legally by an obstetrical nurse practitioner (Marco, 1983). Such findings assist in reassuring the American public that the quality of care of physicians and advanced nurse practitioners is equal.

■ EXERCISE 12–2

Reread your state nurse practice act. Is there a provision for advanced practice in either the act or the board of nursing's rules and regulations? If there is no provision, is the board of nursing working on such a provision (or rules and regulations) to create such a role? How can the board of nursing strengthen the scope of practice for advanced practice nurses?

PRESCRIPTIVE AUTHORITY

Prescriptive authority is central to independent practice by advanced practice nurses. Only 50 years ago, most drugs not classified as narcotics were available as over-the-counter medications, and nurses worked independently with physicians in recommending such medications (Pearson, 1992). This was changed by the 1938 Federal Food, Drug, and Cosmetic Act. The movement away from consumer control to physician control of education strengthened the medical profession by increasing its social privilege and economic power (Pearson, 1992).

Legal issues in this area involve the extent of professional decision making allowed the advanced practice nurse and the range of drugs from which the advanced practice nurse may select. States may allow autonomous prescriptive authority while imposing written protocols or may mandate formularies that dictate which medications may be prescribed. In states with written protocols, nurses frequently are prevented from prescribing a full range of medications, and the scheduled days of therapy are usually short. In such states, it is not uncommon to see an advanced practice nurse prescribe three days of antibiotic therapy as opposed to the more effective 7- to 10-day course of therapy. A written formulary of medications, usually filed with the state board of nursing, is another means of limiting the range of medications that advanced practice nurses can prescribe. Some states further restrict prescriptive authority by requiring physician supervision or direction in the area of medication selection or by restricting prescriptive authority to certain geographic areas (rural or underserved areas) or practice settings (skilled nursing centers).

With the recent passage of the bill in Illinois granting title recognition and prescriptive authority, all 50 states and the District of Columbia allow some degree of prescriptive authority for nurse practitioners. The independence of the nurse practitioners' prescriptive authority varies greatly, and in some states words other than "prescribe" are substituted. In the majority of states, physician collaboration is required for nurses to prescribe. In 17 states and the District of Columbia, nurses have full independent prescriptive authority, including authority for prescribing controlled substances. In one state (Kansas), nurses may "transmit" medication orders. In one state (California), nurses may "furnish" medications. In two states (Georgia and Michigan), physicians may delegate authority to prescribe under protocols, and in one state (Montana), physicians must review a percentage of nurse practitioners' charts as part of a quality assurance program.

A growing number of states also allow prescriptive authority to be extended to clinical nurse specialists. Currently, nine states do not allow clinical nurse specialists to prescribe medications, either independently or with physician supervision. The remaining 41 states and the District of Columbia allow some degree of prescriptive authority, generally mimicking the authority of the nurse practitioner in the same state (Carson, 1997).

Actions needed at state level to improve prescriptive authority include statutory amendments stating that advanced practice nurses may prescribe scheduled and non-scheduled medications without the necessity of a sponsoring physician and that prescriptive authority is included in the advanced practice nurses scope of practice, regardless of the practice setting or area. Amendments to state nurse practice acts should eliminate any language on written protocols, because the primary purpose of such protocols is to limit the prescriptive authority of advanced practice nurses.

ADMITTING PRIVILEGES

Admitting or hospital privileges are becoming more of an issue. *Admitting privileges* are granted by individual facilities, and the extent of the privilege varies from allowing the practitioner to visit patients to permitting direct admission and entries in the medical record. Admitting privileges are facility controlled and no state or federal legislation is involved.

Admitting and hospital privileges are an area of major concern to certified registered nurse anesthetists since their practice setting is primarily the hospital setting. *Antitrust issues* are central and arise when health care professionals seek access to health care facilities controlled by physicians with whom they compete. Because most hospital credentialing committees that vote on extending hospital privileges to qualified practitioners are composed exclusively of physicians, nurse anesthetists must constantly fight this battle.

Antitrust issues arise whenever:

1. There is exclusion of a class (here nurse anesthetists) from membership on the medical or hospital staff.
2. There are questions about the fair market value of a service.
3. There are attempts by one society or association to restrict its members use of a second class of practitioners.

The issue that the courts must decide is whether the antitrust laws can eliminate professional group boycotts motivated by anticompetition interests, while preserving legitimate professional self-regulation aimed at maintaining the competence and professional conduct of a particular profession.

The courts are now beginning to assist advanced practice nurses to secure hospital privileges (*Bahn v. NME Hospitals*, 1987, and *Wrable v. Community Memorial Hospital*, 1987). However, these issues may need to be addressed on the local level rather than the state and federal levels. Perhaps the biggest hurdle to overcome is the prevailing practice of allowing advanced practice nurses to admit patients to an institution under the name of a supervising physician. This practice decreases the autonomy of the advanced practice nurse while ensuring that only physicians are credentialed by the institution.

REIMBURSEMENT ISSUES

Reimbursement issues and practices are a major stumbling block to expanded practice. Several issues come under this heading, including equal pay for equal services, direct reimbursement by third-party payors, and the range of services for which reimbursement will be paid. Advanced practice nurses will not be able to practice independently until these issues are addressed and solved.

Reimbursement for advanced practice nurses is affected by state and federal regulations. To secure equitable reimbursement for advanced practice, nurses must work for change at the federal and state levels. Federal action is needed to expand reimbursement to all services provided by advanced practice nurses, to eliminate regulations that narrowly circumscribe direct reimbursement, and to require that the same services are compensated by the same payment. State regulations are needed to prevent health insurance or health care service plans from discriminating against advanced practice nurses and to extend Medicaid reimbursement to advanced practice nurses' services.

■ EXERCISE 12–3

Investigate reimbursement issues and prescriptive authority for advanced practice nurses within your state. How do these two issues affect the overall ability of nurse practitioners to start their own practice? Which of these two issues has the most impact on nurses in your area?

DIRECT ACCESS TO PATIENT POPULATIONS

Physicians have traditionally been the gatekeepers of the health care delivery system. *Direct access* to alternate providers, such as advanced practice nurses, has been curtailed by medicine, regulators, and accreditors, including state health departments and the Joint Commission on Accreditation of Healthcare Organizations. Nurses have only recently taken definitive action for discharge planning, including when the patient is released from the health care facility.

Some of the current proposals for allowing advanced practice nurses direct access to patient populations concern managed care corporations. Today, managed care corporations retain the power of the physician as the gatekeeper, but negotiations for advanced practice nurses in these corporations is advancing in some areas of the country. These negotiations are being undertaken in light of the current research on patient outcomes and who provides more optimal services in relationship to cost containment and patient satisfaction. Such research needs to continue if advanced practice nurses are to be allowed more direct access to patients.

STATUTE OF LIMITATIONS

Statutes of limitations dictate that actions must be heard within a prescribed number of years or be barred from ever being heard. Most states impose a two-year limitation on medical malpractice suits, although some states have a one-year limit. Whatever the jurisdiction, there seems to be the same statute of limitations for all health care providers in the state.

■ EXERCISE 12—4

Are there differences in the application of ethical principles for advanced practice nursing? The legal system teaches that the standards of care are different for nurses with greater education and experience. Is this also true for ethics? Take a single ethical principle and show how it is the same or different for staff nurses as opposed to advanced practice nurses.

SUMMARY

The major legal challenges involving advanced practice nurses have centered on scope of practice, standards of care, and malpractice issues. Legal issues that must be addressed in the future if advanced practice nurses are to be allowed to fully practice include issues directed at reimbursement, prescriptive authority, admitting privileges, and direct access to patient populations. For advanced practice nurses to function to their full potential and provide the quality, compassionate care demanded by the American public, nurses must mount campaigns for change at state and federal levels. Advanced practice nurses must be enabled to deliver independent health care services to all parts of the United States, rural and urban, in all practice settings, and must be compensated fully for their services. This will ensure that America's underserved and forgotten patients also receive the quality health care to which they are entitled.

AFTER COMPLETING THIS CHAPTER, YOU SHOULD BE ABLE TO

- Define the roles of advanced practice nurses, including nurse anesthetists, nurse midwives, advanced nurse practitioners, and clinical nurse specialists.

GUIDELINES: NURSING IN EXPANDED PRACTICE ROLES

1. The nurse in an expanded practice role must first recognize that along with the role's increased autonomy also comes increased accountability and liability. While nurses are always accountable for their actions and omissions, the nurse in an expanded practice role adopts a higher standard of care for the services and actions performed.

2. Function and accept patients and responsibilities within your field of expertise and within your allowable scope of practice. Review carefully the state nurse practice act, medical practice act, pharmacy act, and public health laws for scope-of-practice issues. Review and understand the rules and regulations promulgated by the state board of nursing for allowable scope of practice.

3. Understand the allowable scope of practice if your state requires that you function under the delegatory language of the state medical practice act. Be sure that you do not exceed any physician-delegated responsibilities.

4. Ensure that you have obtained valid informed consent and have obtained such consent from the proper person(s) before proceeding to care for or treat a particular client. As with physician malpractice suits, this area is frequently cited in nursing malpractice suits.

5. Be sure the client knows of your status as a nurse in an expanded role and understands that you are not a physician. Impersonation of a physician is fraud and opens you to licensure suspension or revocation as well as to other civil lawsuits.

6. Seek assistance from other specialists and physicians when circumstances exceed your scope of knowledge and expertise. Failure to refer the patient to a physician or more qualified advanced nurse practitioner when your skills are exceeded or when complications arise has been the basis of previous lawsuits. The failure to refer in a timely manner may place you in the position of acting beyond the allowable scope of practice for your expanded role.

7. Do not practice independently unless your state recognizes independent practice by the advanced nurse practitioner. Many states require a supervising or collaborating physician, and you may not exceed the bounds of that supervision or collaborative role.

8. Maintain your current skills and continue to broaden your knowledge and skills through continuing education and advanced nursing degrees. Maintain your certification or seek certification through appropriate associations as proof of your qualifications, knowledge base, and skills in a defined functional or clinical area of nursing.

9. Document carefully and accurately any nursing care given. Legible and dependable nursing records are vital if a nurse functioning in an expanded nursing role hopes to successfully defend a future lawsuit.

- Describe the legal constraints to advanced professional practice encountered by nurses educationally and clinically competent to perform these roles, including:
  Scope of practice
  Malpractice issues
  Standards of care
  Prescriptive authority
  Hospital or admitting privileges
  Reimbursement issues
  Direct access to patient populations

- Analyze means to overcome these legal constraints.
- Compare and contrast the current status of advanced nursing practice with that role in the future.

APPLY YOUR LEGAL KNOWLEDGE

- How does the state nurse practice act affect the role of advanced nursing practice within a given state?
- Are there areas in which advanced nursing practice is making more of an impact than others? Do these correspond with the primary purposes of advanced nursing practice?
- What must professional nursing do to ensure that advanced nursing practice is fully utilized by persons most needing these professionals' care?
- Why is advanced practice nursing vital to the continued growth of the discipline of nursing?

YOU BE THE JUDGE

Mary Webb brought suit against Brian Arnold, an anesthesiologist, and his professional corporation; Cecilia Morales, a certified registered nurse anesthetist employed by the professional corporation; and M. Michael Pullman, an ophthalmologist, and his corporation, alleging negligence in the performance of cataract surgery. Evidence showed that during the surgery a cataract was to be removed from the patient's right eye and a new lens inserted. Ms. Morales was responsible for administering the anesthetic agents during the surgery and for setting up the anesthesia machine and equipment before the procedure began.

Ms. Morales testified that she followed her usual preoperative procedures that morning, which included checking the anesthesia cannister to ensure that it contained a sufficient amount of Forane, the principal anesthetic agent used during this procedure. The chart she prepared to document her activities during the surgery stated "anesthesia machine checked out and working" prior to the start of the procedure. Dr. Pullman stated that approximately 15 minutes after he started the procedure, as he was viewing the patient's eye through a microscope and preparing to insert the lens implant, he saw the patient's eye move and felt her head rise slightly. Dr. Pullman testified that he informed Morales that the patient was "anesthetic light" and that in response Morales replied that the problem had arisen because there was no more Forane. Dr. Pullman further testified that he watch Morales refill the cannister with an "aqua-greenish" liquid and had to wait three to five minutes for the patient to become stabilized before he could resume the procedure. He then noted that the patient had experienced a loss of vitreous humor, which had extruded through the incision. As a result, he could not insert the lens, but was instead compelled to perform a vitrectomy to correct the extrusion.

It is undisputed that after the surgery, the patient developed a swelling of nerve fiber in the back of the eye which led to loss of vision. The cause of this occurrence, however, was contested at trial level, with the parties in complete disagreement on the critical question of whether the anesthetic was depleted during the surgery and whether the patient became "anesthetically light" during the operation. The jury rendered a verdict in favor of the surgeon and his professional corporation, and against Arnold, Morales, and their professional corporation. The latter three defendants appealed.

Legal Questions

1. Did Ms. Morales fall below an acceptable standard of care while delivering anesthesia to this patient?
2. What was the standard of care used to judge whether she was negligent or not?
3. What other evidence do you need to find either for or against Ms. Morales?
4. How would you decide the outcome of this case?

REFERENCES

Adams v. Kreuger, 856 P.2d 864 (Idaho, 1993).

American Association of Nurse Anesthetists (1998). *Nurse Anesthesia and the American Association of Nurse Anesthetists.* Park Ridge, IL: Author.

American Nurses Association (1976). *Congress for Nursing Practice: The Scope of Nursing Practice. Description of Practice: Clinical Nurse Specialist.* Kansas City, MO: Author.

Azzolino v. Dingfelder, 322 S.E.2d 567 (N.C. Ct. App., 1994).

Bahn v. NME Hospitals, 669 F. Supp. 998 (E.D. Cal., 1987).

Bellegie v. Board of Nurse Examiners, 685 S.W.2d 431 (Tex. Ct. App.–Austin, 1985).

Carson, W. (1997). *States which Recognize Clinical Nurse Specialists in Advanced Practice.* Washington, DC: American Nurses Association.

Chalmers-Francis v. Nelson, 6 Cal.2d 402 (1936).

Cohen v. State Board of Medicine, 676 A.2d 1277 (Pa. Cmwlth., 1996).

Fein v. Permanente Medical Group, 38 Cal.3d 137 (1985).

Flanagan, L. (1998). Nurse practitioners: Growing competition for family physicians? *Family Practice Management* 10(10), 1–8.

Goodliffe v. Parish Anesthesia Associates, 769 So.2d 769 (La. App., 1995).

Georgopoulos, B. S., and Christman, L. (1970). The clinical nurse specialist: A role model. *American Journal of Nursing* 70(5), 1030–1039.

Gugino v. Harvard Community Health Plan et al., 403 N.E.2d 1166 (Massachusetts, 1983).

Harris v. State through Huey P. Long Hospital, 371 So.2d 1221 (Louisiana, 1979).

Hendry v. United States, 418 F.2d 744 (2d Cir., 1969).

Hernicz v. State of Florida, Department of Professional Regulation, 390 So.2d 194 (Fla. Dis. Ct. App. 1980).

Inglis, A. D., and Kjervik, D. K. (1993). Empowerment of advanced practice nurses: Regulation reform needed to increase access to care. *Journal of Law, Medicine, and Ethics* 21, 193–205.

Jenkins v. Payne, 465 S.E.2d 795 (Virginia, 1996).

Lane v. Otis, 412 So.2d 254 (Alabama, 1982).

Mannino, M. J. (1982). *The Nurse Anesthetist and the Law.* New York: Grune & Stratton.

Marco C. (1983). Can a nurse practitioner testify against a physician? *Legal Aspects of Medical Practice* 11, 2.

Moses, E. B. (1992). *The Registered Nurse Population. Findings from the National Sample Survey of Registered Nurses, March 1992.* U.S. Department of Health and Human Services, Public Health Service, Division of Nursing, Health Resources and Services Administration.

Olson v. Bolstad, 161 Minn. 419, 201 N.W. 918 (1925).

Paris v. Kreitz, 331 S.E.2d 234 (North Carolina, 1985).

Pearson, L. J. (1992). 1992–1993 update: How each state stands on legislative issues affecting advanced nursing practice. *The Nurse Practitioner: The American Journal of Primary Health Care,* 18(1), 23–38.

People v. Arendt, 60 Ill. App. 89 (1894).

Public Law, 105-33, 1997.

Ray v. Anesthesia Associates of Mobile, 674 So.2d 525 (Alabama, 1995).

Reverby, S. M. (1987). *Ordered to Care: The Dilemma of American Nursing, 1850–1945.* Cambridge, MA: Cambridge University Press.

Ruggiero v. State Department of Health, 643 N.Y.S.2d 698 (N.Y. App., 1996).

Rules and Regulations (1998). *Federal Register,* 63 (211), 58871–58876.

Safriet, B. J. (1992). Health care dollars and regulatory sense: The role of advanced practice nursing. *Yale Journal on Regulation* 9, 417–487.

Samii v. Baystate Medical Center, 395 N.E.2d 455 (Massachusetts, 1979).

Sermchief v. Gonzales, 660 S.W.2d 683 (Mo. en banc, 1983).

Stevens, R. (1971). *American Medicine and the Public Interest.* New Haven: Yale University Press.

Tatro v. State of Texas, 703 F.2d 823 (5th Cir., 1983).

Topp v. Logan, 554 N.E.2d 454 (Ill. App. Ct. 1 Dist., 1990).

Whitney v. Day, M.D. and Hurley Hospital, 300 N.W.2d 380 (Ct. App.–Mich., 1981).

Wrable v. Community Memorial Hospital, 205 J.J. Super 428 (1985), aff'd. 517 A.2d. 470 (October 22, 1986), cert. denied, 526 A.2d 210 (April 28, 1987).

thirteen

Nursing in Acute Care Settings

■ PREVIEW

The previous chapter concerned nurses in advanced practice roles—those recognized by their state nurse practice acts and state boards of nursing to practice within expanded nursing roles. This chapter concerns the nurse practicing within acute care settings, performing daily more highly skilled tasks and having responsibility for increasingly more acutely ill patients. Gone are the days when sophisticated machines were seen only in critical care areas or emergency centers. Patients on general medical and surgical units may have ventilators, central intravenous lines, and chest tubes, as well as a variety of other machines and devices, and clinical patients may have dialysis lines and permanent central catheters. Thus, employees who work in acute care settings are encountering the need for greater skills as well as facing potentially more liability. This chapter addresses issues arising within acute care settings, giving guides on competent, quality health care delivery.

■ KEY CONCEPTS

patient safety	restraints	failure to adequately assess,
psychiatric and vulnerable patients	medication errors	monitor, and communicate
suicide prevention	technology and equipment	failure to act as a patient advocate

ACUTE CARE NURSING

The past 30 years have witnessed dramatic changes within the nurse's role in acute care settings. Three decades ago, it was easy to define the practice of medicine and the practice of nursing, and to articulate the difference between the two professions. Today, the roles are becoming masked with the advent of:

1. Critical care units.
2. Intermediate care units.
3. Advanced nursing skills within specialized units such as the operating room, postanesthesia care unit, labor and delivery units, and emergency centers.
4. Advanced nursing knowledge, technology, and equipment.

Today's nurse must assume responsibility and accountability for patient care that requires knowledge of complex illnesses and use of highly sophisticated machinery.

For example, an emergency department nurse may be assigned the role of triage coordinator in patient selection. This role involves performing a thorough assessment of patients, formulating initial nursing diagnoses, and making decisions concerning which patient will be seen immediately and which patients can wait to be seen by medical personnel. Should a patient be misclassified, serious injury could result due to a delay in initiating therapy.

Other examples of increased accountability and responsibility include the use of complex technological skills within labor and delivery units and the postpartum monitoring of maternity patients and newborns. Even psychiatric skills and knowledge have greatly expanded in the past few decades, and patients are returning to home programs and community-based living centers for their major therapies.

Nurses can best avoid potential liability by giving safe and competent nursing care, while recognizing potential problems, identifying the risk areas in individual practice, and remaining current in new technology, nursing diagnoses, and the latest institution policies and procedures. The following sections list types of incidents that are encountered frequently in acute care nursing.

PATIENT SAFETY

One of the most important responsibilities of nurses today is in ensuring *patient safety* needs. This responsibility includes protecting patients against falls, protecting patients from injuring themselves or others in the clinical setting, ensuring that medication errors do not occur, and protecting patients from faulty equipment or unsafe conditions. Examples of how nurses ensure such safety measures include inspecting siderails to see that they are functional and in the raised position for elderly or confused patients, foreseeing risks to patient safety (e.g., slick or wet floors), and restraining patients as indicated.

Given the complexities of individuals and society, nurses today are encountering hostile patients in greater numbers. Patients falling in this category typically have unrealistic expectations of their treatment plans and may be described as hostile, angry, or noncompliant. Although nurses have often thought of these patients as merely "difficult" and "challenging," such patients also present a safety hazard and increase the potential of liability for the nurses who care for them.

Spend additional time, not less time, with such patients, and show them that they are important. Attempt to understand their anger, but do not become part of it by showing hostility in return. Know the institution's policy on dealing with violent patients, and diffuse the situation according to the policy. Attend seminars on preventing violence in the workplace, and practice techniques for diffusing such situations. Document the patients' complaints or noncompliance and interventions taken to resolve the situation. Consult with colleagues about the best approach to take, and ensure that the entire health care team is reinforcing the approach selected.

Should patients have a serious violent episode, follow these simple rules:

1. Position oneself at least four arm lengths away and to the side of patients, to ensure that they do not feel threatened.

2. Keep hands in sight and maintain eye contact.
3. Avoid touching, pointing, challenging, or interrupting the patient.
4. When speaking, talk softly and address the person by name.
5. Request permission to ask questions.
6. Acknowledge the patient's feelings, and express regret without assigning blame.
7. Show empathy and offer solutions that address the patient's concerns.
8. Remain calm and professional (Bartlett and Rehmar, 1997).

PSYCHIATRIC AND VULNERABLE PATIENTS

Patients with serious mental illnesses occupy more acute care beds than those with any other illness (National Alliance for the Mentally Ill, 1994). With these types of statistics, nurses in all acute care settings must know how to recognize patients with psychiatric or emotional disturbances and meet their special needs. Because caring for these *psychiatric and vulnerable patients* presents unique issues, nurses must know what legal risks are involved and how to minimize them while maximizing nursing care.

The law has long recognized psychiatric patients as part of the group of vulnerable persons, along with children, the elderly, the imprisoned, and the mentally challenged. Persons falling within the category of vulnerable do so because they are often unable to recognize their unique circumstances, and because they are frequently unable to speak for themselves, thus asserting their rights in health care settings. Several issues arise with these patients.

Suicide Prevention

Nurses have obligations related to *suicide prevention.* Not all self-destructive and depressed patients will be hospitalized on psychiatric units, and some patients respond to hospitalization with depression and suicidal thoughts, particularly the elderly, the recently anesthetized, and postpartum patients. Nurses should listen carefully to comments spoken by patients, because nearly all suicidal patients have some ambivalence and give some warning clues before self-destructive behavior is evident. Once identified as a potential suicidal or self-destructive patient, the duty of care owed the patient increases, as the foreseeable consequences of not meeting the duty of care required is obvious. Identification of such patients offers nurses the opportunity to counsel them, alert psychiatric clinical nurse specialists or psychiatric intervenors that they are at risk for self-destruction, and implement precautions while they are recovering. Above all, the nurse should treat these patients and their families with concern, consistency, and caring behaviors.

Nurses should have an understanding of which patients are more likely to become self-destructive. Older patients are more likely to commit suicide than younger patients, although the younger patients may be more verbal. Women make more suicide attempts, but men, by a two to one ratio, are more likely to be successful in their attempts. Most successful suicide patients have a previous history of suicide attempts or prior hospitalization for self-destruction.

Once identified, nurses have a legal responsibility to protect the patient. The court in *Winger v. Franciscan Medical Center* (1998) held that a hospital and its staff must exercise reasonable care to protect suicidal patients from self-harm. This is true whether the patient had been voluntarily or involuntarily admitted.

The adolescent patient in this case had a history of suicide attempts. He had been admitted to the facility five times in the five months prior to his death. He told the nurses when he was voluntarily admitted the fifth time that he had held back taking his Elavil and then had taken an overdose. He stated that it was his intent to "sink so low again that he would get suicidal." The nurse's admitting note indicated a plan of care to monitor the patient and prevent self-harm. However, the patient was improperly placed on close supervision and not on suicide precaution.

Hospital policy mandated that potentially suicidal patients be placed on suicide precaution. The hospital's definition of a suicidal patient included a patient who had discussed death or the uselessness of life or one who had been admitted for an apparent suicide attempt. A potentially suicidal patient on suicide precaution was not allowed unmonitored access to the restroom or allowed to have objects such as belts, shoelaces, or phone cords that could be used for self-harm.

Two days after his voluntary admission for aggressive electric shock therapy for his depression, the patient expressed doubts to a nurse that the planned therapy would relieve his depression, saying that he felt bad and hopeless all the time, and that he could not go on living this way much longer. Still, he was kept on close supervision and was not transferred to suicide precaution.

In the middle of the night, the patient stuffed clothes into his bed to make it appear as if he were still in bed, then hanged himself in his bathroom. The court ruled that the parents had legal grounds for a wrongful death lawsuit against the hospital and the attending psychiatrist.

In analyzing the case, the court decided that the patient's suicidal actions were foreseeable and that the conduct of the patient's caregivers was not a reasonable response to his circumstances. Health care professionals in these circumstances must adhere to the standard of care toward their patients that would be followed by other members of their profession under similar circumstances.

Note the importance of the ability to foresee conclusions in finding liability against health care providers. In *Mounts v. St. David's Pavilion* (1997), the court expressed its deepest sympathies to the parents of a young woman who had committed suicide by hanging herself from the shower in her room while in a psychiatric hospital. At the same time, the court ruled that the evidence did not support a wrongful death claim against the facility. The court disagreed with the allegation that the hospital was negligent in the design and construction of the shower curtain rod in the bathroom.

The court also ruled that the hospital was not negligent in its management of her suicide risk. The patient had cut her wrists with a piece of glass. She was placed on close suicide watch for two days, and then placed on stepped-down 30-minute checks. Her therapist believed that her suicide risk was an impulsive pattern of acting out and that she did not have the potential for deliberately formulating and carrying out a suicide plan. There was a no-harm contract signed by the patient when the suicide precautions were stepped down. It was believed that the stepped-down suicide precautions and the explicit decision to leave the shower curtain in the bathroom would promote trust and thereby decrease the potential for her to act out self-destructively.

With the benefit of hindsight, the court recognized that the staff's assessment of this patient's situation was not correct. However, according to the court, a psychiatric hospital is required by law to take reasonable measures in light of its best professional judgment as to the foreseeability of the patient's doing self-harm and is not judged before the law by perfect hindsight.

Hindsight, though, may be closely related to foresight, and the court will rule in favor of patients and their families when untoward events are foreseeable. In *Bossley v. Dallas County Memorial Health and Mental Retardation* (1995), the court held that the purpose for having locked double doors between the outside and the psychiatric unit was to prevent patients from merely walking out of the facility, and that both doors should be kept locked. When a patient is allowed to escape due to the fact that one door is "unlocked during daytime hours," a patient bent on escaping could overcome the staff member when the only locked door is unlocked by that staff member. Such an event is foreseeable.

A case that extends the reasoning regarding foreseeability and hindsight as used in *Mounts* is *Phillip v. University Medical Center* (1998). The outpatient alcohol and drug abuse clinic was on the ground floor of the same building that housed an outpatient mental health clinic. Two men, both drunk, walked into the alcohol and drug abuse clinic, seeking help for the drinking problem of one of the men. They were seen together by a counselor.

The man seeking help admitted to the screening counselor that he had had suicidal thoughts three weeks earlier. He denied current suicidal and homicidal ideation. The court was satisfied that the counselor would have made sure the patient received an immediate psychological evaluation at the mental health clinic in the same building if he had expressed current suicidal thoughts.

The counselor determined that the man needed detoxification and an inpatient substance abuse program. The counselor gave him information on three facilities with detoxification capability and inpatient programs. The man indicated that he would follow up with the one that was nearest his home.

At this point, the court determined that the outpatient clinic had fulfilled its legal duty to the man. The clinic initiated no further contact with the patient after he voiced his intent to go to the detoxification center and admit himself, and the court ruled that the clinic had no legal duty to follow up and see if he was admitted.

The man was never actually admitted to the detoxification center as planned. When he called the center, there was no bed available, and the patient agreed to be placed on the waiting list. The center then lost his paperwork and placed him at the bottom of the waiting list. He shot himself 10 days after his initial screening with the counselor named in this suit. In the family lawsuit that was subsequently filed, the court ruled that the clinic that screened him was not responsible for his suicide.

Should the nurse identify such a patient or potential patient, there are several nursing interventions that might be initiated. Although not an exhaustive list, some of the more obvious nursing interventions include:

1. Close supervision of the patient by staff or family members.
2. Removal of potentially dangerous objects from the patient's bedside and room.
3. Ensuring that the patient takes all medications when given so that there can be no accumulation of medications to be taken all at once.
4. Transferring the patient closer to the nurses' station or to another unit as needed for closer observation and frequent checks.

5. Transferring a rooming-in infant back to the nursery since postpartum depression may be seen not as self-destruction, but as destructive behaviors aimed at neonates.
6. Ensuring that windows in the patient's room cannot be opened or opened only partially.
7. Notifying the physician promptly of changes in the patient's condition and administering medications as needed to prevent further depression or self-destruction.
8. Restraining the patient as indicated.

Warning of Intent to Harm

Failure to warn of a patient's dangerous propensities when the victim is identifiable has long been accepted as a liability-producing situation by courts of law (*Tarasoff v. The Regents of the University of California*, 1976). Several recent cases have reaffirmed this principle, including *Shepard v. State Department of Mental Health* (1998), *Bishop v. South Carolina Department of Mental Health* (1998), and *Rocca v. Southern Hills Counseling Center, Inc.* (1996).

Shepard held that a state psychiatric facility has a responsibility to foreseeable victims of a patient's known violent propensities not to release the patient prematurely. In that case, the patient shot and killed his wife and children, and then shot himself four days after being released from a state psychiatric facility. One of the evaluating physicians had made a written recommendation that the patient was not to have guns around after his release. However, this recommendation was not communicated to the patient's wife when the patient was released.

In *Bishop*, the issue surrounded medical confidentiality and the exception to such confidentiality when there is an identifiable person against whom a patient has verbalized a threat or intention to do bodily harm. In this case, during her involuntary psychiatric stay, a patient verbalized an intention to harm her children after her release. Nonetheless, the state hospital did not contact the grandmother, who had custody of the children, to warn her of their mother's threats. Nor was the grandmother warned of the mother's impending release.

The mother went to the grandmother's house and asked to see her 3-year-old child. The grandmother let her into the home, let her see the child, and left her alone with the child. The child's body was marked up with a felt-tip marker, including the vaginal area, but no medical evidence of sexual violation could be detected.

The court dismissed the case, holding that the grandmother, who knew the history of her daughter, was negligent in leaving the mother alone with the 3-year old, and that her action was the causative factor of the child's harm. The court also said in its findings that a mental health worker may have to warn the intended victim, or warn others to warn the victim, or notify the police where the victim lives, or do anything else reasonably necessary for the person's protection. Even though it dismissed the hospital from the suit, the hospital, in this case, had a responsibility to warn the grandmother that the mother had verbalized a threat against her children and should have warned the grandmother of the impending release.

Rocca directly addressed the issue of medical confidentiality. The court held that a mental health facility, whose staff made the choice to inform the attorney representing the person standing accused of murdering a patient's daughter that the patient had voiced an intention to kill that person, had acted appropriately. The patient alleged in the lawsuit that the facility had breached its duty of medical confidentiality and thus was guilty of malpractice. According to the court, however, the preservation of medical confidentiality is a less important social issue than the prevention of violent criminal actions by patients who have revealed to caregivers the intention to commit such acts.

Turner v. Jordan (1997) extended the duty to warn to staff members per se. In that case, the Supreme Court of Tennessee ruled that a violent patient's attending physician has a duty to the nurses working on the psychiatric unit to see that measures are taken to control the patient for the nurses' safety. According to the court, a psychiatrist's first responsibility is to evaluate whether the patient poses a danger to nurses and other staff who will be working with the patient.

In this case, the psychiatrist already knew the patient well. The patient had been on the unit five times during the manic phase of his long-term bipolar illness. Three of those times, the patient had been adjudged to pose a danger to himself and to others and had been held and treated involuntarily. When the patient came in voluntarily this time, he told the emergency center resident that he had not been taking his lithium. The resident assessed the patient as disorganized, grandiose, and delusional. The patient was admitted to bring his lithium level into therapeutic range.

The psychiatrist wrote a note less that one hour after admission that the patient was aggressive, grandiose, intimidating, combative, and dangerous. The psychiatrist's plan, such as it was, was to wait for the patient to leave against medical advice. Later that same evening, the patient brutally attacked a staff nurse.

The court ruled that nurses have the legal right to expect that a psychiatrist will frankly inform them about a patient's level of dangerousness. This psychiatrist should have ordered medications for the patient and should have restrained and/or secluded him for the nurses' protection, or taken immediate steps to transfer the patient into a more secure setting that could properly handle a dangerous patient as well as meet the patient's treatment needs.

Failure to Protect from Harm

A variant application of duty to warn involves the failure to protect from harm. This need to protect occurs in instances when patients, because of their vulnerable state and their inability to distinguish potentially harmful situations, must be protected by health care providers. A case that illustrates this concept was first tried at the appellate level with liability held against the nurse and then reversed by the Supreme Court in Minnesota.

In *Wall v. Fairview Hospital and Healthcare Services* (1997), the nurse saw patients with her employer, a psychiatrist; sat in on therapy sessions with patients and took notes; and saw patients by herself to administer and monitor medications. The nurse knew that the psychiatrist had begun a personal and sexual relationship with at least one female patient that lasted in excess of four years. Two other patients were the individuals who brought this lawsuit. The nurse did not know that the psychiatrist was abusing these two patients, but the court ruled that it did not make any difference.

The court ruled that it was the duty of the nurse, under the law, to report a physician who physically, emotionally, verbally, or sexually abused a vulnerable patient. The nurse admitted that she understood this duty, but thought that a "vulnerable adult" was one who was receiving inpatient mental health treatment. The court stated that "vulnerable" means an adult who is unlikely or unable to report abuse. A patient in therapy for mental health illness is by law a vulnerable patient. This is especially true for patients with mutiple personalities. A therapist could call up one of the patient's personalities (as this psychiatrist had done), abuse the person as that personality, intimidate or deceive that personality to remain silent, then summon back another personality before ending the session.

The nurse in this case was also liable for not reporting the physician's obvious alcohol and cocaine impairment. This became relevant in the patients' civil lawsuit, because this impairment clouded his judgment and furthered his abuse of his patients. Every licensed health care professional has a strict legal duty to promptly report abuse of a vulnerable adult to the proper authorities.

Following the decision of the Court of Appeals of Minnesota, the Supreme Court of Minnesota reversed the judgment against the nurse (1998). The Supreme Court upheld the general definition of abuse to include nontherapeutic conduct that produces or could be expected to produce pain, injury, mental or emotional distress, and, more specifically, any sexual contact between the caregiver and a vulnerable patient.

The Supreme Court explained that the nurse in question had no actual knowledge that the two patients were being sexually abused. The nurse heard one of the third patient's alternative personalities accuse the psychiatrist of abuse during a therapy session. However, according to the court, that did not mean there was probable cause to report abuse of other patients.

The nurse was aware that there were "boundary violations" by the psychiatrist with respect to the two patients who were abused; that is, the nurse knew that he had taken both of them out for ice cream. But that boundary violation, standing alone, did not give rise to a duty to report that the patients whose boundaries are being violated are being sexually abused.

The Supreme Court also noted that knowing the psychiatrist had an alcohol problem did not mean that the nurse had probable cause for reporting sexual abuse of the patients. There are rules for reporting substance abuse. But failure to report substance abuse is not a relevant factor in a lawsuit against a nurse for failure to report sexual abuse of patients. Reasonable cause means more than a suspicion of abuse or knowledge of the opportunity for abuse. Reasonable cause means grounds for belief supported by factual circumstances that would lead a cautious person to conclude that abuse is taking place.

Courts have also ruled that staff members have a duty to protect patients from harm, especially when vulnerable persons are left in circumstances in which they could be harmed. In *Laman v. Big Spring State Hospital* (1998), a mental health patient was given a sedative and soon went to sleep. The nurses left the patient, a newly admitted delusional patient, alone and totally unattended. The room where she was left was on the men's side of the hall. The door to the room was left unlocked, and the room was accessible to entry from the men's hallway. The patient was raped by a male patient as she slept. The court found liability against the staff for negligence.

In *Genoa v. State of New York* (1998), a patient who, if procedure had been followed, should have been observed every 30 minutes was left alone for a two and one-half hour interval. During that time, she was raped by another patient. This patient, like the patient in *Laman*, was heavily sedated and asleep in a room other than the one assigned to her. The staff was found negligent for its lack of supervision of the patient.

False Imprisonment/Wrongful Commitment

Psychiatric patients may voluntarily admit themselves for treatment, or, in the case of persons unable to judge what is best for them, the state may involuntarily hospitalize the patient. Case law abounds yearly on the issue of whether the patient should or should not have been detained and whether the patient had the competency to make a rational decision. Some case examples may help clarify these issues.

In *Application of Anthony M. v. Sanchez* (1996), the court concluded that the patient's continued involuntary psychiatric commitment was justified. The court concluded that the patient not only suffered from a mental illness, but presented a substantial threat of harm to himself and to others, and was in need of continued treatment and structured care. The patient, while confined to the hospital, threatened a nurse who was carrying a hypodermic needle. He screamed at her that he would take the needle from her and poke out her eyes.

The patient often screamed at the top of his lungs that he was going to kill anyone trying to keep him at the hospital and that, after his release, he was going to come back and "get his revenge." There were other outbursts of aggression in which the patient hurled verbal expletives at the staff. He also masturbated in front of female staff members.

Additionally, there were problems with medication compliance on the part of the patient. He was known to try to avoid taking his medications that were being administered to control his anxiety and impulsiveness, while calmly taking other medications without incident. In trying to devise an aftercare plan for the patient, no appropriate caregiver could be found. The only family member willing to take him into her household had significant health problems and had no ability to exert any manner of control on the patient.

The court was also mindful that the patient had a criminal record for rape. Just because the patient could remain stable for a few days in a secure and controlled hospital environment did not mean that his release was appropriate, and the court ruled that the involuntary commitment was justified.

Copeland v. Northwestern Memorial Hospital (1997) held that when a patient comes in voluntarily for mental health reasons, a nurse can and must obtain a full history. The history must include why the person is seeking treatment. If the patient voluntarily discloses that he or she has just committed a crime, the nurse can take appropriate safety measures and notify the police. The nurse and the hospital are not to be held liable in a civil lawsuit for damages if the authorities decide to come to the hospital and arrest the patient for the criminal activity he or she has voluntarily disclosed, while the patient is still choosing to remain voluntarily for assessment and treatment.

The nurse was not engaged in a custodial interrogation and was not in a position to violate the patient's civil or constitutional rights. Custodial interrogation is defined as initiated by law enforcement officials after they have taken the person into police custody or deprived the person of liberty in a significant fashion.

When the nurse in this case questioned the patient about the circumstances leading up to his coming to the hospital seeking a psychiatric admission, the patient volunteered that he must have just committed an armed robbery during his blackout to get the $1,400 he found he had with him to go on his cocaine binge. At this point, the nurse properly summoned the hospital security guard to sit with the patient, who was still free to go, while she spoke with the physician and called the police. Once voluntarily admitted, the patient was placed in a locked observation room, but was still free to ask to leave and did not have to answer the physician's questions. The court held that the nurse, physicians, and the hospital did not arrest, detain, or interrogate the patient or violate his constitutional rights. Similar conclusions were reached in *S. P. v. City of Takoma Park* (1998).

In *Heater v. Southwood Psychiatric Center* (1996), the court extended the ruling to note that even when there are grounds to hold a person for psychiatric reasons, the law still requires a full court hearing before powerful antipsychotic medication can be given to the person against his or her will. Ativan, ordered only to relieve agitation, can be given without first going to court for authorization. The court in *In re Dorothy W.* (1998) allowed medications for severe paranoid schizophrenia to be given after a court ruling was requested.

An Iowa court (*In the Interest of "J.P.,"* 1998) delineated the criteria for involuntary commitment. They include:

1. A mental illness.
2. The lack of sufficient judgment to make responsible decisions with respect to the person's hospitalization or treatment, due to the mental illness.
3. The likelihood of inflicting serious physical or emotional harm on self or others, or the inability to satisfy the person's own basic physical needs, if allowed to remain at liberty.

The court further noted that all three criteria must exist in order to hold a patient involuntarily for psychiatric treatment. "The law is essentially the same in all jurisdictions, due to the United States Supreme Court's nationwide standards for the constitutionality of state mental-health laws" (*Legal Eagle Eye Newsletter,* 1998, p. 4).

RESTRAINTS

Restraints, both physical and chemical, are used daily in many hospital settings, from the critical care unit to the psychiatric unit. Physical restraints assist in preventing patient falls, discourage patients from disconnecting vital equipment or intravenous and feeding lines, and prevent patients from harming either themselves or others. Chemical restraints also prevent patients from disconnecting vital, life-sustaining equipment; assist in preventing hostile and impaired patients from hurting themselves or others; and allow staff to care for all patients on a given unit.

But restraints are not without serious side effects and harm. Physical restraints can cause skin impairment, impaired respiratory status, strangulation, neurological damage, and death. Chemical restraints may result in increased drowsiness, respiratory distress, hemodynamic instability, decreased competency and judgment, and confusion.

All hospitals have policies and procedures outlining when and how restraints are to be used and the nursing care that must be documented on restrained individuals. Because of the inappropriate use of restraints, many hospitals insist on securing a physician's order before applying restraints, and federal law prohibits chemical restraints in certain nursing home patients.

In the past, failing to raise siderails for elderly patients was synonymous with substandard care. However, research is now showing that elderly patients are more likely to fall and suffer injuries when siderails are used. Less intrusive interventions, such as asking patients to call for assistance, keeping night-lights on to reorient the patient to unfamiliar surroundings, and placing mattresses on floors to break a possible fall, may be more effective ways of preventing falls in the elderly, especially an elderly patient whose mind sometimes wanders. Thus, many institutions are reevaluating and rewriting their policies on the use of restraints.

Case law consistently has held that siderails on stretchers and gurneys must be in the raised and locked position. Patients using such devices are either in the process of being transported or are under constant supervision. That differs greatly from the patient who is in a hospital room on a general medical or surgical floor.

Examples of patients harmed because they were not properly restrained can still be found in current case law. In *Swann v. Len-Care Rest Home, Inc.* (1997), a group living facility provided the same type of care that might be found in an individual's home, but did not provide direct, one-to-one personal care for the residents. The resident's granddaughter visited regularly and requested that the patient, as she became more confused and her general condition deteriorated, be restrained because she had a tendency to stand up unassisted when unattended. When the granddaughter found the grandmother up, wandering and unattended, she would bring the need for restraints to the staff's attention.

At the family's urging, the resident's physician wrote and signed an order for restraints as needed and wrote a separate letter to management requesting that the resident be restrained when unassisted. The resident fell, sustained a serious head injury, and sued the facility. At trial, it was noted that this was the resident's third fall, all occurring while she was unrestrained and unassisted. The court ruled that she should have been restrained while in her chair and unattended.

Another case that upheld the application of restraints is *St. Elizabeth's Hospital v. Graham* (1994). In that case, a patient suffered comminuted, depressed, and basilar skull fractures. Following a craniotomy, he was transferred to the neurological intensive care unit. While there, he was placed in a recliner chair, without restraints, and fell with such force that he was found on the floor, disoriented and bleeding from his ear. The fall caused further brain injury, and the family sued. At trial, it was disclosed that the patient had nearly fallen out of the same chair the day before, while his mother was visiting, and that she had requested the nurses to restrain her son to prevent injury. A neurologist testified that the nurses had failed to exercise due care in not restraining him, as Graham was experiencing postoperative confusion, problems with coordination, and mild combativeness. He further testified that using a Posey vest restraint would have assisted in preventing injury to this patient, and the court agreed.

The Joint Commission for the Accreditation of Healthcare Organizations (JCAHO) sets forth guidelines on the use of restraints, which the individual institution policy and procedure manual should reflect. These recommendations include:

1. The decision to use physical restraints should be based on the patient's condition at that moment, rather than on a prior history of violent behavior, the fact that he had previously discontinued feeding tubes, or what might happen if the patient becomes confused.
2. Whenever possible, attempt alternative, less restrictive approaches first. For example, use a lap tray rather than physical restraints while the patient is sitting in a chair to support and prevent slipping.

3. If restraints are necessary, choose the least restrictive device to restrict the patient. Do not use four restraints if soft wrist restraints are sufficient.

4. Document frequent assessments of the patient, including the removal of restraints for short periods of time. Documentation should include how one assessed circulation, whether the patient was offered food or hydration, and assistance with elimination, such as assisting the patient to the bathroom, providing a bed pan, or the fact that the patient had an indwelling catheter. Most institutions have a specialized form to document nursing interventions while a patient is restrained.

5. Obtain an order for the restraints, even if it is after the restraints have been applied. Remember, the patient's safety comes first. Do what is necessary to protect the patient, and then follow institution policy.

6. The order must include the date and time that restraints were ordered, the type of restraint to be used, the purpose, and a specific short-term time limit, defined as 24 hours or less.

7. For psychiatric patients, the patient may not be restrained for longer than four hours for adults, two hours for adolescents, and one hour for a child under nine years of age. After this initial period, a licensed practitioner must reassess the patient and continue the restraints as needed, up to 24 hours. If a psychiatric patient requires hospitalization for medical illness and conditions, the parameters change to that of the patient's primary clinical issue.

8. The order for restraints cannot be renewed without reassessment of the patient. Vague orders, such as "restrain until no longer agitated," are not acceptable. If restraints are still required after assessment, a new order must be written.

When using restraints, it is vital to follow hospital policy and procedure, documenting adequately why the patient was restrained, how he or she was restrained, how patient safety needs were met during the time restraints were used, and the removal or continuance of restraints. In documentation, record what type of patient behavior necessitated the restraints, including ineffective methods of restraint that may have been used and the exact type of restraint finally applied, such as soft wrist restraints, kerlix hand restraints, or a Posey vest or belt. The date and time of application of restraints should be noted, as well as the patient's response to the restraints. Patient safety needs, such as skin integrity, circulation in the restrained extremities, respiratory status, nutrition and elimination needs, and elevation of the patient's head prior to feeding should be noted according to the hospital policy. Also document the need for continued restraint and periodic assessments to ascertain when restraints may be removed.

Perhaps part of the difficulty in complying with patient restraint standards is a basic misunderstanding of what constitutes restraints and how nurses document the use of various devices. The rate of hospital compliance with restraints is about 50% (Kobs, 1997). Belts, vests, wrist ties, leathers, and siderails may all be restraints, but some can also serve other purposes. For example, a vest restraint may prevent a patient from falling, or its purpose may be to help an elderly patient maintain correct alignment and support while in a chair. Similarly, one could reason that soft wrist restraints are preventative in patients with endotracheal tubes who are ventilator-dependent, as their purpose is to prevent harm, and a possible respiratory arrest, if the endotracheal tube is removed prematurely. In both instances, documentation of why the device is used is the key to whether the device is a restraint or is being used for some other purpose.

If restraints as applied are not effective, chemical restraints may augment the physical restraints. For example, the ventilator-dependent patient with adult respiratory distress syndrome may be physically restrained to prevent the accidental dislodgment of an endotracheal tube and chemically restrained to allow the ventilator to regulate respiratory rate and tidal volume. Or chemical restraints may be used without physical restraints, as in patients in whom sedation alone is effective.

A newer trend in restraints is to use a bed occupancy monitor or similar device so that personnel are alerted immediately when a patient is no longer in bed. Although it may not prevent the patient from falling, the device will ensure that assistance is provided immediately. Since there are some patients who can successfully free themselves from all restraints, courts will look to how quickly and effectively the patient was treated after falling. Bed occupancy monitors greatly aid in early intervention and assistance.

■ EXERCISE 13—1

Review your institution policies and procedures for chemical and physical restraints. How does the current policy requiring documentation adhere to the above recommendations for documentation of restraints? Are there separate forms for documenting the continuous assessment of patients who are restrained? If not, develop a form that would assist nurses in accurately documenting such patient care. If there is a form, does it allow for accurate and continuous charting? How would you adapt the form?

GUIDELINES: CHEMICAL AND PHYSICAL RESTRAINTS

1. Involve the patient and family in the decision regarding the need for restraints. This allows the nurse to explain the purpose of the restraints, why they are needed, and care that will be given while the person is restrained.
2. Document the reason for the restraint, any explanation given to the patient and family, and measures undertaken to ensure the continuing safety of the patient. This includes circulation checks, range of motion exercises, meeting nutritional and hydration needs, and assessing frequently for the continuing need for the restraint.
3. Document a thorough assessment of the extremity to be restrained before applying the restraining devices. This will protect you against allegations that the restraint caused physical harm to the patient if your assessment shows that the skin was bruised or broken prior to applying the restraint.
4. Document your continuing assessment of the restrained extremity according to hospital policy and the removal of restraints for short periods of time, if that is part of your policy.
5. Document the continuing need for restraints and the reasons necessitating the restraints if possible. For example, if a certain medication is causing the patient confusion, document the discontinuance of the medication.

MEDICATION ERRORS

Researchers predict that 770,000 hospital patients experience an adverse drug event yearly, and that almost half are preventable, such as those due to miscalculations, drug interactions, or drug allergies (Clinical News, 1997). *Medication errors* are difficult to defend because they are most often easily averted. Take the time needed to recheck the medication, the dosage, route of administration, time of administration, patient to whom the medication is to be given, and desired effects as well as potential side effects. Schools of nursing most often teach these precautions as the "five rights" of medication administration:

1. Right patient
2. Right medication
3. Right dose
4. Right route
5. Right time

Most medication errors fall into one of the following categories.

Incorrect Patient

Institution policy and procedure manuals insist that nurses check patient identification bands frequently, even if the nurse is sure of the patient's identification. Such policies exist to prevent giving a medication to other than the patient for whom the medication was intended and to prevent harmful side effects of the medication in the patient. In *Demers v. United States* (1990), the plaintiff's husband was admitted to the hospital for the implantation of a pacemaker. Subsequent to the procedure, the patient was administered Cardizem, a medication intended for another patient in the unit, resulting in his premature demise.

Incorrect Dosage or Incorrect Route of Administration

More commonly, nurses administer medications in wrong doses or by a route other than that ordered. Such errors can stem from the nurse's lack of knowledge about the medication. For example, a decedent suffered a cardiac arrest when a nurse administered an overdose of lidocaine (*Dessauer v. Memorial General Hospital,* 1981). In that case, the nurse, who normally worked on the obstetrical unit, had been floated to the emergency room, where she gave a dosage of 800 mg of intravenous (IV) lidocaine rather an the ordered 50 mg. Additional case law in this area of incorrect dosage includes *Wingstrom v. Evanston Hospital* (1992), in which 2 g of IV lidocaine were substituted for a 100-mg dosage; *Van Hyning v. Hamilton Hospital* (1994), in which a solution of 99% acetic acid was substituted for a 5% solution during surgery to remove genital warts; *Gallimore v. Children's Hospital Medical Center* (1992), in which the nurse substituted 200 mg of IV gentamicin for an ordered 30-mg dosage; and *Sharrow v. Archer* (1983), which again concerned an overdosage of IV lidocaine. In this latter case, the nurse also altered the patient's record at the direction of the attending physician, and the plaintiffs recovered damages for both malpractice and fraud.

Improper Injection Technique

Biggs v. United States (1987) illustrates this cause of action. In *Biggs,* the patient claimed that the nurse had used incorrect technique in administering an intramuscular injection. The injection, if given 3 to 4 inches above the knee as was claimed, could have resulted in nerve damage and would have been contrary to nursing standards of care. Because the patient exhibited signs and symptoms of nerve damage, the court remanded the case back to trial level on the issue of nursing malpractice.

Incorrect Time of Administration

Giving medications at wrong time intervals may cause patients serious injury. In an older case illustrating this point, a Utah nurse failed to give an antipsychotic medication as ordered, and the patient subsequently jumped from the hospital window and was permanently paralyzed. In finding for the plaintiff, the court stressed the importance of timely giving ordered medications and the need to understand the actions and desired effects of such medications so that timely administration would occur (*Farrow v. Health Services, et al.,* 1979).

Standards of care require nurses not only to be able to administer medications correctly, but to understand the pharmaceutical actions of the medications, potential side effects, and contraindications. Nurses must also understand the interactions of medications because most patients receive more than three medications during a 24-hour period, and they must properly question the prescribing physician before administering the medication. Nurses should reverify orders for medications if the order is illegible or if any portion of required information is omitted, such as the route of administration.

Failure to Note Patient Allergies

When nurses administer medications to which patient have already disclosed an allergy, the court will typically find against the nurse and the hospital. A recent case illustrates this point. In *Bazel v. Mabee* (1998), Betadine was used as the antiseptic agent on a surgical site following coronary artery bypass surgery. The Betadine was used before and after the procedure to secure venous material for the bypass graft, even though the patient had noted such an allergy on admission. The court found the hospital liable for his subsequent debridement and skin grafts.

■ EXERCISE 13–2

You are the medication nurse for a busy medical–surgical unit. After giving a patient her medication, she complains of itching and slight shortness of breath, and you notice obvious signs of an allergic reaction on her skin. Should the patient decide to later file suit and name you in the case, could you be held liable for the allergic response and subsequent harm to the patient? What would be your best defense against liability in such a suit?

PATIENT FALLS

Patient falls remain second to medication errors in untoward events that may happen to patients. Patient falls are among the top 10 incidents that cause or create the potential for serious patient injury or death, according to the JCAHO (1998). Patient falls are also among the most common types of cases that are filed against health care providers.

Some falls will result in liability to health care workers, but for some falls the court finds no liability against health care workers. For example, in *Parker v. Centenary Heritage Manor Nursing Home, et al.* (1996), the patient was 80 years of age, had a history of falls, and required a great deal of assistance with his activities of daily living. A few days after his admission to the nursing home, he fell and cut his head. The nursing home notified the family that he was being transferred to the local hospital for treatment. While in the hospital, the patient fell again and suffered a broken hip, requiring surgical intervention. Four days later, he had a massive myocardial infarction and died.

The family sued, alleging that both health care facilities had been negligent in his care. The nursing home settled out of court, and the case against the hospital went to trial. The family alleged that the nursing staff in the emergency center failed to properly restrain and monitor Mr. Parker. They claimed that they were notified of the fall, and that the nurse told them one of the siderails on the stretcher had not been raised. No notation of whether the siderails were up was made in the patient's medical record. Mr. Parker had been left unattended, a breach of the standard of care since the patient was neither alert nor oriented, alleged the family.

The emergency center nurse testified that when the patient was admitted, he was placed on a stretcher in the treatment room, with the siderails up, the bed in the lowest position, and the wheels locked. The nurse also testified that, before leaving Mr. Parker alone, he and the patient had a conversation about the patient's work as a farmer and about his fall at the nursing home. Just prior to leaving the patient, the nurse instructed a nursing assistant to check on the patient. The nursing assistant corroborated the nurse's testimony that the siderails were up and said that Mr. Parker was lucid and coherent. The hospital record also showed that Mr. Parker had a perfect score on the two Glasgow Coma Scale readings that were done.

The court found for the hospital, based on the evidence and the credibility of the witnesses. It was reasonable for the jury to find that the bed rails were up and that the patient's mental status was appropriate. An opposite holding occurred in *Bellamy v. Central Valley General Hospital* (1996), in which the court found that the patient was left alone, the locks were not set on the stretcher, and the siderails were not raised.

In a second 1996 case, *Romaro v. Marks*, the patient was ordered to remain in bed, on strict bedrest, for 24 hours. The patient testified that she was aware of the orders, but she got up to use the bathroom without calling the nursing staff. She fell as she returned to bed from the bathroom. The court dismissed the case, stating that the nursing staff had no obligation for keeping the patient in bed, beyond making sure that she understood the physician's instructions.

When a patient falls, the first duty of care is to the patient. Notify the patient's physician and management personnel after the patient has been fully assessed for injuries. Give the patient's physician a brief description of what happened, and a full description of the patient's condition. The emphasis should be on treatment to prevent further injury. Most institutions require that the patient's family also be notified of the fall. In some states, the law requires that patient's families be informed of falls in residential treatment centers and long-term care facilities.

Carefully document the patient's condition, treatments or tests performed to prevent further injury or done to ascertain the full extend of the injury, who was notified, and when they were notified.

TECHNOLOGY AND EQUIPMENT

Advances in *technology and equipment* have created special problems of liability for nurses. In addition to assessing and monitoring the patient, the nurse must also know the capabilities, limitations, hazards, and safety features of numerous machines and devices. As Aiken and Catalano (1994) note, most equipment injuries occur not because of unfamiliarity with the equipment, but because of carelessness or misuse of equipment. Thus, nurses should carefully follow manufacturers' recommendations for use of equipment and refrain from making modifications to the equipment.

Nursing negligence associated with improper use of equipment can arise in a variety of ways. First, after learning the correct use of machinery, the nurse is expected to conform with the manufacturers' recommendations and hospital policy and protocols (Killian, 1990). In *Stark v. Children's Orthopedic Hospital and Medical Center* (1990), the nurse mistakenly plugged heart monitor leads into a live power cord rather than the heart monitor. Luckily, the child survived. Liability was averted because of extenuating circumstances with the child's parents.

More recent cases include *Dent v. Memorial Hospital of Adel, Inc.* (1997), in which the court ruled that the hospital's nursing staff has a duty to see that a pediatric apnea monitor is switched "on" and to respond rapidly and competently if the alarm sounds. In *Chin v. St. Barnabas Medical Center* (1998), the surgeon attached an "unclipped" hose to an exhaust port on a surgical apparatus, thinking it was the suction line, causing the death of a hysteroscopy patient. Neither of the nurses who assisted during the procedure knew how the apparatus functioned or which port was the suction and which was the exhaust line. In *Karl v. Armstrong* (1997), a thermal injury during a laparoscopy caused the patient to suffer colon and small bowel burns, resulting in a permanent colostomy and removal of 16 inches of her ileum.

Liability can result from using defective or unsafe equipment, and nurses have a duty to make a reasonable inspection of equipment and refrain from using equipment that is defective or not working properly (Tammelleo, 1990). In *Beltran v. Downey Community Hospital* (1992), a patient recovering from disk surgery reported that her bed folded into a V, causing her pain and necessitating a second surgical procedure. In investigating the patient's complaint, counsel discovered that the previous patient to have used the bed stated that the same thing had happened to her and that the nursing personnel had refused to change the bed or have the bed repaired. Although this case was settled in favor of the hospital because it was shown in court that the bed could not move in the way described, the case does indicate that nurses could be found liable for failure to reasonably inspect equipment and refrain from using defective equipment. The *Beltran* case may have been avoided had the nursing personnel alerted maintenance when the first patient complained of the folding of the bed.

Nurses are also expected to give quality, competent care despite equipment failures and faulty equipment. An older case illustrates this point. In *Rose v. Hakim* (1971) an infant, who had sustained a cardiac arrest during surgery, required the use of a hypothermia unit in a pediatric intensive care unit. The continuous-readout thermometer on the hypothermia unit was faulty, and the nurse caring for the child failed to verify the thermometer's accuracy or use ancillary cooling measures such as medications, ice packs, or alcohol sponge baths. The infant suffered a grand mal seizure and a respiratory arrest, and was placed on a ventilator for respiratory assistance. When the infant showed signs of poor air exchange on the ventilator, the nurse corrected an obvious kink in the ventilator tubing, but failed to check oxygen concentration and tidal volume delivery. The court held that the infant's subsequent injuries were due primarily to negligent actions and omissions by the nursing personnel, and secondarily to the defective equipment.

Finally, nurses may have a legal duty to assess the equipment's appropriateness. In *Hall v. Arthur* (1998), the surgeon implanted an artificial material during an anterior cervical diskectomy and fusion surgery, rather than bone harvested from the patient's hip or from the tissue bank. Eventually, the patient required a second operation, removing the implant and using the patient's bone. The court ruled that the hospital was also liable because the nurse ordered the synthetic implant without having the unusual request reviewed by the appropriate managers, as was the hospital's policy, and because the product's original package insert specifically contraindicated its use for spinal procedures.

Nurses, through the risk management department, may also have a duty to evaluate whether institutions are following the Safe Medical Devices Act of 1990. Under this law, all medical device–related adverse incidents must be reported to manufacturers and, in cases of death, to the Food and Drug Administration, within 10 working days. The purpose of the law is to investigate and take action the first time an event occurs to prevent reoccurrence and harm to subsequent patients.

FAILURE TO ADEQUATELY ASSESS, MONITOR, AND COMMUNICATE

Nurses are frequently told that their most important duty is that of communication— whether to physicians, other staff members, or through written documentation. Communication is vital, but one must have something to communicate. Perhaps equally important is the nurse's role in assessing and monitoring patients, then in communicating to others.

Failure to adequately assess, monitor, and communicate can occur in all aspects of nursing and in all hospital units. This same failure can occur with all types of nursing procedures and skills, from the simplest to more complex procedures and skills.

Failure to Monitor

Failure to monitor blood pressure and respirations was the cause of action in *Barton v. AMI Park Place Hospital, et al.* (1992). In that case, a high school student was involved in an automobile accident and admitted to the hospital with right upper quadrant pain.

Over the course of seven hours, he bled to death, and his parents brought suit for negligence in monitoring his deteriorating condition and for failure to provide necessary care to stop the bleeding.

Failure to monitor for compartment syndrome in orthopedic cases is a common malpractice allegation. In *Pirkov-Middaugh v. Gillette Children's Hospital* (1991), a 4 year old developed compartment syndrome following hip surgery. Evidence at trial showed that:

1. The nurses had not monitored for compartment syndrome and did not have the equipment needed to test quickly for compartment syndrome.
2. The nurses did not know what equipment was needed.
3. Neither the nurses nor the physicians even knew where the needed equipment was located.

Too often, nurses fail to monitor adequately because of lack of knowledge of potential complications or fail to notify physicians when the patient's condition changes.

Failure to monitor was also the holding in *Stringer v. Katzell* (1996). The patient suffered permanent eighth cranial nerve damage when the staff failed to monitor gentamicin levels in a pediatric patient.

Failure to Assess and Monitor

The failure to assess and monitor is a frequent holding in obstetrical cases. In *Fairfax Hospital System, Inc. v. McCarty* (1992), a labor and delivery nurse was found liable for failure to monitor during a 10-minute period after fetal distress had become apparent. A similar cause of action occurred in *Dobrzenieck v. University Hospital of Cleveland* (1984) when a 36-week preeclampsia patient was admitted for observation. Within two hours, a monitor indicated fetal distress, which went undetected by the nurse and was therefore not reported to the attending physician. Four hours later, the infant was delivered by cesarean section and resuscitated.

Failure to Communicate with Interdisciplinary Health Care Members

Nurses have a responsibility to communicate with interdisciplinary health care members, particularly if there is a change in patient status. In *Seal v. Bogalusa Community Medical Center* (1995), a patient was admitted to an acute care hospital and then transferred to another facility for cardiac angiography, following which she developed renal failure. She began dialysis treatments and was admitted to a skilled nursing unit. On admission to the skilled nursing unit, the physician wrote orders for an immediate consult with a nephrologist and for daily blood chemistry studies.

The blood chemistry studies were done daily as ordered. However, the laboratory results, which indicated a rising potassium level, were only recorded in the medical record by the nurses and were not reported to the physician. The patient was not scheduled for dialysis on the skilled nursing unit as she had been in the acute care facility.

Three days after admission, the patient began to experience nausea. The nurses called the physician, who ordered an antiemetic medication to be given. The patient continued to deteriorate and, since she had a valid do-not-resuscitate order in her medical record, she died within a week of her admission to the skilled nursing unit.

The court ruled that the nurses were negligent for failing to communicate the laboratory results to the attending physician, as was the attending physician for failing to ascertain the laboratory results he had ordered, in light of the patient's admitting diagnosis of acute renal failure. The court also found fault with the nursing staff for failure to consult a nephrologist, as ordered. The court reasoned that had the nephrologist been consulted, the laboratory results would have been closely monitored and hemodialysis restarted.

The failure to communicate medically significant changes to the patient's physician also resulted in liability in *Critchfield v. McNamara* (1995). Here, expert witnesses testified that the nursing personnel should have reported the findings of muscle tone abnormality, lethargy, and the presence of contractions. The significant changes in neurological condition were not recognized, and significant brain injury occurred.

Wingo v. Rockford Memorial Hospital (1997) illustrates the need for nurses to communicate signs and symptoms to physicians unambiguously. Here, a patient was sent home on the physician's belief that a rupture of the membranes in a term pregnancy had sealed over and that labor contractions had ceased. When the physician called to check on the patient who had been admitted with initial rupture of the membranes and irregular contractions, the nurse reported that there was "no change" in the patient's condition. The nurse, held the court, must take responsibility for reporting in a manner that will be understood by the physician, as well as assessing the patient's physical signs accurately.

In *Nguyen v. Tama* (1997), the court reached an opposite conclusion when the nurse accurately communicated assessment data to the physician and even requested that the patient's urine be checked for protein and that magnesium sulfate be started. The fact that the physician did not follow through on these suggestions was immaterial on the part of the nurse. The court in *Rampe v. Community General Hospital of Suffolk County* (1997) ruled that nurses must keep phoning the physician to report that late decelerations are continuing to occur until the physician has physically arrived at the institution and taken charge of the situation.

A case vividly illustrating the need to assess, monitor, and communicate and then to document that these were performed is *O'Donnell v. Holy Family Hospital* (1997). In that case, the labor and delivery nurses noted carefully the specific time that the monitoring strips began to show fetal distress and that the physician was informed and there to look at the strips and assess the patient within a six-minute time frame. The nurses noted the exact time the cesarean section was decided upon, when the anesthetist and neonatologist were called, when the mother was prepped for surgery, and the exact time the initial incision was made. All of these events occurred within an acceptable 30-minute time frame.

Based on the notes at delivery, the court, through expert testimony, was able to conclude that the fetus was essentially born dead, with the airways so hopelessly obstructed in utero that the child could not be brought back to life. Although this was a tragedy, it did not result from failure to assess or to monitor the mother and the unborn child.

The opposite conclusion was reached by the courts in *Conerly v. State of Louisiana* (1997). At 11:45 P.M., the patient, who was 38 weeks pregnant, was admitted, placed on a monitor, and checked once or twice during the night. When the monitoring strips were checked by the resident at 6:00 A.M., they showed fetal distress. The residents then decided what actions to take, and a cesarean section was performed after two and one-half hours. The child was born with severe complications, and the parents were awarded $3,000,000 in damages.

Failure to Communicate with Patients

Obstetrical nurses must also be attentive to communication of relevant patient data. In *Bryant v. John Doe Hospital and John Doe, M.D.* (1992), the patient had two hours of late decelerations, but the nurse failed to communicate these late decelerations to anyone. Sometimes, though, the physician fails to listen to the nurse. In a separate case that same year, the nurses did notify the physician of fetal distress on the monitor, and one nurse even begged him to do an immediate cesarean section to no avail. The physician continued to order drugs to further induce labor and was absent when the woman finally delivered a profoundly retarded neonate (*Herron v. Northwest Community Hospital*, 1992).

The importance of nursing communications cannot be overemphasized because treatment decisions may be made based on those communications or lack of communications. In *Lopez v. Southwest Community Health Service* (1992), a woman who was 28 weeks pregnant experienced pain at home and called the physician's office. She was instructed to go to the hospital, and the physician's nurse called the hospital to inform them of the impending admission and that the patient was in labor. Two nurses worked with her in the hospital. The first nurse failed to examine her, and the second nurse, after doing a pelvic examination, determined that she was 10 cm dilated and that the membranes were bulging. When the physician was notified of these results, he ruptured the membranes and delivered the baby, who is now a quadriplegic, deaf, blind, and brain damaged.

Neither of the nurses questioned the patient or her mother when they arrived at the hospital. Neither did a history of the patient, and they must have not talked with her. If they had, they would have known that neither the patient nor her mother believed that she was in labor but were concerned about her persistent pains. And the physician would not have delivered the child had he not listened to the nurses.

Other cases reflect this failure to listen to patients and what they are trying to tell the staff. In *Parker v. Bullock County Hospital Authority* (1990), the patient fell while taking a shower in the hospital. The patient had had surgery, and she told the nurse when the nurse helped her to the shower that she was dizzy and lightheaded, but the nurse left her unattended to take her shower, obviously ignoring her statement.

What nurses fail to communicate is equally important. Several cases have held nurses directly liable for the failure to communicate pertinent patient data or for not informing the primary health care provider in a timely manner. In one case, a 6-year-old boy lost the use of his hand because the nurse had written an accurate assessment in the nursing notes but failed to bring that same data to the attention of the attending physician before permanent injury occurred (Mandell, 1993).

The duty to communicate is not directed exclusively to nurses. In *Rixey v. West Paces Ferry Hospital, Inc.* (1990), the court held that physicians have a duty to alert nurses to the fact that they should anticipate a significant change in the patient's condition and a possible medical emergency. In this case, a 24-year-old patient was admitted for shortness of breath and chest tightness. The x-ray indicated air in the subcutaneous neck tissues and mediastinum, and the patient was intubated and placed on a ventilator. The physician, however, failed to tell the staff about the air seen on the x-ray and the possibility of a tension pneumothorax developing. The physician left the facility, and the patient subsequently arrested and could not be successfully resuscitated.

In the postanesthesia care unit (PACU), the primary responsibility of nurses is to monitor patients. Cases such as *Torbert v. Befeler* (1985) and *Sanchez v. Bay General Hospital*

(1981) show the tragedy that can occur rapidly when patients are not adequately assessed in the PACU environment. In *Torbert*, the patient began having premature ventricular contractions (PVCs) after anesthesia was started but before the surgical procedure was begun. A consulting cardiologist was called, and the patient was given IV lidocaine and cleared for surgery. While in the PACU, the patient continued to have PVCs, and she arrested three hours after surgery, suffering hypoxic brain damage and death. The family brought suit for failure to closely monitor the patient. The patient had been given lidocaine approximately 45 minutes before her arrest, but the primary nurses caring for her were assisting another patient and the arrest went undetected for some 10 minutes.

In *Sanchez*, the patient had undergone an elective laminectomy and had vomited upon admission to the PACU. Even though the patient's vital signs were taken and recorded every 15 minutes, the various nurses caring for her failed to note the obvious changes in her vital signs or that she was having difficulty breathing. The patient then went into cardiac arrest, and none of the PACU nurses were able to perform cardiopulmonary resuscitation. On review of her record, the court noted that:

1. There was no suctioning equipment ordered for the patient, even though she had been vomiting on admission and during her stay in the PACU.
2. No comparison was made of vital signs in the recovery room, although there had been a significant change in vital signs between admission and the time of the arrest.
3. Vital signs were not taken more frequently after the arrest.
4. No neurological examination of the patient had been performed.
5. No physician was notified of deteriorating vital signs.
6. The nurses failed to note that she had an atrial catheter, although they had used it as an IV.
7. No report was made to the oncoming shift of the patient's deteriorating condition.

A third case in this area had similar results. Following gallbladder surgery, a 27-year-old male was taken to the PACU. He was conscious, thrashing about, and attempting to remove his oral airway. Upon admission to the PACU, the anesthesiologist requested that the admitting nurse monitor the patient frequently because he had just received sufentanil, a potent respiratory depressant. The admitting nurse immediately asked a second nurse to monitor the patient, neglecting to tell the second nurse about the sufentanil injection, and then the admitting nurse left the PACU. When the admitting nurse returned, the patient was alone and his respiratory rate was 8 or less. Shortly after the nurse's return, the anesthesiologist returned, asked about the patient, and was assured that the patient was fine. However, when the anesthesiologist approached the patient's bedside, the patient was in full respiratory arrest. The court found that the sole negligence and cause of the respiratory arrest was the nurse's failure to monitor (*Eyoma v. Falso*, 1991).

A case that extends the duty of health care providers to warn patients of danger of contact with persons at risk is *Troxel v. A. I. Dupont Institute* (1996). In *Troxel*, a mother and her newborn infant were diagnosed with cytomegalovirus (CMV). Despite their diagnosis, the mother and child were visited at home by a friend who assisted with feeding and bathing the infant and with changing diapers. The friend herself had just become pregnant. Six months after she began visiting the mother and baby, the friend discovered that CMV is highly contagious and poses a special threat to pregnant women. She also learned that she herself was probably infected with CMV. Her infant was born three months later. The friend's infant died from CMV, having been affected in utero. The friend filed suit against the medical facility that diagnosed and treated her friend and her friend's infant, claiming damages for her infant's death and for her own infection.

The court held that health care professionals have the legal duty to warn their patients who have highly contagious diseases, such as CMV, hepatitis C, and human immunodeficiency virus (HIV), of the possibility of spreading their diseases to others in certain specific circumstances, and to point out to their patients examples of persons they might encounter who are particularly at risk of contracting their diseases from them.

Assessment and monitoring allow the nurse to use the nursing assessment of the patient to prevent harm or deterioration of the patient's status, while notifying the physician, and to make appropriate nursing diagnoses based on the assessment. One of the better case examples in this area is *Lunsford v. Board of Nurse Examiners* (1983). Ms. Lunsford was a registered nurse who failed to fully assess a potential heart attack patient and thereby failed to initiate appropriate nursing interventions. No medical diagnosis of a myocardial infarction, pulmonary embolism, or pulmonary edema was needed for Lunsford to take vital signs, to listen for cardiac and breath sounds, and to assess for diaphoresis, shortness of breath, and an abnormal cardiac rhythm. Had such steps been taken, she could have communicated and intervened with the hospital physician and seen that the patient received proper care. Ms. Lunsford was the triage nurse on the day of this occurrence. Because of her failure to follow acceptable standards of care, to assess and monitor the patient, her license was suspended, and she settled out of court in the subsequent civil lawsuit.

Communicating with the Culturally and Ethnically Diverse

Some of the issues concerned with communication involve working with culturally and ethnically diverse patients and health care workers. English is not the primary language for many Americans today, and this may result in communication difficulties. There is some limited case law to support not hiring personnel because of their inability to communicate effectively with the public, an essential requirement of jobs in which the individual interfaces with people daily (*Fragante v. City and County of Honolulu, et al.*, 1989), and in refusing to allow nurses to converse in their native language as opposed to English (*Dimaranan v. Pomona Valley Medical Center, et al.*, 1991). In *Dimaranan*, the hospital prohibited nurses on a maternity unit from conversing in their native Filipino dialect, because such conversations had created differential treatment for the nurse who spoke the dialect and adversely affected worker morale and supervision. The court further stated that this language restriction did not violate the nurses' civil rights because it was motivated by a desire to eliminate dissension that could have compromised patient safety and quality health care delivery.

There is also limited case law showing the harm that can occur when English is not the primary language for the patient. In *Nevarez v. New York City Health and Hospitals Corporation* (1997), a patient who did not speak English was brought into the hospital by her brother. She was having labor contractions and was bleeding. The brother brought her to the information desk, rather than to the emergency center. The information desk staff phoned the physician, who told them to have her wait for his arrival, which occurred some three hours later.

She was in labor with a difficult breech presentation, requiring transfer by ambulance to a second facility for a cesarean section. The baby was born with severe hypoxic brain damage and the mother was awarded $10,000,000 in damages.

The court found that the patient should have been sent to the emergency center, even though the physician requested that she wait there. Additionally, if the patient had been able to better describe her distress or if the facility had provided a translator, the patient would have been able to make herself understood and she would have been timely seen in the emergency center.

Because of this diversity, state laws, JCAHO standards, and the American Hospital Association Bill of Rights for Patients have included provisions for ensuring that patient rights means also being able to meet their communication needs, particularly if patients do not speak English or speak it so brokenly that they are unable to express themselves or understand what is said to them. To prevent such a happening, most institutions now provide interpreters for non-English speaking patients, and nurses must make reasonable efforts to ensure that patients understand care issues and discharge education and instructions.

Nurses should document who was used as the interpreter—family member or hospital-provided interpreter—instructions given, and means of ensuring that the patient understood the instructions or conversations. Means that may be employed to ensure comprehension include having the patient repeat the material back to the nurse or asking questions and requiring that the patient respond. As more non-English speaking patients enter the health care delivery system, the profession may see additional causes of action based on their noncomprehension and failure to follow instructions because they never understood the instructions.

■ EXERCISE 13–3

A patient, admitted for minor surgery, tells you that he is having some chest discomfort and shortness of breath. The patient, a known cardiac patient, had nitroglycerin prescribed for chest pain, and you give him the ordered medication, then go back to the task you were doing when he called for assistance. You do not notify the physician of the chest discomfort, nor do you check back with the patient to see if the medication eased the pain or had any effect at all. Later in the day, during a preoperative visit by the nurse anesthetist, the nurse anesthetist asks about the patient's status and recent cardiac history and again you say nothing. If the patient suffers a massive heart attack during surgery the next morning, could liability for failure to assess, monitor, and communicate be found against you? What would you plead as your best defense in such a case?

FAILURE TO ACT AS A PATIENT ADVOCATE

As the profession develops, it has become apparent that nurses owe a higher duty to patients than merely following physician's orders. Professional nurses serve in the role of patient advocate, developing and implementing nursing diagnoses and exercising good patient judgment as they monitor the care given to patients by physicians as well as peers. The failure to function in this independent role has long been recognized by the courts as a *failure to act as a patient advocate,* and court decisions continue to emphasize this vital function of nursing.

The professional nurse has a duty to report medical care or medical orders that jeopardize the care of patients. In *Catron v. The Poor Sisters of St. Francis* (1982), a patient was admitted for an unintentional drug overdosage. While in the hospital, the patient had been intubated via a nasotracheal tube for several days before its removal. He then had a tracheostomy to prevent respiratory failure. The patient brought this cause of action due to inability to speak in a normal voice after removal of the endotracheal tube and tracheostomy.

The hospital defended the case by asserting that it was medical judgment when to remove an endotracheal tube and how long one could remain in place without causing the patient harm. The court, in finding against the hospital and nursing staff, held that while a hospital is usually not liable for nurses following physicians' orders, an exception exists when the nurses know that the practice does not follow usual procedure. The nurses had an affirmative duty to report this deviation to their supervisors.

Thus, nurses have a duty not only to question incomplete and illegible orders, but to also question orders that deviate from the usual standards of practice and to inform hospital administration, via nursing supervisors and midmanagement nurses, of such deviations. Fiesta (1994) suggests that this affirmative duty involves not only questions of competence or inappropriate medical decisions, but also the reporting of "bizarre and disruptive behavior or conduct which may be a symptom of impairment" (p. 15).

But contrast the preceding case with *Dixon v. Freuman* (1991). In this case, the physician ordered the removal of a Foley catheter, and the nurses removed the catheter per hospital policy. When the patient brought suit that the catheter should not have been removed, the court held that, in the absence of proof that the order to remove the catheter was "clearly contraindicated by normal practice," the nurses and hospital could not be held liable for the subsequent fistula.

The duty to serve as a patient advocate may also require nurses to directly disobey physicians' orders. In *Cruzbinsky v. Doctors' Hospital* (1983), a circulating nurse was ordered by the physician to leave the operating room before the patient had been sent to the PACU. Although the nurse initially questioned the order, she finally left at the doctor's insistence. After her departure, the patient arrested, suffering significant permanent damage. The patient then brought suit against the hospital and nurse for abandonment.

The court held that the nurse had a duty to remain with the patient, following the hospital policy and procedure manual, even if the physician was insistent and "yelling at her." The court further concluded that this abandonment was so obvious that no expert witness was needed for the jury to conclude that abandonment had occurred.

Premature patient discharge is another area in which nurses have a duty to be the patient's advocate. Court cases such as *Wickline v. State of California* (1986) and *Wilson v. Blue Cross of Southern California* (1992) speak to the harm that can befall patients if discharged from acute care settings before they are sufficiently improved or stabilized. In the first case, the patient lost her leg due to infection and in the second case, a psychiatric patient committed suicide after his early discharge. Although these two cases were directed at physicians and utilization reviewers, there seems little doubt that the courts would also extend such holdings to nurses who failed to serve as patient advocate, speaking directly to the involved physicians and to nursing supervisors, when patients are discharged inappropriately. In *Koeniquer v. Eckrich* (1988), it was the court's holding that nurses do have a duty to question a physician's discharge orders or to delay the discharge if they believe that the discharge violates acceptable standards of care.

Patient Education

The issue of early discharge also addresses the crucial need for early and ongoing discharge planning and education of patients. In a home health care case, *Ready v. Personal Care Health Services* (1991), a child was discharged from home health care services, developed pneumonia, and died. The parents brought suit, in part, for the failure of the nurses to adequately address potential complications and to educate the parents about the possibility of such life-threatening conditions.

Nurses have a duty to protect patients, to question orders that are inappropriate or likely to cause harm to the patient, and to provide adequate, early discharge education. If directly speaking with the attending physician does not result in the desired outcome, then nurses have a duty to inform their supervisors and midmanagement personnel so that other means of providing safe and competent health care may be obtained. Communication is vital and interventions taken on behalf of patients should be promptly and adequately charted in the patient record.

GUIDELINES: ACTING AS A PATIENT ADVOCATE

1. Nurses should be aware of hospital policies and protocols, as well as acceptable standards of care. Question physicians when orders are contrary to the acceptable standard of care or you believe following the order could cause patient harm. Do not be intimidated into following orders, but use your independent judgment. If physicians persist or refuse to change the order, consult nursing supervisory personnel.

2. In emergency situations in which the nurse believes that following the physician's order could result in harm to the patient, the nurse should disobey the order, ensure patient safety and appropriate nursing care, then notify nursing supervisors and administrative supervisors.

3. If the patient is discharged early and such early discharge could cause direct harm to the patient, voice your concern to the attending physician and nursing supervisor. Remember, you have a duty to attempt to prevent such early discharges.

4. Discharge planning and instruction must begin early—when the patient is admitted—and be completed before the patient's discharge. Include in your teaching potential complications for which the patient/family member must be alert and what to do if signs and symptoms of complications arise. Give the patient written instructions if available and carefully document carefully your instructions in the patient's medical record.

5. The patient is your priority concern, and nurses have an affirmative duty to serve as patient advocates.

■ **EXERCISE 13—4**

Mr. Jones, a newly diagnosed insulin-dependent diabetic, is to receive discharge planning about his condition. You are the diabetic coordinator for the hospital and have developed a wonderful diabetic teaching protocol. Dr. Smith, one of the good old boys, tells you not to teach his patient anything. "He's my patient and I'll teach him what he needs to know. I do not want you interfering in my patient's care, not now or ever." How would you proceed in this instance? Does Dr. Smith have the final say about his patients in all aspects of their care? What if Mr. Jones later filed a lawsuit because of your failure to teach and he suffers significant harm?

What are the ethical principles involved in working with this physician? With the patient? Can the nurse ethically not teach the patient about his diabetes, merely because the physician does not want the patient taught by the discharge nurse? If Mr. Jones should later develop complications from his lack of patient education, what ethical implications would that have for the nurse?

SUMMARY

Potential lawsuits for nursing malpractice can arise from almost any act or failure to act that results in injury to a given patient. This chapter has stressed the more commonly occurring areas of nursing liability, giving guidelines, nursing interventions, and current case law examples for the nurse to implement and understand in avoiding future litigation in these areas. As the acuity of inpatient care increases, so will the potential for liability. The growing trend of courts in assessing nurses' liability for malpractice will also continue as standards of care are redefined and professional autonomy is recognized.

AFTER COMPLETING THIS CHAPTER, YOU SHOULD BE ABLE TO

- Describe the changing health care environment that has created increased responsibility in staff nurses.
- Describe uniquenesses to the care of psychiatric and vulnerable patients.
- Differentiate two types of restraints, and describe the difference between those restraints, including nursing management of the restrained patient.
- Describe the nurses responsibility in medication errors and five means to avoid such errors.
- Analyze the potential liability for nurses when using technologic advances and specialized equipment.
- Compare and contrast the nurses responsibility for assessing, monitoring, and communicating in clinical settings.
- Describe the role of the nurse as a patient advocate.

APPLY YOUR LEGAL KNOWLEDGE

- If a patient falls and suffers injury, is the nurse always liable? What defenses could the nurse argue in his or her support?
- What can nurses do to prevent medication errors?
- Are there areas of the hospital in which potential liability as a staff nurse is greater? What can the staff nurses on that unit do to prevent potential lawsuits?
- How do communications prevent lawsuits? What must be communicated and to whom?
- Are there ever times when the nurse cannot be the patient's advocate? Give examples to support your answer.

YOU BE THE JUDGE

On June 25, Roger Treinis was admitted to Deepdale General Hospital for surgery to repair a torn Achilles tendon. Although his blood pressure was elevated, he was certified for surgery by his primary physician. Given antihypertensives both before and during surgery, his blood presure remained elevated while he was in the postanesthesia care unit (PACU). The attending physician ordered the nursing staff to begin administering by titration the medication nitroprusside (Nipride). The nurses refused, citing hospital policy and procedure that prohibited administering Nipride to patients not admitted to the intensive care unit (ICU).

The attending physician then ordered that Treinis be transferred from the PACU to the ICU, but no beds were available for about an hour. Other antihypertensives were given to the patient during this hour, and his blood pressure improved slightly. Once transferred to the ICU, a Nipride drip was immediately begun, but it failed to control his elevating blood pressure. A cardiologist ordered additional medications, but Treinis's condition deteriorated. When he developed respiratory distress, the patient was intubated and placed on a ventilator.

Treinis died 16 hours after admission to the ICU. An autopsy attributed his death to a rare, previously undiagnosed tumor and massive heart failure. Mr. Treinis's wife sued for wrongful death and negligence. The hospital filed a summary motion, which was denied, and the hospital appealed.

Legal Questions

1. Did negligence or malpractice cause this patient's death.
2. Was the nursing staff at fault for having refused to begin the Nipride drip in the PACU?
3. How significant is hospital policy and procedure?
4. Did the nurses' compliance with hospital policy and procedure cause this patient's death?
5. How would you decide this case?

REFERENCES

Aiken, T. D., and Catalano, J. T. (1994). *Legal, Ethical, and Political Issues in Nursing.* Philadelphia: F. A. Davis Company.

Application of Anthony M. v. Sanchez, 645 N.Y.S.2d 23 (N.Y. App., 1996).

Bartlett, E. E., and Rehmar, M. I. (1997). *The Difficult Patient: How to Reduce Your Liability Risk.* Rockville, MD: EBA Publications.

Barton v. AMI Park Place Hospital, et al., No. 909-066318 (Texas, 1992).

Bazel v. Mabee, 576 N.W.2d 385 (Iowa App., 1998).

Bellamy v. Central Valley General Hospital, 57 Cal. Rptr.2d 894 (Cal. App., 1996).

Beltran v. Downey Community Hospital (1992). *Medical Malpractice Verdicts, Settlements, and Experts* 8(5), 30.

Biggs v. United States, 655 F. Supp. 1093 (W.D. La., 1987).

Bishop v. South Carolina Department of Mental Health, 502 S.E.2d 78 (South Carolina, 1998).

Bossley v. Dallas County Memorial Health and Mental Retardation, 934 S.W.2d 689 (Tex. App., 1995).

Bryant v. John Doe Hospital and John Doe, M.D. (1992). *Medical Malpractice Verdicts, Settlements, and Experts* 8(1), 35.

Catron v. The Poor Sisters of St. Francis, 435 N.E.2d 305 (Indiana, 1982).

Chin v. St. Barnabas Medical Center, 711 A.2d 352 (N.J. Super. A.D., 1998).

Clinical News (1997). *American Journal of Nursing* 97(4), 10.

Conerly v. State of Louisiana, 690 So.2d 980 (La. App., 1997).

Copeland v. Northwestern Memorial Hospital, 964 F. Supp. 1225 (N.D. Ill., 1997).

Critchfield v. McNamara, 32 N.W.2d 287 (Nebraska, 1995).

Cruzbinsky v. Doctors' Hospital, 188 Cal. Rptr. 685 (Cal. App., 1983).

Demers v. United States (1990). *Medical Malpractice: Verdicts, Settlements, and Experts* 6(3), 34.

Dent v. Memorial Hospital of Adel, Inc., 490 S.E.2d 509 (Ga. App., 1997).

Dessauer v. Memorial General Hospital, 628 P.2d 337 (N.M. Ct. App., 1981).

Dimaranan v. Pomona Valley Medical Center, et al., 775 F. Supp. 338 (C.D. Cal., 1991).

Dixon v. Freuman, 573 N.Y.S.2d (New York, 1991).

Dobrzenieck v. University Hospital of Cleveland, #17843 (Cyahoga City Ct. of Common Pleas, May 22, 1984).

Eyoma v. Falso, 589 A.2d 653 (N.J., 1991).

Fairfax Hospital System, Inc. v. McCarty, 419 S.E.2d 621 (Va., 1992).

Farrow v. Health Services, et al., 604 P.2d 474 (Utah, 1979).

Fiesta, J. (1994). Failing to act like a professional. *Nursing Management,* 24(7), 15–17.

Fragante v. City and County of Honolulu, et al., 888 F.2d 591 (9th Cir., 1989).

Gallimore v. Children's Hospital Medical Center, WL37742 (Ohio App. 1 Dist., 1992).

Genoa v. State of New York, 679 N.Y.S.2d 539 (N.Y. Ct. Cl., 1998).

Hall v. Arthur, 141 F.3d 844 (8th Cir., 1998).

Heater v. Southwood Psychiatric Center, 49 Cal. Rptr.2d 880 (Cal. App., 1996).

Herron v. Northwest Community Hospital (1992). Emergency Medical Associates et al. *Medical Malpractice Verdicts, Settlements, and Experts,* 8(10), 33.

In re Dorothy W., 692 N.E.2d 388 (Ill. App., 1998).

In the Interest of "J.P.," 574 N.W.2d 340 (Iowa, 1998).

Involuntary psychiatric commitment: Court reviews legal criteria for holding patient (1998). *Legal Eagle Eye Newsletter for the Nursing Profession,* 6(5), 4.

Joint Commission for the Accreditation of Healthcare Organizations (1998). *Sentinel Event Statistics.* Oakbrook Terrace, IL: Author.

Karl v. Armstrong, No. 92-7084 (Hillsborough County, Fla., 1997).

Killian, W. H. (1990). Equipment mishaps may result in lawsuits. *The American Nurse,* 22(3), 34.

Kobs, A. (1997). Patient Restraints and JCAHO Compliance. *Journal of Nursing Management,* 28(1), 14–15.

Koeniquer v. Eckrich, 422 N.W.2d 600 (South Dakota, 1988).

Laman v. Big Spring State Hospital, 970 S.W.2d 670 (Tex. App., 1998).

Lopez v. Southwest Community Health Service, 833 P.2d 1183 (New Mexico, 1992).

Lunsford v. Board of Nurse Examiners, 648 S.W.2d 391 (Tex. Civ. App.–Austin, 1983).

Mandell, M. (1993). What you don't say can hurt you. *American Journal of Nursing* 93(8), 15–16.

Mounts v. St. David's Pavilion, 957 S.W.2d 661 (Tex. App., 1997).

National Alliance for the Mentally Ill (1994). *Mental Illness: Information for Writers.* Arlington, VA: Author.

Nevarez v. New York City Health and Hospitals Corporation, 663 N.Y.S.2d 190 (N.Y. App., 1997).

Nguyen v. Tama, 688 A.2d 1103 (N.J. Super., 1997).

O'Donnell v. Holy Family Hospital, 682 N.E.2d 386 (Ill. App., 1997).

Parker v. Bullock County Hospital Authority, (1990). A9OAO 762 *Medical Malpractice: Verdicts, Settlements, and Experts* 6(10), 28.

Parker v. Centenary Heritage Manor Nursing Home, et al., 677 So.2d 568 (La. App., 1996).

Phillip v. University Medical Center, 714 So.2d 742 (La. App., 1998).

Pirkov-Middaugh v. Gillette Children's Hospital, No. C9-91-526 (Minnesota, 1991).

Rampe v. Community General Hospital of Suffolk County, 660 N.Y.S.2d 206 (N.Y. App., 1997).

Ready v. Personal Care Health Services, #842472 (California, 1991).

Rixey v. West Paces Ferry Hospital, Inc., 916 F.2d 608 (Georgia, 1990).

Rocca v. Southern Hills Counseling Center, Inc., 671 N.E.2d 913 (Ind. App., 1996).

Romaro v. Marks, 647 N.Y.S.2d 272 (N.Y. Sep., 1996).

Rose v. Hakim, 335 F. Supp. 1121 (D.C.C., 1971).

Safe Medical Devices Act of 1990, 21 U.S.C., 306i.

Sanchez v. Bay General Hospital, 172 Cal. Rptr. 342 (Cal. App., 1981).

Seal v. Bogalusa Community Medical Center, 665 S.W.2d 42 (La. App., 1995).

Sharrow v. Archer, 658 P.2d 1331 (Alaska, 1983).

Shepard v. State Department of Mental Health, 957 P.2d 553 (Okla. Civ. App., 1998).

S. P. v. City of Takoma Park, 134 F.3d 260 (4th Cir., 1998).

Stark v. Children's Orthopedic Hospital and Medical Center (1990). #87-2-12416-9. *Medical Malpractice: Verdicts, Settlements and Experts* 9(10), 28.

St. Elizabeth's Hospital v. Graham, 883 S.W.2d 433 (Tex. App., 1994).

Stringer v. Katzell, 647 So.2d 193 (Fla. App., 1996).

Swann v. Len-Care Rest Home, Inc., 490 S.E.2d 572 (N.C. App., 1997).

Tammelleo, D. (1990). Who's to blame for faulty equipment? *RN* 17(5), 67–72.

Tarasoff v. The Regents of the University of California, 554 P.2d 347 (California, 1976).

Torbert v. Befeler, No. L-17463-81, Union Cty. Sup. Ct. (April 25, 1985).

Troxel v. A. I. Dupont Institute, 675 A.2d 314 (Pa. Super., 1996).

Turner v. Jordan, 957 S.W.2d 815 (Tennessee, 1997).

Van Hyning v. Hamilton Hospital (1994). *Medical Malpractice: Verdicts, Settlements, and Experts* 10(9), 24.

Wall v. Fairview Hospital and Healthcare Services, 568 N.W.2d 194 (Minn. App., 1997), cert. granted, 584 N.W.2d 395 (Minnesota, 1998).

Wickline v. State of California, 192 Cal. App.3d 1630, 239 Cal. Rptr. 810 (1986).
Wilson v. Blue Cross of Southern California, 222 Cal. App.3d 660, 271, Cal. Rptr. 876 (1992).
Winger v. Franciscan Medical Center, 701 N.E.2d 813 (Ill. App., 1998).
Wingo v. Rockford Memorial Hospital, 686 N.E.2d 722 (Ill. App., 1997).
Wingstrom v. Evanston Hospital, WL 97934 (N.D. Ill., 1992).

fourteen

Employment Laws: Corporate Liability Issues

■ PREVIEW

Whenever a nurse is employed by another, be it a hospital, clinic, or physician, the employing entity accepts potential liability for the nurse-employee. The nurse becomes the employer's representative and, because of their special legal status, conveys potential liability to the employer. Never, though, does the nurse convey all liability to the employer. Each individual is ultimately responsible for his or her actions.

As nurses become more independent of the hospital setting, whether becoming entrepreneurs, freelancing as consultants and educational specialists, or entering into partnerships with other health care providers, understanding and knowing aspects of contract law become more imperative. Some hospital nurses have had formal, written contracts, although the majority of nurses working in non–collective bargaining states and institutions are truly better classified as at-will employees.

This chapter discusses theories of corporate liability and a variety of employment laws. This chapter also outlines contract law, defining the various aspects of formal and informal contracts, and concludes with a discussion of legal issues involved in contract law.

■ KEY CONCEPTS

vicarious liability
respondeat superior
borrowed servant doctrine
dual servant doctrine
corporate liability
negligent hiring and retention
ostensible authority
independent contractor
personal liability
indemnification
Equal Employment Opportunity
   Commission (EEOC)
1964 Civil Rights Act
Federal Tort Claims Act of 1946
Age Discrimination in Employment
   Act of 1967

affirmative action
Equal Pay Act
Occupational Safety and Health
   Act of 1970 (OSHA)
employment-at-will
wrongful discharge
collective bargaining
   (labor relations)
National Labor Relations
   Act (NLRA)
Family and Medical Leave Act
   of 1993
contract
statute of frauds
formal contract

oral contract
expressed contract
implied contract
contract termination
breach
monetary damages
injunction
specific performance
mediation
arbitration
fact finding
summary jury trial
contract negotiation

THEORIES OF VICARIOUS LIABILITY

Vicarious liability, or *substituted liability,* is the term used to describe the instance in which one party is responsible for the actions of another. The law allows substituted liability to prevent further injustice to the injured party and to encourage employers to maintain employee competence. If the injured parties could sue only the nurse who harmed them, the injured person might not be able to be fully compensated monetarily, unless, of course, the nurse is independently wealthy. Making the employer liable increases the chances that money will be available to cover the damages incurred. It also encourages the employer to hire and retain safe practitioners.

Vicarious liability is not a shift in liability, but an extension of liability to allow justice to be fairly distributed. Vicarious liability extends liability to include the employer, but never to the extent that personal and individual liability is lost.

Respondeat Superior

Respondeat superior, "let the master respond" or "let the master answer," is the old common law principle of substituted liability based on a master–servant relationship. While nurses may disagree with a master–servant relationship, the courts have found similar elements: (1) The employer controls the actions of the employee; and (2) substituted liability applies only to actions within the scope and course of employment. The effect of this doctrine is that the employer is given responsibility and accountability for an employee's negligent actions and that the injured party may recover damages from the employer or employing institution.

The rationale for such recovery lies in a benefit burden analysis. Employers, standing to reap the benefits of the employees' activities, must also bear the burden of the employees' errors. Employers have an obligation to see that those they hire perform duties and tasks in a safe and competent manner. As the court said in *Hunter v. Allis-Chambers Corporation, Engine Division* (1986): "An employer is directly liable for torts caused by his employees against others. The employer could have prevented these torts by reasonable care in hiring, supervising, and, if necessary, firing the tortfeasor" (at 1419).

The leading case for respondeat superior in health care is *Duling v. Bluefield Sanitarium, Inc.* (1965). In that case, a 13 year old was admitted to the hospital with a diagnosis of rheumatic heart disease. At 7:00 P.M. on the evening of her admission, Nancy Duling was seen by the attending physician, and he told her mother that the child could easily develop heart failure. The physician explained to Mrs. Duling the signs and symptoms to be alert for, and to notify the nursing staff immediately if she observed any of those signs and symptoms in Nancy.

Shortly after the physician left, Nancy began exhibiting signs of failure, and Mrs. Duling notified the staff. The nurses did not check Nancy and, in spite of frequently pleas for help and an obvious deterioration in Nancy's condition, the nurses waited over six hours before adequately assessing the patient. By that time, Nancy's condition was so serious that subsequent treatment failed to save her life.

The issue at court was whether the hospital was liable for the negligence of the nursing staff for failure to provide competent nursing care. The court enumerated the hospital's standard of care thusly: "A private hospital, conducted for profit, owes to its patients such reasonable care and attention for their safety as their mental and physical condition, if known, may require. The care exercised should be commensurate with the known inability of the patient to care for himself" (at 759). Thus, the court found that the hospital was liable for the care provided (or not provided) by its employees.

This reliance on the doctrine of respondeat superior stems from the nurses' responsibility to act according to standards of care and from the employment relationship with the hospital wherein the nurse provides care and meets not only legal standards, but also hospital mandates.

Scope and Course of Employment

Two hurdles that the injured party must pass before the principle of respondeat superior is allowed are:

1. The injured party must show that the employer had control over the employee.
2. The negligent act must have occurred within the course and scope of the employee's employment.

The first element is fairly straightforward and is usually shown by proving employment status. The second element is more difficult, because the injured party must show that the actions were those for which the nurse was hired and that they occurred during the course of work.

Courts tend to decide scope and course of business on a case-by-case basis. The first factor that courts of law consistently determine is foreseeability of the action. Should the employer have been able to foresee that an employee could perform a certain action as he or she did? Various case decisions indicate that most activities undertaken by employees will be held foreseeable for the purpose of finding employer liability. For example, the court in *Robertson v. Bethlehem Steel Corporation* (1990) held that if employees acted within the scope of their employment and their actions were in connection with the employer's business, the plaintiff could recover. *Biconi v. Pay 'N Pak Stores, Inc.* (1990) extended the scope and course of employment to intentional torts as well as negligent torts.

Some of the other factors consistently analyzed by courts include:

1. Usual place of employment.
2. Whether the act's purpose, in whole or in part, was in furtherance of the employer's business.
3. The extent to which the act was similar or different from authorized acts of the employer.
4. The extent to which the act was a departure from the employer's customary methods.
5. The extent to which the employer should have expected such an act to occur. (*American Jurisprudence*, 1992).

Two examples may help. In the first example, Nurse A allows Mr. Jones to fall as she is assisting him back to bed. Mr. Jones is a patient in the intensive care unit who had hip surgery two days prior to this incident. Liability would extend to the hospital, as the hospital policy and procedure manual mandates that she properly assess the patient and obtain adequate help before assisting the patient either to or from his bed. Note, however, that if Nurse A failed to assist Mr. Jones in the manner prescribed by hospital policy, the hospital would have cause to argue that this action was not performed according to the master–servant doctrine.

In the second example, Nurse A is in the hospital for the sole purpose of collecting her paycheck. Nurse B, a coworker in the intensive care unit, asks Nurse A to put Mr. Jones back to bed so that Nurse B can finish her charting and then join Nurse A for lunch. Mr. Jones subsequently falls. Nurse A would be solely accountable for her actions, as she was not within the course and scope of her employment at the time of Mr. Jones's fall. The hospital may still be held accountable, however, through the actions of Nurse B, also a hospital employee.

Actions that would be outside the course and scope of employment include the rendering of voluntary health services, either at the scene of an accident or as part of a community health drive, and the giving of health-related advice on a voluntary basis, for example, to a neighbor or friend. Additionally, performing actions that are reserved for physicians or advanced practice nurses is not considered within the scope of employment for staff nurses.

Note that the nursing supervisor is also an employee of the hospital, not the employer. While the nursing supervisor may be liable if there is a negligent act by an employee of the hospital, the supervisor's liability is incurred because of a failure to perform the supervisory duties in a competent manner, for example, as a reasonably prudent nursing supervisor would.

The doctrine of respondeat superior applies equally to acts of omission as well as commission. In the landmark decision of *Darling v. Charleston Community Memorial Hospital* (1965), the nurses and thus the hospital were found liable for their failure to notify the medical staff or the chief of the medical service when the attending physician failed to deliver proper medical care to James Darling.

In *Darling,* the patient had undergone a cast procedure to set a broken bone in the patient's leg. The nurses assigned to care for Mr. Darling subsequent to the cast application assessed his recovery accurately: The circulation to his casted extremity was sluggish, he continued to require ever-increasing amounts of pain medications, and there was a foul odor coming from the cast site. Numerous nurses charted their observations and continued to apprise the attending physician of the patient's symptoms. The attending physician responded to their assessments by ordering increased amounts of pain medications and increasing the antibiotic therapy for Mr. Darling. Ultimately, James Darling was transferred to a second hospital, and, despite aggressive therapy, the physicians were unable to save the leg.

The court, in finding against the nurses and the hospital, stated that it is not sufficient to merely apprise the attending physician of a deterioration in a patient's condition. Hospital staff have a further duty to inform others in authority positions so that the patient may receive competent care. In the case described, the chief of staff or the hospital medical committee could have intervened had they known of James Darling's substandard medical care.

When a lawsuit is filed using the master–servant or respondeat superior doctrine, both the hospital and the nurse are sued. Often, the hospital will attempt to claim that the nurse was acting outside the scope of his or her employment to avoid liability. Thus, nurses must first show that they were within the scope of employment at the time of the incident. Also, some suits are filed against the employer without naming the nurse as a defendant. The employer may still be held liable because of the employer–employee relationship.

■ EXERCISE 14—1

Judy Jones, an employee of Doctor Doe, and Beth Smith, an employee of Doctor Roe, are friends, and both of their offices are in the same building. One day, as the nurses are leaving the building for lunch, they notice an elderly lady in obvious respiratory distress. Judy recognizes the lady as a patient of Doctor Doe and immediately runs back to the office to get him. Meanwhile, Beth Smith, in attempting to help the patient, injures the elderly lady. The patient subsequently dies, and her estate sues Doctor Doe and Doctor Roe, claiming negligence on the part of Beth Smith. Are the physicians negligent under the doctrine of respondeat superior? Is anyone at fault? Will the family be able to recover damages?

Borrowed Servant and Dual Servant Doctrines

The *borrowed servant doctrine* is a special application of the doctrine of respondeat superior. A borrowed servant is one who, while in the general employment of another, is subject to the right to direct and control the details of the servant's particular activities. This right to direct and control must be more than a mere cooperation with the suggestions of an authority figure. The borrowed servant doctrine applies when one employer lends completely the services or skills of an employee to another employer, and the key to this doctrine is the right or manner of control.

The borrowed servant doctrine's usual application in nursing occurs when the nurse-employee comes under the direct supervision and control of a physician, and the employer-hospital would not be liable for negligent or intentional torts of the nurse while the nurse is under the direct control and supervision of the directing physician. The directing physician becomes liable under the doctrine of respondeat superior if the injured party can prove exclusive control and course and scope of employment. The right to control, said the court in *Harris v. Miller* (1994), is not presumed because the surgeon is in charge during the operation, but must be proven during the course of the trial.

Traditionally, the borrowed servant doctrine applies to situations within the operating room or to cardiopulmonary resuscitation and is sometimes referred to as the *captain of the ship doctrine*. The name and application refer to situations in which one person and only one person has command, and any negligence incurred will be imputed back to the person in command. The captain of the ship doctrine was first used in a medical malpractice context in 1959 (*McConnell v. Williams*).

The trend in national case law is away from the captain of the ship doctrine. This is reflected by the landmark decision made by the Texas Supreme Court in *Sparger v. Worley Hospital, Inc.* (1977), which concluded that the captain of the ship doctrine is a false application of a specific rule of agency and that one must first determine if the nurses are borrowed servants in deciding liability issues. Recent case law in Kansas, Colorado, and Washington, however, shows that the captain of the ship doctrine is still used in some jurisdictions (*Oberzan v. Smith*, 1994; *Spoor v. Serota*, 1992; and *Van Hook v. Anderson*, 1992). In the *Van Hook* case, there was a mistake made in the sponge count, and the court held that the physician was not liable under the captain of the ship doctrine for the nurse's error in counting the sponges. In fact, the court noted that counting sponges entailed following written hospital policy and procedures and that there was no showing in this case that the surgeon gave orders how or when to count sponges.

A case with a similar result is *Golinski v. Hackensack Medical Center* (1997). In essentially the same fact scenario, the court in this case found that the surgeon, circulating nurse, and surgical technician were all legally responsible for an incorrect sponge count in the operating room. No mention was made of the captain of the ship doctrine, and all three defendants were held equally responsible. A similar conclusion was reached in *Johnson v. Southwest Louisiana Association* (1997). In *Johnson*, the surgeon was held to be 60% liable and the operating room nurses 40% liable for a retained sponge during a hernia repair. No mention was made of the captain of the ship doctrine, and perhaps its application is further deteriorating nationwide.

For the hospital to be relieved of liability, the nurse must be totally following the physician's order. If the nurse is merely taking a short-cut and violating hospital policy, then the hospital usually retains its responsibility and liability. Some courts prefer to enact a *dual servant doctrine,* which allows for vicarious liability to flow to both the employer-hospital and to the physician (*Holger v. Irish,* 1993). A dual servant is one who can be shown to be serving both entities at the same time. For example, circulating nurses in the operating room remain hospital employees, yet strictly follow the orders of the surgeon in charge. In *Holger,* the injured plaintiff had to show that the operating nurses were negligent, and that the nurses were the surgeon's employees or agents or that there were other facts that established the surgeon's supervision and control over the nurses at the time of the incident. As with all vicarious liability situations, the nurse who does not act in a reasonably prudent manner may be held individually negligent along with the employer. A similar finding was seen in *Golinski.*

CORPORATE LIABILITY

The courts have created over the past 15 years what is now known as *corporate liability,* a doctrine that evolved as hospitals became more profitable and competitive. The *Darling* case is the landmark case for corporate liability, placing certain nondelegable duties regarding patient care directly on the hospital corporation. Prior to the *Darling* ruling, hospitals bore no liability for the provision of health care because the facility was considered to be one in which others provided care.

Under this new doctrine, corporations have a direct duty to the public that they serve, ensuring that competent and qualified practitioners will deliver quality health care to consumers. A later court case interpreted *Darling* to include the duty to make a reasonable effort to monitor and oversee the treatment that is prescribed and administered by physicians and nurses practicing within the institution (*Bost v. Riley,* 1980).

All of the hospital's corporate duties have a direct impact on the provision of patient care. The emphasis on the hospital's responsibility for adequate care is apparent. Most of the early case law dealt with the hospital's responsibility to select and delineate clinical privileges of physicians. The hospital, however, has duties to the patient outside of clinical privileges, which include adequate staffing, supervision for education and training of staff members, maintaining the premises in a reasonably safe manner, provision of properly functioning and reasonably updated equipment, reasonable care in the selection and retention of employees, and the duty to meet a national standard of care.

A case that illustrates corporate liability is *Carter v. Hucks-Folliss* (1998). In this case, the issue was whether a hospital could be sued for granting clinical privileges to a physician without considering the physician's board status. The court held that while Joint Commission for the Accreditation of Healthcare Organizations (JCAHO) standards do not require a physician to be board certified in order to obtain clinical privileges, the JCAHO does require the hospital to consider the physician's board status.

In this case, the hospital did not consider the physician's board status before granting clinical privileges. The patient was then injured and brought a lawsuit against the hospital for liability under a corporate liability standard. In holding for the injured patient, the court concluded that legal precedents have established that if a patient suffers harm in an instance in which an accredited health care facility deviates from the standards of its accrediting body, the patient can use that deviation as proof of negligence in a subsequent lawsuit against the hospital.

Negligent Hiring and Retention

The doctrine of *negligent hiring and retention* of employees is often used by injured parties when respondeat superior cannot be applied to the current fact situation. For example, in situations in which nurses were not acting within the course and scope of employment or in which they were acting solely for personal reasons. This doctrine essentially means that the employer can still be held liable if the injured party can show that the employee was incompetent or unsafe for the position and that the employer knew or should have known that the employee was incompetent or unsafe.

Like respondeat superior, negligent hiring and retention is based on the master–servant relationship. An employer is under a duty to exercise reasonable care so as to control employees while acting outside the scope of his employment and to prevent the employee from intentionally harming others. Hospitals are under an affirmative duty to provide adequate numbers of staff as well as adequately educated and skilled staff members.

The hospital's obligation under this doctrine is to monitor or supervise all personnel within the facility, ensuring quality care to patients within the facility. The institution would be liable for substandard care or injury incurred by patients if personnel fail to perform in accordance with acceptable standards of care. Institutions must also periodically review staff competency (*Park North General Hospital v. Hickman,* 1990). A second obligation that institutions have under this doctrine is to investigate physicians' and advanced practice nurses' credentials before allowing them admitting privileges. Most importantly, the doctrine requires that the hospital terminate unqualified practitioners or make available to these practitioners the education and skills needed to competently deliver quality health care to patients.

OSTENSIBLE AUTHORITY

Ostensible authority is an application of agency law and allows a principal to be liable for acts and omissions by independent contractors working within the principal's place of business or at the direction of the principal, and a third party misinterprets the relationship as employer–employee. In health care law, hospitals have been held responsible for actions by independent contractors in suits in which reasonable patients argued that they could not distinguish the hospital employees from the independent contractors.

Ostensible authority is also known as *agency by estoppel,* and, while there is no true agency authority and no agency has been created in respect to an unknowing third party, the court will allow the principal to be held liable to the injured third party (*Corpus Juris Secundum*, 1984). There are four criteria that the courts employ to establish ostensible authority: (1) subjective, (2) inherent function, (3) reliance, and (4) control.

Subjective

This criterion speaks to the extent that third parties see the person as a hospital employee, and it is subject to their interpretation of the relationship. In hospitals in which the emergency center or urgent care physician is an independent contractor working in the hospital facility, the court would look to the subjective interpretation of a patient in assuming that the physician is indeed a hospital employee.

Inherent Function

Here, the courts center their arguments and interpretations on whether the independent contractor is furthering the primary function of the corporation or has a role easily seen as distinguishable from the corporation's primary function. For example, emergency center physicians are contracted to serve the primary function of the hospital in that they are contracted to provide emergency and needed treatment to persons in need in the hospital setting. This is easily distinguished from a contracted food vendor that the hospital contracts to provide food while the hospital cafeteria is renovated.

Reliance

Reliance, akin to the subjective criterion, actually involves the faith that the patient places in the hospital's judgment. If the hospital contracted with Dr. Jones, then the patient assumes that his credentials and skills have been investigated and that he is competent to perform the role of an emergency center physician.

Control

To determine who had the greater control, the independent contractor or the hospital will ascertain the following factors:

1. The extent to which the employer determines the details of the work and work setting
2. Whether the work is supervised by the employer or the independent contractor is free to perform the work in the manner he or she see fit
3. Who supplies the instruments, equipment, and supplies needed to perform the work
4. The actual worksite
5. The method of payment

The more control the corporation has in determining these factors, the more likely it is that the court will find ostensible authority.

THEORIES OF INDEPENDENT LIABILITY

Several legal theories and dictates refer specifically to one's personal responsibilities and liabilities. Such theories serve to make one continually accountable for one's own actions.

Independent Contractor Status

An *independent contractor* is one who arranges with another to perform a service for him or her but who is not under the control or right to control of the second person. In nursing, independent contractor status usually applies to private-duty nurses and to selected advanced practitioner roles. As with ostensible authority, the key issue is control, and neither party may terminate the contract at will. Termination should be a provision of the expressed contract, as should length of contract, dispute resolution, relationship of the parties, duties and responsibilities of the independent contractor, payment schedule, and professional liability insurance (Aiken and Catalano, 1994).

In theory, the classification of this status makes the nurse solely liable for negligent or intentional torts and should relieve the hospital or employer of liability. In application, however, many hospitals have been assessed liability by courts under the doctrine of corporate liability or nondelegable duty. One such case was *Zakbartchenko v. Weinberger* (1993). In that case, a rabbi was held negligent in the performance of a bris. The court ruled that the hospital would be held liable if the child's parent established that they had relied on the availability of the hospital's facility and personnel in deciding to perform the bris at the hospital. Because they could establish reliance, the hospital was also liable to the parents.

The hospital owes certain legal duties to the patient—duties completely independent of any derivative liability such as liability for (1) inadequate facilities, (2) inadequate institutional policies, or (3) improper enforcement of rules and regulations of the JCAHO and other licensing and accrediting bodies.

Personal Liability

Stated simply, the doctrine of *personal liability* makes each individual responsible for his or her own actions. The law does not impose liability on a third party or entity and allow the person primarily at fault to avoid responsibility and accountability; one cannot negate one's responsibility merely because a second or third party also has responsibility.

Neither will the law impose liability on the competent practitioner. The mere fact that a second or third party has liability does not necessarily convey the liability back to the first individual. For example, a team leader assigns a new staff member to care for an uncomplicated patient. The staff member draws a blood sample from the patient in a negligent manner or fails to monitor the patient's vital signs accurately. The new staff member should be capable of performing both tasks competently. The court finds the staff member negligent and therefore liable in a subsequent lawsuit that is filed. The team leader would not share in the liability even though he or she was the person who directly assigned the particular patient's care to this nurse. As a team leader, one has a right to expect that staff members are capable of performing functions normally assigned to staff members. The example changes, however, if the staff member expressed, at the time of the assignment, an inability to competently perform the tasks. Then both the team leader and the assigned nurse could incur liability.

Indemnification

Closely akin to personal liability is the principle of *indemnification,* which allows the employer to recover from the individual personally responsible any damages paid under the doctrine of respondeat superior for the negligent act. Nurses' personal liability for negligent actions makes them subject to this principle after the hospital, via respondeat superior, has paid damages to the injured party. The key to applying this principle is twofold:

1. The employer is at fault in a liability suit only because of the employee's negligence.
2. The employer incurs monetary damages because of the employee's negligence.

The employer can then institute a lawsuit against the negligent employee and recover the amount of damages that the employer paid to the injured party.

Prior to the 1980s, employers seldom instituted such lawsuits. Today, it is more commonplace to see such lawsuits filed, although it is hardly a trend.

■ EXERCISE 14–2

Jose, an 8-year-old boy, was injured while playing basketball with his friends. It was a pleasant summer evening about 10:00 o'clock when he fell, dislocating his shoulder. He was admitted to your hospital, in extreme pain, and seen by the emergency center physician. After what seemed forever, an x-ray was done and the physician told Jose's parents that surgery would be "done first thing in the morning" as there was no anesthetist on call, but that the anesthetist would be there about 8:00 A.M. Jose was sedated and spent a long and painful night at the hospital. Following surgery, he developed a permanent disability of his shoulder and arm due to the delayed surgery. His parents bring suit against the hospital, the emergency center physician, and the anesthetist. What are their grounds for liability, and who will be found liable for Jose's injury?

EMPLOYMENT LAWS

The federal and individual state governments have enacted a cadre of laws regulating employment. To be effective and legally correct, nurses must be familiar with these laws and how individual laws affect the institution and labor relations. Many nurses have come to fear the legal system because of personal experience or the experiences of colleagues. However, much of this concern may be directly attributable to uncertainty with the law or partial knowledge of the law. By understanding and correctly following federal employment laws, nurse-managers may actually lessen their potential liability as they have complied with both federal and state laws. Table 14–1 gives an overview of key federal employment laws.

EQUAL EMPLOYMENT OPPORTUNITY LAWS

Employment discrimination laws seek to prevent discrimination based on gender, age, race, religion, handicap or physical disability, pregnancy, and national origin. In addition, there is a growing body of law preventing or occasionally justifying employment discrimination based on sexual orientation. Discrimination practices include bias in hiring, pro-

TABLE 14–1. SELECTED FEDERAL LABOR LEGISLATION

Year	Legislation	Purpose and Effect
1935	The Wagner Act; National Labor Act	Established many rights in unionization; National Labor Relations Board established
1947	The Taft-Hartley Act	Resulted in more equal balance of power between unions and management
1946	Federal Tort Claims Act	Permitted the U.S. government to be sued for torts of its employees
1962	Executive Order 10988	Public employees could join unions
1963	Equal Pay Act	Made it illegal to pay lower wages to employees based solely on gender
1964	Civil Rights Act	Protected against discrimination due to race, color, creed, national origin, etc.
1967	Age Discrimination Act	Made it illegal for employers to discriminate against older men and women
1974	Wagner Amendments	Allowed nonprofit organizations to join unions; opened unionization in nursing
1990	Americans with Disabilities Act	Sweeping legislation against discrimination against disabled individuals in the workplace
1991	Civil Rights Act	Specifically addresses sexual harassment in the workplace; overrides and modifies previous legislation in this area
1993	Family and Medical Leave Act of 1993	Allows men and women to take medical leaves from their employment to care for a child, spouse, or parent with a serious medical condition, and for the birth or adoption of a child

Adapted from Marquis and Huston, 1994, p. 319.

Marquis, B., and Huston, C. J. *Management Decision-Making for Nurses*, 2nd ed. Philadelphia: JB Lippincott, 1994.

motion, job assignment, termination, compensation, and various types of harassment. The main body of employment discrimination laws is composed of federal and state statutes. Additionally, the U.S. Constitution and some state constitutions provide protection when an employer is a governmental body or the government has taken significant steps to foster the discriminatory practice of the employer. Employment discrimination laws are enforced by the *Equal Employment Opportunity Commission (EEOC)*. Additionally, states have enacted statutes that address employment opportunities and the nurse-manager should consider both when hiring and assigning nursing employees.

The most significant legislation affecting equal employment opportunities today is the amended *1964 Civil Rights Act* (43 Federal Register, 1978), part of the Nineteenth Century Civil Rights Act. Section 703(a) of Title VII makes it illegal for an employer "to refuse to hire, discharge an individual, or otherwise to discriminate against an individual, with respect to his compensation, terms, conditions, or privileges of employment because of the individual's race, color, religion, sex, or national origin." Title VII was also amended by the Equal Opportunities Act of 1972 so that it applies to private institutions with 15 or more employees, state and local governments, labor unions, and employment agencies.

In 1991, the amended Civil Rights Act was signed into law. This act further broadened the issue of sexual harassment in the workplace and supersedes many of the sections of

Title VII. Sections of the new legislation define sexual harassment, its elements, and the employer's responsibilities for harassment in the workplace, especially prevention and corrective action.

The Civil Rights Act is enforced by the EEOC as created in the 1964 act; its powers were broadened in the 1972 Equal Employment Opportunity Act. The primary activity of the EEOC is the processing of complaints of employment discrimination. There are three phases: investigation, conciliation, and litigation. Investigation focuses on determining whether on not Title VII has been violated by the employer. If the EEOC finds "probable cause," an attempt is made to reach an agreement or conciliation between the EEOC, the complainant, and the employer. If conciliation fails, the EEOC may file suit against the employer in federal court or issue to the complainant the right to sue for discrimination.

The EEOC also promulgated written rules and regulations that reflect its interpretation of the laws under its auspices. Included in these written rules and regulations are those relating to staffing practices and those relating to sexual harassment in the workplace. The EEOC defines sexual harassment broadly and this has generally been upheld in the courts. Nurse-managers must realize that it is the duty of employers (management) to prevent employees from sexually harassing other employees. The EEOC issues policies and practices for employers to implement to both sensitize employees to this problem and to prevent its occurrence; nurse-managers should be aware of these policies and practices and seek guidance in implementing them if sexual harassment occurs in their units.

Cases filed alleging gender discrimination include *Auston v. Schubnell* (1997) and *Lynn v. Deaconess Medical Center-West Campus* (1998). In *Auston,* the court found that a male nurse could file a gender discrimination lawsuit, because male nurses are members of a protected class of persons. To succeed with a discrimination case, a male nurse must show that similarly situated female nurses were treated more favorably than he was. Even if differential treatment of a member of a protected class can be shown, the employer still has the option to try to convince the court that there is a legitimate nondiscriminatory reason for the employer's actions. In this case, 53 female nurses and this one male nurse lost their week-end "Baylor" positions when the hospital decided to phase out the "Baylor" positions as part of a cost containment measure.

In *Lynn,* the court upheld the male nurse's gender discrimination lawsuit. This male nurse was terminated after a series of disciplinary "write-ups" for substandard performance. He contended that the treatment of female nurses for substandard performance was different. A female nurse on the same unit, with far more serious instances of substandard performance, was counseled and given numerous "second chances" before being terminated. This, the court said, was discrimination since the court could see no logical reason for the female nurse being treated differently, other than for the mere fact that she was a female.

Several recent cases have been filed alleging race or national origin discrimination (*Sada v. Robert F. Kennedy Medical Center,* 1997; *Lawrence v. University of Texas Medical Branch at Galveston,* 1999; *Peoples v. State of Florida Department of Children and Families,* 1998; and *Thompson v. Olsten Kimberly Qualitycare, Inc.,* 1999). In *Sada,* a Hispanic nurse applied for a job on a unit where she had previously worked as an agency nurse. The nurse was born in Mexico, attended a Catholic school that required fluency in American English, and obtained her nursing degree and prior job experience in Texas. By outward appearances, she did not appear to be of Hispanic origin, and the court emphasized that it makes no difference to what degree someone is perceived or not perceived to be of a minority group in racial discrimination lawsuits.

When she interviewed for the job opening, the unit manager asked her where she was from and learned for the first time that she was from Mexico. The nurse-manager then asked her why she did not just go back to Mexico to work and abruptly ended the job interview. For this court, these facts were more than enough evidence that prejudice was an obvious motivating factor in the nurse's not being offered the job position.

A similar fact situation occurred in *Peoples*. An African-American nurse met all the qualifications for the senior nurse supervisor position. Her qualifications were rejected on four separate occasions and, in each instance, the position was filled with a Caucasian nurse. The court found that the facility's selection process made no sense as a fair method for assessing candidates objectively as promotion decisions were based on short interviews, without considering the applicant's resume, employment history, or references. It appeared to the court that the decisions were made in advance of the interviews, and that race could not be disregarded as a factor. The court ruled that the subjective process for evaluating nurses for job promotion was a pretext for biased choices and ordered the institution to change its practices and keep race out of the promotion evaluation process.

Thompson involved a Korean-American nurse who sued for national origin discrimination when she was terminated for failure to adequately care for a home health care client. The court conceded that the facility had never fired a Caucasian nurse for the same failure of care, but stated that all the Caucasian nurses had been past their probationary period when the substandard care occurred. For the Korean-American nurse, the failure to give appropriate care was not an isolated instance and the facility was within its jurisdiction in terminating the nurse for cause.

Lawrence presents a reverse discrimination lawsuit. Two candidates applied for the same position, and the facility awarded the position to the minority candidate. While conceding that Caucasian nurses may sue for reverse discrimination, the facts of the case did not support such a conclusion. The minority candidate hired for the position had superior qualification for the position and thus was the better candidate.

Individuals have brought suit for religious discrimination (*Thomas v. St. Francis Hospital and Medical Center*, 1998, and *E.E.O.C. v. Allendale Nursing Center*, 1998). In *Thomas*, the court ruled that a hospital cannot discriminate against an employee for the employee's religious beliefs, but the hospital can insist that employees not preach their beliefs to patients. The hospital then has the right to take disciplinary action against the employee for refusal to comply. In *Allendale Nursing Center*, the court held that employees must obtain Social Security numbers even if it is against the employee's religious beliefs.

Discrimination suits can center around veterans' rights. *Tarin v. County of Los Angeles* (1997) involved a lawsuit brought by a nurse who had been called up for active duty during Desert Storm. She was then restored to her former civilian nursing position as required by the Veterans Reemployment Rights Act. The nurse later filed an application for promotion to a more desirable nursing position. Following an unfairly low performance rating on the required evaluation for the promotion, the nurse brought suit claiming discrimination. At trial, she was able to show that the supervisor completing the evaluation gave the low scores because she was angry about the nurse's being absent during her military service and thus gave no credit for her performance while in the military. The court held that this nurse had a valid discrimination suit.

A final potential source of discrimination occurs with the pregnant worker. In *Center for Behavioral Health, Rhode Island, Inc. v. Barros* (1998), the court held that it is unlawful for an employer to discriminate against an employee on the basis of gender and that basis of gender includes pregnancy, childbirth, and other related medical conditions. In this case, the nurse's progressive disciplinary process changed drastically after she informed her supervisor that she was pregnant. The court concluded that the abrupt change in how these matters were handled after she became pregnant could support only one conclusion: She was a victim of discrimination. This right to be free from unequal treatment was also supported by the court in *Duncan v. Children's National Medical Center* (1997).

There are a number of bases on which employers may seek exceptions to Title VII. For example, it is lawful to make employment decisions on the basis of national origin, religion, and gender (never race or color) if such decisions are necessary for the normal operation of the business, though the courts have viewed this exception very narrowly. The U.S. District Court for the Southern District of Florida upheld the right of a hospital to create a "women-friendly" environment on the obstetrical/gynecological unit without inferring that the hospital discriminates against male nurses (*Wheatley v. Baptist Hospital of Miami, Inc.*, 1998). Promotions and layoffs based on bona fide seniority or merit systems are also permissible (*Firefighters Local 1784 v. Scotts*, 1984) as are exceptions based on business necessity (*Herrero v. St. Louis University Hospital*, 1997).

In *Herrero*, a 63-year-old woman of Filipino origin was terminated due to the elimination of her position. She sued for employment discrimination, but the court could find no evidence that her termination was based on race, nationality, age, or gender discrimination. Rather, the court said, this was a bona fide reduction of force, based on economic necessity and guided by business judgment. The layoffs were based strictly on job classification, employment status, prior job experience, seniority, and licensure and/or certification.

A final option for persons who have endured intolerable conditions at work caused by illegal acts of discrimination is to resign. Once the individual has resigned, he may file a claim of *constructive discharge*. To claim constructive discharge, the employee must prove that the employer deliberately created intolerable working conditions with the intention of forcing the employee to quit. Courts do not give the benefit of the doubt to employees who are unreasonably sensitive to their working conditions. Constructive discharge occurs only when a reasonable employee would find the conditions intolerable. An employee who is scrutinized and reprimanded more than others does not have unreasonable working conditions, merely because the job is less enjoyable and the employee experiences added stress (*French v. Eagle Nursing Home, Inc.*, 1997).

Courts allow suits under a constructive discharge cause of action very judiciously. In *Yearous v. Niobrara County Memorial Hospital* (1997), the court defined intolerable conditions as working conditions, when viewed objectively, that are so difficult that a reasonable person would feel compelled to resign. In other words, the employee must have absolutely no other choice but to quit. In this case, the court found that the hospital had used questionable judgment in hiring a new director, but that the nurses had also exercised questionable judgment by taking an inflexible "either she goes or we go" stance. When the nurses resigned, there was still the option of whether or not to leave the employment position, and the hospital board was requesting that they rescind their resignations and that the board would try to resolve the problems within internal channels. Thus, they were not constructively discharged.

FEDERAL TORTS CLAIMS ACT OF 1946

The *Federal Tort Claims Act of 1946* was enacted to allow patients and persons with claims against federal workers to be able to sue the U.S. government. Prior to that time, the government was immune, even if negligent actions of its employees caused injury or loss of property to nongovernmental individuals. After the enactment of this law, the government is substituted as the defendant in civil actions filed to recover damages against federal employees, and the Federal Tort Claims Act is the sole remedy available to a patient injured by a federal employee providing health care.

Under this act, the court first establishes whether the individual was an employee or an independent contractor with the government. This is done because greater liability exposure occurs with employees than with independent contractors. For example, in *Broussard v. United States* (1993), the court held that no negligence had occurred on the part of the defendant because the physician was an independent contractor at the time of the injury. There was a contract between the government facility and the physicians that the physicians would assume full responsibility and accountability for their own actions. In *Bird v. United States* (1991), the ruling had been just the opposite and a nurse anesthetist was considered a government employee because the nurse was under the same control and supervision as a regularly employed governmental employee.

AGE DISCRIMINATION IN EMPLOYMENT ACT OF 1967

The outcome of the *Age Discrimination in Employment Act of 1967* was that it became illegal for employers, unions, and employment agencies to discriminate against older men and women. The prohibited practices are nearly identical to those outlined in Title VII of the Civil Rights Act. The Age Discrimination in Employment Act of 1967, in a 1986 amendment, prohibits discrimination over the age of 40. The practical outcome of this act has been that mandatory retirement is no longer seen in the American workplace.

Some of the practices that are prohibited under the Age Discrimination in Employment Act include placing older nurses in positions that are being phased out merely as a means of easing the worker out of a job and forcing older workers to waive their rights as part of a termination program. Termination programs include early retirement and reduction-in-force efforts. Waivers were part of the amendments to the Age Discrimination in Employment Act. Known as the *Older Workers Benefit Protection Act*, it mandates that waivers must be written in such a manner that employees understand their options and that employees be given 21 days to decide whether to sign the waiver.

As with Title VII, there are some exceptions to this act. Reasonable factors, other than age, may be used when terminations become necessary. Such reasonable factors could be a performance evaluation system and some limited occupational qualifications, for example, tedious physical demands of a specific job.

As the nursing community ages (the current average age of the employed registered nurse in the United States is 44.4 years), the number of age discrimination cases will also rise. This is especially true as the health care industry continues to downsize and employ more cost-cutting measures. A recent case in this area of the law is *Trkula v. South Hills Health System* (1996). In *Trkula*, the plaintiff was a 59-year-old director of facilities. He was told that his position was eliminated and that he was to leave immediately. In the lawsuit, the plaintiff showed that only two other employees were terminated from this same department and that they, too, were 59 years of age or older.

The evidence at trial showed that approximately a year before his termination, the health care facility had hired a new vice president, who was in his 30s. A key decision maker, the vice president had written "60 years old" next to the plaintiff's name on a list of company employees when considering possible employee terminations. He also wrote "retirement/goes" next to the name of another employee who was terminated at the same time as the plaintiff. When questioned, the vice president was unable to explain these notations. The defendant health care facility argued that the hospital-wide cost-cutting needs could be met in the plaintiff's department only by a reduction in force, and that it was a coincidence that this affected two of the three oldest employees in the department. The court found in favor of the plaintiff and awarded him $261,000 in lost past wages and $176,000 in loss of future wages. The award for past wages was doubled because the court also found "willfulness" on the part of the defendant.

Goodhouse v. Magnolia Hospital (1996) presents a similar fact scenario. In *Goodhouse*, a 53-year-old nurse was terminated under a reduction-in-force program. She had been employed by the hospital for 23 years during two separate periods. During 1993, the hospital allegedly lost over a million dollars in revenue, and 61 full-time positions were eliminated. The plaintiff had been the director of admissions for 14 years at the time of her termination, and she applied for a clinical nursing position. The hospital refused to rehire her because she had not been in clinical nursing for those 14 years.

The issue at court was the necessity of the reduction-in-force program and the motive for discharge. A former administrator testified that the revenue resulting in the reduction-in-force program was higher than the previous year's revenue. There was also evidence that the chairman of the board had told another employee that the hospital planned to lay off "older employees." Additional evidence was presented that supported the fact that the plaintiff was never told she needed to take a refresher course, even though the hospital contended that it did not rehire her because she had taken no refresher course. The court awarded $50,000 in lost wages and ordered her reinstatement. They also awarded her $50,000 in punitive damages.

In a case that supported the employer's discharge of a 61-year-old nurse, the court upheld the employer's right to terminate an employee for deficiencies in job performance despite a long period of ongoing attempts at correction and improvement. In *Ziegler v. Beverly Enterprises-Minnesota, Inc.* (1998), the court outlined the factor needed to prevail in an age discrimination lawsuit. "To file a wrongful discharge lawsuit for age discrimination, an employee must:

1. Be 40 to 70 years old.
2. Perform her job up to her employer's expectations.
3. Be discharged.
4. Be replaced by a substantially younger person" (at 674).

REHABILITATION ACT OF 1973

The purpose of the Rehabilitation Act of 1973 is "to promote and expand employment opportunities in the public and private sectors for handicapped individuals," through the elimination of discrimination and affirmative action programs. Employers covered by the act include agencies of the federal government and employers receiving federal contracts in excess of $2,500 or federal financial assistance. The Department of Labor enforces Section 793 of the act, which refers to employment under federal contracts, and the Department of Justice enforces Section 794 of the act, which refers to organizations receiving federal assistance. The EEOC enforces the act against federal employees, and individual federal agencies promulgate regulation pertaining to the employment of the disabled.

AFFIRMATIVE ACTION

The policy of *affirmative action* (AA) differs from the policy of equal *employment opportunity* (EEO). Centers for affirmative action enhance employment opportunities of protected groups of people, whereas EEO is concerned with utilizing employment practices that do not discriminate against or impair the employment opportunities of protected groups. Thus, AA can be seen in conjunction with several federal employment laws. For example, in conjunction with the Vietnam Era Veteran's Readjustment Act of 1974, AA requires that employers with government contracts take steps to enhance the employment opportunities of disabled veterans and other veterans of the Vietnam era.

EQUAL PAY ACT OF 1963

The *Equal Pay Act* makes it illegal to pay lower wages to employees of one gender when the jobs:

1. Require equal skill in experience, training, education, and ability.
2. Require equal effort in mental or physical exertion.
3. Are of equal responsibility and accountability.
4. Are performed under similar working conditions.

Courts have held that unequal pay may be legal if based on seniority, merit, incentive systems, and a factor other than gender. The main cases filed under this law in the area of nursing have been by nonprofessionals.

OCCUPATIONAL SAFETY AND HEALTH ACT

The *Occupational Safety and Health Act of 1970 (OSHA)* was enacted to assure that healthful and safe working conditions would exist in the workplace. Among other provisions, the law requires isolation procedures, the placarding of areas containing ionizing radiation, proper grounding of electrical equipment, protective storage of flammable and combustible liquids, and now the gloving of all personnel when handling bodily fluids. The statute provides that if no federal standard has been established, state statutes prevail. Nurse-managers should know the relevant OSHA laws for the institution and their specific area. Frequent review of new additions to the law must also be undertaken, especially in this era of acquired immune deficiency syndrome (AIDS) and infectious diseases, and care must be taken to ensure that necessary gloves and equipment as specified are available on each unit.

Violence in the workplace is one issue that OSHA is beginning to address in its rules. Violence is perhaps the greatest hidden health and safety threat in the workplace today, and nurses—the largest group of health care professionals—are most at risk of assault at work. In 1996, OSHA developed voluntary guidelines to protect health care workers and consumers, but not all employers have instituted them. Additionally, only four states to date have sponsored legislation that would increase penalties against persons convicted of assaulting health care workers (Minnesota, New Hampshire, Ohio, and Washington).

Latex allergies and needle-stick injuries are other areas that OSHA is beginning to address. A bulletin regarding latex allergies was recently released, and the U.S. Congress continues to attempt to pass legislation in this area. Several bills were introduced in the last Congressional term regarding needle-stick injuries, and OSHA is pursuing a three-pronged attack to help minimize the risk of occupational exposure to bloodborne diseases due to needle-stick injuries.

The first measure is a revised record-keeping rule that all injuries resulting from contaminated needles and sharps be recorded on OSHA logs, which are currently used by employers to record injuries and illnesses. Second, OSHA will revise the bloodborne pathogens compliance directive during the latter part of 1999 to reflect the newer and safer technologies now available. Finally, the agency will take steps to amend the bloodborne pathogens standards by placing needle-stick and sharps injuries on its regulatory agenda during Fall 1999. These lattter provisions were part of the Fiscal Year 1999 Omnibus Appropriations Bill, signed into law by President Clinton on October 21, 1998.

On November 5, 1999, OSHA published the *Bloodborne Pathogens Standard Compliance Directive*, which provides instructions for OSHA compliance officers (inspectors) when they inspect health care institutions to cite employers for failing to evaluate, purchase, and implement safer needles and other safer sharps devices. Even if the employers are using safer devices, they may still be fined if they are not continuing to evaluate and purchase devices that are demonstrated to reduce injuries in the workplace. OSHA will also conduct additional inspections in response to complaints for noncompliance with the new standards. The new standards do not call for additional compliance officers or enforcement programs, but are seen as a positive move toward better protection for health care deliverers (Nawar, 2000).

EMPLOYMENT-AT-WILL AND WRONGFUL DISCHARGE

Historically, the employment relationship has been considered as a "free will" relationship. Employees were free to take or not take a job at will, and employers were free to hire, retain, or discharge employees for any reason. Many laws, some federal but predominantly state, have been slowly eroding this at-will employment relationship. Evolving case law provides at least three exceptions to the broad doctrine of *employment-at-will.*

The first exception is a public policy exception. This exception involves cases in which an employee is discharged in direct conflict with established public policy (Twomey, 1986). Examples of such discharge include discharging an employee for serving on a jury, for reporting an employer's illegal actions (better known as "whistle blowing"), and for filing a workers' compensation claim.

Several cases attest to the number of termination for retaliation causes of action against health care employees. Often called "whistle blowing" cases, the health care workers are terminated for speaking out about unsafe practices, for violations of federal laws, and for filing lawsuits against the employers. In *Reich v. Skyline Terrace, Inc.* (1997), the court stated that a nurse cannot be fired for reporting violations of OSHA guidelines, specifically the lack of protective gloves for patient care activities. In *Hausman v. St. Croix Care Center* (1997), the nurse was allowed to sue for illegal termination when she was fired for reporting patient care violations in a nursing home setting. In this case, the patient care violations involved abuse and neglect of the residents of the home. The court noted in *Hausman* that some employees are legally obligated to report such violations because they can lose their licenses to practice and face legal prosecution for failure to report such abuse and neglect. A similar finding was made in *Paradis v. Montrose Memorial Hospital* (1998).

Contrast these cases, though, with *Prince v. St. John Medical Center* (1998). In *Prince,* the nurse's complaint was about being the only nurse on duty in the nursery during the night shift and about being made charge nurse without certification. The court ruled that the hospital had violated no law, regulation, or public policy simply by making staffing decisions that went against its own internal staffing guidelines. Strictly speaking, this was not a "whistle blower" case, and there was no right to sue over the nurse's termination. This was not a case of reporting matters of public concern. A similar holding occurred in *Witham v. Baptist Health Care of Oklahoma, Inc.* (1996). In that case, the court held that there was no right to sue for violation of free speech because the employee was not speaking out on a matter of concern to the public, but was focusing his remarks on internal operations of the facility. Allowing such a case would undermine the employer's right to carry out its operations effectively and efficiently without dissent.

Walborn v. Erie County Care Facility (1998) upheld the right of a nurse to sue when she was terminated for bringing a discrimination suit against her employer; employers are banned from retaliating aginst an employee who files or assists another with a discrimination claim. The court in *Koehler v. Hunter Care Centers, Inc.* (1998) allowed the nurse to sue for unlawful discharge after she had reported a violation of the law by a coworker. The coworker had falsified her time records. Interestingly, the court said that one who reports a violation of a law, either to management or to law enforcement officials, cannot be made a victim of retaliation for having made such a report.

The second exception involves situations in which there is an implied contract and the concept of **wrongful discharge.** The courts have generally treated employee handbooks, company policies, and oral statements made at the time of employment as "framing the employment relationship" (*Toussaint v. Blue Cross and Blue Shield,* 1980). In that case, the court held that a statement in the company's policy handbook that stated an employee would be discharged only for "good cause" provided an enforceable contract between the employer and employee.

Courts will uphold the rights of employees who are discharged in violation of the hospital's policy. In *Chicarello v. Employment Security Division, Department of Labor* (1996), the court held that an employee has the right to expect an employer to follow its own employment policies for progressive discipline procedures. For example, the court pointed out, if an employee is to be warned for two unexcused absences and fired only after two warnings, the employee cannot be terminated any sooner than that time period for excessive absenteeism. Employees have the right to have the employer's job performance expectations known to them, the right to have unsatisfactory job performance pointed out, and the right to make necessary corrections before being subject to discipline. Then, and only then, can the employer terminate the employee.

Note, however, that the courts also enforce the policies presented in employee handbooks. In *Watkins v. Unemployment Compensation Board of Review* (1997), an employee was terminated for refusing to attend a counseling session. Under the guidelines that had been set out in the employee handbook, an employee's attendance at such a session was mandatory. The employee walked out before his supervisor was finished speaking with him and was terminated. The court ruled that the firing was justified on grounds of willful insubordination.

A more recent case in this area of the law has a very different holding than *Toussaint*, and may be signaling a change to this exception. In *Pavilascak v. Bridgeport Hospital* (1998), a licensed practical nurse accepted employment with the defendant hospital and received a copy of the employee handbook, acknowledging in writing that she had received the handbook. She worked in various units at the hospital over the next five years, with her final position as a scrub nurse in the operating arena of the obstetrical unit. During her time at the facility, she received favorable performance evaluations, merit raises, and bonuses.

She was terminated in 1991 after two significant events. The first occurred when a laparotomy sponge was left inside a patient after a cesarean section. Both she and the circulating nurse received written warnings. The second event occurred when the nurse left the sterile environment of a cesarean section to prepare for another operation scheduled to take place shortly after the first operation. This, according to the nurse, was standard procedure for the hospital. She had been instructed to remain in the first operating arena, but left to set up the second sterile field. She was then ordered to return to the first operating room, but, by the time she returned, the operation had been completed.

Three days after the second event, she received a written notice that she had breached accepted standards by leaving the first operation. According to the nurse, this written notice resulted from a personality conflict with her supervisor. She left on vacation and, when she returned, was notified that she had been terminated, effective immediately.

The licensed practical nurse sued the hospital, claiming breach of an express contract, breach of an implied contract, and negligent infliction of emotional distress. She also made a claim of promissory estoppel, claiming that she had been promised that she could not be discharged without cause, and that she had reasonably relied on that promise to her detriment, even though the hospital did not have a written contract with her. At trial level, the nurse prevailed on the grounds of promissory estoppel and negligent infliction of emotional distress. The hospital prevailed on the issue of alleged breach of an implied and an expressed contract. Both sides appealed the ruling.

The appellate court ruled in favor of the hospital on all counts, rejecting the nurse's causes of action. The appellate court rejected the finding that the hospital had made a promise to the nurse upon which she reasonably relied. Since the hospital's manual permitted the hospital to discharge employees "with or without cause, at any time," it was illogical to infer that the hospital had made a "clear and definite promise that the nurse would have employment as long as she adequately or satisfactorily performed her job" (*Pavilascak v. Bridgeport Hospital*, 1998, at 585).

The nurse had appealed on the causes of breach of contract. Since the nurse had not produced a written contract between herself and the hospital, there was no breach of an expressed contract. The nurse argued that the hospital's benefit plan, pension plan, wage increases, and periodic performance reviews constituted an implied contract that she would not be discharged except for just cause. This argument was rejected by the court.

In retrospect, this case seems to indicate that there is little the individual nurse can do regarding arbitrary discharge. Having a signed contract is a beginning point. Contracts are discussed in greater detail later in this chapter.

The third exception is a "good faith and fair dealing" exception. The purpose of this exception is to prevent unfair or malicious terminations, and the exception is used sparingly by the courts. In *Fortune v. National Cash Register Company* (1977), an employee was discharged just before a final contract was signed between his employer and another company, for which the employee would have received a large commission. The court held that he was discharged, in bad faith, solely to prevent the paying of his commission by National Cash Register.

Nurses are urged to know their respective state law concerning this growing area of the law. Midlevel management nurses and those in higher management positions should also review institution documents, especially employee handbooks and recruiting brochures, for unwanted statements implying job security or other unintentional promises. Managers are also cautioned not to say anything during the preemployment negations and interviews that might be construed as implying job security or other unintentional promises to the potential employee.

COLLECTIVE BARGAINING

Collective bargaining, also called *labor relations,* is the joining together of employees for the purpose of increasing their ability to influence the employer and improve working conditions. Usually, the employer is referred to as management, and the employees, even professionals, are labor. Those persons involved in the hiring, firing, scheduling, disciplining, or evaluating of employers are considered management and may not be included in a collective bargaining unit. Those in management could form their own group but are not protected under these laws. Nurse-managers may or may not be part of management; if they have hiring and firing authority, then they are part of management.

Collective bargaining is defined and protected by the **National Labor Relations Act (NLRA)** and its amendments. The National Labor Relations Board (NLRB) oversees the act and those who come under its auspices. The NLRB ensures that employees are able to choose freely whether they want to be represented by a particular bargaining unit and it serves to prevent or remedy any violation of the labor laws.

Collective bargaining is relatively new to nurses. *Executive Order 10988* in 1962 made it possible for public employees to join collective bargaining units, and nonprofit health care organizations have been subject to these laws only since 1974 with an Amendment to the Wagner Act. The American Nurses Association has long supported the right of nurses to bargain collectively. Since 1946, the American Nurses Association through its state constituent associations has collectively represented the interests of nurses within the individual states. Two of the main reasons proposed for this support are:

1. Collective bargaining allows for achieving the basic elements of professional status.
2. Collective bargaining allows a mechanism for nurses to resolve conflicts within the workplace setting, thereby enhancing quality of care to patients.

Collective bargaining is a power strategy based on the premise that there is increased power in numbers. Collective bargaining assists in the following areas:

1. Basic economic issues as salary, shift differentials, overtime pay, length of the work day, vacation time, sick leave, lunch breaks, health insurance, and severance pay.
2. Unfair or arbitrary treatment as scheduling, staffing, rotating shifts, on-call, transfers, seniority rights, and posting of job openings.
3. Maintenance and promotion of professional practice as acceptable standards of care, other quality of care issues, and adequate staffing ratios.

Issues against collective bargaining by professionals include the charges of unprofessionalism, unethical behavior especially when faced with a strike situation, that it is divisive, and that job security is actually endangered because of the concept of a closed shop (everyone must join the union). Most health care unions are open shops, allowing nurses to either join the union or not. All of these issues have many sides that can be argued; many nurses now acknowledge that they have progressed because of collective bargaining and unionization.

The process of unionization is a complex one. Table 14–2 highlights some of the terms used in unionization and collective bargaining. Organizing is the first phase, and a labor organization is formed, called an *organizing council.* This proceeds to NLRB-supervised elections when enough written interest has been expressed to warrant the formulation of a recognized union. This election period is normally tense and both management and union officials attempt to influence the vote in their favor.

If the election is successful for the union and the bargaining agent is certified by the NLRB, a contract negotiation period is begun. Each side appoints a spokesperson and good faith bargaining is mandated by law for both sides. During this phase, there may be stalemates, mediation, and binding arbitration. The arbitrator is a neutral party whose

 GUIDELINES: TIMETABLE FOR CALLING A STRIKE

1. Make sure that you are following the most recent federal guidelines; check the current status of the law before proceeding, and be sure to comply with all procedural requirements of the act.
2. The party wishing to end or modify a contract must notify the opposition 90 days prior to the contract expiration date.
3. If within 30 days of notification the two sides cannot agree, notification of the dispute must be given to the Federal Mediation and Conciliation service and its corresponding state agency.
4. This federal agency will appoint a mediator within 30 days and, if needed, an inquiry board.
5. The mediator or inquiry board makes its recommendations within 15 days after appointment.
6. Fifteen days after the preceding recommendations, if the parties still cannot agree, the employees may plan to strike, and a strike vote by union members is conducted.
7. With the majority of employees voting to strike, the union must give 10 days' notice of the scheduled strike, giving to management the exact day, time, and place of the strike. (*Note:* No strike may be scheduled before the contract actually expires.)

TABLE 14–2. COLLECTIVE BARGAINING TERMS

Arbitration	The terminal step in the grievance process during which an impartial third party attempts to come to a reasonable solution taking into consideration both management and labor issues; may be either a voluntary or a government enforced compulsory process; this person has the final power of decision making in the dispute.
Closed shop	Synonymous with union shop.
Collective bargaining	The relations between employers and labor; employers act through their management representatives and labor acts through its union representatives.
Conciliation and mediation	These are synonymous terms describing the activity of a third party to assist the disputants reach an acceptable agreement; this individual has no final power of decision making as does the arbitrator.
Free Speech	Under Public Law 101, Section 8, the "expression of any views, argument, or dissemination thereof, whether in written, printed, graphic, or visual form, shall not constitute or be evident of unfair labor practice under any provision of this Act, if such expression contains no threat of reprisal or force or promise of benefit."
Grievance	Process undertaken when the perception exists on the part of a union member that management has failed in some way to meet the terms of the labor agreement.
Lockout	Consists of closing a place of business by management in the course of a labor dispute for the purpose of forcing employees to accept management terms.
National Labor Relations Board	Formed to implement the Wagner Act and serves to (1) determine who should be the official bargaining unit when a new unit is formed and who should be in the unit and (2) adjudicate unfair labor changes.
Open shop	Also known as an agency shop; employees are not required to join a union, although they may if they so desire and one exists within the workplace.
Professionals	Have the a right to be represented by a labor union; cannot belong to a union that also represents nonprofessionals unless a majority of the professionals vote for inclusion into the nonprofessional unit.
Strike	A concerted withholding of labor supply in order to bring economic pressure upon management and force management to grant employee demands.
Supervisors	Someone who has the authority to hire, fire, transfer, and promote employees; supervisors are excluded from protection under the Taft-Hartley Act and cannot be represented by a union.
Union shop	Also known as a closed shop; all employees are required to join the union and to pay dues.

purpose is to be fair to both sides; the arbitrator's solution and recommendations are binding to both sides, so often the two sides are more likely to negotiate for small favors.

If the two sides cannot agree and are unwilling to call for arbitration, work stoppages by employees and lockouts by management can occur. With 10 days' notice, the union can then proceed to a strike. Usually, ratification of the agreement is reached since no side wants a strike and negotiations take on added fervor during work stoppages and lockouts.

Once ratified, collective bargaining does not end but enters the enforcement stage. Grievances can be brought by either management or employees if there are disputes and complaints. Grievances typically can be solved without further steps being taken, but there are specific provisions for resolution, including arbitration.

From a management position, there are several things that nurse-managers and upper-level management can do to prevent unionization. Since most unions form because of real or perceived disagreement with management, a well-rounded, high-quality, effective leadership team is needed to prevent dissatisfaction from becoming rampant. Some suggestions for management include:

1. Provide opportunity for participation in organization decision making; a participative approach may extend to unit self-governance.
2. Maintain salaries in relationship with the education required and the responsibility given.
3. Treat professionals as true professionals; this entails affording respect, trust, and value to all professionals in the organization.
4. Develop, implement, and refine a grievance procedure. This ensures that staff members have direction when they feel dissatisfied and prevents dissatisfaction from becoming so overwhelming that unionization is the only foreseeable answer.
5. Conduct timely and regular surveys and meetings to allow staff an opportunity to express their feelings and views. Open channels of communications are crucial in maintaining positive working relationships.

Once the contract has been accepted and nurse-managers are managing and leading within a union framework, there are some things that they must know and remember. First, know and understand the contract provisions. A thorough understanding and following of the contract can prevent most grievances. Second, treat all persons being supervised with equal respect and consideration, both union and nonunion members. This will prevent a charge of discrimination and should serve to maintain morale. Third, should an issue arise, perform as a professional, be nondefensive, and do not crumble under the pressure. Admit wrong statements or decisions and negotiate a better solution to the problem, assuring that the institution goals will be upheld. If necessary, seek assistance from upper management, especially if the conflict cannot be immediately resolved. And, fifth, continue to expand personal knowledge of management principles through either formal education or continuing education, and practice those principles.

CASE LAW AND THE NATIONAL LABOR RELATIONS BOARD IN THE 1990S

On March 10, 1993, the Sixth Circuit Court held that staff nurses, including licensed practice nurses (LPNs) at a nursing home facility, were supervisors under the definition of the NLRA and therefore were not entitled to the act's protections (*National Labor Relations Board v. Health Care and Retirement Corporation of America*, 1994). The case was granted review by the Supreme Court to determine whether the duties of nurses in directing the activities of lesser skilled employees qualify the nurses as supervisors.

The facts of the case are relatively uncomplicated. The LPNs had brought action, alleging that they were disciplined by the nursing home for engaging in protected conduct for the purpose of collective bargaining. The four LPNs involved in the initial action were staff nurses whose primary responsibilities involved monitoring the work of nurses aides, evaluating the aides' performances, and resolving their grievances. Based on the LPNs' job description, the corporation asserted that these nurses were supervisors and therefore not within the protection of the NLRB because employers cannot be compelled to negotiate with representatives of supervisors. The act defines *supervisor* as "any individual having authority, in the interest of the employer, to hire, transfer, suspend, lay off, recall, promote, discharge, assign, reward, or discipline other employees, or responsibility to direct them, or to adjust their grievances, or effectively to recommend such action, if in connection with the foregoing the exercise of such authority is not of a merely routine or clerical nature, but requires the use of independent judgment" (29 *USCA*, Section 152[11], 1935).

The nurses (through the NLRB) argued that since the primary focus of staff nurses is to exercise their own professional skills to care for patients, the staff nurse does not operate in the interest of the employer's interests. They further argued that the direction of the nursing assistants' work by staff nurses is given routinely in the connection with the treatment of patients to ensure that quality care is provided to all patients within their care units. There is no evidence that the staff nurses' direction of employees' work goes into personal authority, which more directly promotes the interests of the employer and is not motivated by patient care needs. The administrative law judge who heard the case initially agreed with this statutory argument and held that the protective provisions of the act did cover staff nurses.

But the Supreme Court, on May 23, 1994, disagreed. Justice Kennedy, writing for the court, criticized the NLRB's insistence on the interest of the employer as the test for determining whether staff nurses are supervisors. He concluded that when staff nurses exercise professional responsibilities by caring for a patient, they act in the interest of the nursing home, whose business is patient care.

The NLRB further argued that the health care profession should be treated differently from other professions because the concern over divided loyalty between supervisors and subordinate employees played no role in health care professions. Nurses, the Board argued, would not divide loyalty between subordinates and the employer, but nurses would place their professional responsibility to care for patients above any loyalty. The court also rejected this argument.

The court's decision is most important in treating the health care profession as other professions. Interns, resident, salaried physicians, and nurses can be classified as supervisors in the future, overturning the longstanding precedents of the NLRB which held that health professionals were covered by the NLRA. Any professional who uses independent judgment and is employed by an employer subject to the NLRA could be exempted from the protections of the act because of their supervisory status.

Ultimately, the court concluded that it was "up to Congress to carve out an exception for the health care providers, including nurses, should Congress not wish for such nurses to be considered supervisors" (*National Labor Relations Board v. Health Care and Retirement Corporation of America*, 1994, at 1556). Indeed, the court further stated, Congress had made no attempt to carve nurses or health care professionals out of the NLRA's definition of supervisor in the 1974 amendments. Perhaps Congress did not specify this action as it was satisfied with the NLRB's careful avoidance of applying the definition to health care professionals whose activities were directed at quality patient care. If nurses and other health care professionals wish to change this current status, new legislation will need to be enacted in Congress.

Interestingly, a further decision by the NLRB, reached in late February 1996, once more serves to confuse the issue. The decision reached in *Providence Alaska Medical Center v. National Labor Relations Board* (1996) recognizes that the judgment used by registered nurses in monitoring and assessing patients is part of the professional role, rather than part of any statutory supervision as defined by the National Labor Relations Act. This decision paves the way for the nurses of Providence Hospital to organize and to be represented by the Alaska Nurses Association as the bargaining agent.

This decision and its companion decision, ruling that licensed practical nurses in a New York nursing home oversee the work of certified nursing assistants in a routine manner without using the independent type of judgment necessary to be a statutory supervisor, has implications for a number of cases currently before the NLRB (Ketter, 1996). The final outcome of these two decisions will almost assuredly be played out in court in the years to come.

FAMILY AND MEDICAL LEAVE ACT OF 1993

The *Family and Medical Leave Act of 1993* was signed into law in February 1993, becoming effective upon its enactment. The law was passed due to the large number of single-parent and two-parent households in which the single parent or both parents are employed full-time, placing job security and parenting at odds. The law was also passed due to the aging population of the United States and the demands that aging parents place on their working children. The act attempts to balance the demands of the workplace with the demands of the family, allowing employed individuals to take leaves for medical reasons. Such medical reasons include the birth or adoption of a child and the care of a child, spouse, or parent who has a serious health problem. Essentially, the act provides job security for unpaid leave while the employee is caring for a new infant or other family health care needs. The act is gender-neutral and allows both men and women the same leave provisions.

To be eligible under this law, the facility must employ at last 50 persons for each working day during each of 20 or more calendar days in the current or preceding year. To be eligible to for leave, the employee must have worked for at least 12 months and worked at least 1,250 hours during the preceding 12-month period.

Although its title suggests otherwise, the act does not distinguish between family leave and medical leave per se. The act merely speaks of leave. Family leave is available due to an addition in the household, whether through the birth of a natural child or the placement of a child through adoption or foster care. The leave must be taken within 12 months of the birth or placement. Intermittent leave may be taken, if agreeable to both the employer and employee. The employee may take up to 12 weeks of leave, which is unpaid. The act allows the employee to elect, or the employer to require, that the employee use all or part of any paid vacation, personal leave, or family leave as part of the 12 work weeks of family leave provided under the act. The employee who plans to use leave under the act must give the employer 30 days' notice prior to the date that the leave begins or such notice as is practical.

Medical leave may be taken to care for a spouse, son, daughter, or parent of the employee, when that person has a serious medical condition. Employees are also permitted to use medical leave for their own serious health condition. The amount of medical leave is 12 weeks during any 12-month period. Medical leave may be taken intermittently or on a reduced leave schedule when medically necessary. An employee can elect or an employer may require that the employee use vacation, personal, medical, or sick leave as part of the 12 weeks of leave available. Sick leave may be used for medical leave, but not as part of family leave available under the act. The 30 days requirement for notification also applies to medical leave, unless impractical to do so. In such an instance, the employee must give as much notice as is practical.

In a recent case filed under the Family and Medical Leave Act, the court redefined one purpose of the act (*Jeremy v. Northwest Ohio Development Center,* 1999). The court stated that a substance abuse disorder fits the legal definition of a serious health condition and that employees can use their right under the Family and Medical Leave Act to pursue treatment for a substance abuse disorder under the care of a health care provider. Absences from work caused by abuse of alcohol or other substances, apart from ongoing treatment, are not protected by the Family and Medical Leave Act.

Wallace v. Comprehealth, Inc. (1998) illustrates how the Family and Medical Leave Act affects the Americans with Disabilities Act. In dismissing the case against the health care facility, the court said that an employee's perception or misperception that a supervisor has an unsupportive attitude is not a violation of the Family and Medical Leave Act. It is a violation of the act to deny leave or to treat an employee adversely in anticiaption of future need for family leave. In addition, the Americans with Disabilities Act prohibits employers from taking adverse action because the employer knows that an employee had a relationship or association with a disabled person. The court also noted that a supervisor can violate the Americans with Disabilities Act by acting on the assumption that an employee cannot perform the job expectations because of preoccupation with a family member's illness.

The court ruled in *Santos v. Shields Health Group* (1998) that when the employee extends leave under the Family and Medical Leave Act beyond the 12-week limit, the facility can terminate the employee. The court in this case ruled that the employee did have a serious medical condition and was entitled to leave under the act. However, at the end of the 12 weeks, the employee must be ready and able to return to work.

In *Kaylor v. Fannin Regional Hospital, Inc.* (1996), an employee who had a serious medical condition gave his employer two days' notice before a scheduled appointment with his physician. The employee had scheduled the appointment six weeks in advance. He was disciplined for an unexcused absence by his employer and brought this lawsuit. The court ruled that under the Family and Medical Leave Act, his appointment could be treated as an unexcused absence since he failed to give the mandatory 30 days' notice.

The court ruled in *Hopson v. Quitman County Hospital and Nursing Home, Inc.* (1997) that if there had been a change of circumstances, the court would have upheld the shorter notification period. In this case, the court ruled that an unexpected change, such as a major change in the employee's insurance coverage, making it necessary to schedule a procedure at once, was a change of circumstances that allowed the employee to give as much notice as was practical, rather than the mandated 30 days' notice.

■ EXERCISE 14–3

You are the supervisor in a hospital that has collective bargaining for its professional staff. A staff member requests vacation for the next two weekends. There is a family wedding out of state the first weekend. Her mother is having surgery on the Friday of the second week, and she has promised to help take care of her mother that weekend. Do you schedule the staff member for the vacation? What if the contract is silent as to how many weekends a worker must work during a four-week period?

Using the MORAL model, resolve the ethical issues involved in this scenario. How do the legal and ethical resolutions differ?

DUTY OWED THE EMPLOYER

Professional nurses owe the employer and themselves the highest standards or qualities of the profession. These include:

1. Maintaining the standards of their state nurse practice act.
2. Continuously upgrading their skills and education through mandatory or voluntary continuing education.
3. Being a patient care advocate as needed to ensure quality care to all patients.
4. Recognizing and applying legal principles as they apply to all areas of patient care.

CONTRACT PRINCIPLES

A *contract* is a legally binding agreement made between two or more persons to do or to refrain from doing certain actions. Every contract, to be enforceable by law, must have four essential features:

1. There must be *promises* or *agreements* made between two or more persons or entities for the performance of an action or restraint from certain actions. Most nursing contracts specify the conditions and performances that the nurse will undertake, but contracts may also be made to prevent certain actions.
2. There must be *mutual understanding* of the terms and meaning of the contract by all parties to the contract.
3. There must be *compensation* in the form of something of value in exchange for the action or inaction expressed by the contract terms. Usually, this compensation is in monetary terms such as a specified salary or dollar amount per hour earned wage, but other items of value may be seen as compensation.
4. The contract must fulfill a *lawful* purpose. There can be no enforceable contract for illegal acts or fraud.

Legal Elements of a Contract

Legally, contracts have four elements:

1. *Offer:* The person or the entity (a hospital or home health care agency) extends an offer to someone to be hired or with whom they will have a contractual relationship. The person extending the offer is the *offeror,* and the person to whom the contract is extended is the *offeree.*
2. *Acceptance:* The actual acceptance of or agreeing to the terms and conditions of the contract creates the contract. Acceptance may be in written form or verbal. Contracts may also be accepted by the beginning performance of the offeree, for example, when the nurse shows up promptly on the first day of work in a new position.

Exceptions to verbal acceptance have been created by the law. The ***statute of frauds*** is the legal principle that states that a contract does not need to be written to be enforceable. Exceptions to this statute include agreements involving marriage, the sale of land or interests in land, the sale of goods over a certain dollar figure, suretyship (agreements to pay or perform actions in the event that the principal is unable to meet his or her obligations), and agreements that cannot be performed within a 12-month period.

3. *Consideration:* This element concerns the economic costs of an agreement. Consideration is what is negotiated between offeror and offeree. Often, consideration is seen as the salary figure or dollar figure per hour worked, but consideration may also include a set fee per unit of work or other objects of value.

4. *Consent* (sometimes referred to as *mutuality of agreement and obligation*): This element involves the mutual assent to the agreement, or actions that lead the parties to the contract to reasonably believe that an agreement has been reached. As with acceptance, the beginning performance by the offeree would indicate to both parties consent to the contract.

Consent also involves the competency of the parties to the contract to enter into a valid contract. Issues that courts of law evaluate in determining competency include the age of the parties (adults versus those under the age of majority) and the mental capacity to understand the terms and meanings of the contract.

Additional issues that may be considered include the *legality* or *lawful purpose* of the contract. Courts of laws will not enforce contracts made for other than lawful purposes. Contracts that provide for criminal or tortious actions or actions opposed to public policy will not be enforced. Thus, the entire range of criminal and tort law is incorporated into this element.

TYPES OF CONTRACTS

A ***formal contract*** is one that is required by law to be in writing. To prevent fraudulent practices, all states have statutes of fraud requiring certain contracts to be in written form. Some formal contracts also require that they be written under seal, stamped with an official seal, or written on a special imprinted paper. All other contracts are considered *simple contracts,* whether written or oral.

An ***oral contract*** is equally binding as a written contract, though the terms of the contract may be more difficult to prove in courts of law. The terms of the contract are subject to memory and interpretation and often there is a change in personnel during the term of the contract, causing new interpretations of the contract. For these reasons, most contracts are written and include language that the contract survives the employment of the original signors.

An ***expressed contract*** concerns terms and conditions that were specifically negotiated or discussed during the creation of the contract. These expressed terms may be either oral or written, and both parties to the contract have an opportunity to either question or renegotiate the expressed terms at the time of entering the contract. ***Implied contracts*** concern terms or conditions of the contract that each side anticipated were a part of the contract but that were never actually expressed or discussed. Most expressed contracts have some implied provisions as well. For example, the nurse is expected to perform quality, safe nursing care and to follow the policies and procedures of the hospital even though such expectations were not explicitly written or verbalized, and the employer is expected to provide a safe worksite for the employee and to have the necessary supplies and equipment to ensure competent nursing care.

Pavilascak v. Bridgeport Hospital (1998), discussed earlier in this chapter, involved a cause of action for breach of both an expressed and an implied contract. Both causes of actions were rejected by the court. Since there was no written contract with between the nurse and the employer, the court said there was no breach of an expressed contract. The nurse argued that the company's benefit plan, wage increases, pension plan, and periodic performance reviews created an implied contract that the nurse would not be discharged except for just cause. This argument was also rejected.

Individual contracts are negotiated between a single individual and the offeror, whereas *collective contracts* are those negotiated by collective bargaining units for the benefit of the unit. Most individual contracts are informally offered and accepted, whereas collective contracts are negotiated formally, specifying all particulars of the contract, and accepted in writing.

■ EXERCISE 14—4

Obtain a copy of the contract used in your health care facility, if one exists. What terms are expressed, and which terms affecting nursing practice are silent? How would you negotiate the contract differently, or try to negotiate differently, if you were the professional nurse who was to sign the contract?

TERMINATION OF A CONTRACT

Contract termination signifies that the terms of the contract have been fulfilled or that the parties to the contract agree to the contract's end. Sometimes the term *released* from a contract is used to indicate the ending point of the contract. A release implies that the contract has not been completely fulfilled, but that there has been no breach of the contract. In individual employment contracts with health care agencies, the offeree traditionally writes a letter of resignation and the employer-offeror releases the employee from any further obligations under the terms of the contract.

A second means of terminating a contract is by **breach,** which is essentially the failure of one or both of the parties to abide by the agreement and to meet the contract obligations. For example, if an employee agrees to work at a health care facility for a period of no less that 12 months in return for a sign-on bonus and leaves the institution after 8 months, the employee has breached the contract. Remedies for breach of a contract include monetary damages, injunctions, and specific performance.

Monetary damages are the usual remedy for breach of contractual obligations. Because the underlying goal in breach of contract suits is to place damaged or injured parties in as good a position as they would have been if the provisions of the contract had been fulfilled, the court allows injured parties to be compensated monetarily. In the preceding example, the nurse may be required to pay back the entire sign-on bonus previously received or a prorated portion of it.

If the employer is the person breaching the terms of the contract, the employee wrongfully discharged may bring suit for lost salary and other economic benefits that had been agreed upon by the terms of the contract. The injured employee may also ask for reinstatement as well as monetary damages.

The injured party may request an *injunction,* which is a court order requiring a person to refrain from doing a specific act. The hospital in the preceding example may ask the court to issue an injunction against the nurse, preventing him or her from working at another health care facility for the remainder of the contract term. Although injunctions are not often requested, injured parties may seek injunctive relief, particularly if the business concerns a specialty trade or craft. Injunctions may also be obtained to prevent a former employee from contacting individuals served by the business. In a company that has spent years building an established clientele, the company may seek an injunction preventing the former employee from contacting, either directly or indirectly, any of the persons doing business with the previous employer.

A recent Louisiana case illustrates this concept (*Nursing Enterprises, Inc. v. Marr,* 1998). A nurse worked for a nursing staffing agency developing new business relationships with client hospitals and other providers. She also recruited staff nurses, attempting to match their backgrounds and career goals with the clients' needs.

A dispute with her employer over a promotion resulted in her tendering her resignation. After tendering her resignation, but before it became effective, she, her husband, and a nurse-partner leased office space, set up new phone lines, and had an attorney draw up and file articles of incorporation for a new nursing staffing agency. The new agency was successful from the start. The former employer sued and won injunctive relief and an award of compensation for lost business from the trial court.

At the appellate level, the court held that it is not unfair competition for a former employee to enter into competition with a former employer. It is unfair competition, and grounds for a successful lawsuit, for an employee to copy or remove confidential information that belongs to the employer. Files and records are the employer's personal property and the information in the files and records is protected as trade secrets.

However, an employee is free to use the general knowledge of the employer's business practices the employee carries away in his or her mind. The employee is also free to go to phone books and directories for potential client information, even if that yields essentially the same client names as the former employer's client base. According to the court, the law strongly favors business competition.

Specific performance is enforcement by the court to comply with the terms of the contract. The court could force the breaching employee to work the remainder of the four months of his or her contract, having already received the sign-on bonus. Again, this is seldom sought as a remedy by the injured party because morale and work performance become problematic when workers are forced to stay in jobs or positions after they have either left or announced their decision to leave.

ALTERNATIVE DISPUTE RESOLUTIONS

Nurses are frequently reluctant to challenge contract disputes in courts of law because of perceived harm to their reputation and the time that such suits take from their personal and professional lives. Because of such concerns, there are now alternative means of resolving contract disputes. The contract as signed should have a provision that alternative dispute resolution processes will be used as needed.

Mediation

Mediation allows the disputing parties to resolve differences while maintaining a professional relationship. Mediators are neutral third parties who facilitate disputes by assisting both parties to identify their specific needs and concerns and work toward an agreeable solution. Costs of using mediators are usually shared by the parties, and several consultants offer this service.

Arbitration

Arbitration involves the selection of a neutral third-party arbitrator who is knowledgeable in the area of contention and who renders a decision and award. Often used in employment contract disputes, this neutral third party is knowledgeable about working conditions, terms of employment contracts, and factors leading to such disputes. He or she is empowered to make final decisions, and that decision is usually binding to both sides of the dispute, although the parties can agree in advance that the decision will not be binding. Arbitration is used with collective bargaining disputes, and both sides must realize that the arbitrator's decision, unlike the mediator's decision, becomes binding on both sides of the dispute.

Fact Finding

The *fact finding* alternative dispute resolution process is normally reserved for complex multistate and multiparty disputes. Again, a neutral party is employed to sort out the various facts of the dispute and to assist the parties in knowing all the facts of the dispute, from the perspective of all the parties to the dispute.

Summary Jury Trial

A *summary jury trial* is an abbreviated, privately held trial that may be used to give both sides of the dispute an indication of the strengths and weaknesses of their case and the potential outcome should they decide to seek trial resolution.

NURSES AND CONTRACTS

Understanding contracts may not significantly alter one's nursing care, but such an understanding can aid nurses in their decision to accept a position and can increase job security and satisfaction by giving nurses some control within the work setting. Remember, however, that nurses must be satisfied with all the terms of the contract before accepting it. Nurses' bargaining power is in knowing exactly what they want in the work setting and in negotiating for it before the contract is accepted. There is no negotiating power once the contract is accepted. *Contract negotiation* is therefore an important skill for nurses.

Nurses can negotiate for individual employment contracts with health care facilities, as individual consultants for educational purposes, consultants to improve effective management principles in a given facility, and as independent contractors. As the numbers of options increase for the self-employed nurse, contracts will become more vital and prolific. Such self-employment contracts should specifically state the relationship of the parties, duties and responsibilities of the parties, payment schedule, professional liability insurance payment, length of contract, and dispute resolution provisions.

Nurses may also contract with other agencies during the course of operating a privately owned business. For example, a nurse or group of nurses may decide to open a home health care agency. They will need contracts for employees hired as direct patient caregivers, for clerical workers, for space rentals for the agency, for other agencies that deal with the home health care agency such as durable medical suppliers and suppliers of supplies and tangibles, and for the clients that are served by the agency. The terms, both expressed and implied, must be understood, and the home health care agency must ensure that all provisions are expressly contracted. Nurses entering such formal, multiparty contracts are encouraged to seek legal representation for all contract negotiations, particularly as state laws vary. There are a variety of nursing consultants who specialize in this area of the law and a variety of law firms that offer this expertise.

■ EXERCISE 14–5

Imagine that you are negotiating a contract for work as an independent contractor to review legal cases for a large law firm specializing in medical malpractice law. What provisions would you insist be included in the contract? Are there other terms that you would like to see negotiated in the contract? What is the advantage of being an independent contractor versus a part-time employee in this type of work?

CONTRACTS THAT ARISE AFTER EMPLOYMENT

Courts have held that contracts may arise after employment, even in states with employment-at-will doctrines and absence of collective bargaining units. Statements in employee manuals or handbooks may serve to create a valid contract and prevent the discharge of an employee, just as oral statements made to entice a person to take the position may create contract language.

In *Sides v. Duke* (1985), a nurse moved from Michigan to North Carolina, accepting a position from which she was told she could be discharged only for cause, and incompetency was specified as the sole cause for discharge. While at the health care setting, she refused to administer a medication that she believed would injure a patient and, indeed, the patient was injured after another nurse gave the medication. During that patient's malpractice suit against the hospital and physician, Ms. Sides was told not to tell the whole truth by the defendants and their counsel. When Ms. Sides testified to the true matter, she was discharged by the hospital.

In her suit for wrongful discharge, she argued two theories of law: contract and tort. She successfully convinced the jury that the move from Michigan to North Carolina in

GUIDELINES: NEGOTIATING AN INDIVIDUAL EMPLOYMENT CONTRACT

Before accepting a contract with a potential employer:

1. Address employment practices and ensure that you are aware of the following:
   a. Exact work hours and schedules
   b. Time off, including individual days off, vacation time, and sick leave
   c. Float policies
   d. Mandatory or requested days off without pay
   e. Accruement of vacation and sick time
   f. Periodic evaluations, including purpose and by whom
   g. Style of nursing care, as primary or team nursing
   h. Philosophy of nursing
   i. Status of the institution as a collective bargaining unit or employment-at-will
   j. Classification of nurses as Staff Nurse I, II, or III, and how to advance from one level to the next
   k. Orientation time and educational expectations
   l. Number of required hours of continuing education per year
   m. Leaves of absence such as bereavement, medical, jury duty, and personal leaves
   n. Seniority and how it is accrued, how it affects temporary and permanent work reductions, and how it is lost
   o. Grievance procedures
   p. Existence of clinical ladder programs, qualifications, and when the employee becomes eligible to apply for such programs
   q. Use of private car for transportation, as applicable.
2. Understand the payment scale in the following areas:
   a. Base salary
   b. Differentials for evening and night-shift work; charge nurse responsibilities; working specific units as intensive or intermediate care; weekend shift work, holiday pay; and salary differences for degrees, certification, and/or years of experience
   c. Raises, either as cost of living or merit
   d. Number of paid holidays per year and restrictions on when they may be taken
   e. Change in base scale for clinical ladder positions
   f. Reimbursement for use of private car as applicable
3. Ask about benefits and who pays the cost of such benefits for the following:
   a. Group hospitalization, vision, and dental plans
   b. Term life insurance policies
   c. Retirement plan
   d. Parking
   e. Savings programs and employer-sponsored credit union
   f. Conversion of accrued sick leave and vacation time to terminal pay
   g. Professional liability insurance
   h. Child care facilities
   i. Housing
   j. Formal education reimbursement programs
   k. Insurance for private car as needed to see patients in home settings

addition to the statement that she could be discharged only for incompetency created an employment contract. Her expectations, based on the employer's statements, changed an at-will employment to a contractual employment.

Some courts have also held that employee handbooks create a contractual relationship by language that offers continued employment. Coupling with the employee's continued work converts that offer to a formal contract (Aiken and Catalano, 1994).

SUMMARY

There are a variety of legal issues that arise when one employs others in a corporation. Issues of direct corporate liability, through negligent hiring and firing, ostensible agency, and the borrowed servant doctrine, as well as vicarious liability, may overwhelm nurses in management positions. This chapter has reviewed these concepts and employment laws. The next chapter explores more thoroughly how these concepts directly affect nurses in management roles.

Contracts serve as a basis for employment relationships between businesses and the personnel they employ. Contracts also serve as a basis for independent practice by nurses and be contracts for self-employment, contracts for consultant roles, or contracts for nurse executive positions. An understanding and appreciation of this area of the law is needed to ensure that the contract effectively protects the professional nurse.

AFTER COMPLETING THIS CHAPTER, YOU SHOULD BE ABLE TO

- Describe the doctrines of respondeat superior, ostensible authority, corporate negligence, and direct corporate liability.
- Describe federal and state employment laws that affect the delivery of health care in the United States.
- Define and discuss the role of the individual contractor in the health care delivery system.
- Define and describe indemnification from a corporate perspective.
- Describe the employer's obligation to nurse-employees and the professional nurse's obligations to the employing agency.
- Define and describe the principles of and terms used in contract law.
- Describe the four elements of a valid contract.
- Define the statue of frauds and its relationship to contract law.
- Define types of contracts and give examples when each type would be used.
- Describe three remedies for breach of contract law.
- Describe the purpose of alternative dispute resolutions and give four means by which resolutions may be performed.
- Describe how contracts may arise after employment.

APPLY YOUR LEGAL KNOWLEDGE

- How are hospitals liable for acts of individual nurses, even if no lawsuit is brought against the individual nurse?
- Can an institution be held liable for the actions of independent contractors?
- What questions on employment questionnaires or during employment interviews is the nurse allowed not to answer and should never have been asked?
- How does the doctrine of indemnification further the concept that individuals are ultimately responsible for their own actions?
- What are the advantages of having all nursing contracts in writing as opposed to oral agreements?
- Why would one include alternative dispute resolutions in a contract, and when would these provisions be used?
- How does having a formal contract with the employing hospital assist staff nurses in the delivery of competent, safe nursing care?
- What are three advantages for nurses in understanding contract law?

YOU BE THE JUDGE

Charlotte Butler sought treatment for relief of the chronic pain she began to experience in her left chest and rib cage area after undergoing surgery, radiation, and chemotherapy treatments for breast cancer. She was referred by her oncologist to Dr. Kim, a member of the Fulton Anesthesia Associates and an anesthesiologist working as an independent contractor at South Fulton Medical Center, Inc. Dr. Kim administered epidural steroid injections to Butler on January 20, 1988, and February 17, 1989. In September 1989, when the steroid injection failed to give long-term relief, Dr. Kim gave Butler a thoracic sympathetic (neurolytic) block which, unlike the two previous steroid injections, was an injection of the nerve-destroying agent phenol. In January 1990, Dr. Kim performed a second neurolytic block on Butler, following this procedure almost immediately, in February 1990, with a third neurolytic block.

In August 1990, Butler called Dr. Kim requesting additional treatment for her pain. Although the informed consent form filled out by the hospital nursing staff and signed by Butler identified this last procedure as an "epidural steroid injection," Dr. Kim actually administered a fourth neurolytic block using the agent phenol. This last injection was administered to close to Butler's spinal column, with the phenol penetrating the spinal column, and rendering Butler a ventilator-dependent C1 quadriplegic.

Butler settled her claim against Dr. Kim, and subsequently filed suit against South Fulton Medical Center, Inc. alleging that the hospital was negligent in two ways:

1. The hospital's nursing staff did not fulfill their duties and obligations with regard to the obtaining of consent forms from Butler.
2. The hospital failed to adequately supervise Dr. Kim in that it allowed him to perform sympathetic neurolytic blocks without the requisite credentials.

The trial court granted South Fulton Medical Center. Inc.'s motion for summary judgment as to Butler's claim that it had negligently hired and supervised Dr. Kim. They dismissed her cause of action against the hospital nursing staff for failing to identify the correct procedure on the informed consent form. It was significant that Butler noted in her deposition that she never read any of the consent forms before she signed them. Also significant was the fact that Dr. Kim never told her anything specific about any of the procedures he performed in his effort to relieve her chronic pain and that Butler candidly admitted that she did not know the difference in the various procedures that were performed, but that she was relying on Dr. Kim to select the procedure that was "right for her."

Legal Questions

1. Was Butler correct in her assertion that the hospital had a duty to supervise Dr. Kim?
2. Did the hospital have an obligation to ascertain that Dr. Kim was able to perform the procedures he performed within the hospital?
3. What does the status of independent contractor mean, given the facts of this case.
4. How would you decide this case?

REFERENCES

Aiken, T. D., and Catalano, J. T. (1994). *Legal, Ethical, and Political Issues in Nursing.* Philadelphia: F. A. Davis Company.

American Jurisprudence (1992). 4A Agency.

Auston v. Schubnell, 116 F.3d 251 (7th Cir., 1997).

Biconi v. Pay 'N Pak Stores, Inc., 746 F. Supp. 1 (D. Oregon, 1990).

Bird v. United States, 949 F.2d 1079 (10th Cir., 1991).

Bost v. Riley, 262 S.E.2d 391 (N.C. App., 1980), 51 ALR 4th 235 (1990).

Broussard v. United States, 989 F.2d 171 (Texas, 1993).

Carter v. Hucks-Folliss, 505 S.E.2d 177 (N.C. App., 1998).

Center for Behavioral Health, Rhode Island, Inc., v. Barros, 710 A.2d 680 (Rhode Island, 1998).

Chicarello v. Employment Security Division, Department of Labor, 930 P.2d 170 (New Mexico, 1996).

Civil Rights Act, 43 Fed. Reg. 1978, Section 703 et. seq, 1964.

Corpus Juris Secundum (1984). 2A Agency, Sections 1–59.

Darling v. Charleston Community Memorial Hospital, 211 N.E.2d 253 (Illinois, 1965), cert. den'd, 383 U.S. 946 (1966).

Duling v. Bluefield Sanitarium, Inc., 142 S.E.2d 754 (West Virginia, 1965).

Duncan v. Children's National Medical Center, 702 A.2d 207 (D.C. App., 1997).

E.E.O.C. v. Allendale Nursing Center, 996 F. Supp. 712 (W.D. Mich., 1998).

Executive Order 10988, 1962.

Firefighters Local 1784 v. Scotts, 467 U.S. 561, 34 FEP Cases 1702, 1984.

Fortune v. National Cash Register Company, 272 Mass. 96, 264 N.E.2d 1251 (1977). 42 USC Section 12101 et. seq. (1990).

French v. Eagle Nursing Home, Inc., 973 F. Supp. 870 (D. Minn., 1997).

Golinski v. Hackensack Medical Center, 690 A.2d 147 (N.J. Super., 1997).

Goodhouse v. Magnolia Hospital, 92 F.3d 248 (5th Cir., 1996).

Harris v. Miller, No. 345A91, 1994 N.C. LEXIS 16 (January 28, 1994).

Hausman v. St. Croix Care Center, 571 N.W.2d 393 (Wisconsin, 1997).

Herrero v. St. Louis University Hospital, 109 F.3d 481 (8th Cir., 1997).

Holger v. Irish, 851 P.2d 1122, 316 Or. 402 (Oregon, 1993).

Hopson v. Quitman County Hospital and Nursing Home, Inc., 119 F.3d 363 (5th Cir., 1997).

Hunter v. Allis-Chambers Corporation, Engine Division, 797 F.2d 1417 (Cir. App. 7, 1986).

Jeremy v. Northwest Ohio Development Center, 33 F. Supp.2d 635 (N.D. Ohio, 1999).

Johnson v. Southwest Louisiana Association, 693 S.W.2d 1195 (La. App., 1997).

Kaylor v. Fannin Regional Hospital, Inc., 946 F. Supp. 988 (N.D. Ga., 1996).

Ketter, J. (1996). Nurses score victory in NLRB decision. *The American Nurse* 28(1), 1, 6.

Koehler v. Hunter Care Centers, Inc., 6 F. Supp.2d 1237 (D. Kan., 1998).

Lawrence v. University of Texas Medical Branch at Galveston, 163 F.3d 309 (5th Cir., 1999).

Lynn v. Deaconess Medical Center-West Campus, 160 F.3d 484 (8th Cir., 1998).

McConnell v. Williams, 361 Pa. 355, 65 A.2d 243 (1959).

National Labor Relations Act (July 5, 1935) Ch. 372, 49 Stat. 449.

National Labor Relations Board v. Health Care and Retirement Corporation of America, 987 F.2d 1256 (6th Cir., 1993), cert. granted 62 U.S.L.W. 3244 (U. S. Oct. 5, 1993), 114 S. Crt. 1178 (1994).

Nawar, M. (2000). Two new weapons released in battle against needlesticks. *The American Nurse* 32(1), 23.

Nursing Enterprises, Inc. v. Marr, 719 So.2d 524 (La. App., 1998).

Oberzan v. Smith, 869 P.2d 682, 254 Kan. 846 (Kansas, 1994).

Paradis v. Montrose Memorial Hospital, 157 F.3d 815 (10th Cir., 1998).

Park North General Hospital v. Hickman, 703 S.W.2d 262 (1985), 51 ALR 4th 235 (1990).

Pavilascak v. Bridgeport Hospital, 48 Conn. App. 580 (1998).

Peoples v. State of Florida Department of Children and Families, 24 F. Supp.2d 1268 (N.D. Fla., 1998).

Prince v. St. John Medical Center, 957 P.2d 563 (Okla. Civ. App., 1998).

Providence Alaska Medical Center v. National Labor Relations Board, 121 F.3d 548 (9th Cir., 1996).

Public Law 93-360 (1974) Section 2(5) 88 Stat. 395.

Public Law 103-3 (February 5, 1993).

Reich v. Skyline Terrace, Inc., 977 F. Supp 1141 (N.D. Okla., 1997).

Robertson v. Bethlehem Steel Corporation, 912 F.2d 184 (Cir. App. 7, 1990).

Sada v. Robert F. Kennedy Medical Center, 65 Cal. Rptr.2d 112 (Cal. App., 1997).

Santos v. Shields Health Group, 996 F. Supp. 87 (D. Mass., 1998).

Sides v. Duke, 74 N. C. App.3d 331, 328 S.E.2d 818 (North Carolina, 1985).

Sparger v. Worley Hospital, Inc., 547 S.W.2d 582 (Texas, 1977).

Spoor v. Serota, 852 P.2d 1292 (Colorado, 1992), cert. den'd.

Tarin v. County of Los Angeles, 123 F.3d 1259 (9th Cir., 1997).

Thomas v. St. Francis Hospital and Medical Center, 990 F. Supp. 81 (D. Conn., 1998).

Thompson v. Olsten Kimberly Qualitycare, Inc., 33 F. Supp.2d 806 (D. Minn., 1999).

Toussaint v. Blue Cross and Blue Shield, 408 Mich. 579, 292 N.W.2d 880 (1980).

Trkula v. South Hills Health System, Case 94-12870 (Pennsylvania, 1996).

Twomey, D. P. (1986). *A Concise Guide to Employment Laws: EEO and OSHA.* Cincnnati: South-Western Publishing Company.

Walborn v. Erie County Care Facility, 150 F.3d 584 (6th Cir., 1998).

Wallace v. Comprehealth, Inc., 36 F. Supp.2d 892 (E.D. Mo., 1998).

Watkins v. Unemployment Compensation Board of Review, 689 A.2d 1019 (Pa. Cmwlth, 1997).

Wheatley v. Baptist Hospital of Miami, Inc., 16 F. Supp.2d 1356 (S.D. Fla., 1998).

Withiam v. Baptist Health Care of Oklahoma, Inc., 98 F.3d 581 (10th Cir., 1996).

Van Hook v. Anderson, 824 P.2d 509, 64 Wash. 353 (Wash. App., 1992).

Yearous v. Niobrara County Memorial Hospital, 128 F.3d 1351 (10th Cir., 1997).

Zakbartchenko v. Weinberger, 605 N.Y.S. 205 (New York, 1993).

Ziegler v. Beverly Enterprises-Minnesota, Inc., 133 F.3d 671 (8th Cir., 1998).

fifteen

Nursing Administration and the Nurse-Manager

■ PREVIEW

The role of the professional nurse has expanded to include increased expertise, specialization, autonomy, and accountability. Paternalistic attitudes of the past in which physicians and hospitals assumed responsibility for action of employees are no longer the norm. Though the doctrine of respondeat superior still exists, more and more individuals are being held accountable for their own actions. Those nurses in nursing administration must develop an increased understanding of the changing legal climate and of their responsibilities. This chapter explains key concepts underlying nursing management, including supervision of others, the temporary reassignment of nurses to units other than those with which they have primary expertise, unlicensed assistive personnel issues, and the cases involving human immunodeficiency virus (HIV) patients and nurses form a nursing management perspective.

■ KEY CONCEPTS

personal liability	effective discipline	ostensible authority
vicarious or substituted liability	duty to orient, educate, and evaluate	(apparent agency)
respondeat superior	failure to warn	unlicensed assistive personnel
indemnification	hiring practices	(UAP)
corporate liability	adequate staffing	policies and procedures
malpractice	float staff	
delegation	agency personnel	

LIABILITY: PERSONAL, VICARIOUS AND CORPORATE

Personal liability defines each person's responsibility and accountability for individual actions or omissions. Even if others can be shown to be liable for a patient injury, all individuals retain personal accountability for their own actions. The law sometimes allows other parties to be liable for certain causes of negligence. Known as *vicarious or substituted liability,* the doctrine of *respondeat superior* (let the master answer) makes employers accountable for the negligence of their employees. The rationale underlying the doctrine is that the employee would not have been in a position to have caused the wrongdoing unless hired by the employer and that the injured party will be allowed to suffer a double wrong merely because most employees are unable to pay damages for their wrongdoings. Nurse-managers can best avoid these issues by ensuring that the staff members they supervise know and follow hospital policy and procedure and deliver competent nursing care.

Often, nurses believe that the doctrine of vicarious liability shields them from personal liability—that the institution may be sued but not individual nurses. Patients injured due to substandard care have the right to sue both the institution and the nurse. The institution has the right under indemnification to sue the nurse for damages paid an injured patient. The principle of *indemnification* is applicable when the employer is held liable based solely on the actions of the negligent staff member, and the employer pays monetary damages because of the employee's negligent actions.

Corporate liability is a newer trend in the law and essentially holds that the institution has the responsibility and accountability for maintaining an environment that ensures quality health care delivery for consumers. Corporate liability thus refers to issues that are beyond an individual employee's control. Corporate liability issues include negligent hiring and firing issues, a duty to maintain safety in the physical environment, and maintenance of a qualified, competent, and adequate staff in sufficient numbers to care for patients. Under corporate liability, the corporate entity is accountable for impaired employees and physicians when there is reason to suspect that problems exist.

Nurse-managers play a key role in assisting the institution to avoid corporate liability. For example, the nurse-manager is normally delegated the duty to ensure that staff remain competent and qualified, that personnel within their supervision have current licensure, to alert corporate management if staffing levels are dangerously low or there is an incorrect mix of staff for the acuity of the patients requiring care, and that incompetent, illegal, or unethical practices are reported to the proper persons or agencies.

A recent case that illustrates the principal of corporate liability is *Roach v. Kelly Health Care et al.* (1997). In *Roach*, the agency used certified nursing assistants rather than home health aides to provide care to the clients it served. The certified nursing assistants received 60 hours of training that emphasized caring for patients in institutionalized settings under direct supervision. Home health aides received not only the 60 hours of training that emphasized patients in institutional settings, but an additional 60 hours that emphasized home care of individuals.

One of the clients that the agency served was an 87-year-old widow who was confused and had fallen at home. Care was provided on a 24-hour basis by the home health service. The aide caring for her had not checked on the client for a five-hour period and found the widow on the floor with her face against a baseboard heater. The widow sustained severe head, face, and neck burns. Although the agency argued that their staff were qualified to care for this patient, the court held that home health aides were required in caring for such a complex client. The court noted in their holding that the agency had not complied with regulations mandating conferences every second week, nor had they complied with weekly telephone conferences as mandated. The court also held that the nursing supervisor did not have direct supervisory responsibility as she was totally unaware that there were any problems arising from the care of this client.

Gess v. United States (1996) illustrates the need of the corporation to be accountable when staff exhibit suspicious behavior and to take necessary action to safeguard patients. In that case, a medical technician, who had a history of psychiatric hospitalizations and reports of domestic violent behavior, was tried for injecting newborn infants with lidocaine. He was in a position to care for infants in the newborn nursery, and he was always the first on the unit to initiate the process of resuscitation, albeit unsuccessfully in some cases. The subsequent criminal investigation revealed that he had injected one new mother and 11 newborns with lidocaine or similar medications.

The court held that there was an obvious pattern to these adverse patient care incidents that should have alerted the hospital that the incidents were neither random nor isolated. The court emphasized that health care institutions have a responsibility to discover and eliminate the cause of such incidents before significant damage has been done. Quality assurance, through the follow-up to incident reports, is one mechanism that alert institutions about suspicious patterns and persons in adverse patient care situations, such as this pattern of ongoing intentional criminal misconduct.

Courts also impose corporate liability on institutions for failing to act when a physician is incompetent or impaired. A Pennsylvania anesthesiologist was sentenced to 10 years in prison for stealing narcotics from patients who had surgical procedures performed. During the three months that he worked at the hospital, several patients complained of unbearable pain, including full sensation at the beginning of surgical procedures. The institution noted that this one physician requested more narcotics than did other anesthesiologists, and that he could not fully account for some of the medications that he received for patients under his care. The hospital knew that the anesthesiologist had abused drugs in the past and that he had successfully completed a drug rehabilitation program.

Acting on reasonable suspicion based on these patient complaints, the laboratory analyzed blood samples from two preoperative patients and found that they had only trace amounts of narcotics in their blood. A urine sample was obtained from the anesthesiologist, which tested positive for narcotics. He was suspended and later arrested when he reentered the institution using a retained key. He confessed and admitted that he had previously been arrested in California, New York, Ohio, and Massachusetts for various crimes, including drug possession, kidnapping, and assaulting a police officer. The court held the institution responsible under a corporate liability cause of action for not having done a criminal background check on this physician, especially given his history of drug abuse. The hospital claimed that a criminal background check was not part of their credentialing policy and thus none was requested (*Health Risk Management*, 1997).

CAUSES OF MALPRACTICE FOR NURSE-MANAGERS

Nursing managers are charged with maintaining a standard of competent nursing care within the institution. Several potential sources of liability for *malpractice* among nurse-managers may be identified. These causes of action include negligent hiring, negligent retention of incompetent or impaired employees, inappropriate assigning of staff, failure to delegate wisely, failure to supervise and train staff, and failure to warn potential employees of potential problems with previously employed staff. Once identified, guidelines to prevent or avoid these pitfalls can then be developed.

Delegation and Supervision

The field of nursing management involves supervision of a variety of personnel, including professional staff, who directly provide nursing care to patients. The nurse-manager remains personally liable for the reasonable exercise of delegation and supervision activities. The failure to delegate and supervise within acceptable standards of professional nursing practice may be seen as malpractice. Additionally, in a newer trend in the law, failure to delegate and supervise within acceptable standards, may extend to direct corporate liability for the institution.

Delegation involves the transfer of responsibility for the performance of tasks and skills without the transfer of accountability for the ultimate outcome. Nurse-managers may delegate duties to staff nurses, but they retain accountability for the adequate completion of the delegated duties.

Note, however, that nurse-managers are not liable merely because they have a supervisory function. The degree of knowledge concerning the skills and competencies of those one supervises is of paramount importance. The doctrine of "knew or should have known" becomes a legal standard in delegating tasks to licensed individuals whom one supervises. If it can be shown that the nurse-manager delegated tasks appropriately, and had no reason to believe that the licensed nurse was anything but competent to perform the task, then the nurse-manager has no personal liability. But the converse is also true. If it can be shown that the nurse-manager was aware of incompetencies in a given employee or that the assigned task was outside the employee's capabilities, then the nurse-manager becomes potentially liable for the subsequent injury to a patient.

Nurse-managers have a duty to ensure that staff members under their supervision are practicing in a competent manner. The nurse-manager must be aware of nurses' knowledge, skills, and competencies and that they maintain their competencies. Knowingly allowing a staff member to function below the acceptable standard of care opens both the nurse-manager as well as the institution to potential liability.

In a recent case (*Sparks Regional Medical Center v. Smith,* 1998), the Court of Appeals in Arkansas upheld an $80,000 civil judgment against a hospital in favor of a female medical–surgical patient who was sexually assaulted by a male nurse. The court awarded the monetary damages for extreme psychological trauma, anxiety, distress, and depression.

The court noted in their finding that before this particular incident, the male nurse was caught in the room of two female psychiatric patients having a sexual conversation with them. He was only verbally warned and was not restricted from contact with vulnerable patients, nor was an effort made to monitor his activities more closely. This, said the court, was negligence in supervising an employee to the detriment of a patient's safety. The court also found the hospital liable under the doctrine of vicarious liability.

Some means of ensuring continued competency are continuing education programs and assigning the staff member to work with a second staff member to improve technical skills. Another method is to require the nurse in question to attend additional courses at area institutions of higher education. This latter means of increasing nursing proficiency may be used to improve the nurse's knowledge of pharmaceutical agents or to increase the nurse's knowledge and skills in health and physical assessment techniques.

Effective discipline is a vital part of the nurse-manager's role in supervision and delegation. Effective supervision assists persons to perform at their best, improving in areas in which their performance requires improvement and ensuring an acceptable level of competent productivity within the unit. The best means for nurse-managers to assist staff in reaching such acceptable levels of output is through setting firm standards for all work and establishing a formal discipline plan to be used when performance fails to meet these preset standards.

Some guidelines for creating such an effective discipline plan are:

1. Set firm work rules and performance standards, communicating them to everyone before any disciplinary action is needed.
2. Design a progressive discipline system that is fair to all concerned and provides an opportunity for employee improvement.
3. Be consistent in applying the disciplinary rules. Once beginning the process, follow the progressive discipline plan exactly.
4. Investigate all facts and circumstances leading to the disciplinary action, making complete and detailed notes.
5. Document carefully and completely all employment actions.
6. Review the employee's work record and all the facts before determining that action must be taken.
7. Give the employee an opportunity to rebut the allegations.
8. Show the staff member the documentation on reprimands and other disciplinary actions, and ask the employee to sign as acknowledgment. If the employee refuses, include a note to that effect in the documentation.

Duty to Orient, Educate, and Evaluate

Most health care facilities have continuing education departments whose function it is to orient nurses new to the institution, and to supply in-service education for new equipment, procedures, and interventions. Nonetheless, nurse-managers have a *duty to orient, educate, and evaluate.* They are responsible for the daily evaluation of whether nurses are performing competent care. The key to meeting this expectation is *reasonableness.* Nurse-managers should ensure that they promptly respond to all allegations, whether by patients, staff, or other health care personnel, of incompetent or questionable nursing care. Nurse-mangers should thoroughly investigate, recommend alternatives for correcting the situation, and include follow-up evaluations in nurses' records, showing that the nurses are competent to care for patients within clinical settings.

A Texas case, *St. Paul Medical Center v. Cecil* (1992), concerned allegations that the hospital was negligent in retaining, supervising, and assigning a nurse. In that case, a term obstetrical patient presented at St. Paul Medical Center, stating that her "water had broken." The nurse checked the patient by means of a pelvic examination and assessed the patient's vital signs, fetal heart tones, and contractions.

An hour later, the patient was again assessed, this time by a resident, and he determined that the membranes had ruptured and that meconium was present. Another hour passed, and the nurse attached an external fetal monitor and recorded the printout. During the third hour after admission, the resident attached an internal fetal monitor, whose printout showed severe fetal hypoxia, bradycardia, and more meconium was observed. Telling the nurse to alert the attending physician of the need for an immediate cesarean section, there was still an hour delay before a severely brain damaged infant was delivered.

One issue that arose in the defense of the nurse-defendant concerned evaluations that had been written about the nurse's performance three months before this incident arose. At that time, the nurse had been rated as an unsatisfactory employee who sometimes fell asleep while on duty, had difficulty in using electronic fetal monitors, and was reluctant to seek the supervisor's advice or consult with the supervisor when problems arose concerning labor and delivery issues. No subsequent evaluations could be found to support that any of these problems had been addressed or that any had been resolved. The court found the hospital and the nurse both liable to the patient. Liability was averted on the part of the physician as he settled out of court prior to the start of the trial.

One of the many lessons to be learned from this case is the importance of following through on incompetent staff members, either with reassignment to less critical areas of the institution, retraining so that the nurse can safely perform staff nursing skills and intervene in an appropriate and timely manner, or by discharging the nurse. The second lesson is the importance of reevaluation and ensuring that current evaluations show the improved competency of the nurse in question.

Two more recent case examples in this area of the law are *Healthcare Trust v. Cantrell* (1997) and *Bunn-Penn v. Southern Regional Medical Corporation* (1997). In *Healthcare Trust*, a surgical technician was involved. At the time of the incident in question, surgical technicians were not subject to mandatory licensing or certification under state law. The court, however, looked for guidance to the then-current version of *Standards and Recommended Practices for Perioperative Nursing*, published by the American Organization of Operating Room Nurses (AORN). This publication was accepted by the court as evidence of the legal standard of care. The court believed that the publication established a necessity for surgical personnel to have specific training in the tasks and procedures they were asked to perform.

Specifically, the surgical technician should not have been allowed to hold retractors in a pediatric hip arthroplasty. Never having been educated for that task with pediatric patients, the technician was not aware of the risk to the sciatic nerve that could result from even the slightest deviation from the surgeon's manual positioning of the retractor. Assignments, said the court, of surgical personnel to specific tasks and specific procedures in the operating arena must be based on their individual qualifications. It is negligence for a surgical facility to permit a surgical technician to perform tasks for which the technician does not have specific training. It is also negligence for a surgical facility to assign a surgical technician to a procedure with which the technician is unfamiliar. Training and familiarity with procedures performed on adults is not directly transferable to pediatric situations. Surgical technicians must be cleared, and it must be documented before the fact that they are competently trained for the specific tasks and procedures in question.

Note, however, that *Bunn-Penn* illustrates what must be done to prevent liability on the part of the nurse-manager. In that case, a male emergency center technician was accused of sexually assaulting a female patient in the emergency center. Nurses had complained to the nurse-manager that the male technician seemed too eager to assist female patients who were undressing, and that he stayed too long with female patients while they were undressing. The nurse-manager herself noted that he seemed eager to assist female patients on and off bedpans. The hospital's practice was that a male caregiver was to help a female patient with this latter task only when extra assistance was needed due to the size of a particular patient.

The nurse-manager spoke to the technician about these issues. She indicated that how he had acted was not appropriate caregiving as well as what he needed to do in the future about such issues. She continued to monitor his actions and noted no further evidence of inappropriate care involving female patients until the incident occurred that was the foundation for this lawsuit.

The court ruled that the nurse-manager was the supervisor at the hospital who was directly responsible for the technician's conduct on the job. She fulfilled her duty, held the court, by counseling the technician, informing him of appropriate care measures, and by monitoring him to ascertain that his inappropriate actions had ceased. She had also acted promptly when complaints by other staff members surfaced. The nurse-manager was justified in believing that all of her and the other staff nurses' concerns over this employee's inappropriate behavior had been resolved.

Issues concerning delegation and unlicensed assistive personnel are covered in detail later in this chapter.

Failure to Warn

A newer area of potential liability for nurse managers in the area of *failure to warn* potential employers of staff incompetence or impairment. Information about suspected addictions, violent behavior, and incompetency of staff members is of vital importance to subsequent employers. If the institution has sufficient information and suspicion on which to discharge an employee or force a letter of resignation, then subsequent employers should be aware of those issues.

One means that courts have used to address this issue is through a *qualified privilege* to certain communications. As a general rule, qualified privilege concerns communications made in good faith between persons or entities with a need to know. Most states now recognize this qualified privilege and allow previous employees to give factual, objective information to subsequent employers (Trudeau, 1992). Chapter 7 should be reviewed for more information on this defense.

Hiring Practices

Nurse-managers participate in the hiring of new employees. To avoid potential liability in this area, the nurse-manager must be conversant with effective *hiring practices* and careful of potential pitfalls. One such pitfall is representations made about the position during the interview that may later lead to a breach of express or implied contract claims. Such representations usually occur in prehiring interviews, in contract negotiations, in letters offering the position to an individual, or in employee handbooks. Representations may be made about future wages, benefit increases, terms of employment, or cause-for-termination standards.

Employee handbooks frequently create enforceable rights about specific disciplinary procedures. In *Daldulav v. St. Mary Nazareth Hospital Center* (1987), the court ruled that an employee handbook or other policy statement creates enforceable contractual rights if the traditional requirements for contract formation are presented. These elements include a policy statement containing a promise clear enough for the employee to reasonably believe it to be an offer, with acceptance of the employee's beginning or continuing to work after learning of its existence. In a later case, *Karnes v. Doctor's Hospital* (1990), the court disagreed with this ruling, stating that the employee handbook did not create an express or implied contract. In that case, the employee stated that she was aware of the at-will employment and had not read the handbook. The lesson seems to be ensuring that language in the handbook does not constitute expressed conditions or the court will treat it as contractual.

Oral comments made during the interview may also be seen as binding on the employer, particularly those promising continued employment. Thus, during oral negotiations, the nurse-manager should:

1. Avoid making promises about career opportunities.
2. Use words such as "possible," "potential," and "maybe" when describing career opportunities.
3. Refrain from predicting future pay raises or benefits, and refer to past pay raises as merely a guide.
4. Use words such as "now" and "presently" when referring to benefits.
5. Note that all employee benefit plans are subject to change.

■ EXERCISE 15—1

Review your institution for employee handbooks, given either to new employees or to all employees during a calendar year. Does the handbook contain specific enough terms that you would argue creates a duty on the part of the institution? For example, "the employee will be given three disciplinary warnings before termination" could be seen as creating such a duty. Are there other examples? How would you initiate change in the handbook so that language creating a duty is completely eliminated?

STAFFING ISSUES

Three different issues arise under the general term *staffing*:

1. Adequate numbers of staff members in a time of advancing patient acuity and limited resources.
2. Floating staff from one unit to another.
3. Using temporary or "agency" staff to augment hospital staffing.

Adequate Numbers of Staff

Accreditation standards, namely the Joint Commission for the Accreditation of Healthcare Organizations (JCAHO) and the Community Health Accreditation Program (CHAP), as well as other state and federal standards, mandate that health care institutions must provide *adequate staffing* with qualified personnel. This includes not only numbers of staff, but also the legal status of the staff member and the staffing mx. For instance, some areas of the institution must have greater percentages of registered nurses (RNs) than licensed practical nurses/licensed vocational nurses (LPNs/LVNs) such as critical care areas, postanesthesia care areas, and emergency centers, whereas other areas may have equal or lower percentages of RNs to LPN/LVNs or nursing assistants, such as the general floor areas and some long-term care areas. Whether short staffing or understaffing does exist in a given situation depends on a careful, objective analysis of the number of patients, amount of care required by each patient, and the number and classification/type of staff members (Fiesta, 1994). Courts will determine whether understaffing indeed existed on an individual case-to-case basis.

Although the institution is ultimately accountable for staffing issues, nurse-managers may also incur some potential liability because they directly oversee numbers of personnel assigned to a unit on a given shift. Courts have traditionally looked to the constant exercise of professional judgment, rather than a reliance on concrete rules in times of short staffing. This means that using judgment to ensure patient safety and quality care is more important than ensuring that each unit has the exact nurse-to-patient ratio. For nurse-manager liability to occur, it must be shown that the resultant patient injury was directly due to the "short staffing" and not due to the inappropriate or incompetent actions of an individual staff member. Remember, staffing problems never cancel the institution's obligation to maintain a reasonable standard of care.

California is the first state to adopt legislation that mandates fixed nurse-to-patient ratios (*Legislative Network for Nurses*, 1999). Current California regulations require set nurse-to-patient ratios only for critical care units and neonatal intensive care units. The new law does not specify a minimum nurse-to-patient ratio, but instead requires the state Department of Health Services to set such standards. The legislation goes into effect January 1, 2002, giving hospitals a chance to adapt to the legislation and meet staffing requirements.

In a Georgia case, a hospital was sued for negligence to provide adequate staffing. The case concerned the ability of the emergency center staff members to adequately diagnose and intervene appropriately with a patient who suffered a myocardial infarction. The court concluded that the hospital was required to provide staff competent to exercise a reasonable degree of care and skill when delivering health care to patients (*Harrell v. Louis Smith Memorial Hospital*, 1990).

Guidelines for nurse-managers in short-staffing issues include alerting hospital administrators and upper-level managers of concerns. First, though, nurse-managers must have done whatever was under their control to have alleviated the circumstances, such as approving overtime for adequate coverage, reassigning personnel among those areas they supervise, and restricting new admissions to the area. This includes listening to staff members about their competencies, patients who require special expertise and unique care, and what is reasonable to ensure the safety of patients. This may also involve soliciting such information from staff members because some staff members may be reticent to volunteer such needed information.

Second, remember that nurse-managers have a legal duty to notify the chief operating officer, either directly or indirectly, when understaffing endangers patient welfare. One way of notifying the chief operating officer is through formal nursing channels, for example, by notifying the nurse-manager's direct supervisor. Upper management must then decide how to alleviate the short staffing, either on a short-term or long-term basis. Appropriate measures could be closing a certain unit or units, restricting elective surgeries, or hiring new staff members. Once nurse-managers can show that they acted appropriately, used sound judgment given the circumstances, and alerted their supervisors of the seriousness of the situation, then the institution becomes potentially solely liable for staffing issues.

If the hospital has no collective bargaining contracts, the employment is considered to be at-will employment. The hospital is free to set the terms and conditions of employment, including numbers of hours worked and when the hours will be worked. The federal Fair Labor Standards Act, which governs employment conditions, and most state labor laws do not restrict the number of hours that nurses can work in a given pay period or week. Additionally, under employment-at-will, workers can be terminated at any time and for any reason, including failure to follow a direct order, such as mandatory overtime.

One means that nurse-managers in employment-at-will states use is insisting that nurses work mandatory overtime as a means of alleviating short staffing. A recent New York licensure case illustrates what can happen when such mandatory overtime is requested. In *Husbert v. Commissioner of Education* (1992), a nurse was notified by the supervisor that one of the day-shift nurses would be required to work an extra shift due to staff shortage. Under the hospital's mandatory overtime policy, the nurse with the least seniority was required to stay. The RN informed the supervisor that she would stay, but left after an hour, informing no one that she was leaving. Twenty-nine patients were left with no RN supervision, though there were nurse's aides and orderlies. Many of the patients were elderly, suffering from multiple illnesses and requiring multiple intravenous injections. Three of the patients were intubated and ventilator-dependent.

The case was brought before the hearing panel, who found that the policy was appropriate, that the nurse was aware of the policy, and that a true emergency understaffing issue existed on the day of the occurrence. The panel found that the nurse had abandoned the patients, and her license was suspended for one year. Because there had been no reasonable notice given to the nursing supervisor, the supervisor had no opportunity to find a replacement nurse. When she left the floor, the RN had informed the staff that she was going to see the supervisor and that she should be paged if an emergency arose.

The case illustrates nurse's responsibility to the hospital for assisting in times of short staffing by providing reasonable patient care in as safe a manner as possible. For a variety of reasons, management is reluctant to resort to such mandatory overtime, because it is demoralizing to staff and can lead to increased absenteeism, burnout, and turnover of staff. More importantly, mandatory overtime also may be dangerous from a patient perspective, because mistakes and oversights occur more often when one is overworked and tired.

Staff nurses also have some responsibilities to ensure that understaffing does not persist. First, nurses should discuss the issues and concerns with the nurse-manager, either individually or collectively. Nurses may also fill out Assignment Under Protest forms, which are available at some hospitals or state nursing associations, or which they themselves have created. Document specific problems related to the understaffing, such as not being able to timely administer medications, failure to adequately teach patients about their home instructions, or failure to perform ordered treatments. Document in a factual manner, citing numbers of patients, acuity levels, numbers and mix of staff, and specific examples of what actually occurred, not what could have occurred. Also, list positive actions that can be implemented to alleviate the shortage, both short-term and long-term as applicable. Work together with management in a constructive and positive manner to resolve chronic understaffing issues.

Float Staff

Float staff—staff that are rotated from unit to unit—is the second issue that concerns overall staffing. Institutions have a duty to ensure that all areas of the institution are adequately staffed. Units temporarily overstaffed either due to low patient census or a lower patient acuity ratio usually float staff to units less well staffed. Floating nurses to areas with which they have less familiarity and expertise can increase potential liability for the nurse-manager, but to leave another area understaffed can also increase potential liability. Floating nurses from one area to another can also create problems for the nurse who is floated. Accepting the float assignment places the nurse in jeopardy of caring for patients for which one is not fully qualified, and rejecting the assignment places one at risk of disciplinary actions.

Winkelman v. Beloit Memorial Hospital (1992) illustrates this point. Ms. Winkelman sued the hospital for wrongful discharge after she was terminated for refusing to float to the hospital's postoperative and geriatric care area. For 16 years, she had worked exclusively in the newborn nursery, an arrangement that the hospital had approved when she was hired, and had honored all the years she worked in the nursery. The hospital, however, also had a policy that nurses would be floated as needed to maintain quality nursing care in all units of the hospital.

When asked to float to an adult unit, Winkelman immediately contacted her supervisor and explained the working arrangement that she had with the institution. She explained that she had never been floated before, that she was unqualified to float to an adult unit, and that floating would place patients, her license, and the hospital at risk.

According to Winkelman, she was given three options: float as requested, find a replacement nurse to float, or take an unexcused absence from the institution and go home. She chose the latter option. The supervisor maintained at trial that only the first two options were made available to Winkelman, and that there was no option to take an unexcused absence. Later, based on these actions, the hospital insisted that Winkelman had voluntarily resigned and, despite her objections, refused to reinstate her.

She sued and eventually recovered $40,000 in lost wages. The court found that she had been terminated for refusing to float, noting that in this instance the refusal to float was an appropriate action based on her education and experience. The court noted in the ruling that "the sick should be given care only by those who are in fact qualified to do so . . . . licensure does not itself confer a particular qualification" (at 215).

Before floating staff from one area to another, the nurse-manager should consider staff expertise, patient care delivery systems, and patient care requirements. Nurses should be floated to units as comparable to their own unit as possible. From a legal perspective, the nursing care delivered by the float staff need not be perfect, but it must be consistent with that provided by a reasonably prudent nurse with similar skills and expertise under similar circumstances. This requires the nurse-manager to match the nurse's home unit and float unit as closely as possible or to consider negotiating with another nurse-manager to cross-float the nurse. For example, a manager might float a critical care nurse to an intermediate care unit and float an intermediate care unit nurse to the floor unit. Or the manager might consider floating the general floor nurse to the postpartum floor and floating a postpartum floor nurse to labor and delivery.

Open communications regarding staff limitations and concerns as well as creative solutions for staffing can alleviate some of the potential liability involved and create better morale among the float nurses. A newer option is to cross-train nurses within the institution so that nurses are familiar with two or three areas and can competently float to areas in which they have been cross-trained.

Staff nurses have a responsibility to the employer to float to other units in times of need or overstaffing on their primary unit. This includes taking advantage of the opportunity to orient to other units in the institution so that, when floated to that unit, the nurse will already know unit policies and procedures and be more apt to give quality nursing care. A New Mexico case reiterates the employee's responsibility. In *David W. Francis v. Memorial General Hospital* (1986), an intensive care nurse refused to float to an orthopedic unit because he did not feel qualified to act as charge nurse on that unit. The hospital offered to orient him, but he declined and was later terminated at the institution. The court sided with the employer, noting that the employee's unwillingness to orient or even try working with hospital administration undermined his case.

Agency Personnel

The use of temporary or *agency personnel* has created increased liability concerns among nurse-managers. Until recently, most jurisdictions held that such personnel were considered to be independent contractors and that the institution was not liable for their actions, although their primary employment agency did retain potential liability. Some jurisdictions still follow this principle. Other courts have begun to hold the institution liable under the principle of apparent agency or ostensible authority.

Ostensible authority (or *apparent agency*) refers to the doctrine whereby a principal becomes accountable for the actions of his agent. Apparent agency is created when a person (agent) holds himself/herself out as acting in behalf of the principal. In issues concerning agency nurses, the patient is unable to ascertain if the nurse works directly for the hospital (has a valid employment contract) or is working for a different employer. At law, lack of actual authority is no defense. This principle applies when it can be shown that the reasonable patient believed that the health care worker was an employee of the institution. If it appears to the reasonable patient that this worker is an employee of the institution, then the law will consider the worker as an employee for the purposes of corporate and vicarious liability.

Some other courts are using the *borrowed servant* doctrine in cases involving agency staff. With this doctrine, the special master or hospital must have complete control and direction of the servant (nurse), and the general master (employment agency) must have the exclusive right to discharge the employee. Usually, the hospital can be shown to have complete supervisory control over agency nurses while they are in the hospital setting, including assigning them to specific units, assigning patients to their direct care, and making them accountable for following hospital polices and procedures. The agency retains accountability for paying the nurse's wages, furnishing unemployment benefits, and requiring the nurse to maintain validation forms regarding clinical skills.

Whether the agency providing the nurse shares in the liability should patients be injured depends, in large part, on the nature of the relationship with the hospital and agency and the language and words used in their written agreement. In *Hansen v. Caring Professional, Inc.* (1997), a patient had a jugular venous catheter. The catheter became dislodged, presumably while the agency nurse was assisting the patient to sit up in bed, and air entered into her brain. The patient suffered permanent brain injury caused by the bolus of air. Although the nursing staffing agency had provided the temporary nurse to

GUIDELINES: FLOAT NURSES

The responsibilities of a nurse temporarily assigned to another unit include:

1. Before accepting a patient assignment, state any hesitancy that you might have about it to appropriate persons (direct supervisor, nurse-manager, or team leader). Make your objections clear and specific. Follow your verbal hesitancies with a written memo to your supervisor, and make a photocopy of the memo for your records. In the written memo, state ways in which you would feel more comfortable in the reassignment, for example, a formal orientation period or more specific knowledge of the nursing routine for the new unit.
2. State your qualifications and skills concerning assessment skills, performance of routine procedures, and the like to the appropriate charge person. Thoroughly understand the patient assignment before accepting it, because once accepted, you are legally accountable for the nursing care of the patients and could be charged with abandonment if you choose to leave before the next shift of nurses arrives.
3. Identify your immediate resource person, and ask any questions you might have about the assignment, orders, routine procedures, and the like. Resource persons might be the charge nurse, a physician, a team member, or an interdisciplinary staff person.
4. Recognize and give yourself credit for your strengths as well as enumerating your weaknesses. Ask for help only if truly needed, remembering that you are capable of routine nursing procedures and assessments.
5. Remember that much of the case law concerning float nurses concerns the broad area of medications. Double check references, call the pharmacist, or contact your direct supervisor prior to administering any medication about which you are unsure. If there are numerous unfamiliar medications to be given to several patients, arrange to perform more routine nursing procedures for the patients while another nurse who is familiar with the medications, unit, and patients administers all the medications.

The responsibilities of the charge nurse to whose unit a nurse is temporarily reassigned include:

1. Thoroughly assess the qualifications of the reassigned nurse. Ask specific questions so that you may competently make patient assignments. Offer to orient the assigned nurse to the unit, and start with the more critical policies and procedures first.
2. Make the patient assignments carefully. Refrain from taking advantage of the float nurse by overloading the float nurse or by assigning difficult patients merely because this nurse is not a permanent member of your staff. The float nurse may later decide to ask for permanent assignment to your unit based on your fairness and management style.
3. Continue to reassess the reassigned nurse. Offer assistance as needed, and follow behind the float nurse as much as possible to reassure yourself that competent patient care is being delivered.
4. Keep your immediate supervisor apprised of changes within the unit or in patient status. Whether additional help is available or not, you may escape potential liability as you correctly assess the situation and ask for help when it is needed.
5. Reassign patients as dictated by changes in their status or in the number of patients because of admissions to the unit.
6. Run interference as much as possible to assure all the nurses on the unit that you are continually balancing the needs of the patients with the individual demands and needs of the nursing staff.
7. Be aware that much of the case law in this area involves medication errors. Be constantly available as a resource person, and ask questions to ascertain that the float person understands proper dosages, administration routes and potential side effects. Alternately, give the medications yourself, and allow the float nurse to assume other responsibilities of direct and indirect patient care.
8. Nurses who feel appreciated often perform to higher expectations. Give float nurses reassurance that they are doing a good or great job, how much they are appreciated, and how much the staff appreciates the extra hands (Kidner, 1999).

the hospital, the court said that the agency had no right to control the manner of the nurse's work, nor the time, place, or scope of her practice.

The contract between the nurse and the agency described her as an "independent contractor." Indeed, the nurse was responsible for all of her own expenses, none of her income was withheld by the agency, and she was exclusively supervised by the hospital. Part of the evidence produced at trial clearly showed that she had received a Form 1099 to document her earning as an independent contractor from her agency, and not a W-2 form as an employee. Therefore, the court ruled that the agency could not be held accountable for the nurse's alleged malpractice, because no employer–employee relationship had been established.

A different outcome occurred in *Gallegos v. Presbyterian Healthcare Services, Inc., Lloyd's Professional Healthcare Services, Inc., and Speller* (1995). A New Mexico court returned a $166,323 verdict against the hospital, a nurse's aide, and the aide's employment agency after an elderly patient fell and broke her hip. While being cared for by the nurse's aide, who had no prior hospital experience, the patient fell. The hip was surgically repaired and the patient underwent two weeks of rehabilitation. The patient died two months after the fall, either from consequences of the fall or her underlying pathology.

The family filed suit, alleging negligence, wrongful death, and reckless hiring and retention of the aide, who had no previous training as an aide. The trial judge dismissed the wrongful death claim, since it could not be determined to what degree the fall had hastened her death. A nurse testifying for the family stated that the fall would not have occurred if the aide had been trained properly and had experience working as an aide. The jury allocated 45% of the liability to the hospital who supervised the aide at the time of the fall, 50% of the liability to the aide's employment agency for their failure to verify her training or lack of training as an aide, and 5% of the liability to the aide herself.

This newer trend of the law makes it imperative that the nurse-manager consider temporary workers' skills, competencies, and knowledge when delegating tasks and supervising their actions. If there is reason to suspect that the temporary worker is incompetent, the nurse-manager must convey this fact to the agency. The nurse-manager must also either send the temporary worker home or reassign the worker to other duties and areas. Screening procedures, the same as those used with new institution employees, should also be performed with temporary workers.

Additional areas that nurse-managers should stress when using agency or temporary personnel include ensuring that the temporary staff member is given a brief but thorough orientation to institution policies and procedures, is made aware of resource materials within the institution, and is made aware of documentation procedures. It is also advisable that nurse-managers assign a resource person to the temporary staff member. This resource person serves in the role of mentor for the agency nurse and serves to prevent potential problems that could arise merely because the agency staff member does not know the institution routine or is unaware of where to turn for assistance. This resource person also serves as a mentor for critical decision making for the agency nurse.

■ EXERCISE 15–2

Terry Sanchez, an agency nurse floated to labor and delivery, was informed that a patient of Dr. Kwan—a 38-week pregnant patient—was on her way to the hospital. Dr.

GUIDELINES: STAFFING ISSUES

1. When you first realize that a unit will be understaffed, try to get qualified help immediately. Options include asking nurses to work overtime, coming in on a day off, floating nurses from other units, and employing temporary agency nurses.
2. Keep a record of all requests for additional staffing in a log or journal. This ensures an accurate record of what transpired should litigation develop as a result of staffing. While such a record may not prevent some liability, it will show what steps were taken and how you attempted to address the problem.
3. Make frequent visits to the understaffed unit, assessing the situation and working with the charge nurse to set priorities. Transferring patients to other units may be a viable option, depending on the specialty of the understaffed unit and staffing in other units.
4. If you use an agency nurse, assign him or her to fully staffed units and float one of that units staff to the understaffed unit. The staff RN will probably be more help for the understaffed unit, particularly since he or she knows the hospital policies and procedures and needs to ask fewer questions.
5. Pitch in and help as you can. This includes nursing as well as clerical tasks. Reassign ancillary personnel to also assist with clerical and non-nursing tasks, further freeing nursing staff to meet high-priority tasks.
6. Plan ahead for potential understaffing. When hiring new personnel, ascertain if they can assist with additional work time. Even four hours would be an assistance in times of short staffing, and nurses may be willing to help if they are not required to work a full eight- or twelve-hour shift. Orient new employees to at least two units, so that you have more leverage in times of short staffing on one unit.
7. Talk to management about establishing a nursing resource pool or per diem nursing staff. These nurses would be knowledgeable about the hospital's policies and procedures, could be oriented to a variety of units, and are then available for just such emergencies.

Kwan had a standing order that all his patients were to have fetal monitors. Terry, after placing the monitor on the patient, failed to note that the patient indicated a pattern consistent with fetal distress. Dr. Kwan, arriving 45 minutes later, looked at the monitor and ordered an immediate cesarean section, but the child was born severely brain damaged. In the subsequent suit against the hospital, Dr. Kwan, and Terry Sanchez, who would be found liable and why? Which of the defendants could show absence of liability and why?

UNLICENSED ASSISTIVE PERSONNEL

As management struggles to become more cost-effective and provide for better patient outcomes, the issue of alternative patient care providers has been addressed by health care facilities. Many institutions have now employed what has come to be called the *un-licensed assistive personnel (UAP):* persons not authorized under respective nurse practice acts to provide direct patient care. Legal concerns about these UAPs abound.

One of the first questions that arises concerns licensure questions of RNs and LPNs/LVNs. Remember, only licensed persons are granted that license and only they retain or lose it. A variety of unlicensed personnel have functioned in health care institutions for years without this question arising, including orderlies, nursing aides, nursing students from a variety of programs, and clerical workers. These persons work under the auspices and license of the institution, not the professional nurse.

Second, there should be an institution mechanism for consistent and adequate orientation and training of UAPs. This will be established by nursing administration, taking into consideration how these persons will be used by the institution and where their services are most needed. Patient care responsibilities should be well delineated and UAPs must be taught when to inform other personnel of patient data (e.g., vital signs) or untoward happenings. Additionally, nurses should know that they have a responsibility to inquire about expected outcomes, such as asking about the blood pressure readings for a patient scheduled to receive potent vasopressor medications or the heart rate in a patient being treated for cardiac palpitations.

Should untoward patient outcomes occur and a lawsuit be filed for negligence against the health care providers, issues that will arise include the responsible delegation and supervision of UAPs. Once educated to the skills and tasks needed, professional nurses will be responsible for the safe delegation of tasks, including follow-up to ensure that those tasks were performed and the adequate supervision of UAPs. These are the same issues that professional nurses face daily and are not exclusive to UAPs.

Supervision is one of the keys to ensuring that proper delegation with UAPs result in positive and competent patient care. Supervision is the "active process of directing, guiding, and influencing the outcome of an individual's performance of an activity" (American Nurses Association Task Force on Unlicensed Assistive Personnel, 1994, p. 3). Supervision is interpersonal and goal directed. It requires that staff nurses understand their own scope of practice, role dimensions, and job descriptions as well as the scope of practice, role dimensions, and job descriptions of UAPs, from legal, ethical, and organizational perspectives. It involves a thorough understanding of the skill sets and contributions that UAPs bring to care delivery in all clinical settings. Finally, supervision involves an appreciation of the division of effort that allows the professional nurse more time to attend to the nursing needs of complex patients and interdisciplinary collaboration.

Supervision is a means to achieve understood and desired goals. Supervision involves appreciation of teamwork, appropriate assignment of duties, assessment of and provision for ongoing learning needs of UAPs, and oversight of performance with timely feedback to UAPs to ensure quality outcomes.

Effective supervision strategies when working with UAPs include:

1. Know the UAP's role expectations, competencies, strengths, and weaknesses well.
2. Allocate sufficient time for supervision, making rounds, opportunities for the UAP to bring issues and concerns to the staff nurse, and evaluation of the progress of care delivery.
3. Develop and maintain clear channels of communication, including being available to UAPs as needed.
4. Adhere to patient care and work performance standards.
5. Give timely feedback, both positive and negative, and make time for sharing formative information with UAPs.

A second issue is that professional nurses must ensure that tasks as delegated to UAPs are within a delegable scope of practice and that tasks requiring licensure are not delegated to UAPs. Once delegated, the nurse must ensure that the action was performed and performed correctly.

A case example in which communications would have improved the delegation of the task and a better patient outcome is *A. O. v. Department of Health and Rehabilitation* (1997). An aide was told by the charge nurse to bathe several nursing home patients. He bathed one, and then got a second patient into the shower chair. There were no towels left where he had found them earlier, so he asked the nurse where more towels were to be found.

The nurse informed him it was his job, not hers, to look for towels. The aide pushed the patient back into her room, still in the shower chair with a belt secured around her waist. He assumed incorrectly that the nurse knew he was looking for towels, and would keep an eye on the patient. On his return, he found the patient on the floor of her room, having sustained a fractured wrist. The aide was disciplined by state authority for neglect of a patient.

The District Court of Appeals disagreed with this discipline. Leaving this patient alone for a brief period of time is not neglect as defined by the law, the justices held. Close monitoring of the patient had not been ordered, thus it was not neglect to leave the patient alone briefly while the aide was searching for bath towels. It could not reasonably be expected, before the fact, that this patient would suffer harm while being left alone, so the aide cannot be held responsible for her unfortunate injury.

Note that this outcome could have been prevented if communication had been enhanced between the nurse and the aide. The patient would have been more closely watched if the aide had communicated this to the nurse, and perhaps he would have been more inclined to openly communicate if the nurse had not responded so sarcastically to his request concerning the location of additional bath towels.

Lack of communication also resulted in patient injury in *Milazzo v. Olsten Home Health Care, Inc.* (1998). In this case, the patient had a shunt placed to divert fluid that had been building up in her cranium and causing hypertrophic encehalitis. Because she was two days postoperative, the neurological assessment was to be performed at the beginning of the shift, and only during the shift if the patient's condition changed. The nurse performed the night assessment, finding the patient fully intact. The nurse also checked on the patient every two hours during the night, but did not awaken the patient. The nurse checked with the sitter whom the family had hired and was reassured that the patient was "doing fine."

The sitter had twice helped the patient up to the bathroom during the night. The first time the patient remained neurologically intact, but the second time the patient was leaning to one side so badly that she could not stand. The sitter summoned two aides to help her get the patient back to bed, but neither the sitter nor the aides informed the nurse of the change in the patient's condition.

The patient had a one-sided fluid retention in the shunt, causing permanent paralysis. The court found that the sitter's actions were the direct cause of the injury and not the nurse's action or those of the aides. The court relied on the communication between the sitter and the nurse at the beginning of the shift, emphasizing the need to inform the nurse if there were any changes, small or significant. The aides were not part of this conversation, since it was not foreseen that they would be involved in the patient's direct care. The sitter had an obligation to inform the nurse, in a timely manner, of the change in the patient's condition so that emergency measures could be taken. A similar finding was held in *Molden v. Mississippi State Department of Health* (1998).

GUIDELINES: DELEGATION

Actions that may be delegated include those that have:

1. A low potential for harm.
2. Minimum complexity of nursing activity.
3. Minimum required problem solving and innovation.
4. High predictability of outcome.
5. Ample opportunity for patient interaction with the staff nurse.
6. Adequate RN ability to supervise the delegated activity and its outcome.

The nurse who delegates the action is responsible for:

1. Using a thoughtful decision-making process in deciding to delegate.
2. Providing clear and specific directions.
3. Individualizing the plan of care to meet the patient's unique needs.
4. Communicating the method of performance, expected outcomes, and parameters.
5. Supervising performance of the task.
6. Evaluating the patient outcome.

The person receiving the delegation is responsible for:

1. Demonstrating competence to perform the specific task.
2. Asking questions if directions are not understood.
3. Following directions from the RN.
4. Following established protocols and guidelines.
5. Reporting observations and activities to the delegating staff member.

The employer, nurse-manager, or supervisor is responsible for:

1. Providing adequate staffing and other resources needed for safe and effective patient care.
2. Following up on every report of concern for safe staffing or concern for safe practice and taking steps to correct situations which prevent safe or effective care.
3. Providing education and orientation to all employees, including education on delegation (Minnesota Nurses Association, 1997).

As health care attempts to restructure and contain cost, it is conceivable that a variety of nurses will be used in new and innovative ways. In a recently reported pilot project, LVNs, working in consultation with RNs, were found to be capable and competent in giving selected routine, low-risk telephone instruction in an ambulatory care setting (Buccini and Ridings, 1994). Such creative, innovative ideas may be used with UAPs. The important points to be remembered are that UAPs are not to be delegated tasks that require a license and that they are to perform the delegated tasks in a competent manner.

When deciding to use UAPs in patient care units, nursing management should consider the following factors:

1. The type of UAP support being planned and whether it will be primarily supportive or patient care delivery
2. Previous experience and credentials the UAPs need to be eligible for employment

3. Who will be responsible for supervising the UAPs and whether each of these potential supervisors understand both the role and the limitations of UAPs
4. The type of staff mix that will be used in the institution
5. How professional and nonprofessional staff have been included in the work redesign efforts
6. The specific tasks or responsibilities to be delegated
7. How the institution's policies, procedures, job descriptions, and performance evaluations match with these revised roles and expectations
8. How these changes will be announced to other health care providers in the institution
9. The types of communications to be available for staff to make their concerns known
10. The types of evaluations to be done to assess the effectiveness of UAPs (Blouin and Brent, 1995a).

A case that exemplifies the appropriate use of UAPs is *Hunter v. Bossier Medical Center* (1998). In *Hunter*, the physician's orders to ambulate a postoperative diskectomy and spinal fusion patient were carried out by two nursing aides, because it was Sunday and no physical therapists were on duty. The two aides had 26 years of experience between them.

The patient was walked to the nurses' station and back up the hall, with one aide assisting him on each side. When he was back in his room, one aide held him against the wall while the other aide changed the bed linens. When he said he felt faint, the aide followed standard protocol and procedure by leaning the patient against her chest and allowing him to slide in a gentle manner to the floor. One aide immediately summoned the nurse for help, and the other aide took his vital signs, asked him if he was all right, and assessed him for external injuries. Then the three of them put him back to bed.

The physician was promptly notified of the patient's fall, and x-rays were done. There was no evidence that the position of the bone graft had slipped. The court ruled that this same technique of assisting a patient to the floor during ambulation is widely taught to licensed and nonlicensed personnel and is a proper method for safely assisting a patient who is about to fall. The court also noted that it was fully documented in the patient's record that this method had been used, apparently successfully averting injury to the patient. Thus, even though the patient continues to suffer back pain, the actions of the nurses were appropriate, and there was no liability found on the part of the nurses or the hospital.

HIV CASES AND NURSE-MANAGER CONCERNS

The rise of HIV and acquired immune deficiency syndrome (AIDS) has affected the role and responsibility of nurse-managers. Failure to monitor and recognize potential problems can lead to issues of liability for both the individual nurse-manager and the institution. There are also ramifications for the patients involved as well as the nursing staff.

Courts have consistently recognized legally protected interests in antidiscrimination, privacy and confidentiality, and workplace safety in deciding these cases (Blouin and Brent, 1995b). Appellate courts continue to wrestle with conflicting interests in deciding these cases, and many involve health care settings and staff. Nurse administrators must remain alert to potential for conflicts and weigh the varying interests carefully. If a threat to patient safety emerges, the first concern should be patient safety.

Two cases have arisen in the past few years that have direct implications for nurse-managers. Both cases involved workplace safety and discrimination issues, but from very different perspectives.

In *Armstrong v. Flowers Hospital* (1994), a pregnant nurse held that she had been terminated for refusal to care for an HIV-positive patient and that this was unlawful discrimination, forcing her to choose between her unborn child and her nursing position. The case had been granted summary judgment at the trial level in favor of the defendant hospital, and the nurse appealed. The appellate court concurred with the trial court, but the analysis of the case by the court may assist nurse-managers.

The nurse in this suit was a home health care nurse, with previous nursing experience in a newborn nursery. She was assigned approximately 25 patients, visiting them in their homes and providing nursing care to them. After being employed by the home health care division for about four months, she was informed that she was being assigned an HIV-positive patient, recently diagnosed with crypotococcal meningitis. The patient would require approximately four hours of care per day, he had problems with nausea and vomiting, and it would be necessary for her to draw blood samples. She was to be provided sharps containers for used needles and special bags for contaminated materials.

This new patient assignment came at a time when she had just learned of her pregnancy and she had never before, to her knowledge, taken care of an HIV-positive patient. Part of her concern came from her diagnosis of gestational diabetes, which she believed would cause her immune system to be weakened, and part of her fear was because she was in the first trimester of her pregnancy, the most vulnerable time frame for the fetus. The nurse voiced her concerns to her supervisor and was told that she was in the best position to care for this patient. There was also a division policy that stated that refusal to care for a patient could be grounds for termination. After the administrator met with the supervisor, the nurse decided that she would refuse this assignment and chose to be terminated rather than resign.

The hospital and the home health care division shared some policies and some were different. The AIDS universal precautions policies were identical, but a number of written policies, for example, restricting pregnant nurses from working with hepatitis B patients, patients with active herpetic lesions, or patients receiving bronchial or interstitial irradiation pertained only to the hospital. After talking to a nursing supervisor at the hospital, the nurse also maintained that the hospital had an unwritten policy of assigning or attempting to assign isolation patients to nonpregnant nurses.

The nurse argued that her termination was based on her pregnancy, a direct violation of the Civil Rights Act of 1964, with its 1978 amendment pertaining directly to pregnancy discrimination. The purpose of the act was to ensure that employees who provided disability benefits to their employers also provided these benefits to pregnant employees unable to work because of their pregnancy and to prevent differential treatment of the pregnant employee.

Using a *disparate treatment* claim, the nurse first tried to show that she, as a pregnant employee, suffered from differential application of work or disciplinary rules because of the different policies at the hospital and the home health care division. Intent to discriminate must be shown by the plaintiff. The court rejected that argument because the nurse was treated no differently than other pregnant nurses in the home health division.

The second theory, *disparate impact,* involves employment policies that appear to be neutral but fall more harshly or disproportionately on one group of employees and cannot be justified by a business necessity. Intent to discriminate is not necessary with this cause of action. The emphasis in on the effect of the policy and not its intent.

The nurse's argument under this approach was that she was placed in the difficult position of choosing between her fetus and her job, a choice placed only on pregnant employees. The court was unsympathetic with this approach. Although the court acknowledged that the nurse had offered evidence that a pregnant employee is more susceptible to contagious diseases than a nonpregnant employee and that contagious diseases may be communicated by the mother to her fetus, the court could find no evidence presented that these risks were comparable to any risk for which the hospital or the home health care division made an accommodation to the pregnant employee.

The plaintiff also argued that an employer must make the decision easier by offering alternative work. To the contrary, held the court, an employer normally is prohibited from deciding what course of action is best for pregnant employees. The court further contended that the plaintiff was, in reality, arguing for preferential treatment of pregnant workers. The preferential treatment would consist of accommodation of the pregnant employee's concerns with respect to the risks for herself and her unborn child through rescheduling of nursing assignments at the expense of nonpregnant workers, who would have no right to refuse the assignment. The Pregnancy Discrimination Act does not require preferential treatment.

This case is unusual in its application. Previous discrimination suits had dealt with health care workers and patients who are HIV positive, and this appeared as one of the first cases in which a person had argued that the requirement to attend to an individual who is HIV positive constitutes discrimination. Because of the widespread fear of HIV and AIDS, individuals who are concerned about exposure to virus in the workplace are projected to continue to bring future lawsuits.

This case should be helpful to nursing managers and administration for a number of reasons. First, the policy that the hospital and home health care division had did not discriminate against pregnant workers. A reverse policy would have been almost impossible to defend from a discrimination perspective. The court said that "Title VII (of the Civil Rights Act) does not require employers to treat employees with kindness" (*Armstrong v. Flowers Hospital,* 1994, at 1317). Second, the policies of the two entities were identical with respect to treatment of patients who are HIV positive. If the policies had differed, the court might have looked more closely at the accommodation of the pregnant worker by one entity and not the other. At it was, there was no discrimination or differential treatment of the pregnant worker by either entity.

Third, the home health care division was consistent in its application of the rule regarding treatment of all patients. Additional factors that allowed the hospital to prevail were the timely introduction of materials relating to universal precautions during the nurse's orientation and the rationale for assigning the HIV-positive patient to her care. She was the most available to care for the patient at the present time. Finally, the supervisor and administrator discussed the nurse's options with her and left the decision to her. There was no appearance of callous indifference in this instance.

Interestingly, the court seemed to take note of the fact that the nurse had not consulted her primary physician about the increased risk of infection to herself or her fetus, nor did she inquire about the availability of gowns, masks, and other items that would further protect her while caring for the patient. This lack of inquiry served to show the court that she had already made up her mind and was not open to alternative approaches.

Nurse-managers should hesitate before making assignments that accommodate pregnant nurses and serve to single them out as a class. Preferential treatment of pregnant nurses may not pass legal scrutiny and may place the hospital in a discrimination suit by male nurses, since this opens the way for a gender-based discrimination charge.

The second case that affects this area of the law is *Ramirez v. Oklahoma Department of Mental Health* (1994). In that case, an HIV-positive mental health aide was accused of rough treatment of a mental patient. Specifically, the aide had grabbed her tightly and dug his fingernails into her skin, causing contusions and abrasions. The patient was examined and the injuries noted. The examining psychiatrist and other team members were all aware of the HIV status of the aide and that the patient was now at risk of infection. The team members filed a patient grievance with their superiors in the Department of Mental Health (DMH).

Less than two months later, all members filing the grievance received notices of proposed adverse personnel actions against them for failure to follow the DMH policies regarding discrimination against individuals with AIDS and for misconduct in using the wrong form to report the alleged misconduct. Two members of the team were either terminated (the psychiatrist) or transferred (the nurse), with the transfer affecting her seniority and promotion prospects.

These two members of the team brought this action against the DMH, claiming that the defendants wrongfully took personnel actions against them in retaliation for their having exercised their freedom of speech to report an incident of patient abuse and possible lethal infection. They requested monetary damages and reinstatement to their prior positions. The lower court granted the defendant's motion to dismiss and the appellate court reversed that decision.

The court first addressed the issue of governmental immunity, rejecting that in part because the aide was not a governmental official and in part because the attorneys and hearing officers for the defendant violated clearly established rights. The court then addressed the First Amendment freedom of speech contention, and concluded that the nurse and psychiatrist correctly expressed their First Amendment rights consistent with their professional duties and ethics. The court then stated that the issue of the right of a public employee as a citizen to express comments on matters of public concern and the right of a governmental entity to ensure the efficiency of the public services it performs had to be balanced. This latter concern included the retaliation cause of action brought by the two members of the mental health team. The court found that the timing of the adverse personnel actions, plus the giving of seemingly inconsequential reasons for disciplinary action (the filing of the wrong grievance form), and a secret agreement between the attorney for the DMH and the aide to discipline the team members in exchange for the aide's not filing suit supported the inference of a retaliatory action.

Although the major concern of the hospital seemed to be liability to the aide—and such concern is understandable given the various legal protections given to individuals who are HIV positive—the court concerned itself with workplace safety issues in general and the safety of patient in particular. In the event that the two collide, the court clearly believed that patient safety should prevail. In this case, the threat was an actual one since the patient had suffered abrasions and contusions at the hands of an HIV-positive aide. Had the danger to the patient been only a potential one (e.g., the handling of a patient who did not pose a risk for the transfer of HIV), the court might well have found in favor of protecting the employee against possible discrimination. The lesson for the nurse-manager seems to be to err on the side of safety, particularly in the face of clear-cut danger.

Personnel actions should continue to be handled carefully, with impartial investigation and confidentiality. Personnel matters must be handled with tact, impartial procedures, and rationales given for actions taken.

■ EXERCISE 15—3

How are personnel policies concerning HIV-positive status handled in your institution? Is there a written policy, outlining the need for confidentiality, grievance procedures, and procedures for refusing patient assignments if such assignments will potentially harm the HIV-positive worker?

What kinds of ethical issues are raised by workers and patients who are HIV positive or have AIDS? Are these issues easily resolved? Using the nurse in the *Armstrong* case, resolve that dilemma from an ethical perspective by using the MORAL model.

POLICIES AND PROCEDURES

Risk management is a process that identifies, analyzes, and treats potential hazards within a given setting. The object of risk management is to identify potential hazards and to eliminate them before anyone is harmed or disabled. *Gess v. United States* (1996), cited earlier in this chapter, illustrates this vital role of the health care agencies in preventing harm. In *Gess,* the court noted that the actions of Gess should have leaped from the incident reports had anyone been closely monitoring the reports. His was the name that was common on all the reports; in fact, he was the very first person to begin resuscitation efforts in the majority of the patients involved. He was, the court concluded, the only commonality to all the reports, and the hospital should have noted this immediately. The very purpose of quality assurance, held that court, is to be alert for suspicious patterns in adverse patient situations and take corrective actions. A good starting point is to match up the personnel on duty with the incidents, and then to look at what is known about their backgrounds and to monitor their actions.

Written *policies and procedures* fall within the scope of risk management activities and are a requirement of JCAHO. These documents set standards of care for the institution and direct practice. They must be clearly stated, well delineated, and based on current practice. Nurse-managers should review the policies and procedures frequently for compliance and timeliness. If policies are outdated or absent, request that the appropriate person or committee either update or initiate the policy.

SUMMARY

In the area of management, it is important to remember that nurse-managers are both employees and employers. As a manager, the nurse has an obligation to be aware of pertinent laws and litigation that affect what managers may or may not do. As employees, nurse-managers have many of the same rights as staff nurses. The effective manager will balance these two concepts to enhance patient care delivery.

AFTER COMPLETING THIS CHAPTER, YOU SHOULD BE ABLE TO

- Compare and contrast the doctrines of respondeat superior, vicarious liability, and personal liability from a nursing management perspective.
- Define three separate issues concerning temporary staffing from the aspect of legal liability.
- Define and evaluate the role of unlicensed assistive personnel in relationship to professional accountability.
- Describe the significance of the cases involving HIV patients and nurses on the role of the nurse-manager.
- Describe the goals of risk management.

APPLY YOUR LEGAL KNOWLEDGE

- What are the most common potential legal liabilities for nurse administration and nurse-managers in health care settings?
- How can these areas of potential liability be minimized or avoided?
- Is there a role for ancillary personnel within the current health care delivery system?
- How do the newer cases involving HIV patients and nurses impact supervisory personnel? Do these cases begin to answer the issues that must be addressed?
- How are the guidelines for effective delegation used in various clinical settings?

YOU BE THE JUDGE

James R. Brown arrived at DeKalb Medical Center emergency center at about 8:30 P.M. on October 20, 1992. He was suffering from a swollen tongue and difficulty breathing. Emergency center personnel medicated him, and called his attending physician, Dr. Feingold. Dr. Alturi, who was covering that evening for Dr. Feingold, arrived at about 11 P.M. She determined that Brown was most likely suffering an allergic reaction to Zestril, an antihypertensive agent, and directed his wife to go home and call in a list of all the medications the patient was taking to the nurse in the emergency center. She also noted that Brown was to have nothing by mouth.

Instead of calling in as requested, Mrs. Brown brought her husband's medications back to the nurses' station. At around 4:00 A.M. Simmons, a nurse in the emergency department, gave Mr. Brown his daily dosage of Zestril. He claimed he did so at Dr. Alturi's oral direction. Dr. Alturi testified that she had given no such order, but her initials appear next to a notation in the chart that the medication had been given. Dr. Feingold saw the patient later in the day and discharged him, even though he was aware that Brown had had another dose of Zestril. Brown was to see Feingold the next day at Feingold's office.

At around 5:00 A.M. on October 22, Brown had a fatal allergic reaction. Mrs. Brown sued the hospital, Drs. Feingold and Alturi, Simmons, and StarMed Staffing, Simmons's agency service. At trial, the relationship that the agency had with the hospital regarding agency staff clearly showed that the agency paid Simmons's wages, furnished health and unemployment insurance, and required him to abide by their rules. The hospital had full supervisory control over Simmons, including the right to discharge him if his performance did not meet their expectations.

The trial court granted summary judgment to StarMed Staffing on the grounds that Simmons was the hospital's borrowed servant at the time of the occurrence. The hospital contended that Simmons was Dr. Alturi's borrowed servant, and thus the charge against them should be dismissed.

Legal Questions

1. Was Simmons a borrowed servant under the definition of a borrowed servant?
2. If he was a borrowed servant, whose borrowed servant was he, or could he be a borrowed servant to two entities simultaneously?
3. How would you decide this case?

REFERENCES

American Nurses Association Task Force on Unliscensed Assistive Personnel (1994). *Registered Professional Nurses and Unlicensed Assistive Personnel.* Washington, DC: American Nurses Association.

A. O. v. Department of Health and Rehabilitation, 696 So.2d 1358 (Fla. App., 1997).

Armstrong v. Flowers Hospital, 33 F.3d 1308 (11th Cir., 1994).

Blouin, A. S., and Brent, N. J. (1995a). Unlicensed assistive personnel: Legal considerations. *Nursing Management* 23(11), 7–8, 21.

Blouin, A. S., and Brent, N. J. (1995b). Legal concerns related to workers with HIV or AIDS. *Nursing Management* 25(1), 17–18.

Buccini, R., and Ridings, L. (1994). Using licensed vocational nurses to provide telephone patient instructions in a health maintenance organization. *Journal of Nursing Administration* 24(1), 27–33.

Bunn-Penn v. Southern Regional Medical Corporation, 488 S.E.2d 747 (Ga. App., 1997).

California staffing bill signed into law: Nurses happy, hospitals disappointed. (1999). *Legislative Network for Nurses* 16(21), 163.

Daldulav v. St. Mary Nazareth Hospital Center, Docket No. 62737 (Illinois, 1987).

David W. Francis v. Memorial General Hospital, 726 P.2d 852 (N.M., 1986).

Fiesta, J. (1994). Legal update for nurses. Part II: Assigning, delegating, and staffing. *Nursing Management* 24(2), 14–16.

Gallegos v. Presbyterian Healthcare Services, Inc., Lloyd's Professional Healthcare Serivces, Inc., and Speller, Bernalillo County District Court, Case #CV 95-228 (N.M. D.C., 1995).

Gess v. United States, 952 F. Supp. 1529 (M.D. Ala., 1996).

Hansen v. Caring Professionals, Inc., 676 N.E.2d 1349 (Ill. App., 1997).

Harrell v. Louis Smith Memorial Hospital, 397 S.E.2d 746 (Georgia, 1990).

Healthcare Trust v. Cantrell, 689 So.2d 822 (Alabama, 1997).

Hunter v. Bossier Medical Center, 718 So.2d 636, (La. App., 1998).

Husbert v. Commissioner of Education, 591 N.Y.S. 99 (New York, 1992).

Karnes v. Doctor's Hospital, 555 N.E.2d 280 (Ohio, 1990).

Kidner, M. A. (1999). *How to keep float nurses from sinking.* RN 62(9), 35–39.

Milazzo v. Olsten Home Health Care, Inc., 708 So.2d 1108 (La. App., 1998).

Minnesota Nurses Association (1997). Position paper: Delegation and Supervision of Nursing Activities. St. Paul, MN: Author.

Molden v. Mississippi State Department of Health, 730 So.2d 28 (Mississippi, 1998).

Ramirez v. Oklahoma Department of Mental Health, 10 IER Cases 102 (10th Cir., 1994).

Roach v. Kelly Health Care et al., 742 P.2d 1190 (Oregon, 1997).

Sparks Regional Medical Center v. Smith, 976 S.W.2d 396 (Ark. App., 1998).

St. Paul Medical Center v. Cecil, 842 S.W.2d 809 (Texas, 1992).

Theft of drugs is serious problem, putting patients and hospitals at risk (1997). *Health Risk Management* 19(4), 41.

Trudeau, S. (1992). *Hospital Law Newsletter.* March, pp. 3–4.

Winkelman v. Beloit Memorial Hospital, 168 Wisc.2d 12, 484 N.W.2d 211 (Wisconsin, 1992).

sixteen

Ambulatory Care Nursing

■ INTRODUCTION

The health care delivery trend toward more careful management of scarce health care resources has placed new emphasis on primary prevention and led to increased opportunities for professionals in traditional ambulatory care settings. These ambulatory settings include traditional clinics, freestanding surgicenters, nurse-managed and -run clinics, telenursing, and parish nursing, among other innovate settings for advanced quality health care. This chapter explores legal issues involved in such settings and the concept of violence in health care, and includes nurses who donate their services, either through disaster nursing or volunteer services.

■ KEY CONCEPTS

ambulatory care nursing	telenursing	volunteer services
risk management	telemedicine	disaster nursing
telehealth	violence	donating health-related advice

AMBULATORY CARE NURSING

Ambulatory care nursing describes practice settings in nursing outside the traditional acute care and long-term care settings, including physicians' offices, nurse-based practices, wellness programs, freestanding clinics, and health maintenance organizations. Numbers of professional nurses employed in such settings increased by 137% from 1980 to 1996 (Moses, 1996). At the same time, in an effort to maximize inpatient dollars, traditional ambulatory settings and community-based settings have been managing more seriously ill persons, those with complex and often multisystem diagnoses. As more clients are cared for in ambulatory settings, more professional nurses, skilled in the role necessary for this practice arena, are required.

The American Academy of Ambulatory Care Nursing Practice Standards defines ambulatory care nurses as nurses "specialized in health care delivery that is uniquely respon-

363

sive to the needs of patients who seek care on an intermittent basis which may continue over time and involve multiple disciplines" (1993, p. 6). The standards note that such nurses value:

1. Shared responsibility among patients, families, and health care team members.
2. Education for patients and families.
3. Continuity of care.
4. Cost effectiveness.
5. Patient advocacy (1993, p. 8).

One of the issues that arises with ambulatory nursing concerns the level of professional nursing performance. One author has suggested that roles for this professional are more technical and less demanding than the roles of hospital-based nurses, including merely escorting patients to examination rooms and preparing patients for the physician or nurse practitioner (Smith, 1999). Such roles may be envisioned, as approximately 75% of the activities performed by staff nurses in ambulatory care settings are non-nursing activities (Pinkney-Atkinson and Robertson, 1993). Perhaps, though, these less demanding roles are reflective of the transition between more traditional inpatient roles and the continually evolving roles in ambulatory care settings. There appear to be several roles in which nurses can excel in this care setting.

Risk Management

Risk management is the process that identifies, analyzes, and treats potential hazards within a specific setting. The object of risk management is to identify potential hazards and to eliminate them before anyone is harmed. Often confused with quality management with its emphasis on individual patient care problems, risk management relies on data from prior patient incidents and errors, analyzes and evaluates the data, then designs means to prevent or minimize losses in the future. The functions of risk management are to:

1. Define situations that place the entity at some financial risk.
2. Determine the frequency of those situations that have occurred.
3. Intervene and investigate identified events.
4. Identify potential risks that exist and opportunities to improve patient care.

All nurses participate in an organization's risk management program. Administration develops a philosophy that encourages safe, competent patient care. Administration also provides an atmosphere that encourages the prompt identification and control of risks within the setting.

Administrative personnel achieve these goals in a variety of ways. One of the first priorities is the identification of which types of services will be performed in the setting. A freestanding setting, such as a nurse-run clinic or surgicenter, must determine which services can be performed safely without the immediate availability of a full-service acute care institution. Second, administrative personnel will have in place the procedure to be followed when patients experiencing unanticipated complications require transfer to institutions offering a full range of services, including intensive care services, if they are required.

Administrative personnel are responsible for ensuring that all persons who work at the ambulatory setting are licensed as required and qualified to perform within their job description. This is normally accomplished through the facility's credentialing committee and yearly review and evaluation of licensed personnel. Administrative personnel are also accountable for the supervision and education of those who work in the setting. Regular educational programs are offered regarding the safe and effective use of new and regularly used equipment, with mandatory attendance that is documented. Educational programs are also offered concerning competent nursing care and effective patient education.

Courts have, in recent years, carved out a duty to orient, educate, and evaluate for nurse-managers and administrators, in all practice settings. This duty incorporates the daily evaluation of nurses performing in a competent manner, as well as those orienting new personnel. In larger centers, continuing education may be done by specialized staff, and in smaller centers, continuing education becomes the responsibility of administrative staff.

The key to meeting these expectations is reasonableness. Nursing risk managers meet risk management expectation by thoroughly investigating all allegations of incompetent or questionable nursing care, by recommending alternatives for correcting situations, and by including follow-up evaluations in nurses' records, showing that the nurses are competent to care for patients within the ambulatory setting.

A case that enforces this responsibility is *St. Paul Medical Center v. Cecil* (1992). In that case, a term obstetrical patient presented to the hospital, stating that "her water had broken." The nurse assessed the patient and also performed a vaginal examination. An hour later, the patient was reassessed, this time by a medical resident, who determined that the membranes had ruptured and that meconium was present. During the third hour after admission, the resident attached an internal monitor, whose printout showed severe fetal hypoxia and bradycardia, and more meconium was observed. Telling the nurse to alert the attending physician of the need for an immediate cesarean section, there was still an hour delay before a severely brain injured infant was born.

An issue that arose in the defense of the nurse-defendant concerned evaluations that had been written about the nurse's performance three months before this incident arose. At that time, the nurse had been rated as an unsatisfactory employee who sometimes fell asleep while on duty, had difficulty in using electronic fetal monitors, and was reluctant to seek advice or consult with the supervisory nurse when problems arose concerning labor and delivery issues. No subsequent evaluation could be found to support that any of these problems had been addressed or that any had been resolved. The court found both the hospital and the nurse liable to the patient.

Lessons to be learned from this case include the importance of following through on incompetent staff members, whether by reassigning them to less critical areas of the facility, by reeducating the nurse so that safe performance of nursing skills can occur, or by discharging the nurse. A second lesson is the need for reevaluation and assurance that current evaluations show the improved competency of the nurse in question.

A second case that illustrates the need to orient and document such orientation and conpetency to perform required tasks is *Healthtrust v. Cantrell* (1997). There, the issue concerned the adequate training of operating room personnel prior to their performing required tasks. To protect itself from liability, the court concluded, a surgical facility should document, before the fact, that personnel have been properly trained for the specific tasks they will be performing and that they are familiar with the specific procedures to which they will be assigned.

Staff nurses in ambulatory care settings also actively participate in risk management programs. They participate through their attendance and attention at continuing education programs, adherence to facility policy and procedure manuals, prompt reporting of identified risks and potential hazards in the environment and about patient care equipment, and in continually ensuring the competency of their patient care.

■ EXERCISE 16—1

Explain the risk management program at an ambulatory setting in which you have clinical experience. If no formal program exists, how is risk management assured by the agency? What types of issues has the risk management program addressed?

Patient Education

While important in all health care settings, the emphasis on prevention of disease and the promotion of health stresses the need for patient education in all ambulatory settings. This is particularly true as most patients continue to seek care at ambulatory settings over long periods of time and are involved with a variety of interdisciplinary health care members. The major emphasis thus is on quality patient education and patient compliance with a course of therapy. Included in the concept of patient education is the entire issue of discharge planning.

To be an effective educator, nurses must remain current on their knowledge of disease processes, therapies and medications to manage these processes, complications that could occur during the course of treatment, and innovative educational models. It is not enough that nurses are knowledgeable about the latest medical treatments or interactions of medications. Nurses must be effective educators, blending teaching styles to the learner needs and objectives, incorporating educational models into their presentations and discussions, and using culturally competent models with a diversity of clients and family members. Staff in-service education programs in the ambulatory setting should include programs on educational models, how the learner is best able to learn, assessment of learner readiness, and evaluation of learner objectives. Merely understanding the medical concepts and newer technologies does not make one an effective teacher. The teacher role also requires intense study and adaptation.

Telehealth/Telemedicine/Telenursing

Telehealth is the use of telecommunications technologies for the provision of long-distance clinical health care, patient and professional education, and health administration. Because telehealth services are widely varied, constantly changing, and the technology complex, the concept is difficult to grasp without some basic definitions.

Telecommunications encompass the transmission of information from one site to another, using a variety of equipment to transmit information in the form of signals, signs, words, or pictures by cable, radio, telephone systems, cable television programing, facsimile transmissions, satellite paging systems, and electronic mail. Telehealth is the use of telecommunications equipment and communications networks for transferring medical health information between participants at different locations. Telehealth can be found in nearly every area of health care, from emergency medical response systems to hospitals and home care, and can be used for direct patient care, patient and health practitioner education, and health services administration. Equipment used in telehealth includes computers, telephones, monitors, and telecommunications networks connecting two or more sites.

Telehealth systems permit the provision of care in situations in which a face-to-face meeting between health care provider and patient is not possible, or would be accomplished only at great cost. *Telenursing,* a subset of telehealth, allows a nurse to deliver care through a telecommunications system. Most nurses already use simple forms of telenursing by telephoning a patient status report to another nurse or by making a phone call to an ambulatory surgical patient to assess discharge status. Other examples of telenursing include home health visits via telecommunications for monitoring and educating patients.

Telemedicine, another subset of telehealth, allows clinicians to provide care via telecommunications. Many telemedicine subspecialties are already recognized, including teleradiology, telepathology, and teleoncology. *Telepresence* combines robotics and virtual reality to allow a surgeon equipped with special gloves and proper video and audio equipment to manipulate surgical instruments at remote sites. Research in telepresence is vital to both the military and civilian health centers, especially for the care of individuals in remote areas of the world.

Video teleconferencing transmits sounds and images between two or more sites, allowing participants to interact. Health care providers at various sites can discuss a patient's status, or a health care provider at a remote site can consult with a patient and family members, or educators at multiple sites can discuss new innovations and interventions.

The concept of telehealth is not new; it dates back to the 1950s when closed circuit audio and video transmission at larger medical conventions allowed participants in several rooms to simultaneously participate in a presentation. By 1965, surgery to replace a defective aortic valve was performed in Texas and transmitted via the Communications Satellite Corporation's "Early Bird" satellite to the Geneva University Medical School in Switzerland.

Since 1990, there has been renewed interest in telehealth for two primary reasons. First, the quality of computers and telecommunications technology has greatly improved. Second, problems that have persistently plagued the health care delivery system in the country such as inadequate access to health care; uneven distribution of health care providers in large, metropolitan areas as opposed to smaller, rural communities; quality management; and escalating costs can be alleviated through the effective usage of telehealth.

Today, a variety of innovative projects are emerging to facilitate consultations among professionals, diagnosing and assessing disease states, interviewing patients, taking patient histories, and prescribing medications and therapies. Some of the projects include:

1. Mobile telehealth applications, ensuring that patients' real-time vital signs data and video images of patients are transmitted during ambulance travel.
2. Educational and emotional support programs for families with high-risk newborns are being done through a hospital monitoring system that allows parents to watch their babies' care from home on a television monitor and receive guidance from hospital staff after discharge.
3. Systems for monitoring child abuse, which establish an around-the-clock monitoring system between the hospital emergency center and child protective team clinicians.

Heralded as the next wave in health care because of its potential to speed access to care and extend services to the underserved, at least 416 rural hospitals have telehealth programs available today and another 564 facilities have plans to establish programs within the next 2 years (Office of Rural Health Policy, 1997). Today, at the Medical College of Georgia Telemedicine Center, both the health care provider and the patient sit in front of cameras mounted on top of computers at their respective locations. They can see, hear, and talk to one another in real time, allowing health care delivery to occur at the site of the patient in rural Georgia (Granade, 1997).

Legal issues with telehealth and telenursing are varied and have the potential to escalate as the entire field continues to expand. Security and confidentiality issues abound since telehealth allows the transmission of patient information electronically. The federal government, recognizing the potential for lack of privacy in transmitted telecommunications, charged the Computer Sciences and Telecommuncations Board (CSTB) with studying the privacy and security of electronic health data. The CSTB has declared that the protection of patient data requires both organizational and technical measures. Organization measures include the imposition of penalties when employees fail to maintain security rules. Technical measures that would prevent unauthorized use include:

1. Access controls that limit practitioners to information that is necessary for their job or direct patient care.
2. Audit trails that maintain records of who has access to specific data and patients' files.
3. Firewalls, which encompass a software feature that prevents hackers from unauthorized use of patients' files and data.
4. Encryption, a mechanism for coding information so that it can be read only by those for whom it is intended and who have the "key" to decode the information.

This issue is also partially addressed by the Health Insurance Portability and Accountability Act of 1997.

A second issue is licensure, either within single states or with a single license that allows nurses to be licensed in one jurisdiction and practice in several jurisdictions. The impetus for multistate licensure seems to be telenursing, since nurses will be in one location and the patients they treat, counsel, or educate will potentially be in any of the 50 states. This issue, though addressed by boards of nursing and nursing organizations, is far from resolution.

A third legal issue involves practice standards, especially as nurses from multiple states are involved in the care of patients through telenursing. In 1999, the American Nurses Association developed the following core principles* for telehealth:

1. The basic standards of professional conduct governing each health care profession are not altered by the use of telehealth technologies to deliver health care, conduct research, or provide education. Developed by each profession, these standards focus in part on the practitioner's responsibility to provide ethical and high-quality care.
2. A health care system or health care practitioner cannot use telehealth as a vehicle for providing services that are not otherwise legally or professionally authorized.

*Source: American Nurses Publishing of the American Nurses Foundation from *Managed Care: Nursing's Blueprint for Action* (1999), p. 16. Used with permission.

3. Services provided via telehealth must adhere to basic assurance of quality and professional health care in accordance with each health care discipline's clinical standards. Each health care discipline must examine how telehealth affects or changes its patterns of care delivery and what modification to existing clinical standards are required.
4. The use of telehealth technologies does not require additional licensure.
5. Each health care profession is responsible for developing its own processes for ensuring competencies in the delivery of health care through the use of telehealth technologies.
6. Practice guidelines and clinical guidelines in the area of telehealth should be developed based on empirical evidence, when available, and on professional consensus among all involved health care disciplines. The development of these guidelines may include collaboration with governmental agencies.
7. The integrity and therapeutic value of the client–health care practitioner relationship should be maintained and not diminished by the use of telehealth technology.
8. Confidentiality of client visits, client health records, and the integrity of information in a health care information system are essential.
9. Documentation requirements for telehealth services must be developed that ensure documentation of each client encounter with recommendations and treatments, communication with other health care providers as appropriate, and adequate protections for client confidentiality.
10. All clients directly involved in a telehealth encounter must be informed about the process, the attendant risks and benefits, and their rights and responsibilities. Clients must provide adequate informed consent.
11. The safety of clients and practitioners must be ensured. Safe hardware and software, combined with demonstrated user competency, are essential components of safe telehealth practice.
12. A systematic and comprehensive research agenda must be developed and supported by governmental agencies and health care professions for the ongoing assessment of telehealth services (American Nurses Association, 1999).

To date, case law involving telenursing has centered on advice given by nurses to patients who telephone for health care advice. For example, in *McCrystal v. Trumbull Memorial Hospital* (1996), the nurse who took the patient's phone call and her nursing supervisor both failed to assess the patient's situation correctly and failed to give the patient correct advice. The patient was pregnant with her fourth child. She had carried three other pregnancies to full term, but each of them had been delivered by cesarean section. She came to the emergency room believing she was in labor, but was reassured that she was not. Six days later, she came back in the morning to the same hospital emergency room believing that she was in labor, and again was sent home. She returned that same afternoon, was examined, and again reassured that she was not in labor.

When the patient returned home, she began to experience vaginal bleeding. She phoned the woman's care clinic at another hospital and spoke with the nurse. The nurse, before giving any specific advice, spoke with her nursing supervisor. The nurse and her supervisor both agreed that it was not necessary for the woman to return to the emergency room. They both assured her that she should stay home and wait for the bleeding to stop.

The woman phoned her physician and received the same advice from him. Later that day, the woman went to the emergency center anyway. During the cesarean delivery of

GUIDELINES: TELENURSING

1. Because privacy and confidentiality are to be afforded all patients, previously established confidentiality and privacy protections of health information must be used with telenursing and reviewed often to ensure that these protections are adequate and used by all personnel.
2. Informed consent should be obtained from all patients before using telenursing, including risks and benefits. Risks include images that may not be as clear as what one would be able to detect were the patient in a more traditional health care setting, and the limitations on some of the finer aspects of physical assessment, such as the use of smell and touch. Benefits include availability of services to patients in distant and hard-to-reach places as well as not having to travel far distances in order to receive quality health care.
3. Remember to ask patients if information concerning them can be shared with others, for example, by telecommunicating data and images of the patient to other health care providers. Patients should also be informed if others outside the health care team will be involved in the telecommunications, such as observers and technical staff.
4. Telenursing should augment health care delivery, not substitute for established, competent nursing care.
5. Adhere to agency policies and protocols regarding telenursing, especially in the use of telephone triage or counseling via telecommunications. Remember, too, that assessment of patients via telephone is dependent on information as relayed by family members and patients. If you are uncertain about the patient's symptoms or have any doubts that the patient should be seen, err on the side of caution and advise the patient or family member to call 911 or go to an emergency center immediately.
6. Document all data used to decide on the care needed for patients, as well as care given or education taught patients.

the child, it was discovered that her uterus had ruptured along the old incision line from a previous cesarean operation. The child had already experienced serious brain damage from lack of oxygen.

The court held that both nurses were negligent. They failed to make a correct assessment. They believed that the bleeding was some minor spotting from the previous vaginal examination and failed to listen to her description of her complaints or explore the full history of the situation. The physician was also negligent, said the court. A similar conclusion was reached in *Starkey v. St. Rita's Medical Center* (1997), when the nurse correctly assessed that the patient was having a myocardial infarction, but failed to advise the patient and his wife of the gravity of a myocardial infarction and said he could wait until later to seek treatment.

In *Havard v. Children's Clinic of Southwestern Louisiana, Inc.* (1998), a 13-year-old's grandmother withheld the girl's morning insulin injection because the granddaughter was sick at home from school and was vomiting. As a child, the 13-year-old had once become hypoglycemic after getting insulin while nauseated and vomiting. The grandmother called the clinic and asked to speak with the child's physician, but he was unavailable. The grandmother told the nurse the girl was diabetic, and had not had her morning insulin. She asked for a prescription for Phenergan suppositories to stop the vomiting.

The nurse said she would check the chart and see if she could send the suppositories. The nurse had the suppositories delivered, apparently without checking the chart or consulting the physician. The girl was taken to the emergency room that night and died in the intensive care unit early the following morning from diabetic ketoacidosis. The family sued the clinic and was awarded a $183,000 verdict, which was reduced by 20% for the grandmother's negligence in withholding the morning insulin and ignoring two elevated blood sugar levels later in the afternoon.

The Court of Appeals upheld the jury's verdict, awarding an additional $10,000. The court ruled that the nurse was negligent in her assessment of the child and her treatment of the child's condition.

Violence

Because of the prevalence of physical and psychological *violence* in society, nurses frequently care for the victims, the perpetrators, and the witnesses of physical and psychological violence. Additionally, nurses are also at risk for experiencing violence in the workplace. According to the Bureau of Labor Statistics (1998), almost two-thirds (64%) of nonfatal workplace assaults occur in hospitals, nursing homes, and residential care facilities. Verbal abuse is even greater, with more nurses now reporting abuse from patients and family members, both in formal settings and in ambulatory settings.

No one knows the full extent of the problem, because many employers do not maintain such files and actively discourage staff from reporting incidents. Similarly, many cases of violence and abuse outside formal health care settings are also not reported, because the victims fear greater violence if they come forward, and because of shame and guilt.

Nursing organizations are now beginning to recognize all types of violence, especially domestic violence, as a major public health threat, one with high incidence and prevalence that requires significant health care interventions. The reduction of violence is targeted as one of the major goals of the U.S. National Health Plan in Healthy People 2000. Often, domestic violence is first noted by nurses in ambulatory settings.

Domestic violence affects a significant proportion of the U.S. population either as direct victims or as witnesses of abuse directed toward spouses or partners, children, and elders. Maltreatment of children affects nearly three million children annually and results in the deaths of more than three children every day (McCurdy and Daro, 1994). Between two and four million women are physically battered every year by partners or former partners (U.S. Public Health Service, 1991). The mistreatment of elders is estimated to affect about 1.1 million individuals annually (American Nurses Association, 1998). As much as 35% of the adult population in the United States reports having witnessed a man beating his wife or girlfriend (Centers for Disease Control and Prevention, 1998).

In addition to immediate physical, emotional, and psychological injury, the sequelae of such abuse are often serious and lifelong. Long-term effects include permanent disabilities, sexually transmitted diseases, and complications of pregnancy and birth, including low-birth-weight babies. Mental health effects include depression, post-traumatic stress disorder, alcohol and drug abuse, and suicide.

In view of the pervasive nature of violence as a major health problem, the American Association of Colleges of Nursing (ACCN) recommends that nurses in all nursing programs understand both the magnitude of the problem and are taught about violence, including clinical experience regarding domestic violence. They recommend that the curricula include:

1. Acknowledgment of the scope of the problem.
2. Assessment skills related to the identification and documentation of abuse and its health effects.
3. Interventions to reduce vulnerability and increase safety, especially of women, children, and elders.
4. Cultural competence in dealing with violence as a health care problem.
5. Legal and ethical issues in treating and reporting violence.
6. Activities to prevent domestic violence (American Association of Colleges of Nursing, 1999, p. 2).

To meet the legal and ethical issues involved in domestic violence, nurses must be aware of state and national legal mandates regarding domestic violence, including mandatory reporting laws. Such mandatory laws include reporting of child abuse and elder abuse in all states. Nurses must also become more cognizant about the appropriate methods for collection and documentation of data so that both the patient and the provider are protected. The entire field of forensic nursing is a testament to the importance of this collection and documentation of data. Nurses must also be aware of confidentiality issues and the individual's right to remain silent. Unfortunately, the abused adult woman or man is not protected as are children and the elderly, presumably because they can "speak for themselves." Thus, they are not considered vulnerable under the law.

Nurses are also becoming better informed about how to approach the issue of abuse with potential victims, asking questions in a way that promotes honest answers rather than mere silence. Nurses, especially those in clinic settings, are also becoming more comfortable addressing the issues, rather than avoiding the hard questions as was so often done in the past. Educational offerings are being made available to all nurses about addressing potential victims of violence. As newer assessment tools are developed, it is hoped that all nurses, in all clinical settings, will address this most pressing public health issue.

Finally, patient education concerning the victim's rights, possible safe harbors, and better career opportunities for adult victims is slowly beginning to make changes in the lives of these individuals. As nurses become better educated about violence and more comfortable speaking with potential victims about violence, the education opportunities for these victims is also increasing.

■ EXERCISE 16–2

Research the statistics concerning domestic violence in your geographic area. How does it differ from the national statistics as noted in the preceding paragraphs? What is being done by local health agencies to reduce such incidents of violence? How can you affect the staggering statistics in your everyday clinical practice?

GUIDELINES: NURSING VICTIMS OF VIOLENCE

1. Understand the immense prevalence of violence in the United States today, especially the silence of its victims. Merely because the individual does not report attacks of violence does not mean that they are not occurring.
2. Enroll in formal and informal courses to better understand the vast impact of violence in the community. An alternative approach to such courses are the numerous articles, many with continuing education credit, that are now appearing in many of the nursing journals. Learn as much as you can about the issue and how to assess patients for incidents of violence.
3. Include questions about the possibility of violence in all assessments of patients, even if they do not appear to be victims of violence. Remember, psychological violence leaves no physical scars, and patients may be able to hide their emotional scars during the short time of assessment. Additionally, the more you include such gentle questions in assessment, the more comfortable you will be with them and the less likely you will be to fail to assess the incidence of violence.
4. Learn all you can about community resources for the victims of violence so that you can fully assist patients when they ask for help. You can also include such community resources in your discussions with patients who request no assistance, hopefully so that they will know their options should they need them.
5. Educate all patients about the subtleties of violence as many patients do not know that violent behavior affects much more than merely physical behaviors. Help individuals to understand how they can help better their situation, including formal educational opportunities, programs to enhance self-image and self-worth, support groups for victims of violence, and preparing in advance an escape plan, as applicable.

VOLUNTEER SERVICES

Many health care providers routinely provide *volunteer services,* usually as a vital part of community services. Volunteer status may also arise when one agrees to care for a sick neighbor or a family member. Remember, the nurse may also be donating professional services and nursing skills when helping to conduct a hypertension screening program or presenting a lecture on juvenile diabetes for the local Parent–Teacher Association.

There are several points to remember about volunteer status:

1. The legal status may not be well defined since donated services do not fall within the auspices of the state nurse practice act. Most nurse practice acts apply only to compensated services, so the strict rules and regulations generated by the state board of nurse examiners do not apply to donated services.
2. Responsibilities and professional actions do not change. The nurse is still a professional and owes a minimum standard of care to patients or clients. The standard of care for a professional nurse remains the same under most circumstances.
3. The fact that services are donated does not exempt the nurse from a possible lawsuit or from the standard of the reasonably prudent nurse. The state nurse practice act still guides one's professional responsibilities.

4. The state board of nursing may subject the nurse to disciplinary action should the care delivered fall below minimum standards. This is true even if no ancillary civil action is filed against the nurse.

5. The nurse–patient relationship is initiated when care is first given to the patient. Once established, the same duty of care owed a hospital or paying patient is owed this patient (*Lunsford v. Board of Nurse Examiners*, 1983).

To protect oneself legally, follow this basic advice.

1. Never administer any treatment or medication without first obtaining a doctor's order or, in the majority of jurisdictions, without a valid standing order. This is true even if the medication is an over-the-counter drug. Professional nurses are responsible for knowing indications, mechanisms of action, contraindications, dosages, adverse reactions, and drug interactions for all medications that they give to patients.

2. Reread carefully one's professional liability insurance policy. Does it cover gratuitous services? Depending on the type of services volunteered (e.g., to a large group as opposed to volunteering to care for a sick relative) and the number of lawsuits filed against nurses in the given geographic area, the nurse may want to increase the dollar amount of the policy. Nurses might also want to increase the coverage limits if they frequently volunteer professional services and come in contact during the donated work with large numbers of persons.

3. A system of record keeping should be initiated and accurate records maintained. Even though there is no formal chart, the records may prove to be invaluable should a lawsuit be filed later. The notes will help to refresh the defendant's memory and may make him or her a more reliable witness.

 ## GUIDELINES: VOLUNTEERING PROFESSIONAL SERVICES

COMMUNITY/NEIGHBORHOOD SERVICES

Before donating professional services:

1. Reread your nurse practice act to see if such free services are covered by the nurse practice act.
2. Check your professional liability insurance policy to ensure that you are covered financially should such services result in a malpractice suit being filed against you.
3. Consider carefully the impact of your decision on public relations and the nursing community should you refuse.

If you decide to volunteer your professional services

1. Stay within the confines of nursing scope of practice.
2. Refrain from crossing into a medical scope of practice; do not make medical diagnoses or distribute medical therapies and treatments.
3. Maintain the same standard of care you would maintain if you were a paid employee.
4. Keep accurate notes for your personal files.
5. Use this opportunity wisely to expand the positive image of nursing to the public at large.

GUIDELINES: DISASTER SITUATIONS

1. Be prepared. Know in advance your capabilities and what to do should a disaster occur. Know the limits of your professional liability policy and the provisions of your nurse practice act.
2. Maintain at least an emergency standard of care. Perform functions that you are qualified and skilled to do, even if they are outside your normal nursing actions, when instructed to do so by those in authority.
3. Allow for needed rest periods. If you are so exhausted that you cannot make valid judgments, no one benefits from your care or presence.
4. Make notes and record happenings as quickly as possible after rendering nursing care. These notes and records will help to refresh your memory as needed.

4. Know the state's Good Samaritan laws. Many states fail to cover nurses for voluntary work done outside of an emergency or away from an accident scene.
5. Above all, one should know the provisions of the nurse practice act. Understand standards of care, and perform to that minimal level or better at all times. If the purpose of the donated services is the better education of the public, as with a mass hypertension screening program, carefully review with the sponsoring agency what the questionnaire should say and the types of questions normally asked. Such review will allow the professional nurse to answer the questions and to conduct the mass learning program at an optimal standard-of-care level.

DISASTER NURSING

Some broad guidelines may be applied to *disaster nursing,* in which a nurse either volunteers or is compensated for aid given during a disaster. The standard of care in a time of a disaster usually becomes similar to the standard of care given in emergency situations. Once having decided to render aid, the level of skill and competency is that which a reasonably prudent nurse practitioner would do under the same or similar conditions. If the practitioner meets or excels these standards, there is no negligence.

A second consideration concerns assuming duties that one ordinarily does not assume. In a true disaster, the professional nurse may be asked to perform actions usually reserved for interns and residents or for nurses with advanced education and skills. Provided that the nurse has the knowledge and skills required to perform the actions competently, he or she is permitted to give such substituted care. An emergency exception to either the nurse practice act or other statutory or common laws will allow the expanded scope of practice in emergency settings.

Health care providers, once committed to aiding those injured in a disaster, have a duty to give safe, competent care. But they cannot meet the standards of safe and competent care if they are physically or emotionally exhausted. Allow time for needed rest. The quality of nurses' work will greatly increase if they are able to reach sound decisions, and the probability of a negligent action will be diminished.

DONATING HEALTH-RELATED ADVICE

Every health care practitioner has been asked at some time for health-related advice. It may have been at a fashionable party, at the grocery store, or over the telephone. Although unlikely, a lawsuit could be filed if the advice given falls below the accepted nursing and community standard or actually endangers the person's life and future health.

As with volunteer services, nurses must make a decision about *donating health-related advice.* There is no mandatory duty to do so, but once started the nurse has a duty to give competent and safe advice. There is no duty under the state nurse practice act, because most nurse practice acts exclude gratuitous actions.

The advice that is given must reflect accepted nursing and community standards and be as current as possible. The nurse should be as open and honest as possible. If the nurse is not sure of the best advice to give or if the person seeking advice asks about a field of nursing in which the nurse has no expertise, it is advisable to avoid giving advice. It is perfectly acceptable to have a specialty area (e.g., cancer or pediatric nursing) and to be unfamiliar with other fields of nursing (e.g., neurological or rehabilitative nursing). There is no liability incurred if the nurse honestly refrains from giving advice, but there may be liability if the nurse guesses and gives incorrect information.

The advice given should be within the scope of nursing practice. Even though freely given, the nurse may not make a medical diagnosis or interfere with the physician–patient relationship. Instead, the nurse should make general statements such as "From what you have described, it could be a mild stroke or a prestroke condition. You should make an appointment and see your doctor as soon as possible," or "I'm not sure. It's been a long time since I had any experience with sick children." Such statements prevent problems with scope-of-practice issues. Likewise, a statement such as "I don't know the doctor you mentioned. I always see Bob Smith" prevents charges that the nurse recommended changing physicians or that the nurse advised ignoring the primary physician's advice.

Another factor to consider concerns a possible nurse–patient relationship and the reliance of the other person in adhering to the health-related advice given. For example, a neighbor calls and asks a nurse about her son's cut elbow. The son had attempted to catch a ride on the hood of a moving car and fell into the street. The nurse examines the obvious wound and applies a sterile dressing, telling the mother that an antibiotic cream should help prevent an infection and that a doctor's visit at this time is unwarranted. The nurse also questions the son about the fall, asking exactly how he hit the pavement, and he reassures the nurse that he took the full brunt of the fall on his arm and elbow. The next day the mother calls to say that the injured arm looks better, but she is concerned with her son's erratic gait. He is bumping into doors and furniture. Now the nurse's professional advice is to have the son immediately see his physician. The mother's reliance on the nurse for advice demands that the advice is kept current and specific as the situation changes.

This reliance type of relationship seldom follows a casual party or a one-time encounter. Two points to remember are:

1. If health care questions are asked in an informal manner, the answers given must meet the standard of any reasonably prudent nurse.
2. There is no duty to recontact the person to see how or if the advice was implemented.

It is always acceptable to suggest that the person seeking advice consult with his or her own physician. For example, "If it were me, I would see my doctor immediately" is an appropriate response. The law does not require that nurses make such a suggestion if, in their professional judgment, such a suggestion is not necessary or if a reasonably prudent nurse would likewise not make the suggestion. Similarly, the law does not place liability if the person seeking advice fails to follow the advice. The person asking advice can choose to ignore advice given.

One final word of caution: Always refrain from reassuring the person who has asked about a particular disease or symptom that there is nothing to worry about. Reassurance is appropriate only if the condition is indeed minor. As a general rule, ask yourself the following question: If you were at your regular employment and a patient asked the same question, how would you answer it? That very same answer should be given to the person asking for free health care advice.

■ EXERCISE 16—3

Your next-door neighbor knocks on your door late one night, stating that his wife has fallen and hit her head, and asking that you come to see her. When you arrive, you find her conscious, inebriated, and bleeding from a 4-cm gash over her left eyebrow. You help her bandage the cut, and advise that she seek medical advice, particularly since she hit her head on a sharp object and was dazed and unconscious for about a five-minute period.

The next day you discover that the neighbor has not sought medical advice and is lightheaded and somewhat unsure on her feet. She still refuses to see a doctor or to go to the local emergency center. What are your potential legal liabilities if further harm comes

GUIDELINES: HEALTH-RELATED ADVICE

1. Before the situation ever arises, reread both the state nurse practice act and your professional liability insurance policy to see if you are covered financially and if the nurse practice act covers such free advice.
2. If you decide to give advice:
   a. Give only current, up-to-date advice.
   b. Stay within the nursing scope of practice and refrain from medical diagnoses and treatments.
   c. Refrain from suggesting that the physician currently being seen is wrong in his or her advice.
   d. Refrain from false reassurance.
   e. Keep a personal written account of your advice.
3. If you are unsure of what to say or how the advice will be taken, suggest that the person seeking advice see his or her own physician, or state that you are unqualified to answer. You will not be sued for advice not given, but you can be sued for incorrect or potentially harmful advice.

to the neighbor? Are you liable? If yes, what would the neighbor's cause of action be against you? Does the husband also have any reason to name you in a lawsuit?

What are the ethical implications of this scenario? Do you have an ethical obligation to see that the patient seeks additional assistance, such as assistance regarding her alcohol intake?

SUMMARY

The field of ambulatory nursing, though not a new concept, evolved into a major practice area during the 1990s, with the advent of newer technologies, more effective use of health care dollars in acute care settings, and increased incorporation of primary health care. This arena is projected to grow equally rapidly into the next millennium as telehealth and ambulatory practice sites evolve and expand. The issue of domestic violence will hopefully be better addressed as nurses understand its prevalence and expand their practice to include issues of violence in all patient encounters.

AFTER COMPLETING THIS CHAPTER, YOU SHOULD BE ABLE TO

- Describe the area of ambulatory nursing, including its emergence, the role of risk management, and the focus of patient education in ambulatory nursing.
- Discuss the field of telehealth and telenursing, including potential for growth as well as legal issues involved in delivery of health care via telehealth.
- Analyze violence as it exists today in the United States from a nursing perspective and potential interventions to lessen its impact on victims.
- Describe the nurse's legal liabilities when volunteering nursing services, including:
  a. Disaster nursing services.
  b. Donating health-related advice to consumers.

APPLY YOUR LEGAL KNOWLEDGE

- How will the legal issues involved in telehealth continue to expand, and what can nursing as a profession do to address these potential issues?
- Give three reasons why ambulatory nursing will expand as a practice arena in the next century, and what nursing must do to prepare for its expansion?
- How can nursing as a profession affect the issue of domestic violence?
- Give three reasons why nurses should donate their services and three reasons why they should not.

YOU BE THE JUDGE

Mrs. Crum, on behalf of her deceased husband, Gary Crum, filed the following lawsuit. During the evening hours of December 19, 1996, Gary began experiencing symptoms "including feeling agitated and upset, nausea, and an urgent need, but inability, to vomit." Gary was 42 years of age. According to the terms of his insurance policy, Gary was required to contact the company, at a specific phone number, and consult with the advisory nurse prior to seeking medical attention. Mrs. Crum testified that at approximately 10:55 P.M., she contacted the advisory nurse on Gary's behalf and informed the nurse of Gary's symptoms and the history of heart trouble in Gary's family. She told the nurse that she wanted to be sure that Gary was not having a heart attack. The advisory nurse told Mrs. Crum that Gary's symptoms were probably due to excess stomach acid and that he would be fine. Mrs. Crum again telephoned at 11:34 P.M. She informed the nurse that Gary was continuing to have symptoms and also that he was experiencing pain in the middle of his chest. According to Mrs. Crum's testimony, the advisory nurse indicated that Gary should sit at a 40-degree angle; that he should drink some milk, which would allow the stomach acids to recede and would help with the discomfort; and that he would be fine in the morning and did not need to go to an emergency room.

At 11:55 P.M., Gary's symptoms had not eased and Mrs. Crum decided to drive Gary to the local emergency department at the local Medical Center. On the way, Gary became nonresponsive. Cardiopulmonary resuscitation was performed when Gary arrived at the medical center at 12:05 A.M. The efforts were not successful, and Gary was pronounced dead at 12:29 A.M. The cause of death, according to the medical examiner, was an acute myocardial infarction.

Mrs. Crum filed suit for wrongful death against both the advisory nurse and the insurance company. Her complaint also included an action against the nurse for practicing medicine without a license.

Legal Questions

1. Was the nurse negligent in the advice she gave Mrs. Crum concerning her husband's condition?
2. Did the nurse render a medical diagnosis of Gary Crum's medical condition, even though she was not trained, qualified, or licensed to practice medicine?
3. Should the advisory nurse have instructed Mrs. Crum to immediately transport Gary to the local emergency center?
4. Does the age of the patient (42 at the time of death) affect the decision of negligence?
5. How would you decide this case?

REFERENCES

American Academy of Ambulatory Care Nursing Standards Revision Task Force (1993). *Ambulatory Care Nursing Administration and Practice Standards* (3rd ed.). Pitman, NJ: Anthony J. Jannetti, Inc.
American Association of Colleges of Nursing (1999). *Violence as a Public Health Problem*. Washington, DC: Author.

American Nurses Association (1999). *Core Principles on Telehealth.* Washington, DC: Author.

American Nurses Association (1998). *Culturally Competent Assessment for Family Violence.* Washington, DC: Author.

Bureau of Labor Statistics (1998). Workplace Violence [pamphlet]. Washington, DC: U.S. Department of Labor.

Centers for Disease Control and Prevention, Office of Women's Health (1998). *Violence and Injury.* Atlanta, GA: Author.

Granade, P. F. (1997). The brave new world of telemedicine. *RN* 7, 59–62.

Havard v. Children's Clinic of Southwestern Louisiana, Inc., 722 So.2d 1178 (La. App., 1998).

Healthtrust v. Cantrell, 689 So.2d 822 (Alabama, 1997).

Lunsford v. Board of Nurse Examiners, 648 S.W.2d 391 (Tex. Civ. App.–Austin, 1983).

McCrystal v. Trumbull Memorial Hospital, 684 N.E.2d 721 (Ohio App., 1996).

McCurdy, D., and Daro, J. (1994). *Current Trends in Child Abuse Reporting and Fatalities: The Results of the 1993 Annual Fifty-State Survey.* Chicago, IL: National Committee to Prevent Child Abuse.

Moses, E. B. (1996). *The Registered Nurse Population: March 1996. Finding from the National Sample Survey of Registered Nurses.* Rockville, MD: Health Resources and Services Administration, Bureau of Health Professions, Division of Nursing.

Office of Rural Health Policy, U.S. Department of Health and Human Services (1997). *Exploratory Evaluation of Rural Applications of Telemedicine.* Rockville, MD: Author.

Pinkney-Atkinson, V. J., and Robertson, B. (1993). Ambulatory nursing: The handmaiden/specialist dichotomy. *Journal of Nursing Administration* 23(9), 50–57.

Smith, R. M. (1999). Ambulatory care nursing courses. *Nurse Educator* 24(4), 45–48.

Starkey v. St. Rita's Medical Center, 690 N.E.2d 57 (Ohio App., 1997).

St. Paul Medical Center v. Cecil, 842 S.W.2d 809 (Texas, 1992).

U.S. Public Health Service (1991). *Healthy People 200: National Health Promotion and Disease Prevention Objectives.* Washington, DC: U.S. Department of Health and Human Services, Public Health Service.

seventeen

Nursing in Managed Care Settings

■ PREVIEW

The continued growth of managed care as a system for health care financing and delivery affords nursing challenges and opportunities. The restructuring of the health care system has resulted in many cost-containment measures, including the silent replacement of the registered nurse (RN) with unlicensed assistive personnel and other ancillary personnel. The decrease in numbers of RNs, particularly those giving bedside care, seems to negate the original goals of managed care as a system of coordinated, seamless services emphasizing prevention and primary care. Within many managed care organizations, nurses have identified opportunities to achieve original managed care goals, ensuring safe, quality health care for patients. They have also learned to avoid many of the potential legal challenges in managed care. This chapter explores potential legal aspects of nursing in managed care organizations.

■ KEY CONCEPTS

managed care	National Committee for Quality	Emergency Medical Treatment
health maintenance organization	Assurance (NCQA)	and Labor Act (EMTALA)
(HMO)	Employment Retirement Income	antitrust laws
preferred provider organization	Security Act of 1974 (ERISA)	patient rights
(PPO)	gag rules	
point-of-service (POS) plan	end-of-year profit sharing	

EMERGENCE OF MANAGED CARE ORGANIZATIONS

Managed care is loosely defined as a health care system that integrates the financing and delivery of health care services to covered individuals, most often by arrangements with selected providers. These systems offer a package of health care benefits, standards for the selection of health care providers, formal programs for ongoing quality assurance and utilization review, and significant financial incentives for its members to use providers and procedures associated with the given plan.

Managed care is generally a prepaid or capitated payment mechanism, which means that a stipulated dollar amount is established to cover the cost of the health care delivered for a person and is paid periodically, usually as monthly or quarterly payments, to a health care provider or a health care plan. The provider or plan is responsible for arranging the delivery of all health care services required by the person under the terms of the contract.

The health care environment has long been changing, and the escalation of costs for health care have continued to soar in the past few decades. Also soaring are the numbers of persons in the United States who are either uninsured or underinsured. These growing numbers of individuals tax individual, employer, and government budgets for health care. In 1998, the number of uninsured Americans was estimated to be 44.3 million. According to a U.S. Census Bureau figure released in 1999, the number of uninsured Americans is up 2.7 million in the past two years, and approximately 48% of the nation's low-wage earners are not covered by insurance. Age distribution of those without health insurance is predominantly in the 18- to 24-year-old-bracket for middle-class Americans, and 18 to 64 for lower-income families. Educational status also plays a factor, with 27% of persons without a high school education lacking health insurance compared to 9% of persons with a college degree lacking health insurance (*Grand Forks Herald,* 1999).

At the end of 1995, approximately 58.2 million Americans were enrolled in managed care health plans (Gabel, 1997). This surge in managed care plans has occurred based on the assumption that managed care plans will lower costs for payors while maintaining an acceptable level of services and quality care for patients.

There are essentially three basic types of managed care plans today. The first type is a *health maintenance organization (HMO),* a comprehensive health care financing and delivery organization that provides or arranges for provision of covered health care services to a specified group of enrollees, at a fixed periodic payment, through a panel of providers. An HMO can be sponsored by the federal government, medical schools, hospitals, employers, labor unions, consumer groups, insurance companies, and hospital medical plans. To be federally qualified as an HMO, the organization must have the following three aspects:

1. An organized system for providing health care in a geographic area
2. An agreed-upon set of basic and supplemental health maintenance and treatment services
3. A voluntary enrolled group of persons

It is now estimated that there are in excess of 500 HMOs in the United States today. Four types of HMOs are common:

1. *Staff model:* A health care model in which providers practice as employees and are usually paid a set salary.
2. *Independent practice association model:* A separate legal entity that contracts with an HMO for a negotiated fee. The health care providers continue in their existing individual or group practices, seeing HMO patients as a part of the practice.
3. *Group model:* A health plan that contracts with a multispecialty group to provide care to plan members. The providers are not employees of the HMO but are employed by the group practice and are paid a negotiated salary.

4. *Network model:* A model that contracts with two or more independent group practices and/or independent practice associations to provide services, and pays a fixed monthly fee per enrolled member.

A second type of HMO is a *preferred provider organization (PPO).* This type of managed care plan involves contracts with independent providers for negotiated, discounted fees for services to members. Usually, the contract provides significantly better benefits for services received from preferred providers, thus encouraging enrollees to use those providers. Enrollees are often allowed benefits for nonparticipating providers' services, usually on an indemnity basis with significant copayments. There are over 900 PPOs in the United States.

The last type of HMO is the *point-of-service (POS) plan,* also known as the HMO–PPO hybrid or open-ended HMO. This last type of HMO provides a set of health care benefits and offers a range of health services, and members are given the option of using either the managed care program or out-of-plan services. This option is given each time the enrollee seeks care. Members usually pay substantially higher premiums, increased deductibles, and coinsurance if they select a provider outside the panel of participating providers. Many plans have this option for the convenience of enrollees who travel and need medical assistance when away from their usual provider.

As the network of managed care has continued to evolve, a system of accreditation for managed care has emerged. The *National Committee for Quality Assurance (NCQA)* is the independent, nonprofit health maintenance organization accrediting agency. The NCQA is composed of independent health quality experts, employers, labor union officials, and consumer representatives. Accreditation is mandated in at least eight states, and more are contemplating through legislative action to mandate accreditation. The NCQA focuses on quality improvement, credentialing, members' rights and responsibilities, utilization management, preventive health services, and medical records. None of these standards currently focus on nursing-specific measures of patient care outcomes.

Many health care experts agree that, at least in theory, managed health care is an effective manner in which to deliver quality health care. Patients receive care through a single, seamless system as they move from wellness to illness and back to wellnesss. Continuity of care, prevention, promotion of wellness, and early intervention are stressed. In reality, though, managed care has become a means of financing health care and not as a system of organizing patient care. Many of the measures currently adopted by managed care companies illustrate this financial concern, including early discharge, gag rules, incentives for cost-saving measures that fail to take into consideration the overall health status of the patient and staff shortages. Such issues, exclusively aimed at cost cutting, have raised several legal issues surrounding managed care.

LEGAL ISSUES SURROUNDING MANAGED CARE

There are several sources of legal issues that arise under the concept of managed care, including Employment Retirement Income Security Act issues, gag rules and end-of-year profit sharing, standards of care, Emergency Treatment and Active Labor Act issues, and antitrust issues.

Employment Retirement Income Security Act

One of the earliest issues to emerge with managed care concerned potential legal liability under the *Federal Employment Retirement Income Security Act of 1974 (ERISA)*. The ERISA amendment ensured uniformity in the regulation of employee benefit plans and avoided conflict with state laws. Because of their role as both insurer and health care provider, ERISA has shielded HMOs from liability for questionable health care. Countless stories of poor medical decisions, untoward patient outcomes, and premature patient demise have been told by patients and families, with the HMOs protected under the ERISA laws. Congress passed the original ERISA amendments to reserve for the federal government the power to enact any laws or regulations that relate to employer-sponsored benefit plans. These benefits have been broadly interpreted by the courts to include pensions, health plans, and other benefits. ERISA also was created to prevent unfounded actions from eroding benefits and to prevent conflicts among state laws. The act leaves to the states the right to regulate commercial health insurance plans. Since states have been very active in this area of the law and the federal government has not, many large employers have established "self-insured" health plans that are not subject to state regulations on health plan rates, benefits, and other protections.

Congress never intended, however, for ERISA to bar lawsuits against HMOs, health insurers, or health plans regarding patient management decisions. There is now a trend away from the idea that all patients' and beneficiaries' lawsuits against health pans are disallowed under the legal doctrine of federal preemption under ERISA. Courts still adhere to the rule that patients and beneficiaries do not have the right to file lawsuits in state or federal courts to challenge benefit schedules, internal management decisions, and financial priorities. Those areas remain off limits.

What is new is a trend toward allowing patients and beneficiaries to sue health plans, insurance companies, and HMOs for acts that can be characterized as medical care decisions rather than administrative matters. A health care professional who prepares a beneficiary's health plan while working for a health insurer, health plan, or HMO and following its rules can commit malpractice and can be sued along with the health insurer, health plan, or HMO, if the health plan falls below acceptable professional standards, said the court in *Moreno v. Health Partners Health Plan* (1998).

States have been active in promoting greater accountability on the part of HMOs to their patients. For example, legislation passed in the summer of 1997 in both Missouri and Texas make managed care providers legally responsible for adverse medical decisions that cause damages to patients. The Missouri law modifies the definition of *health care provider* in the Missouri Code to add HMOs to the definition. Managed care providers are thus considered medical practitioners, and may be liable for treatment decisions and reimbursement denials that result in patient harm. The Texas law, called the Health Care Liability Claims Act, imposes a duty of ordinary care on managed care providers when making treatment decisions. Persons harmed by adverse decisions may sue in state court after exhausting the administrative appeal process as provided for by the Texas Legislature. Other states, including New York, California, Connecticut, and Rhode Island either have bills pending or have passed bills giving similar protections to patients who have been harmed by medical decisions made by HMOs.

Case examples of this newer application of the law can be seen in the following cases. In *McEvoy v. Group Health Cooperative of Eau Claire* (1997), the court held that an HMO may be liable under the same standards as an insurance company for bad faith refusal for out-of-network treatment. This is especially true of the company making such a bad faith use of out-of-network providers when driven by unreasonable and economically motivated judgments.

McEvoy involved a 13-year-old girl covered under a group health cooperative (GHC) plan providing 70 days of coverage for inpatient psychological care. Her GHC physician diagnosed anorexia nervosa and recommended treatment in a non-GHC residential treatment center for patients with eating disorders. GHC approved the plan, but discontinued treatment coverage after six weeks despite strong opposition from the girl's treating physician and an out-of-network psychiatrist, who protested that she was not ready for release. Instead, the HMO approved a weekly outpatient therapy group for compulsive overeaters. The girl immediately relapsed and lost 21 pounds by the time GHC readmitted her to an out-of-plan center less than two months after her initial discharge. The period of coverage ended a week later, and she remained in treatment at her own expense. She filed suit against GHC for breach of contact and bad faith in failing to authorize care.

The Supreme Court of Wisconsin upheld the allegations against the HMO, stating that the purpose of a bad faith tort is to help redress the bargaining inequality between insurance companies and patients, who frequently have little or no ability to influence the terms of their medical coverage. The HMO, said the court, is "under a contractual duty to provide or pay for reasonable services to remedy the subscriber's condition. . . . up to policy limits" (at 404). The court further held that this was not a malpractice issue, because the cooperative made its decision based on administrative, not medical, considerations.

A second case that illustrates the HMO's potential liability for independent decision making is *Fox v. Health Net* (1994). In that case, a jury rendered a $90 million verdict against an HMO for its decision to refuse to cover a needed bone marrow transplant. The patient claimed that the decision was based on a decision made by the HMO medical director, who received a performance bonus that encouraged him to deny payment for expensive procedures and treatments. The court concluded that such end-of-year bonuses that amount to significant amounts of money can alter the decision-making ability of a medical director.

■ **EXERCISE 17–1**

Explore the managed care options in your geographic setting. Are the plans traditional HMOs or some other type of managed care, such as PPO or POS plans. How many enrollees does the plan cover? What are the advantages to the community of having an HMO rather than more traditional insurance coverage to people in the area? What are the disadvantages? How has the quality of health care delivery changed in the past 10 years?

Gag Rules and End-of-Year Profit Sharing

Managed care plans, in order to be financially successful, must restrict patients' choices and redirect health care away from high-cost options and providers. To encourage providers within the HMO to keep costs as minimal as possible, many HMOs initiated *gag rules,* preventing health care providers from offering certain more expensive therapies as options and restricting service to the complaint about which the patient presented to the HMO. Under the gag rule, health care providers are prevented from informing patients about concomitant illnesses or diseases.

End-of-year profit sharing, sometimes called a *performance bonus,* is an incentive given to reward health care providers for keeping costs at a minimum. A certain percentage of profits are distributed at the end of the calendar year to health care providers who did not order expensive tests or who did not prescribe extensive therapy. The more the health care provider assisted the HMO in making a profit, the more profit that is given back to the health care provider.

Both means of keeping costs low have the potential for substandard treatment of patients and would seem to directly conflict with the purpose of HMOs in ensuring preventative care and promoting health at the primary level. Because of the immense harm that can befall patients, many states have now outlawed both gag rules and end-of-year profit sharing.

Standards of Care

Health care providers have a duty to render quality, competent care. This is true whether or not the ERISA laws apply. For example, in *Hand v. Tavera* (1993), a patient presented to an emergency center in considerable distress. The court preempted the case against the HMO based on the ERISA laws, but the patient was still able to prevail against the health care physician. The physician whom the patient initially saw in *Hand* did not have admitting privileges with the hospital. He called the health care plan's on-call primary physician. This second physician, who was the patient's assigned physician, had never met the patient, and failed to order an admission to the hospital. The patient subsequently suffered a stroke in the hospital's parking lot. The court held that when a patient is fully enrolled in a prepaid plan, goes to the emergency center, and the plan's designated physician is consulted, the physician–patient relationship exists and the physician owes the patient a reasonable duty of care, in compliance with established medical standards of care.

A newer case application is *Shannon v. McNulty* (1998). In that case, the patient belonged to an HMO when she became pregnant with her first child. She was given a choice of six different physicians as her primary prenatal care provider, and she chose one of the six. Her HMO membership card instructed her to contact either her chosen primary care provider or the HMO itself if she had questions about her health care. If the subscriber phoned the HMO directly, the subscriber would speak with a telephone triage line staffed by registered nurses employed by the HMO.

The patient saw her primary physician frequently during the pregnancy for abdominal pain and back pain. She was seen in his office on three consecutive days for these complaints. On the third of these three consecutive visits, the physician informed her that she had a fibroid uterus. He did not perform any tests and did not instruct her about the symptoms of preterm labor. The patient called the physician's office several more times in the ensuing days, and he insisted that she was not in labor. The next time the patient called, she could not reach her primary physician and she then called the HMO. A nurse listened only very briefly, then simply told the patient to call her primary physician. On the next two days, the same scenario happened. None of the nurses working on the triage telephone line knew her history or listened long enough to find out that she was in the fifth month of a very difficult pregnancy.

When the patient called the HMO the fourth time, still complaining of back pain, she was put in contact with an in-house orthopedic physician-consultant. He instructed her to drive to the emergency center at West Penn Hospital, a facility one hour away, further from her home than three other hospitals. At the hospital, the patient was treated as an orthopedic patient, since her referral had been through an orthopedic physician-consultant. The patient was allowed to go to the labor and delivery unit for a check-up.

In the labor and delivery unit, it was decided that the patient was in premature labor and, a few hours later, a small preterm infant was delivered. The infant survived for two days before he died due to his extreme prematurity. The patient sued the HMO and her primary physician under a corporate or vicarious liability theory, and the trial court dismissed her suit.

The appeals court, however, upheld her lawsuit and ruled that corporate liability duties are applicable to HMOs. Though providers do not practice medicine, they do involve themselves in decisions affecting their subscribers' medical care. When decisions are made to limit the subscriber's access to treatment, the decision must pass the test of medical reasonableness. There is no reason, said the court, why the duties applicable to hospitals should not equally apply to an HMO when the HMO is performing the same or similar functions as the hospital. When an HMO is providing health care services

GUIDELINES: PRINCIPLES FOR MANAGED CARE: NURSING'S BLUEPRINT FOR ACTION*

1. Every individual has the right to access health care services along the full continuum of care.
2. Consumers are acknowledged as empowered partners in making health care decisions.
3. Quality health care services will be provided in an interdisciplinary, collaborative manner, with registered nurses retaining their essential role in providing and directing health care in all settings.
4. Health care services must be value-based to maximize quality while controlling costs.
5. The health care system must address the health of individuals, families, communities, and populations.
6. Health care services must be provided in a culturally competent and linguistically appropriate manner.
7. Providers, plans, and health care systems must adhere to high standards of ethical behavior.
8. Accountability for quality, cost-effective health care must be shared among health plans, health systems, providers, and consumers.
9. Confidentiality of patient information must be closely safeguarded.
10. While pursuing the reduction of costs in the health care system, the right to a safe and healthful work environment for all health care providers must not be compromised (American Nurses Association, 1998).

*Source: American Nurses Publishing of the American Nurses Foundation from *Managed Care: Nursing's Blueprint for Action* (1999), p.16. Used with permission.

rather than merely paying for services, the HMO should be judged the same as a hospital or other health care provider.

By the same token, the court reasoned, the patient had established a cause of action for vicarious liability. An HMO has a nondelegable duty to select and retain competent primary care providers. Likewise, the HMO provided a medical service in the form of telephone advice nurses. The adequacy of that service and the reasonableness of the patient's use of that service under the circumstances are questions for a jury.

Emergency Medical Treatment and Labor Act

When Congress passed the *Emergency Medical Treatment and Labor Act (EMTALA)* in 1986, they passed legislation that established a unique right in the American health care delivery system—the right of access to medical care regardless of one's ability to pay for that care (Dame, 1998). The need for the law had become paramount because patients were being turned away from hospitals or "dumped" on other hospitals, primarily through the emergency departments of the hospitals, based solely on their inability to pay for health care. To prevent untoward outcomes, Congress passed the EMTALA.

Essentially, the law applies to every health care institution that has a Medicare provider agreement in effect and requires the following:

1. Examination and treatment for emergency medical conditions and women in labor.
2. A medical screening requirement which mandates that whenever a patient comes to the emergency department and requests examination or treatment for a medical condition, the hospital must provide for an appropriate medical screening examination within the capability of the hospital's emergency department, including ancillary services routinely available to the emergency department, to determine whether or not an emergency condition exists.
3. Necessary stabilizing treatment for emergency medical conditions and labor, which means that when the individual comes to the emergency department requesting treatment and the hospital determines that the individual has an emergency medical condition, the hospital must provide either available treatment within the hospital or transfer the individual to another medical facility for treatment.
4. Transfers are restricted until the individual is stable, unless the individual or legally responsible person acting on the individual's behalf, after being informed of the hospital's obligation to treat and the risk of transfer, in writing requests transfer to another facility, or a physician has signed a certificate based on the time of transfer that the medical benefits reasonably expected from the provision of appropriate medical care at another institution outweigh the increased risk to the individual or the unborn child, or a qualified medical person has signed a medical certificate after consultation with the physician and the physician subsequently countersigns the certificate of transfer.
5. An appropriate transfer is defined as a transfer in which the transferring hospital provides the medical treatment within its capability which minimizes risks to the individual's health or the health of the unborn infant, and in which the receiving facility has available space and qualified personnel for the treatment of the individual and has agreed to accept the transfer of the individual and to provide appropriate medical treatment.
6. Emergency medical condition means a medical condition manifesting itself by acute symptoms of sufficient severity (including severe pain) such that the absence of im-

mediate medical attention could reasonably be expected to result in placing the health of the individual or unborn child in serious jeopardy, or serious impairment of bodily functions, or serious dysfunction of any bodily organ or part.

7. Stabilize means, with respect to the medical condition, to provide such treatment of the condition as may be necessary to assure, with reasonable medical probability, that no material deterioration of the condition is likely to result from or occur during the transfer of the individual from the facility or during the delivery of the unborn infant (42 U.S.C., Section 1359dd).

Despite the fact that the law has been in force for over 10 years, cases still arise under the EMTALA. The advent of HMOs, with their cost-cutting measures, has seemed to intensify such cases. There is, however, some clarification of the law and general guidelines presented by the many cases.

Perhaps the earliest challenges to the law concerned patient "dumping" by hospitals. For example, in *Johnson v. University of Chicago* (1990), city fire department paramedics had been called for emergency care of an infant in cardiac arrest. The paramedics contacted the University of Chicago Hospitals telemetry system and were instructed to take the infant to a hospital other than the one five blocks from the infant's home. The telemetry nurse recommended the alternative hospital because the University of Chicago Hospital's pediatric intensive care unit was full and they had no place to admit the child for treatment. The child later died.

The child's parents brought suit, claiming that the hospital had violated the EMTALA requirements. In the court's holding for the hospital that no EMTALA violation had occurred, the court noted that it would reconsider the evidence if it could be shown that the hospital used the telemetry system as part of a "scheme to dump patients" (at 236).

In 1995, the U.S. Court of Appeals in *Eberhardt v. City of Los Angeles* further defined the role of a hospital in treating medical conditions. In this case, the paramedics had responded to a call that a man was experiencing a heroin overdose. They administered Narcan and transported him to a hospital emergency center. At the hospital, the man reported to the triage nurse that he had used cocaine and smoked heroin immediately before the paramedics arrived. He initially refused treatment but was persuaded to let a physician see him. The physician administered additional Narcan, and his examination of the patient revealed that the man's vital signs had returned to normal levels and that the patient was alert and oriented. He advised the man to seek long-term help through a methadone program at another facility.

The patient then removed his own intravenous line and left the hospital. As he was leaving, he stated that he had a feeling of doom and was upset because the hospital had saved his life. The next day he was shot and killed by police as he attacked them with a machete in a disturbed mental state, and his family brought this lawsuit, alleging an EMTALA violation.

The court ruled that the hospital had met its obligations by attending to the patient's acute medical condition with appropriate care to meet his immediate medical needs and that the hospital was not responsible for his death one day later at the hands of the police.

A 1996 case, *Rios v. Baptist Memorial Hospital System,* reiterated the need for the patient to request care in order to qualify under the EMTALA laws. In *Rios,* a patient with his arm in a sling from a recent industrial accident walked through the emergency department with a family member, stopping only to ask for directions to the admitting department. Unable to find the admitting department, they left and went to another hospital. There was no treatment until four days later, when the injury was significantly worse.

The patient sued the first hospital, alleging an EMTALA violation. The court ruled, however, that a patient must first come to the emergency department and present for care before the hospital's obligations under the EMTALA comes into play. This patient and family member requested no treatment but merely asked for directions. Thus, the patient has no basis for a lawsuit.

Courts have also defined when patient screening is appropriate (*Trivette v. North Carolina Baptist Hospital*, 1998). The key, said the court, is uniform treatment of emergency patients with similar signs and symptoms, regardless of the ability to pay. In this case, the patient received a battery of tests, including x-rays, and was admitted to the hospital. The next day, he was seen by his primary medical provider and released. The court said in its conclusion that EMTALA does not concern itself with possible misdiagnosis, but whether the patient has had a proper screening examination and been offered appropriate treatment to stabilize the emergency condition that brought him to the emergency center.

Other cases have discussed the appropriateness of screening examinations. In *Marshall v. East Carroll Parish Hospital Service District* (1998), a hospital was sued for sending a teenager home with what seemed like only an upper respiratory infection. In fact, the young woman had suffered a cerebrovascular accident consistent with a left middle cerebral artery infarction. The teenager's parents sued only the institution, not the nurses or physicians at the facility.

The court noted that EMTALA applies to nursing assessment in the emergency center as well as to the physician's examination and treatment under the general term *appropriate medical screening examination*. The court further noted that when patients sue over a substandard emergency center medical screening examination, the court looks only at whether the patient was given the same screening examination as other patients presenting with similar signs and symptoms. In dismissing this case, the problem for the court was that staff could not show that this patient was treated any differently than other patients coming into the emergency center with the same signs and symptoms.

In dismissing this case, the court expressly discounted the testimony of a nurse who had overheard a heated discussion between the emergency center physician and a second nurse. The second nurse was vehemently arguing with the physician that the teenager should either be admitted or transferred to another facility, rather than being sent home.

Morrison v. Colorado Permanente Medical Group (1997) illustrates that nurses and physicians may be liable for their actions as well as extending liability to their institution for EMTALA violations. In *Morrison*, the patient had presented to the emergency center with elevated vital signs and flank and buttock lesions that the nurse thought were uninfected bedsores. The patient was seen and released, even though he had necrotizing fasciitis/myositis, for which he should have been immediately treated.

This court examined the language regarding stabilizing treatment in deciding that the physician and nurses were in violation of the EMTALA. The patient was not adequately screened and was thus sent home despite the fact that his medical condition was, within reasonable medical probably, likely to deteriorate. The court also reiterated that all patients, whether or not they have insurance or the ability to pay privately for care, have the right to sue for an EMTALA violation.

Brodersen v. Sioux Valley Memorial Hospital (1995) illustrates the requirement that a nurse's assessment may trigger the hospital's duty to provide stabilizing care. In this case, the hospital's policy was for the emergency center charge nurse to oversee initial screening in the emergency center. For patients presenting with chest pain, an electrocardiogram was to be obtained simultaneously with the physician's being notified of the patient's arrival. According to the testimony of two emergency department staff nurses, it was the hospital practice for the nurse to move acutely ill patients to cardiac or intensive care before the emergency center physician saw the patients, if that was warranted by the patient's initial screening and nursing physical assessment.

When this patient, who was on public assistance, was not given an electrocardiogram and was left to be seen by the emergency center physician, with chest pains for which his physician had instructed him to go to the emergency center and with signs of acute myocardial infarction, the court read a discriminatory motive into the nurse's conduct, and ruled that the hospital had indeed violated the EMTALA.

Note that the opposite conclusion can also be triggered by the nurse's actions. In *Fischer v. New York Health and Hospitals Corporation* (1998), a 6-year-old patient was brought in by ambulance with a fever and headache, 18 hours after he was hit in the head with a snowball. The emergency triage nurse saw him at 12:30 A.M. His vital signs were taken, revealing a temperature of 104.6°F. The mother told the nurse of his injury with the snowball and that he had complained of a headache, loss of appetite, and generalized body pain ever since the incident. At 1:00 A.M., he was given 180 mg of Tylenol to reduce his fever.

The nurse was required by the institution policy to categorize each patient as "routine," "high priority, " or "emergent." She classified this patient as "high priority." The patient was seen by the emergency center physician at 1:15 A.M. for a pediatric examination. By 2:20 A.M., the fever was 102.0°F and the patient was sent home.

He returned two days later, was admitted, and a brain scan showed a serious brain abscess. The family sued for an EMTALA violation, which was dismissed by the court. The court reiterated that the key to avoiding EMTALA violations is equal treatment of emergency center patients. Emergency center physicians and nurses must follow the hospital's same standard screening procedures that they would follow for any other patient in the emergency center with the same medical condition. Here, the emergency center had met its obligations to this patient.

Departure from the emergency center's standard screening procedures can trigger liability as *"C. M." v. Tomball Regional Hospital* (1997) illustrates. In this case, the nurse conducted an entire screening for a 15-year-old rape victim in the emergency department waiting room, crowded with 10 to 15 other persons, rather than providing for the emotional support and medical detection screening that was part of the institution's policy manual.

The nurse was told that the teenager had been raped by a 27-year-old man and was in severe pain. The nurse took no vital signs, nor did she ask any questions about the teenager's medical history. There was no physical examination of the teenager. The nurse did ask questions concerning how the rape had occurred, asking if the patient had since bathed. Learning that the girl had taken a bath, the nurse said there was nothing further that the hospital could do for her, and she instructed the girl and her mother to see their private physician. No other instructions were given by the nurse.

The court reported that the mother had repeatedly asked for a physical examination to see if the girl was all right but that the nurse repeatedly said that there was nothing the hospital could do for her. One of the persons in the waiting room knew the victim and quickly spread the news of the alleged rape to those in the neighborhood, causing the mother and child to relocate to a new home and new school district due to emotional trauma. The mother also testified that her daughter became physically ill when discussions arose about seeking medical care, was afraid of any type of medical activity, and would not trust anyone with private information about herself.

The court ruled that the hospital, emergency center physician, and nurse had violated the EMTALA. The court pointed out that the nurse herself had testified that she followed none of the hospital's own rape crisis procedures.

Court cases have also given guidance with patient stabilization prior to transfer. In *Cherukuri v. Shalala, Secretary of the Department of Health and Human Services* (1999), the court determined that medical and nursing personnel at the first hospital were genuinely concerned about the patients' well-being and were trying to respond to an overwhelmingly difficult situation. Several bad automobile accident trauma victims were brought into a rural hospital. The hospital had an emergency department but no trauma center, no equipment for monitoring anesthesia during neurosurgery, and had in place a long-standing policy against attempting such surgery.

Two patients required brain surgery but were also bleeding into their abdomens. The physicians wanted to operate for the internal bleeding, then send the patients to a teaching-trauma center 85 miles away. The on-call anesthesiologist, however, refused to come to the hospital, insisting that the procedure was too risky, and that the patients should be immediately transferred.

The nurses assisted in the initial triage. Then they cared for three less seriously injured patients while the physicians concentrated on the two more serious victims. They monitored the patients' blood pressures, phoned the anesthesiologist repeatedly to try to get him to come in, and tried to get a helicopter. They were forced to use ambulances for the transport. The physicians and nurses communicated with the trauma center during the transport, and the patients suffered no harm during the transport.

Technically speaking, a patient does not have to be stabilized to be transferred from the hospital that first accepted the patient as an emergency case. However, the physician must make a written certification based on the information available at the time of transport that the provision of appropriate medical care at another medical facility outweighs the increased risk to the patient from making the transfer, and only if the receiving institution has agreed to accept transfer of the patient and to provide the patient with appropriate medical treatment. A patient who has been stabilized can be transferred to another hospital without a physician's certification and without an agreement from the other hospital to accept the patient. When a transfer is being contemplated, it is the patient's immediate situation that is paramount and long-term goals are not the primary focus. Here, the court held that these patients were stabilized within the first hospital, so that no EMTALA violation occurred.

Torres Nieves v. Hospital Metropolitano (1998) also held that transfer of a stable patient was appropriate. In this case, the patient was transferred to a public hospital for surgery after being stabilized at a private institution. The court ruled that the private institution did not have to perform surgery on a charity basis, since the patient was stable and could be transferred to a public hospital without deterioration of her condition during or as a result of the transfer. The opposite finding occurred in *Roberts v. Galen of Virginia, Inc.* (1999), when a patient was transferred prematurely to a skilled nursing home. Here, there was a violation of the EMTALA as the patient still needed care at an acute facility, and her medical condition was compromised as a result of the transfer. The court further noted that for a successful lawsuit, the patient did not need to show that the transfer was motivated by financial considerations, only that the transfer was inappropriate.

Lopez-Soto v. Hawayek (1997) further clarified the issue of appropriate transfer when the case involves a newborn infant. The U.S. District Court for Puerto Rico held that the EMTALA does not apply to a baby born in a hospital, if the mother at the time of admission to the hospital had a normal onset and progression of her labor and was not an emergency case when she arrived at the hospital. The baby was born after a normal labor and delivery at a hospital that did not have a neonatal intensive care unit. Her physician ruptured her membranes, noted meconium in the amniotic fluid, and performed a caesarean section. The infant aspirated meconium at birth, and the physician arranged transfer to a second hospital with a neonatal intensive care unit. The baby's father, who had connections with staff members at a third hospital, arranged to have the baby transferred to the third hospital. Due to complications that were not addressed quickly enough at the first hospital, the baby died. The parents sued the first hospital for a EMTALA violation.

The court held that EMTALA did not apply because the baby's emergency arose in the hospital after the mother's nonemergency admission to the hospital. Thus, there was no legal requirement for the hospital to jump through EMTALA hoops in order to transfer this baby to neonatal intensive care at another hospital.

The family appealed the ruling of the District Court in Puerto Rico, and the first Curcuit Court of Appeals reversed the initial decision and ruled that the legal protection afforded by EMTALA does extend to patients who enter the hospital as nonemergency cases, but who experience a medical emergency for the first time while in the hospital. The court did fault the hospital for not stabilizing the baby prior to transfer, that is, for not dealing with the life-threatening pneumothorax and merely transferring the baby to the third hospital (*Lopez-Soto v. Hawayek,* 1999). Courts have also held hospitals responsible for delays in transfer when the patient's medical condition deteriorates as a direct result of the transfer (*Garcia v. Randle-Eastern Ambulance Service, Inc. et al.,* 1998).

Health maintenance organizations have long held that patients must have prior authorization for medical treatment, including emergency treatments. In 1998, a Special Advisory Bulletin was developed by the U.S. Department of Health and Human Services Office of the Inspector General and the Health Care Financing Administration (HCFA) to better define the EMTALA regulations. Specifically, this bulletin was devised to strike down the prior approval by HMOs. Under the section entitled "HCFA has special concerns about the provision of emergency services to enrollees of managed care plans" is the statement that "once a managed care enrollee comes to a hospital that offers emergency services, the hospital must provide the services required under the EMTALA without regard for the patient's insurance status or any prior authorization requirement for such insurance" (*Federal Register,* 1998).

A recent court case (*Barris v. County of Los Angeles,* 1999) upheld this advisory statement when it ruled that prior approval by an HMO is no basis to deny emergency care under the EMTALA. In this case, an infant had an emergency medical condition for which bacterial cultures and antibiotics were necessary before the infant could leave the hospital. Rather than ordering the tests to rule out bacterial sepsis or beginning antibiotic therapy, the physician instructed the parents to take the child to an HMO-operated facility or seek prior authorization from the HMO. When patients are denied proper emergency screening and treatment, they can bring suit successfully for violations of the EMTALA.

■ **EXERCISE 17–2**

Review the policies and procedures for standards of care of emergency and labor patients in your clinical facility. Do the standards define appropriate medical treatment for patients presenting with specific signs and symptoms? Is there a written policy and procedure for the triage nurse's role in the emergency center? How is the assessment of the patient performed and documented? Have there been issues regarding the appropriate screening and care of patients who present to the emergency center requesting treatment?

Antitrust Issues in Managed Care

Health care delivery systems are becoming dominated by large, for-profit centers in most American cities today. Mergers and acquisitions, coupled with the integration of services and insurance, give greater market power to competitors and an opportunity to provide more competent care of patients.

With these mergers and large, for-profit centers come the questions about antitrust and monopolies in the health care industry. *Antitrust laws* contain specific restrictions for exclusive contracts, resisting utilization reviews, and collusion. Antitrust laws do not merely monitor the anticompetitive services of large corporations; they also regulate the practice of health care providers.

Historically, the move toward health care reform has been anchored by three broad promises:

1. Enhanced coordination of clinical services for all eligible enrollees
2. Reduced medical costs and wastes
3. Improved quality of care

The overall goal of America's antitrust laws is to promote competition while creating efficient markets. These antitrust laws apply to all settings and scenarios that limit competition. The laws are based on the premise that larger numbers of individuals and corporations will bring more efficient allocation of resources, improve quality of care, and increase innovation and technology, access, and services to all.

Until the landmark case of *Goldfarb v. Virginia State Bar* in 1975, health professionals were exempt from the antitrust laws due to their "learned profession" status. Since that lawsuit, extensive antitrust litigation has spurred significant changes in the health care delivery system. The Federal Trade Commission (FTC) vigorously challenged the merger of Hospital Corporation of America (HCA) with Hospital Affiliates International (HAI) and Health Care Corporation (HCC) as the possibility existed that such a merger would eliminate healthy sources of competition and make an already concentrated market more conducive to collusion (Furrow et al., 1997). Some of the more likely forms of collusion that could result from such a merger involve:

1. Collective resistance to emerging cost-containment pressures from third-party payers.
2. Conspiracies to boycott certain insurance companies that offer competitive prices.
3. Refusal to undergo utilization review programs or provide information needed by third-party payers.

The court found that the merger violated specific sections of the Clayton Act and of the FTC Act and ordered HCA to divest two of the hospitals that it had acquired. Without such FTC action, the marketplace would have had fewer providers, and the reduced supply may have resulted in increased prices and a decreased quality of services (Furrow et al., 1997).

Lessons for nurses to be learned from antitrust laws and mergers in managed health care include the fact that such factors force nurses to become more valuable in the health care delivery system. For example, nurses must continue to closely examine the new organization's cost-containment measures to prevent the devaluation and compromise of the nursing profession. Reduction in licensed professionals and the silent replacement of registered nurses with unlicensed assistive personnel has forced nursing to relook at the delivery of competent patient care, and has emphasized the role of the professional nurse as patient advocate and patient educator. It has also emphasized the concept of delegation in health care settings, with the result that more efficient and effective nursing care is now being delivered to patients across the United States.

The inclusion of antitrust laws within the entire health care delivery system has also strengthened the use of midlevel practitioners in a variety of clinical settings, both acute care and community settings. This increased utilization of midlevel practitioners has primarily occurred among advanced practice nurses. When one considers the issues that will shape nursing in the future, including universal access to health care, cost containment, patient outcomes, empowered consumers, and the radical realignment of the private sector health care industry (Mundinger, 1994), it is not surprising that the use of all advanced practice nurses is on the rise.

PATIENT RIGHTS

As managed care has continued its measures of cost containment, many health care providers have become increasingly concerned with issues of *patient rights.* Though some of the factors that caused such concerns are now eroding, such as the strict interpretation that consumers were barred from filing suits against HMOs under the ERISA laws, gag rules, end-of-year profit sharing, and patient "dumping" violations, many still fear that individuals have no true rights in managed care settings. Patients frequently cannot select their own practitioner, but must take whoever is available under the health care plan; they have no means of questioning who or what status of person will be caring for them; morbidity rates, infection rates, and rates of complications are not published about individual health care practitioners or settings; and preapproval must be obtained for most health care treatments.

As a response to these issues, the president, the U.S. Congress, and individual state legislatures have been working on a variety of patient rights bills over the past several years. On March 26, 1997, President Clinton appointed the Advisory Commission on Consumer Protection and Quality in the Health Care Industry, charging them to "advise the

President on changes occurring in the health care system and recommend measures as necessary to promote and assure health care quality and value, and protect consumers and workers in the health care system"(Advisory Commission on Consumer Protection and Quality in the Health Care Industry, 1997, p. 1). Part of their charge was to draft a consumer bill of rights.

The committee adopted eight areas of consumer rights:

1. *Information disclosure.* Consumers have the right to receive accurate, easily understood information, and some require assistance in making informed health care decisions about their health plans, professionals, and facilities.
2. *Choice of providers and plans.* Consumers have the right to a choice of health care providers that is sufficient to ensure access to appropriate high-quality health care. Public and private group purchasers should, whenever feasible, offer consumers a choice of high-quality health insurance products. Small employers should be provided with greater assistance in offering their workers and their families a choice of health plans and products.
3. *Access to emergency services.* Consumers have the right to access emergency health care services when and where the need arises. Health plans should provide payment when a consumer presents to an emergency department with acute symptoms of sufficient severity—including severe pain—such that a "prudent layperson" could reasonably expect the absence of medical attention to result in placing that consumer's health in serious jeopardy, serious impairment to bodily function, or serious dysfunction of any bodily organ or part.
4. *Participation in treatment decisions.* Consumers have the right and the responsibility to fully participate in all decisions related to their health care. Consumers who are unable to fully participate in treatment decisions have the right to be represented by parents, guardians, family members, or other conservators.
5. *Respect and nondiscrimination.* Consumers have the right to considerate, respectful care from all members of the health care system at all times and under all circumstances. An environment of mutual respect is essential to maintain a quality health care system. Consumers must not be discriminated against in the delivery of health care services consistent with the benefits covered in their policy or as required by law based on race, ethnicity, national origin, religion, gender, age, mental or physical disability, sexual orientation, genetic information, or source of payment. Consumers who are eligible for coverage under the terms and conditions of a health plan or program or as required by law must not be discriminated against in the marketing and enrollment practices based on the preceding discrimination factors.
6. *Confidentiality of health information.* Consumers have the right to communicate with health care providers in confidence and to have the confidentiality of their individually identifiable health care information protected. Consumers also have the right to review and copy their own medical records and request amendments to their records.
7. *Complaints and appeals.* All consumers have the right to a fair and efficient process for resolving differences with their health plans, health care providers, and the institutions that serve them, including a rigorous system of internal review and an independent system of external review.
8. *Consumer responsibilities.* In a heath care system that protects consumers' rights, it is reasonable to expect and encourage consumers to assume reasonable responsibilities.

Greater individual involvement by consumers in their care increases the likelihood of achieving the best outcomes and helps support a quality improvement, cost-conscious environment. Such responsibilities include taking responsibility for maximizing healthy habits, such as exercising, not smoking, and eating a healthy diet, becoming involved in specific health care decisions, and working collaboratively with health care providers in developing and carrying out agreed-upon treatment plans (Advisory Committee on Consumer Protection, 1997, pp. 1–8).

To date, these recommendations are not fully enforced, though some of the language from this document can be found in the EMTALA act.

The Health Care Financing Administration has also enacted new standards for hospitals that participate in Medicare and Medicaid funding to ensure minimum protection of patients' rights. These standards were published July 2, 1999, and became effective August 2, 1999. The standards include:

1. *Notification of rights.* This section includes informing patients about their rights in advance of furnishing or discontinuing patient care and the establishment of a grievance procedure for prompt resolution of patient grievances.
2. *Exercise of rights in regard to care.* This section allows the patient to participate in the development and implementation of the plan of care, and to make informed decisions about care issues. It also includes the right to formulate advanced directives.
3. *Privacy and safety rights.* Rights under this section include personal privacy, care in a safe setting, and freedom from all forms of abuse or harassment.
4. *Confidentiality of records.* This section includes the right to access the medical record.
5. *Freedom from restraints that are not clinically necessary.* Restraints are both chemical and physical, and the restraint can be used only if needed to improve the patient's well-being and less restrictive interventions have been determined to be ineffective. Restrain orders may not be written as a standing or "PRN" order.
6. *Freedom from seclusion and restraints used in behavior management unless clinically necessary.* This section allows the patient to be free from restraints imposed as a means of coercion, discipline, convenience, or retaliation by staff members. Hospitals must report to HCFA any death that occurs while a patient is restrained or in seclusion, or where it is reasonable to assume that a patient's death is the result of restraint or seclusion (*Federal Register,* 1999, pp. 36069–36089).

Congress continues to work on legislation that would more fully address patients' rights to information about health care providers, staff-to-patient ratios, staffing mix, and other factors that would potentially influence the consumers choice of health care plans and health care providers. Although some states have already passed such legislation, there is currently no federal legislation that gives these rights to all persons in the United States.

■ EXERCISE 17–3

Draft a patients' bill of rights that would address all the issues you feel are ethically important in today's health care environment. If your state already has such a law, read it carefully for its completeness. What more should the bill contain? Review the voting records of major legislators in your state. Would they support such a bill? What would you need to do to assure the bill's passage? Is it ethical not to support such a bill, one primarily designed to afford rights to all patients?

SUMMARY

Issues surrounding managed care will continue to evolve well into the next millennium. Many of those issues will continue to address the three basic needs that may be found in today's health care delivery system: access to health care for all Americans; cost containment and prevention of wastes; and quality, competent provision of care. As the health care delivery system changes, new laws and court challenges to those laws are inevitable, for cutting costs frequently prevents the provision of competent health care to all individuals. The challenge for the future will be how to more effectively manage the issues that are addressed today as well as how to more effectively utilize the health care providers who will be more technically knowledgeable and more technologically competent.

AFTER COMPLETING THIS CHAPTER, YOU SHOULD BE ABLE TO

- Define managed care, including health maintenance organizations, preferred provider organizations, and point-of-service plans
- Distinguish the four models of health maintenance organizations, including:
  Staff model
  Independent practice association model
  Group model
  Network model
- Describe the accreditation of HMOs.
- Discuss the Employment Retirement Income Security Act and its application in managed care settings.
- Describe gag rules and end-of-year profit sharing as means of cost-containment measures in HMOs.
- Discuss the Emergency Medical Treatment and Labor Act and its application in managed care.
- Define antitrust laws and their importance to registered nurses in all practice settings.
- Describe advancement of patient rights in the 1990s.

APPLY YOUR LEGAL KNOWLEDGE

- Why is accreditation an important concept for HMOs? How does accreditation protect consumers?

- How do antitrust laws further practice opportunities for advanced practice nurses? For staff nurses?
- How do you think patient rights will continue to expand in the next century?

YOU BE THE JUDGE

On Monday, May 2, 1991, the hospital admitted Justin Casey, age 3, to the emergency center at 6:30 P.M. with a temperature of 106.5°F. Dr. Hubbird, Justin's pediatrician, then examined the boy. He ordered laboratory tests to be performed and chest x-rays to be taken. These were done promptly as ordered by hospital personnel. By 8:30 P.M., Justin's temperature was 103.2°F.

Dr. Hubbird consulted with Dr. Steven O'Grady, a pediatric intern at the hospital. Dr. Hubbird then concluded that Justin was constipated and recommended that he be taken home. On May 3, 1991, at approximately 4:45 A.M., Justin started convulsing and stopped breathing. An ambulance took Justin to the hospital, where he died at 6:15 A.M. The cause of his death was determined to be meningococcemia.

The parents sued the hospital, alleging that the admitting nurse had violated the EMTALA. The suit alleged that the hospital had not provided an appropriate medical screening as required by the EMTALA, because the admitting nurse had not taken the patient's complete vital signs. The parents' expert witness claimed it is negligence for an emergency center nurse not to include the patient's blood pressure as part of taking vital signs.

The hospital countered this allegation by showing that it had a standard written policy for how the triage nurse was to assess patients in the emergency center. The hospital's policy was that vital signs should be taken on all urgent patients at the time of triage by the nurse, while nonurgent patients could be asked to wait in the lobby until the nurse became available to take vital signs. It was not the hospital's actual practice for its policy regarding vital signs to be interpreted by emergency center nurses to require blood pressures be taken on all pediatric patients at the time of initial triage in the emergency center. The hospital offered the affidavit of its trauma services coordinator regarding its policies and practices.

The trial court found on behalf of the hospital and nurse, and the parents appealed.

Legal Questions

1. Was the blood pressure of this 3-year-old child a material part of the assessment by the nurse?
2. Did her failure to take the child's blood pressure cause the nurse to violate the EMTALA?
3. Did her failure to take the child's blood pressure cause the hospital to have violated the EMTALA?
4. How would you decide this case?

REFERENCES

Advisory Committee on Consumer Protection and Quality in the Health Care Industry (1997). *Consumer Bill of Rights and Responsibilities: Report to the President of the United States.* Washington, DC: U.S. Government Printing Company.

American Nurses Association (1998). *Principles for Managed Care: Nursing's Blueprint for Action.* Washington, DC: Author.

Barris v. County of Los Angeles, 972 P.2d 966 (California, 1999).

Brodersen v. Sioux Valley Memorial Hospital, 902 F. Supp. 931 (N.D. Iowa, 1995).

Cherukuri v. Shalala, Secretary of the Department of Health and Human Services, 175 F.3d 446 (6th Cir., 1999).

"C. M." v. Tomball Regional Hospital, 961 S.W.2d 236 (Tex. App., 1997).

Dame, L. (1998). The Emergency Medical Treatment and Labor Act: The anomalous right to health care. *Health Matrix, Journal of Law-Medicine* 8(1), 3.

Eberhardt v. City of Los Angeles, 62 F.3d 1253 (9th Cir., 1995).

Emergency Medical Treatment and Labor Act (1986). 42 U.S.C. Section 1359dd.

Federal Register (December 7, 1998). Emergency Medical Services: New HCFA advisory bulletin will strike down prior approval by health maintenance organizations, pp. 67486–67489.

Federal Register (July 2, 1999). Patients' rights: Major new conditions of participation for Medicare and Medicaid, pp. 36069–36089.

Fischer v. New York Health and Hospitals Corporation, 989 F. Supp. 444 (E.D.N.Y., 1998).

Fox v. Health Net, No. 216992 (Riverside County Superior Court, 1994).

Furrow, B., et. al. (1997). *Health law: Cases, Materials, and Problems,* 3rd ed. St. Paul, MN: West Publishing Company.

Gabel, J. (1997). Ten ways HMOs have changed during the 1990s. *Health Affairs* 16(3), 134–145.

Garcia v. Randle-Eastern Ambulance Service, Inc. et al., 710 So.2d 74 (Fla. App., 1998).

Goldfarb v. Virginia State Bar, 421 U.S. 773, 95 S. Ct. 2004, 44 L. Ed.2d 572 (1975).

Grand Forks Herald (October 4, 1999). 44.3 million lack insurance. 121(97), 1A.

Hand v. Tavera, No. 04-92-00618CV (4th Cir., September 22, 1993).

Johnson v. University of Chicago, 982 F.2d 230 (7th Cir., 1990).

Lopez-Soto v. Hawayek, 988 F. Supp. 41 (D. Puerto Rico, 1997); reversed 175 F.3d 170 (1st Cir., 1999).

Marshall v. East Carroll Parish Hospital Service District, 134 F.3d 319 (5th Cir., 1998).

McEvoy v. Group Health Cooperative of Eau Claire, 570 N.W.2d 397 (Wisconsin, 1997).

Moreno v. Health Partners Health Plan, 4 F. Supp.2d 888 (D. Ariz., 1998).

Morrison v. Colorado Permanente Medical Group, 983 F. Supp. 937 (D. Colo., 1997).

Mundinger, M. (1994). Health care reform: Will nursing respond? *Nursing and Health Care* 15(1), 28–33.

Rios v. Baptist Memorial Hospital System, 935 S.W.2d 799 (Tex. App., 1996).

Roberts v. Galen of Virginia, Inc., 119 S. Ct. 685, 142 L. Ed. 648 (1999).

Shannon v. McNulty, 718 A.2d 828 (Pa. Super., 1998).

Torres Nieves v. Hospital Metropolitano, 998 F. Supp. 127 (D. Puerto Rico, 1998).

Trivette, v. North Carolina Baptist Hospital, 507 S.E.2d 48 (N.C. App., 1998).

eighteen

Nursing in Community Health Settings

■ PREVIEW

As nursing moves from a more traditional acute care setting, a variety of new and innovative opportunities are opening for professional nursing in a variety of community health settings, including public health nursing, school health nursing, occupational nursing, long-term care nursing, and home health care nursing. All of these opportunities offer new and exciting, more autonomous roles for nursing, and all have some potential liability for the nurses practicing in the roles. This chapter presents potential legal liability for nurses in community settings.

■ KEY CONCEPTS

Social Security Act of 1935	abandonment	occupational health
Public Health Service Act of 1944	refusal of care	school health
community health nurses	agency policy	
home health care	long-term health care	

OVERVIEW OF COMMUNITY HEALTH NURSING

The primary purpose of community health nursing is to promote and maintain the health of aggregates (Miller, 1990). Everything that is done to promote and maintain this health has a basis in law and is subject to legal sanctions of one type or another. Perhaps the best starting point for understanding these legal concepts in community health nursing is to know and understand federal and state laws affecting the implementation of community health nursing.

FEDERAL STATUTES

Few pieces of legislation have affected the health and welfare systems of the United States as have the Social Security Act of 1935 and the Public Health Service Act of 1994, with their respective amendments.

Social Security Act of 1935

The Social Security Act of 1935 was signed into legislation by President Franklin D. Roosevelt, as a result of the Great Depression of 1929. The act was based on European health and welfare practices, and many of its roots can be traced back to early European poor laws.

The *Social Security Act of 1935* provided for the general welfare by establishing a system of federal old-age benefits and by enabling states to make provisions for aged persons, blind persons, dependent and crippled children, maternal and child welfare, public health, and administration of state unemployment compensation laws. Programs were both *contributory*, financed through taxation and individual contributions, and *assistance* or *noncontributory*, financed only through taxation. Historically, contributory programs have offered more comprehensive benefits than assistive programs.

The act has been amended numerous times since its enactment, with the addition of Medicare and Medicaid in 1965 being the most important health programs. The act affects the services that nursing provides to its clients. Through Medicare-reimbursable services, regulations specify which clients nurses see, what type of care is provided, how the care is provided, and how long the care is provided. Medicare benefits have changed greatly since their enactment; alcohol detoxification facility benefits were added in 1980, hospice reimbursements were added in 1983, and a 1990 amendment has allowed Medicare Part B premiums to be paid for eligible beneficiaries.

Nurses must recognize their own personal values and attitudes in relation to the programs under the act and realize that these attitudes and values may cause conflict for them. For example, if the nurse believes that single mothers should not receive monetary support from the government, the nurse may have difficulty working with mothers receiving Aid to Families with Dependent Children (AFDC) assistance or even letting clients know that they are eligible for the services.

Public Health Service Act of 1944

The *Public Health Service Act of 1944* consolidated all existing public health legislation under one law and became the major piece of health legislation for the country. This piece of legislation, through the original act and its amendments, provides a variety of resources and services, including the National Institutes of Health; nursing training acts; traineeships for graduate students in public health; health services for migratory workers; family planning services; health research facilities; and programs and services for the prevention and control of heart disease, cancer, stroke, kidney disease, sudden infant death syndrome, sickle cell anemia, and diabetes. These services are administered by a number of federal and state agencies.

Implications of this broad and comprehensive act are extensive with regard to nursing. The act provides funding for services to at-risk aggregates in the community, such as migratory workers, persons with acquired immune deficiency syndrome (AIDS), tuberculosis, and other communicable diseases, as well as programs for persons with chronic problems, such as heart disease, stroke, kidney disease, and diabetes. This act financially covers at least some aspect of nursing in all acute care, home health care, and institutional settings. It provides funding for nursing education and funding for all levels of disease prevention: primary, secondary, and tertiary.

The amendments to this act have brought about numerous changes over the years since the act's enactment. There are now block grants to states, allowing the individual states to decide which programs are most needed in their territories, and monies remain available for specific programs such as immunizations, family planning, and venereal disease programs. Table 18–1 depicts some of the more important aspects of these two acts.

TABLE 18–1. FEDERALLY LEGISLATED PUBLIC HEALTH LAWS

Title	Purpose of Act
SOCIAL SECURITY ACT AND AMENDMENTS	
Social Security Act of 1935, Titles I–XI	Enabled each state to furnish financial assistance to the aged, needy individuals; additional titles allowed for payments to persons over 65, aid to dependent children, and maternal and child welfare
Old Age and Survivors Amendments of 1939	Provided for payment of insurance benefits to qualifying survivors of workers
Maternal and Child Health and Retardation Act of 1963	Amended the act to assist states and communities in preventing and combating retardation
Social Security Amendments of 1965, Title XIX (Medicaid)	Provided funding to states to establish medical assistance for the needy as defined under the act
Social Security Amendments of 1965, Title XVIII (Medicare)	Established hospital and medical insurance benefits for persons over 65 who are residents of the United States.
Social Security Amendments of 1977 (Health Clinic Services)	Authorizes reimbursement for clinic services in rural areas designated as "health manpower shortage areas"
Tax Equity and Fiscal Responsibility Act of 1982 (DRGs)	Set forth a system of prospective payment for Medicare Services called Diagnostic Related Groups
Child Support Enforcement Acts of 1984	Amended the act to allow mandatory income withholding and other improvements in child support enforcement programs
Family Support Act of 1988	Reformed the system to emphasize work and child support; established child support programs, job opportunities, and basic skills and training programs
Medicare Catastrophic Coverage Act of 1988	Amended act to protect Medicare recipients from from catastrophic health care expenditures
PUBLIC HEALTH SERVICES ACT AND AMENDMENTS	
Public Health Services Act of 1944	Created federally coordinated department to address the public health need of the nation; established the office of the Surgeon General, National Institutes of Health, Bureau of Medical Services, and Bureau of State Services
Special Health Revenue Sharing Act of 1975	Amended the act to revise and extend the health sharing program, providing comprehensive public health services
Omnibus Budget Reconciliation Act of 1981	Consolidated federal assistance to states for social services into a single grant to increase the states' flexibility in using grants to achieve the goals of preventing, reducing, or eliminating dependency; created block grants for social services
Omnibus Budget Reconciliation Act of 1986	Created screens for client eligibility, required signatures to be witnessed after explaining client rights and legal contracts for service, incorporated extensive list of consumer rights for participation of home health agencies in the Medicare program

Source: Data from the *U.S. Code, Congressional and Administrative News* (1935, 1939, 1944, 1963, 1965, 1975, 1977, 1981, 1986, 1987). St. Paul, MN: West Publishing Company.

LEGAL RESPONSIBILITIES OF COMMUNITY HEALTH NURSES

Serving in a variety of settings, *community health nurses* care for persons in need of their services in the clinic (public health nurses), school (school health nurses), home (home health nurses), nursing home (long-term care nurses), and workplace (occupational health nurses). Many of the legal responsibilities of these nurses are slightly different, depending on the setting. For ease of understanding, these various nurses working in the community will be discussed separately.

HOME HEALTH CARE NURSES

Home health care nursing emerged as a key component of health care delivery in the 1990s. These nurses provide care that ranges from assistance with daily living to complex, highly technical nursing skills. And the care is provided in the client's home—a setting where the nurse has little control but many potential risks.

Federal Legislation

Federal legislation sets requirements for all home health care nurses. The 1987 provisions to the Omnibus Budget Reconciliation Act of 1986 substantially changed the federal law relating to participation of home health care agencies in the Medicare program. Clients must be screened for eligibility, and the signatures of clients must be witnessed after client rights and legal contracts for service have been explained to them. Important provisions of the statute include an extensive listing of consumer rights, for example, the right to be fully informed in advance about the care and treatment to be provided by the agency, to be fully informed in advance of any changes in the care or treatment to be provided by the agency that may affect the individual's well-being, and to participate in planning care and treatment or changes in care or treatment. The act also enumerates the right of individuals to confidentiality of clinical records, the right to have one's property treated with respect, and the establishment of a grievance hotline to be established by each state. A separate provision under this act sets strict criteria of qualifications for home health care aides who have a predominant role in direct, hands-on contact with clients. Under this provision, the agency may not use any individual who is not a licensed health care professional, unless the individual has successfully completed a training and competency evaluation program that meets minimum federal standards and the individual is actually competent to provide the services assigned.

In 1987, amendments were also made to the Older Americans Act (Public Law 100-175), which directly affects home health care agencies. These amendments were aimed at developing demonstration projects to strengthen home care consumer protection mechanisms, such as rights of the developmentally disabled person. Since these demonstration projects have been successful, regulations concerning home health care consumer protection and corresponding provider obligations are being developed.

Other federal legislation affecting home health care delivery of services is the Patient Self-Determination Act of 1991. Under this regulation, agencies that receive federal funds (including home health agencies) must inquire whether patients being admitted to their services have executed a living will and/or special directive such as a durable power of attorney for health care. If the patient has such a document, then the agency is obligated to abide by its provisions. If there is no such directive and the patient so desires to complete a directive, the agency must provide guidance on completing such directives.

Newer legislation was enacted in 1998, which became effective February 24, 1999, regarding home health care agencies that participate in the Medicare program. Specifically, this final rule requires that each patient receive from the home health agency a patient-specific, comprehensive assessment that identifies the patient's need for home health and meets the patient's medical, nursing, rehabilitative, social, and discharge planning needs. In addition, the final rule requires that as part of the comprehensive assessment, home health agencies use a standard core assessment data set, the Outcome and Assessment Information Set (OASIS) when evaluating adult, nonmaternity patients (*Federal Register,* 1999). These changes are an integral part of the Administration's efforts to achieve broad-based quality improvements through federal programs and in the measurement of that care.

The data required to be collected on the OASIS include:

1. Clinical record items.
2. Demographics and patient history.
3. Living arrangements.
4. Supportive assistance.
5. Sensory status.
6. Integumentary status.
7. Activities of daily living.
8. Medications.
9. Equipment management.
10. Emergent care.
11. Data items collected at inpatient facility admission or discharge only (Section 484.55).

Under the new standards, the home health agency must continue to comply with physicians' orders. Verbal orders are put into written form, signed, and dated with the receipt of the registered nurse or qualified therapist responsible for furnishing or supervising the ordered services. Verbal orders are accepted only by personnel authorized to do so by applicable state and federal laws and regulations as well as by the home health agency's internal policies (Section 484.18).

The initial assessment visit must be conducted by a registered nurse to determine the immediate care and support needs of the patient and to determine eligibility for Medicare home health benefits, including homebound status, if the patient qualifies for Medicare. The initial assessment visit must be within 48 hours of referral, within 48 hours of the patient's return home, or on the physician-ordered start-of-care date. If the only ordered service is rehabilitative therapy service (speech/language pathology, physical therapy, or occupational therapy), the initial assessment service may be performed by the appropriate skilled rehabilitation professional (Section 484.55).

The comprehensive assessment must be completed within five days after the start of care. The comprehensive assessment must include a review of all medications the patient is currently using in order to identify any potential adverse effects and drug reactions, including ineffective drug therapy, significant side effects, significant drug interactions, duplicate drug therapy, and noncompliance with drug therapy (Section 484.55).

The comprehensive assessment must be updated and revised as frequently as the patient's condition warrants due to a major decline or improvement of the patient's health status, but not less frequently than:

1. Every second calendar month beginning with the start-of-care date.
2. Within 48 hours of a patient's return to home from a hospital admission of 24 hours or more for any reason other than diagnostic tests.
3. At discharge (Section 484.55).

A second part of the final rule, also becoming effective February 24, 1999, requires electronic reporting of data from the OASIS as a condition of particiaption for home health agencies. Specifically, this rule provides guidelines for the electronic transmission of the OASIS data set as well as responsibilities of the state agency or Health Care Financing Administration (HCFA) OASIS contractor in collecting and transmitting this information to HCFA. The final rules set forth mandates concerning the privacy of patient-identifiable information generated by the OASIS (Sections 484.11 and 484.20).

State Legislation

State laws encompass a variety of issues that may arise within home health care settings. The home health care nurse is advised to explore individual state law in such areas as protection of uninsured persons, abused persons, or homeless persons; rights of renters or tenants; and laws that protect individuals from eviction under certain circumstances. All caregivers should be aware of the state abuse laws, knowing how and when to report suspected abuse. (Elder abuse is covered in more detail under the long-term care section of this chapter.) Family law issues, such as the right to decide for another, rights of guardians, and consent to perform procedures on minors or incompetent persons also vary from state to state.

One of the most important state legislative acts is the state nurse practice act. Home health nurses must practice within the scope of their nurse practice act, including all relevant administrative rules and statutes, particularly with respect to standards of practice. Standards of practice or standards of care refer to both state and national standards concerning the minimum degree of care that is to be delivered to the client. Standards of care are established through the nurse practice act, relevant current literature, professional organizations, and agency policy and procedure manuals. Home health care nurses are responsible for ensuring that the client receives quality and competent nursing care.

■ EXERCISE 18–1

You are a community health care nurse and have been assigned to assess a family of six about their potential health care needs. The 42-year-old mother is unemployed and caring for a 2-month-old child, a 5 year old, and an 8 year old. The 8 year old attends an elementary school about six blocks away. There is also a maternal grandmother with insulin-dependent diabetes and congestive heart failure who is unable to be employed outside the home and a 20-year-old daughter who works at a commercial cafeteria. The mother receives AFDC, and she would like to start a home day-care center for additional income. The 20-year-old daughter has been diagnosed with salmonella by stool culture.

What state and federal laws provide guidance for the health care worker in assessing this family group? Where would you find out about applicable laws? Speak with a public health nurse about applicable laws once you have decided which laws fit this case scenario. Were you surprised at the number of laws applicable to this one family group?

Standing Orders

Because of the relative isolation of home health care, nurses should have written standing orders in case of emergencies or unexpected needs of clients. Such standing orders complement verbal orders, and both types of orders should be clarified when used by the home health care nurse. Standing orders should be reviewed and updated on a regular basis and must be signed by the attending physician(s) before being implemented. Some agencies prefer protocols that are jointly written by nursing and medicine. Both standing orders and protocols must be specific about their implementation and approval by agency physicians.

If verbal orders are used, the home health care nurse should document the order, and have the physician cosign the order as soon as practical. If a patient was injured when the nurse relied on a verbal order and no written documentation of the order is evident, the nurse may have difficulty in demonstrating that the physician's written order was accurately followed. The agency should develop a plan by which verbal orders are to be cosigned, such as a system to mail the order to the physician and have the physician mail the signed order back to the agency for inclusion in the client record.

Contract Law

Home health nurses must honor contracts made with clients. Contracts include both the written and oral agreements of understanding made between the agency and the receiver of health care services. Contracts made with clients include the advertised services that are included in agency brochures and advertisements, as well as formal contracts signed by clients and agency staff. Provisions that should be included in all contracts include:

1. Provider's and client's respective roles and responsibilities.
2. Length, type, frequency, and limitations of services.
3. Cost and payment schedules.
4. Provisions for informed client or surrogate consent for specific interventions on both an initial and a continuing basis.

Be careful of promises that one may not be able to meet, such as a provision in a brochure ensuring that clients will be evaluated within 12 hours of contacting the agency.

All of the agency's legal duties to the client stem from the legal relationship formed between the two parties. Thus, the referral as well as initial evaluation periods are crucial. Medicare and Joint Commission for Accreditation of Healthcare Organizations (JCAHO) standards require that a home care agency accept clients based on a reasonable expectation that the patient's medical, nursing, and social needs can be adequately met by the agency in the client's residence. New referrals must be carefully evaluated, from a referring physician aspect as well as a nursing aspect to ensure that:

1. The client is medically stable or that a medically unstable condition, as with the dying client, can be managed.
2. There is a desire for home care.
3. The needs of the client can be safely and effectively met by the home care agency.
4. Satisfactory financial arrangements can be made.

Any deficiencies or inability to provide adequate care should be discussed with both the physician and potential client before entering a contract. Client education and informed consent issues as well as client options and other available resources and services should be discussed and agreed upon before entering the contract.

At the initiation of the contract, clients should be instructed about the availability of 24-hour staffing, how to contact staff at other than routine office hours, and reasons when such 24-hour staff may be needed. Agencies are advised to have written guidelines on the appropriate use of 24-hour staffing and financial responsibilities of the client if such 24-hour staffing is used.

Clients may be transferred or their care terminated by the agency after a formal contract is entered. Before transferring the care of the client, a discussion about the advantages as well as disadvantages should be conducted between the client and agency. Issues such as adverse physical and mental reactions to the transfer must be considered as well as better or more acceptable levels of care by the transferring agency.

Care must be taken to avoid *abandonment* of the client by unilaterally terminating the professional relationship without affording the client reasonable notice and health care services. Two recent cases illustrate a home health agency's commitment to clients.

In *Winkler v. Interim Services, Inc.* (1999), the lawsuit was filed against the home health agency by several elderly and disabled Medicare beneficiaries who had been receiving home health services. The lawsuit alleged that the clients were essentially "dumped" and abandoned as a result of recent changes to Medicare reimbursement rules. They alleged that the agency's refusal to continue to provide medically necessary home health care services was based on the simple fact that the clients were all heavy service users and thus economically undesirable to the agency.

The court found that these clients were terminated when the new reimbursement rules went into effect, without any evaluation, assessment, or documentation that they no longer needed home health services. A home health agency cannot discriminate against Medicare patients who are heavy users of services and are thus economically less desirable. A federal law, the Rehabilitation Act of 1973, gives handicapped persons the right to sue if they are excluded from participation, denied benefits, or subjected to discrimination with respect to any program that receives assistance from the federal government. A federally funded program that serves the less handicapped, while failing to accommodate more severely handicapped persons, is operating in an illegal discriminatory manner.

The court also noted in its finding that the home health agency had a contract with the patients to provide services. Thus, the court said, the agency had no legal right arbitrarily and unilaterally to suspend its own obligations under the contract simply because it was no longer profitable.

Morris v. North Hawaii Community Hospital (1999) involved a patient who was notified by his home health agency that his services were being terminated. He, too, claimed that his service termination was motivated by financial considerations. Caps per patient

Medicare home health benefits were part of the Balanced Budget Act of 1997. The ostensible reason given to the patient for his discharge was that he was no longer "homebound" and thus not eligible for Medicare home health benefits.

The court noted that an individual is considered to be confined to home if the individual has a condition, due to illness or injury, that restricts the ability of the individual to leave his or her home without the assistance of another individual or the aid of a supportive device, such as crutches, a cane, a wheelchair, or a walker, or if the individual has a condition such that leaving the home is medically contraindicated. Although an individual does not have to be bedridden to be considered confined to his home, the condition of the individual should be such that there exists a normal inability to leave home, that leaving home requires considerable and taxing effort by the individual, and that absences of the individual from home are infrequent or of relatively short duration or are attributable to the need to receive medical treatment.

The court then redefined "homebound," based on the condition and care of this patient. He was a 40-year-old quadriplegic who used a motorized wheelchair as the result of an automobile accident. Though he was occasionally seen out of the home, he still qualified as a "homebound" patient given the following facts:

1. He could not leave his bed or home without the aid of at least one other individual, and it required considerable and taxing effort to transfer him from his bed to the wheelchair.
2. He could not leave his home without the use of a wheelchair. Leaving home required at least one and one-half hours of preparation, even for a visit to his physician.
3. His absences from home were infrequent and of relatively short duration, usually for the purpose of physician visits at the clinic or office.

Remember, though, that a contract is a two-way street and that both parties have roles and responsibilities. Agencies do not have perpetual, ongoing responsibilities to provide services in the absence of compensation, nor do agencies need to continue to provide care if the safety of the agency staff is threatened. To avoid liability for client abandonment or dumping, the agency must develop and implement a satisfactory discharge program. Discharge planning should be started with the initial evaluation of the client, and clients should be involved in the plan throughout their care. Potential clients should be made aware of this discharge program before a formal contract is signed.

Confidentiality

As a general rule, home care workers and the agency must treat as confidential any information that becomes known as a direct result of the agency–client relationship. Persons and agencies violating this rule may be held liable for damages to the client.

There are some exceptions to this general rule. One exception is the sharing of information among the various health care providers who are responsible for the client's care, including professional staff members, home health care aides, occupational or physical therapists, social workers, and the like. It is advisable to obtain the client's written provision for such sharing of information at the time of the initial contract. If no provision was made for this sharing of information, then the client should sign a release form, authorizing such release of information. The release form should include exactly what information is to be released, to whom the information is to be given, and the duration of time for which the release is valid. This latter provision may be time-related or event-related.

Other exceptions include the release of information to third-party payors. This will be done by the client or client surrogate because release of this type of information is required before insurance companies and other third-party payors honor requests for payments. The client may also request information from the record, and the agency should have a written policy concerning the release of records to the client or client surrogate. Although the original record is the property of the agency, a copy may be given to clients for their records.

Refusal of Care

An issue of growing concern is clients' right to refuse treatment. Even if clients have previously consented to treatment, they can later withdraw consent. Verbal withdrawal of consent is adequate and the agency staff should immediately communicate such withdrawal of consent to other members of the health care team and document the refusal or withdrawal of consent in the agency record.

Refusal of care is dependent on informed consent. With informed consent, the client must be given sufficient information on which to base an informed choice. Information needed includes the purpose or expected outcome of the treatment or procedure, risks and complications that accompany the treatment or procedure, who is to perform the treatment or procedure, and alternatives to the treatment or procedure. To refuse treatment, patients need this information as well as the potential and realistic expectations of the refusal or withdrawal of consent. Again, documentation of the refusal and the client education must be documented in agency records.

Agency Policies

Home health nurses have a duty to inform themselves about written *agency policies* and procedures, because deviation from these policies may result in substandard care to the client. If the policies are outdated, communicate this to the agency so that there may be changes and more current policies. Additionally, ensure that the policies do not require the nurse to function outside of the scope of nursing practice. The employer's policies and procedures set the standard of care and will be used to show deviation from that standard if a lawsuit develops.

Malpractice and Negligence

One of the major roles of the nurse is to assess and instruct patients and their families. The nurse must be able to identify significant changes in the patient's condition and decide if further medical intervention or hospitalization is required. If changes occur, the home health care nurse must convey clearly any concern and indication for further treatment. While clients have the right to refuse further interventions, nurses must ensure that they or their family members understand the nature and extent of change in their condition. It may be necessary for home health care nurses to contact their supervisor, other family members, and the physician. Because they are working alone in the home setting, it is vital that nurses carefully assess and communicate concerns quickly and appropriately.

In a case that exemplifies negligent training of employees, a home health care aide left a patient unattended in the shower while she did some other work in the patient's home. The patient, disabled and using a shower chair, was unable to control the temperature of the water and was severely scalded. The aide applied ice to the burned areas and attempted to reach her supervisor, who was unavailable at the time. The aide waited before calling an ambulance, and the patient suffered severe third-degree burns over a large portion of her body that required numerous operations and skin grafts (*Loton v. Massachusetts Paramedical, Inc.,* 1989). This case also exemplifies the need to evaluate and call for assistance immediately when needed.

Much of the current case law in this area concerns the duty to train and supervise in the home setting, particularly of home health care aides and nursing staff members. The *Loton* case showed the need to properly train personnel, particularly when the patient is disabled and placed in a position in which harm is likely to occur. In a later case that shows this same need to train and supervise, a home health care aide lost control of a wheelchair on a hill and the 19-year-old quadriplegic was rendered unconscious (*R.W.H. v. W.C.N.S., Inc.,* 1992).

Both of these cases also show the failure to adequately supervise, an issue that is of extreme importance yet difficult to manage, given the isolated nature of home health care nursing. Nursing personnel should institute a system of periodic visits in the home to identify the efficiency and level of care being delivered by the home health care aide as well as other nursing personnel. Patient satisfaction questionnaires may be another means to pinpoint potential trouble areas so that follow-up visits can be made.

Patient Education

The duty to instruct patients is paramount in the home setting, because patients and family members must rely on these instructions when the nurse is not readily available in the setting. The education of the patient and family should include both preventative and self-care information, and the nurse must ensure that the patient or family member has understood the instructions. Asking for return demonstrations or ensuring that questions are answered appropriately are ways of validating patient understanding. Because references may not be available, nurses should refrain from answering questions or providing information until they are sure that the information is correct. Thus, nurses in these settings must remain current in aspects of information that they will be responsible for teaching.

LONG-TERM CARE NURSING

As managed care continues to affect the size and structure of acute care facilities, more nurses are employed by *long-term health care* facilities, including nursing homes, assisted living centers, extended care facilities, day care facilities for adults, and skilled nursing homes. Many of the employees of these agencies are unlicensed assistive personnel (UAPs) and licensed practical or vocational nurses (LPN/LVNs) working with minimal supervision. Thus, liability issues differ from those of acute care settings and are often similar to those of home health agencies.

GUIDELINES: HOME HEALTH CARE NURSING

1. Know areas of the law that pertain to home health care nursing, including federal and state laws, and adhere to the mandates of those laws. Request the agency to provide a continuing education program to ensure that all nurses in the agency are knowledgeable about laws affecting home health care nursing.
2. Practice within the scope of nursing practice. If in doubt, request that the agency clarify the issue before proceeding with the treatment or procedure in question.
3. Obtain permission (consent) before caring for clients in the home. This means being able to discuss with patients or their families the risks and benefits of the proposed procedure or intervention before initiation of the intervention.
4. Honor the patients' right to refuse care, if that is their wish. If the patient has a living will or other advanced directive, honor that document. The patient in the home has the same rights as hospitalized patients to know about such advanced directives and to implement such directives. If the patient refuses care, make sure that refusal is communicated to all members of the health care team.
5. Respect the patient's privacy rights, including confidentiality in the nurse–patient relationship. Release forms must be used if patient information is to be given to other health care agencies or health care providers.
6. Follow standing orders and protocols, particularly in times of emergencies or changes in the patient's status. Verbal orders may be secured as needed, and then signed by the physician as per agency protocol.
7. Client education is one of the responsibilities of the home health care nurse. Answer questions as much as possible and tell patients that you will find out needed information and get back to them. Remember, you are most likely the patient's sole reference in health matters and it is vital that you give correct information.
8. Follow agency policies and initiate change in policies as needed.
9. Document all pertinent information, patient condition, and information concerning teaching and referrals that you may have made. As with other health care settings, the one way to show and remember what was done is through effective and timely documentation.
10. Delegate wisely, supervise effectively, and train personnel in the delivery of competent patient care and how to respond to emergencies. Much of the case law to date in this area of the law has concerned these three vital concepts, so ensure that all three issues are addressed.

The majority of cases filed against nurses and long-term care facilities involve malpractice issues, and the standards of care differ somewhat from the applicable standards as seen in acute care settings. Though the definition and elements remain constant, the application is unique to the circumstances and settings in which the care is provided (Fiesta, 1991).

Falls and Restraints

Similar to acute care settings, falls are the primary reason that lawsuits are filed against long-term care facilities. In this setting, unlike the acute care setting, falls are more preventable and are thus frequently less able to be defended. For example, in *Parker v. Illinois Masonic Warren Barr Pavilion* (1998), an 83-year-old resident fell twice, once in the bathroom in her room and a second time in the hallway.

The first time she fell she was not wearing nonskid slippers. The second time, her nurse came to the room and told her that she was being moved to another room to resolve conflicts between roommates. The resident thought she was to pack her own belongings. She packed them in plastic bags and slung them over the top of her walker, proceeded into the hallway, and fell.

In this particular nursing home, nurses assess each resident's ambulation status on a daily basis, and note whether a resident is "independent" or what degree of assistance is required for ambulation. This particular resident was documented as requiring "standby" assistance, which was not given, because the nurse who told the patient she was being moved neither knew what was noted regarding the resident's ambulation status nor knew what "standby" assistance meant. The nurse testified that she thought it meant the nurse was to assist the patient as the nurse deemed necessary. She also testified that she thought the resident was "independent" in her ambulation status. The court found that the home was liable for this patient's falls, especially since the staff caring for the patient had no knowledge regarding ambulation status.

Similar findings were held by the court in *Abrahams v. King Street Nursing Home, Inc.* (1997). In that case, the resident's family had filed a lawsuit, alleging a preventable fall. The court found for the defense for the following reasons. There was no meaningful evidence presented showing how the defendant nursing home was negligent in its supervision of the care of the resident. The resident's physician had not ordered restraints during the day, and the nursing home's policy was that residents were not to be restrained without a physician's order. Additionally, there was no evidence presented that the resident's condition warranted the application of restraints.

Contrast the preceding cases with *Bates v. Forum Lifecare, Inc. et al.* (1994). In *Bates,* an 86-year-old woman fell at home and was admitted to an acute care facility for fever and possible reinjury of a previously fractured femur. She was treated, then discharged from the acute care facility and admitted to a long-term care facility.

On admission to the long-term care facility, her physician's orders included restraints as needed during her first two days at the home. On the second day, the physician visited the patient, and both the physician and nurse determined that the patient did not require restraints. Shortly after they left the room, the patient fell and fractured her femur. The resultant lawsuit alleged the patient's history of previous falls, her diagnosis of Alzheimer's disease, her advanced age, and the presence of a urinary tract infection as factors indicating the patient's need to be restrained at all times.

The defense maintained that restraints were not indicated because the patient was not agitated, combative, or a danger to herself, staff, or other patients. They also contended that the presence of factors as alleged by the plaintiffs did not mandate the use of restraints. Additionally, the defense produced evidence regarding the medical sequelae that can result from the use of physical restraints, including the limitations of the resident's activity that could become permanent. The court returned a verdict for the defense.

In long-term care settings, the adverse effects of therapies must be evaluated when the best course of therapy for patients is considered. Restricting a patient's mobility can prevent falls but can also force the elderly to live far more restricted lives than their limitations require (Blakeslee, 1988). In settings in which the use of restraints are seldom used, rates of falls have increased, but the incidence of long-term injuries has not changed.

Since the late 1980s, the federal government has discouraged the use of restraint, both physical and chemical, in the elderly, especially in long-term care facilities (Omnibus

Budget Reconciliation Act of 1986). Long-term care administrators and nursing staff continue to explore means to prevent serious injury due to falls while allowing patients the freedom from limitations that is required for them to remain as physically fit as possible for the greatest amount of time.

Providing Quality Care

Due to the length of time residents remain in long-term care facilities, some types of cases become more prominent. Most lawsuits regarding decubitus ulcers arise in long-term care settings or in home care settings. For example, in *Convalescent Services Inc. v. Schultz* (1996), a 77-year-old resident suffered from end-stage Alzheimer's dementia. The patient was bedridden and incontinent, and his extremities were contracted. On admission to the facility, the nursing staff noted a large, reddened area on his coccyx and buttock, classified as a stage I or stage II pressure ulcer. The ulcer worsened as the skin became broken 11 days after admission to the long-term care facility. After a month, the patient was transferred to an acute care hospital for aggressive treatment of the ulcer, which now extended to the bone. He had several surgical procedures and was hospitalized for three months.

The family alleged that the long-term care facility was negligent in the care of the resident, specifically by the failure to:

1. Turn the patient every two hours.
2. Notify the physician when the ulcer worsened.
3. Follow the physician's orders for daily whirlpool therapy.
4. Ensure adequate nutrition.
5. Provide the appropriate mattress to relieve pressure on the ulcer.

The facility alleged that these were merely deficiencies in documentation. The court noted the rapid deterioration of the resident in upholding the verdict that substandard care had been given this resident. Additionally, he had developed new decubitus ulcers during his stay in the facility.

The court awarded punitive damages to the resident, based on a finding of gross negligence by the nursing home staff and administration. In doing so, the court used the previous definition of gross negligence:

1. The act or omission, viewed objectively from the standpoint of the actor, involved an extreme degree of risk, considering the probability and magnitude of the potential harm to others.
2. The actor had actual, subjective awareness of the risk involved, but nevertheless proceeded in conscious indifference to the rights, safety, or welfare of others (*Convalescent Services Inc. v. Schultz*, 1996, at 736).

The court cited the extreme degree of dependency and vulnerability of this resident in determining the seriousness of the risks. Additionally, the facility continued to violate its own policies and procedures in caring for this resident. The facility also allowed the resident to rapidly deteriorate without informing the family of his status. The court held that these actions offended a public sense of justice and properly warranted the imposition of damages both as punishment and as a deterrent to such practices in an effort to ensure quality care for elderly persons in nursing homes.

Providing quality care includes the responsibility to feed residents who cannot safely feed themselves, the court ruled in *Thrasher v. Houston Northwest Medical Investors d/b/a Vila Northwest Convalescent Center* (1997). In that case, a 79-year-old resident with Alzheimer's dementia could not feed herself. Her family brought suit, alleging that the nursing assistants fed her improperly, causing her to choke and aspirate food into her lungs. Additionally, the family alleged that the facility failed to call emergency medical assistance quickly and to adequately oxygenate the resident while waiting for medical assistance to arrive, namely the 911 emergency team. The resident was ultimately admitted to an acute care hospital, where she died 11 days after the aspiration from complications caused by the aspiration and hypoxia.

The defense was able to show that the patient choked because of her difficulty swallowing and not because of improper feeding techniques. They also showed through documentation that the resident was promptly assessed and treated and that she was oxygenated while awaiting the 911 ambulance. The court found for the defense.

The court may also find against the nursing home, however, as it did in *Beverly Enterprises Inc.-Virginia v. Nichols* (1994). The allegation was that the resident, an elderly Alzheimer's dementia patient, died because employees failed to assist her with feeding. The resident's mental capacity was greatly diminished, and she was restrained and unable to eat unassisted. The resident had difficulty with choking prior to admission to the home, and the administrator and nursing staff had been informed by the family of the resident's need for assistance with feeding. During one visit, a relative of the resident noted that no one assisted the resident with eating, but merely left the tray at her bedside.

The following day, an employee placed the dinner tray by the resident, and a nursing assistant who was feeding the resident in the adjacent bed noted that the resident was having difficulty. The aide ran for assistance and returned with the nurse, but the resident had expired. Testimony from the nurse indicated that the resident did need to be spoon-fed, and that if a tray of food was left at the bedside it would have been a mistake. The medical examiner testified that the autopsy revealed that the resident had died of asphyxia. No expert witness was required because the act of negligence clearly fell within the range of the jury's common knowledge and experience. The jury awarded the family $100,000.

Sometimes, the failure to provide quality care is termed negligence of the elderly by the court. The failure of a designated caregiver to meet the needs of the patient is generally accepted as a form of neglect, which is most often unintentional and may stem from a genuine inability to provide care. An example of such neglect occurred in *Chugh v. Axelrod* (1989). The resident, aged 91, was admitted to the nursing home suffering from strokes, organic brain syndrome, arteriosclerosis, and renal failure. Her physician ordered heat lamp treatments for the patient's decubitus ulcers. Instead of the 60- to 75-watt bulb normally used for heat lamp treatments, the LPN used an infrared lamp with 100 watts for the treatment. She placed the lamp two to three feet from the resident's back and buttocks, and left the resident unattended for about 20 minutes. During the time the LPN was away, the patient rolled onto her back, exposing her upper legs to the lamp at about the distance of one foot.

When the nurse noted the burns, she notified the physician. He made no arrangements to see the resident or to have her examined by another physician. Several hours later, the nursing supervisor reached the physician by phone, and he ordered the resident

transferred to an acute care setting. The acute care setting to which he ordered her transferred had no provisions for treatment of burns. The resident was then transferred to an
acute care setting with a burn unit. The resident died four days later of bilateral bron-
chopneumonia caused by the trauma of the burns.

The court found that the physician was negligent for his failure to examine the patient
when he learned of the burns, for his failure to ensure that the resident promptly received adequate treatment, and for subjecting her to an extra transfer by ambulance. On
appeal, the court found that the physician should have understood the severity of the
burns and, at the very least, have had the patient examined.

Liability issues in long-term care facilities differ from liability issues in acute care settings because of the lack of direct physician contact with residents. The need for nursing
staff to adequately assess changes and potential problems and notify the resident's physician or the medical director of the facility is critical. In *State v. Peoples* (1998), the court
held that negligent actions by a director of a nursing home were not criminal negligence,
but would support a finding of civil negligence. In *Peoples,* aides in the nursing home repeatedly told the director that a certain resident was vomiting. The resident vomited 17
times in a 42-hour interval, and the director was notified at home on the first night he
had problems, then again told throughout the day that he was still vomiting, and was
called the second night at home because of the continued vomiting. She neither notified
the resident's physician nor instructed the aides to notify the resident's physician. Even
though the resident died of heart failure related to a lower gastrointestinal bleed, unrelated to his vomiting, the court held that the nurse would be liable for malpractice in a
civil lawsuit. The previously cited case of *Convalescent Services Inc. v. Schultz* (1996) also
included liability for the failure of the nursing staff to notify the resident's physician of a
change in the resident's pressure ulcers.

Involuntary Discharge

Discharge from the nursing home, similar to discharge from home health agencies, may
be permitted under the law. For example, in *Robbins v. Iowa Department of Inspections*
(1997), a nursing home discharged a patient for violent conduct and verbal abuse of
others, specifically running his wheelchair into other residents and restraining their freedom of movement, and for directing abusive language at both residents and staff members. The facility attempted several times to stop the resident's acting out, to no avail,
and the court held that, with proper notice, the home could discharge this resident. In
fact, the court noted that an extended care facility risks liability for keeping a resident
who poses a threat of harm to other residents.

To discharge a resident involuntarily, written notice must be given to the resident, a responsible party, a state agency, or an ombudsman. The resident has the right to social
work counseling and a written plan of care. Residents can also ask the court to oversee
that their rights are being honored or to negate the whole process if they are not honored.

The Nursing Home Reform Act of 1987 applies to nursing home admission practices,
stating that a nursing home must not require a third party to guarantee payment to a facility as a condition of admission or continued stay in the facility. This Act applies
whether the nursing home accepts Medicare and Medicaid applicants or is a private-pay
extended facility. A family member who voluntarily agrees to cosign as a financially re-

sponsible party is entitled to advance written notice before a nursing home can legally discharge the patient. The court in *Podolsky v. First Healthcare Corporation* (1996) held that it is unfair and a deceptive trade practice to allow a family member to sign as such a third-party guarantor without advising that a cosigner is not required for admission, but only gives the cosigner the right to notice if the resident is to be discharged. A later case (*Guardianship of Skrzyniecki,* 1997) held that a nursing home does have the right to take legal action if a resident's guardian exhausts the resident's assets to pay for nursing home care but then neglects to apply for Medicaid or Medicare benefits for the resident.

End-of-Life Care and Patient Education

Residents who are admitted to long-term care facilities have the same rights as all inpatients under the Right to Self-Determination Act of 1990. In fact, a recent study investigating patients' understanding of the benefits and burdens of cardiopulmonary resuscitation, artificial hydration, and nutrition in the elderly concluded that, in general, the elderly perceive more benefit from these interventions than was previously thought (Coppola et al., 1998). This underscores the need for continued patient education about the resident's right to self-determination as well as the benefits of the variety of therapies and treatments that are available to the elderly. Nurses should continue to teach patients about their options, empowering the patient and family members, so that they remain competent decision makers.

■ EXERCISE 18–2

Julia works in the independent living section of a retirement community. Mrs. Chu is a patient who is terminally ill with cancer but is still able to care for herself and performs her own activities of daily living. Mrs. Chu executed a living will just prior to her admission, and her physician has signed a do-not-resuscitate order in the event of her demise. The retirement community has just enacted a new policy, stating that all residents will be resuscitated in the event of a cardiopulmonary arrest, regardless of the resident's wishes? Should Mrs. Chu suddenly experience a cardiopulmonary arrest, what should Julia do? Whose rights prevail in such a situation?

Elder Abuse

The mistreatment of the elderly has prompted a legislative response to the issue, much as was done with child abuse some years ago. All states now have elder abuse laws, designed to protect the older, vulnerable adult from abuse, neglect, and financial exploitation. Though the laws differ from state to state, they generally define vulnerable adults as persons with a mental or physical condition that significantly impairs their ability to care for themselves. Some states also use a specific age, generally 60, though some states do not specify when the person is chronologically considered an elder adult for purposes of the law.

Although definitions vary, the term *abuse* usually includes physical and psychological abuse. Physical abuse means intentional infliction, or allowing someone else to intentionally inflict bodily injury or pain. Examples of such injury or pain include slapping, kicking, biting, pinching, and burning, as well as sexual abuse. Examples may also include the inappropriate use of medications and physical restraints. Psychological abuse includes verbal harassment, intimidation, denigration, and isolation, as well as repeated threats of abandonment or physical harm.

Neglect is the failure of the caregiver to provide the goods, services, or care necessary to maintain the health and safety of the vulnerable adult. Neglect may be a repeated conduct or a single incident that endangers the elder's physical or psychological well-being.

Financial exploitation occurs when family members, friends, or paid caregivers take financial advantage of the person, cleaning out bank accounts, selling possessions, and taking Social Security checks for their own benefit. Financial exploitation also includes the improper or unauthorized use of funds, property, powers of attorney, and guardianships. Exploitation may also include making elderly persons work against their wishes.

The majority of states mandate the reporting of elder abuse, with the minority of states encouraging the reporting of abuse. The standard for reporting is a reasonable belief that a vulnerable person has been, or is likely to be, abused, neglected, or exploited (Stiegel, 1995). Note that one does not need to be certain that abuse has occurred, but have a legitimate basis for suspecting that abuse has or will occur. Reporting is thus done in "good faith." Most states grant immunity from civil and criminal action for reporting, and some prevent employment retaliation for reporting. Since the procedure for reporting and the agency to whom the report is made varies from state to state, nurses are advised to explore their individual state laws regarding elder abuse.

Court cases that have resulted because of elder abuse are increasing. In *In the Interest of E. Z., Dependent Adult* (1998), the court applauded the nurse who reported a case of elder abuse by her caretaker. E. Z. was 96 years of age, suffering from organic brain syndrome and multiple medical conditions, and was living with her grandson. They both subsisted on her Social Security check. On two occasions, a visiting nurse found the woman alone, helpless, and in serious need of attention. The nurse reported the situation to the human services department, so that an emergency court order could be obtained to take the woman to a hospital and then to a nursing home. A guardian ad litem was appointed by the court to represent the woman's interests. The court ruled that she was a victim of dependent adult abuse by her grandson-caretaker, who had apparently abandoned her.

Elder abuse also occurs in some health care settings. In *Hearns v. District of Columbia Department of Consumer and Regulatory Affairs* (1997), the court noted that, pursuant to federal regulations, a nursing facility must not use verbal, mental, sexual, or physical abuse or use corporal punishment or involuntary seclusion. In this case, the aide did not physically harm the resident but did intimidate the resident, and thus it was proper to register this aide as someone who had abused the resident.

A registered nurse testified that she saw the aide talk roughly to the resident, then shake her finger in the resident's face, and grab the resident by the wrist, dragging the resident from the hallway into the resident's room. The court ruled that physical or verbal intimidation of a nursing home resident is an act of violence, even if no actual physical harm comes to the resident. An act of intimidation is considered willful abuse, even if it is intended for the ostensibly beneficial purpose of controlling a resident's behavior for the resident's own benefit.

In *Mueller v. Saint Joseph Medical Center* (1997), the court said that even though elder abuse may have occurred and the plaintiffs had shown extreme deficiencies in the patient's care, under the wording of the California law, the resultant lawsuit would be for health care malpractice rather than elder abuse from professional caretaker.

Abuse can result in criminal charges being brought against the abusers. In *State v. Easton* (1998), two nonlicensed personnel working in a residential care facility were convicted of the felony offense of the willful creation by a custodian of an emergency situation for an incapacitated adult and the misdemeanor of battery, and sentenced to 2 to 10 years in prison.

Their crimes were committed when they tried to restrain a patient residing in the facility where they were employed. The two defendants refused to take directions from an experienced worker who knew how to take down and safely restrain a combative patient. Instead, they taunted and cursed the resident, tore his clothing, and struck him for two and one-half hours while his agitation escalated, apparently trying to intimidate him into behaving and following the rules.

The defendants created the emergency situation because their actions showed they had the willful intent to abuse this resident. Their convictions and sentences were appropriate, said the court.

Sexual abuse can also occur in long-term care settings. In *Dixon Oaks v. Long* (1996), an elderly resident could not walk or get out of bed on her own. The 79-year-old resident had a medical diagnosis of Alzheimer's dementia. Her daughter discovered a large bruise on her mother's buttocks and inner thigh. She was told by the nurse that her mother had fallen a few days earlier, and this was the possible source of the bruise. Two days later, while changing her mother's clothes, the daughter saw severe bruising and swelling in mother's anal and genital area.

The following day, the daughter was contacted by the nursing home and told that a male resident had been caught fondling her mother's genitals. The same male resident had been found kissing and fondling her on more than one occasion. The male resident admitted having sex with the woman, and was arrested and charged with deviant sexual assault.

OCCUPATIONAL HEALTH NURSING

The expansion of practice in the area of *occupational health* nursing has greatly increased the potential for liability. This area of practice is greatly influenced by a variety of federal and state laws, particularly workers' compensation laws, mandatory reporting laws, and occupational safety and health laws. Because of the unique interplay between workers' compensation laws and the doctrine of respondeat superior, nurses in this setting face a higher risk of personal liability than do nurses in most other settings.

State workers' compensation laws mandate the compensation of employees who are injured while at work in accordance with specific compensation schedules. These same laws make this the injured employee's sole remedy against the employer, and thus deny the employee the legal right to sue the employer for damages even if the employer's negligence was the prime cause of the injury.

In a minority of states, employees injured on the job may sue any person, including coworkers, but not their employer, whose negligence caused the resultant injury. In most states, the immunity extended to the employer is also extended to coworkers of the injured employee. Thus, a nurse employed by a company in these states is protected from civil liability in much the same manner as the employer. However, nurses may work as independent contractors within companies and thus are not protected.

Occupational nurses have responsibilities in a variety of areas, including adequate and rapid assessment of clients, communications with other health care providers who are frequently not at the worksite, delivery of nursing interventions using standing orders and protocols, teaching preventative health and safety needs plus the teaching involved with specific diseases and conditions, development of safety programs within the setting, and verification of employees' ability to work. Thus, the job description of the occupational health nurse is of vital importance.

It is also important for these nurses to have specific guidelines, standing orders, and protocols. These written standards give guidance to nurses and serve to prevent greater liability exposure for them. If they were allowed to work under a "do whatever you think is necessary" standard, such a standard would open the nurses to charges of practicing medicine without a license as well as increased malpractice liability. Remember that nurses retain personal accountability for their actions, as well as potentially making other persons liable.

A case that exemplifies some of the nursing responsibilities of this role is *Therrell v. Fonde* (1986). In that case, an employee suffered a crushing hand injury, which was examined by the occupational health nurse. She examined and wrapped the injured hand and gave him an injection of either Vistaril or Demerol. The patient was then directed to wait in the outer waiting room while transportation was being secured. During the patient's hour wait for transportation to arrive, the company-employed physician arrived, was told of the injury, and refused to see the patient.

Eventually, the patient was seen at the health care facility that the company routinely used for its employees, and surgery was performed, resulting in a partial amputation of two fingers and permanent disuse of the index and little finger of his left hand. The suit was brought for negligence, alleging that the company failed to transport promptly and to adequately diagnose and treat his injury, and that such conduct was willful, outrageous, and wanton.

Occupational health nurses may also have some accountability for the action of non–health care providers who render first aid assistance at the worksite. If occupational health care nurses have the responsibility to teach first aid or to ensure that needed supplies for first aid intervention are available, they may incur potential liability. Additionally, they will have potential liability if nurses note that first aid assistance is not being delivered correctly and fail to do anything about the lack of quality first aid assistance.

■ EXERCISE 19–3

Julio Ortis is an occupational health nurse employed in a state that has not granted immunity for coworkers of an employee injured on the job. Dr. Doe is the plant physician, and there are a number of written protocols and standing orders that guide Julio's practice in the absence of the Dr. Doe. A patient presented to the occupational health clinic, during Dr. Doe's absence, was misdiagnosed and negligently treated by Julio, and as a result of the negligent nursing care, the patient suffered permanent and extensive injuries. Who has potential liability in this instance and why? How would the liability change if Dr. Doe was present at the time of the patient's arrival but was unable to see the patient because of a second worker's injuries? Would the liability change in the latter instance? Why or why not?

What ethical principles has the nurse violated in giving negligent care to Julio? Which principles did she uphold in her care? What ethical advice would you give the nurse?

SCHOOL HEALTH NURSING

School health nurses face much of the same type of increased liability issues as occupational health nurses. In most jurisdictions, the school nurse is subjected to the same potential liabilities as other governmental workers, because of the relationship of the school district (employer) to the state. This exposes the nurse to greater potential legal liability for injuries.

Because they work in a nonmedical environment, school nurses must exercise considerable independent judgment and must be able to recognize and treat or know when to seek immediate assistance. This includes the ability to assess the situation quickly, treat the child if appropriate, or make arrangements for the child to be taken for immediate medical attention.

Many children visit the school health nurse for traumatic injuries, and the nurse must be competent to provide an emergency standard of care. If injuries occur after school hours, and they frequently do in schools with competitive sports teams, the nurse will be functioning outside the scope of her employment. Again, the nurse will be held to the standard of the reasonably prudent nurse in an emergency setting.

One court case that exemplifies this need to follow an emergency standard is *Schlussler v. Independent School District No. 200, et al.*, a 1989 Minnesota case. In that case, a child had come to the nurse's office, suffering from an asthmatic attack. The nurse assessed the situation, gave another child's inhaler to this child, and sent the child back to the classroom. After other children came to the office concerned about this child's breathing pattern, the nurse assessed the child and determined that neither supplemental oxygen nor emergency transportation via an ambulance were needed to transport this child to the physician's office. Within minutes after leaving the school, the child collapsed and died following a brief comatose period.

The court, on hearing evidence from nursing and an asthma expert witness, concluded that school nurses have a higher duty of care than hospital nurses to make an assessment of the need for emergency medical services. Although they are not expected to provide medical treatment, they are expected to determine the need for those services and for immediate, safe transportation to emergency medical care. The nurse's action also fell below the acceptable standard of care when she used another child's inhaler for this child.

Actions that could have been performed in this case include competent assessment skills, performance to a standard of care and laws governing prescription medications, better monitoring of the student, adherence to school policy concerning the notification of parents (particularly in a case in which the child has no prescription medications for asthmatic attacks), and consultation with other school health nurses and health care providers to develop written criteria for such emergency conditions.

A case that could greatly affect school nurses is *Cedar Rapids Community School District v. Garret F.* (1999). In that case, the U.S. Supreme Court considered the care of a disabled child in light of the Individuals with Disabilites Education Act (IDEA) (20 U.S.C. Section 1400[c]). The section specifies that to help "assure all children with disabilities have available to them . . . a free appropriate public education which emphasizes special education and related services designed to meet their unique needs," the IDEA authorizes federal financial assistance to states that agree to provide such children with special education and related services as defined by the law (at 993).

Respondent Garret F. is a wheelchair-bound and ventilator-dependent school child who requires, in part, a responsible individual nearby to attend to his physical needs during the school day. The Community School District refused to accept financial responsibility for the services that Garret required, believing they were not legally obligated to provide continuous one-on-one nursing care. The requested services are supporting services because Garret cannot attend school without them and the requested services are not medical services, but rather those that can be provided by registered nurses educated in the care of ventilator-dependent patients.

The Supreme Court held in this case that the school district was obligated to provide these services for Garret F. during school hours. The related services are those that he needs to be assisted to "meaningfully access public schools" as a disabled child. The holding has great implications for school districts, beyond financial implications. Public school nurses will become responsible either as the direct provider of care or indirectly as the coordinator of care to students with respirators, feeding tubes, and other chronic health needs that require services that are not medical services.

SUMMARY

Nursing in community health settings is both fluid and dynamic. As laws continue to evolve in community health care, nurses are cautioned to remain current on state and federal laws as well as on pertinent court decisions within their geographic areas. Treating the client with respect and competent nursing care allows the nurse to remain free from potential liability and encourages the nurse to communicate with the client and family. Remember, people—not events or bad outcomes—bring lawsuits, and the client who feels that the nurse is a caring, trusting individual is less likely to bring suit even if a bad outcome occurs.

AFTER COMPLETING THIS CHAPTER, YOU SHOULD BE ABLE TO

- Describe the provisions of the Social Security Act of 1935 and the Public Health Service Act of 1944, with their respective amendments, and give examples of how each act has changed community health nursing.
- Describe legal responsibilities of community health nurses, including:
  Home health care nurses.
  Long-term care nurses.
  Occupational health nurses.
  School health nurses.

APPLY YOUR LEGAL KNOWLEDGE

- How have the Social Security Act of 1935 and the Public Health Service Act of 1944, with their respective amendments, changed the health care delivery system in the past 10 years?
- What advice should be given to nurses seeking employment as occupational health nurses or school health nurses about their potential legal liability?
- Why is the standard of care different in long-term care and acute care nursing? How does this difference in care standard affect nurses?

YOU BE THE JUDGE

Olsten Home Health Care provides home health care through a managed care delivery network. These services are provided, in part, through a skilled corps of registered nurses. Mrs. Craig initially failed her home health test as given by the agency, but passed it on her second try and was hired by the agency. Pursuant to her employment contract, the first 90 days were considered probationary. During this time period, the employee's actions are evaluated to ensure that the nurse has the necessary skills and judgment for home care. The employee handbook provides that the employee may be terminated during this probationary period without advance notice.

Prior to this employment, Craig had never worked as a home health nurse. As a home health nurse, Craig was responsible for rendering skilled nursing services to the elderly in their homes, including the proper administration of a protime test for patients taking Coumadin. This procedure included the correcting drawing of the patient's blood and prompt delivery of the blood sample to the appropriate agency for analysis. Any delay in delivering the blood sample in a timely manner could prevent the health care provider from adequately caring for the patient, particularly if the Coumadin dose needs to be altered.

On Friday, July 18, 1997, Craig was paged by a supervisor and instructed to draw a particular patient's blood for a protime test. Craig drew the blood and took the sample to the laboratory, where she normally delivered blood samples for analysis. The laboratory technologist advised Craig that the sample could not be accepted, because the patient was a Medicare patient. Once Craig realized that the blood could not be analyzed at the laboratory, she was forced because of the time interval to discard the sample.

Craig testified that she did not know what to do next. She went home and attempted to contact the patient's physician. She knew only that the physician was named Sharp, but did not know his first name. Since the phone book contained several Dr. Sharps, she ceased her efforts to contact him because she "was not going to call all the Dr. Sharps." She did nothing more about the patient's protime test on Friday.

Craig then testified that she contacted Ms. McKarnin, a mentor assigned by the agency to her, on Saturday morning. According to Craig, McKarnin advised her to wait until Monday morning to contact the physician and let him know that the patient's protime had not been done. McKarnin testified that she had not been contacted by Craig until Monday morning about the issue.

On Monday morning, Craig told her immediate supervisor what had happened, received the full name of the patient's doctor, drew another blood sample and delivered it to the correct laboratory for analysis. None of managers from Olsten Home Health Care confronted her about the issue until she was discharged on August 13, 1997.

On August 6, 1997, Craig was given a verbal order to change the dressing on a different patient. According to the supervisor's instructions, Craig was to put a duoderm patch on the patient's wound. Craig claims that she did as instructed, but that she inadvertently wrote in the nurse's notes that she had used a tagaderm dressing on the patient's wound. While conducting a routine review of nurses' notes, her supervisor found the discrepancy and Craig was terminated by the agency on August 13, 1997.

Craig was told that she was being discharged based on her demonstrated lack of judgment skills and failure to follow instructions. Highlighted were the protime issue in July and the dressing change with tagaderm. Craig filed this lawsuit in early December 1997, alleging that the defendant terminated her based on racial issues (she is an African American and her country of origin is Jamaica).

Legal Questions

1. Was the care Craig gave the patients involved negligent?
2. Did she show, by her actions, that she lacked judgment and skills necessary to perform as a home health care nurse?
3. Could her treatment have been racially motivated, given the facts of this case?
4. How would you decide this case?

REFERENCES

Abrahams v. King Street Nursing Home, Inc., 664 N.Y.S.2d 479 (N.Y. App., 1997).
Bates v. Forum Lifecare, Inc. et al., Maricopa County, No. 92-15969 (Arizona, 1994).
Beverly Enterprises Inc.-Virginia v. Nichols, 441 S.E.2d 1 (Virginia, 1994).
Blakeslee, J. A. (1988). Untie the elderly. *American Journal of Nursing* 88(6), 15.
Cedar Rapids Community School District v. Garret F., 119 S. Ct. 992 (1999).
Chugh v. Axelrod, 542 N.Y.S.2d 437 (New York, 1989).
Convalescent Services Inc. v. Schultz, 921 S.W.2d 731 (Texas, 1996).
Coppola, K., et al. (1998). Perceived benefits and burdens of life-sustaining treatment differences among elderly adults, physicians, and young adults. *Journal of Ethics, Law, and Aging* 4(1), 12–16.
Dixon Oaks v. Long, 929 S.W.2d 226 (Missouri, 1996).
Federal Register (January 25, 1999). Home health: HCFA now requires OASIS, electronic reporting for medicare patients. Sections 484.11, 484.20, 484.18, 484.55, 3747–3785.
Fiesta, J. (1991). Nursing home liability. *Nursing Management* 22(4), 26–30.
Guardianship of Skrzyniecki, 691 N.E.2d 1105 (Ohio App., 1997).
Hearns v. District of Columbia Department of Consumer and Regulatory Affairs, 704 A.2d 1181 (D.C. App., 1997).
In the Interest of E. Z., Dependent Adult, 485 N.W.2d 214 (Iowa, 1998).
Loton v. Massachusetts Paramedical, Inc. (Mass. Sup. Ct., 1987). *National Jury Verdict Review and Analysis* (1989).

Miller, T. W. (1990). Political involvement and community health advocacy. In B. S. Spradley (ed.). *Community Health Nursing: Concepts and Practice.* Boston: Little, Brown and Company.

Morris v. North Hawaii Community Hospital, 37 F. Supp.2d 1181 (D. Hawaii, 1999).

Mueller v. Saint Joseph Medical Center, 68 Cal. Rptr.2d 268 (Cal. App., 1997).

Omnibus Budget Reconciliation Act of 1986.

Parker v. Illinois Masonic Warren Barr Pavilion, 701 N.E.2d 190 (Ill. App., 1998).

Podolsky v. First Healthcare Corporation, 58 Cal. Rptr.2d 89 (Cal. App., 1996).

Public Law, 100-175 (1987).

Robbins v. Iowa Department of Inspections, 567 N.W.2d 653 (Iowa, 1997).

R.W.H. v. W.C.N.S., Inc. (1992). No. 88-CV-18315, *Medical Malpractice Verdicts, Settlements and Experts* 6, 34.

Schlussler v. Independent School District No. 200, et al. Case No. MM89-14V, *Minnesota Case Reports* (Minnesota, 1989).

State v. Easton, 510 S.E.2d 465 (West Virginia, 1998).

State v. Peoples, 962 S.W.2d 921 (Mo. App., 1998).

Stiegel, L. A. (1995). *Recommended Guidelines for State Courts Handling Cases Involving Elder Abuse.* Washington, DC: American Bar Association.

Therrell v. Fonde, 495 So.2d 1046 (Alabama, 1986).

Thrasher v. Houston Northwest Medical Investors d/b/a Vila Northwest Convalescent Center (1997). No. 94-15038, *Medical Malpractice Verdicts, Settlements, and Experts* 13(9), 27.

20 U.S.C. Section 1400(c), and 1401 (a)(17).

Winkler v. Interim Services, Inc., 36 F. Supp.2d 1026 (M.D. Tenn., 1999).

nineteen

Nursing in Academic Settings

◼ PREVIEW

Students, including nursing students, frequently ask questions about their rights to an education, their rights to matriculate and graduate, and their rights in disputes concerning clinical settings or clinical grades. Likewise, faculty have rights, including those in the academic setting, academic freedom, and employment rights. Although there may be some overlap between these two entities, legal issues can be separated. This chapter address issues affecting both students and faculty and gives guidelines for effective communication between students and faculty. Employment issues of faculty, including promotion and tenure, are not addressed because they are outside the scope of this book.

◼ KEY CONCEPTS

nursing students	arbitrary treatment	student liability
admission requirements	safe environment	nursing faculty
disciplinary and/or grievance procedures	confidentiality of records	
	standard of care	

NURSING STUDENTS

The rights of *nursing students* are not as comprehensive as those of faculty. Many of the faculty rights are derived from the employer–employee relationship, a relationship that students do not enjoy. Some of the faculty rights are also derived from their professional and licensure status. Students' rights come through statutes and constitutional law, including the right of due process.

Admission Requirements

Applicants have some rights in applying to schools of higher education. Schools are not allowed to discriminate against potential applicants. Areas that are usually concerned with discrimination include race, gender, age, and national origin. States may add other areas under the general category of discrimination. Since the passage of the Americans with Disabilities Act, schools cannot discriminate against the disabled and must make reasonable accommodations that allow disabled students to attend classes. These reasonable accommodations include constructing or remodeling buildings and rooms within buildings to make them wheelchair accessible, providing readers for blind students, providing specialized communication devices for hearing-impaired students, and allowing alternate means of testing for the vision impaired or for students who have learning disabilities.

Admission requirements should be based on the school's or program's mission statement, and all admission requirements must be reasonable. Schools of nursing usually establish health requirements, immunization requirements, professional liability coverage requirements, and prerequisite course requirements. These prerequisite requirements allow students to more quickly move through the beginning nursing courses and may include courses such as chemistry, anatomy and physiology, sociology, and psychology. Health and immunization requirements are established because the students will be functioning in patient settings during the course of their study. In the past, schools denied admission to the visually impaired, hearing impaired, and other disabled students. Now schools are required to make reasonable accommodations for these students, though they may still deny admission if no accommodations are reasonable. For example, the wheelchair-dependent person may be unable to meet clinical requirements.

Professional liability coverage requirements are frequently mandated by clinical agencies with whom the school has formal contracts for on-site clinical practice. Some schools require that students purchase their own professional liability coverage and that they show evidence of such coverage at the beginning of each semester. Other schools purchase "blanket" coverage for all students and faculty while they are in clinical courses. The clinical contracts also mandate specific immunization information, such as proof that students are free from tuberculosis and have completed the hepatitis B series prior to caring for clients in the clinical agency.

Disciplinary and Grievance Procedures

Schools should have written *disciplinary and/or grievance procedures.* One component of these procedures is a *policy on grievances,* outlining the steps the student may elect to take in grade disputes, probation, or suspension from the program. Generally, the courts see the academic institution as having the expertise in handling and deciding grade disputes, and their issues are whether the student was afforded due process rights, if a public institution, and whether the school adhered to its own policies and procedures.

Courts often hold that the *school catalog* creates a contract with the student. The catalog must state what the grading policy is for the institution and what grades must be achieved to be considered passing. Students must have a copy of the catalog or handbook, and the institution must abide by its stated policy.

One of the leading cases in this area is *The University of Texas Health Science Center at Houston, School of Nursing v. Babb* (1982). In that case, the student entered the program under a catalog that stated that each course must be passed with a D or better. The student was advised before the end of the term that she was failing a course and that she should resign from the program and then request readmission. She followed that advice and was subsequently readmitted the following year. During the time before her readmission, the program changed the catalog to read that courses must be passed with a C or better. The student earned two D's during her first semester after admission and brought this action alleging that the school was unfair in changing its policy and that she should be allowed to continue under the catalog requirements in effect when she first entered the program. The court agreed, holding that there was a contract between the student and the school and that the contractual agreement dated from the time she first entered the program. The court further held that schools have the right to change and amend catalogs, but that these amended catalogs cannot cancel contracts previously existing and that the student need only fulfill the requirements of the initial catalog under which the student was admitted.

Today, students are allowed the freedom to elect to follow the provisions of later published catalogs or to continue to follow the provisions as outlined in the catalog under which they were admitted. Students cannot "pick and choose" provisions, but must follow either the first catalog provisions or elect to follow all provisions in the later published catalog.

A more recent case that illustrates the importance courts place on catalog and handbook language is *Bruner v. Petersen* (1997). In Bruner, the student brought suit against the nursing school, alleging that the school breached the contract with the student when Bruner was required to enroll in a critical thinking course before allowing him to re-enroll in a required nursing course that he had failed. The faculty member believed that the reason the student had failed the course was because of inadequate critical thinking skills, as evidenced by his inability to assess and document data and his inability to incorporate data into a "complete clinical picture." The faculty member also identified critical concerns about Bruner's performance, including concerns for patient safety in the area of medication administration, managing patients' changing status and concerns for independent practice and thought processes. Based on these factors, the chair of the school of nursing required that Bruner enroll and successfully complete a critical thinking course, namely English 120.

Bruner argued that the English course was outside the formal degree plan of required courses for an Associate Degree in Nursing at the University of Alaska, and that the school was arbitrary and capricious in its treatment. The court noted in its opinion that the language of the catalog under which the student has enrolled states "the catalog lists required courses for each major and in order to progress within the Associate of Applied Science, Nursing program, students must earn a satisfactory grade of C or higher or P(ass) in all nursing and health science courses" (*Bruner v. Petersen*, 1997, at 46). The student handbook further states that "for students who are unable to earn an acceptable grade in a nursing course during their initial enrollment . . . conditions for re-enrollment will be reviewed on an individual basis by the Chairperson and/or faculty" (*Bruner v. Petersen*, 1997, at 47).

The court carefully noted that nothing in either the catalog or handbook promises that a student's requirements for graduation will be limited to those classes as listed for the nursing major. Rather, the catalog and handbook note that further academic conditions may be imposed on a student who fails to pass a required course. Thus, the court found that the university did comply fully with the provisions of both the catalog and the handbook in finding that the student could be required to complete an English 120 course before re-enrolling in a required nursing course.

In their finding, the court also noted that faculty are best suited to determine how to help a student to succeed and must have the discretion necessary to maintain the curriculum's integrity. Nothing in the provisions of either the catalog or the handbook departed from acceptable academic standards and norms.

One of the more antagonizing decisions for faculty concerns students' lack of competence or minimal competence in the clinical setting. Because evaluations of clinical students are subjective, faculty may be reluctant to place students on probation or to fail the student in the clinical practicum. Case law upholds the faculty member's expertise in accurately evaluating student abilities.

An Ohio case, *Morin v. Cleveland Metro* (1986), exemplifies the court's reluctance to interfere with faculty members' professional judgment, particularly in matters that relate to clinical evaluations. In that case, a student during her final medical–surgical course was observed by the clinical faculty as providing six separate instances of what the faculty believed to be unsafe nursing practices. The student was given instructions and evaluations with each occurrence, and later dismissed from the program based on the unsafe nursing practices, a poor pattern of performances evidenced by previous probation, and failure to meet the school's curriculum requirements. The student subsequently completed her nursing education at another program.

In the court's final analysis, the justices were reluctant to interfere with the professional's judgment as it pertains to subjective clinical grading. As long as the decision is made with clear deliberation and the student is given an opportunity to be heard and to understand the allegations against him or her, judicial interference in academic decision making is minimal. The court also noted that, with each instance of unsafe practice, the student was counseled and an honest attempt was made to assist the student in her learning. There was no indifference on the part of the faculty, nor was there evidence that the faculty member had anything but the patient's ultimate safety and the student's learning as motivating factors.

A further example of the need to allow students the opportunity to rectify behavior is *Clements v. County of Nassau* (1987). In that case, the student failed a required nursing course because she did not "maintain cleanliness" and was allowed to retake the course, passing with a grade of B. During her final clinical course, she failed to maintain sterile procedure when changing a dressing and was unable to recognize the mistake. The faculty recommended that she be allowed to withdraw from the final clinical course and reapply to the program at a later date. Clements appealed that decision and was allowed to repeat the final clinical course; this time she failed again due to patient safety issues. The school dismissed her from the program.

At trial, the court upheld the school's decision, noting that the school had given the student ample warnings of substandard behavior and had provided ample opportunity for her to rectify her behavior. When the student was unable to change her behavior, the school was justified in dismissing her from the program (*Clements v. County of Nassau,* 1987).

Arbitrary Treatment

The courts look very differently if there is evidence of **arbitrary treatment** of students, which includes the lack of clear criteria in the school catalog concerning grading policies, passing grades, or grievance procedures. Students are to receive course syllabi at the beginning of courses, specifying how the final grade will be determined, content of the course, and student expectations. If students can demonstrate that the course syllabus is not followed, particularly in grading procedures, there may be a discrimination charge by the student against the institution.

To avoid such a happening, faculty are required to prepare course syllabi with care, and to follow the syllabus as written and distributed. Documentation through the keeping of anecdotal notes should be encouraged because such documentation assists the faculty member in giving students concrete examples of when and how they either met the course criteria or failed to meet the criteria.

Legal Representation

A New Jersey court recently addressed the issue of legal representation for students when schools dismiss students from accredited programs. In *Hernandez v. Overlook Hospital* (1997), the court held that the student had no right to legal counsel and that the school was not required to have a court reporter for transcription of an academic proceeding. The court stated that graduate or professional schools were the best judge of student performance and the student's ability to master performance of the required curriculum. The case involved a medical resident who had been dismissed as lacking the professional judgment necessary for a second-year resident, difficulty using professionalism and decorum when dealing with other staff members, and failing to properly diagnose and treat patients.

Safe Environment

The school has a responsibility to ensure a *safe environment* to students, and it is reasonable for students to expect that they will have a certain degree of safety on school property. Schools have a responsibility to alert students of unsafe or potentially dangerous situations and to assist in alleviating such situations. For example, if the school administration knows of unsafe or potential dangers and fails to alert students to those dangers, the school may be held liable. In a 1987 case, there had been attacks on students in the campus dormitory and the school was held liable when a subsequent student was attacked because of failure to alert students to the possibility of such attacks (*District of Columbia v. Doe*, 1987).

Delta Tau Delta v. Johnson (1999) expanded this finding to require that there is a "duty of reasonable care" expected of a fraternity, and that a fraternity has the responsibility to protect guests from assault. In that case, a former student at Indiana University at Bloomington, brought suit against the fraternity house for failing to protect her safety when she was sexually assaulted at the fraternity house after a party held in 1990. The courts acknowledged that in finding for the plaintiff that it was setting a new precedent in this area of the law, but cited special circumstances as the reason for this landmark decision. This particular fraternity house had previous instances of assault in the two years previous to the incident that formed the basis of this lawsuit, and, in the month before this particular incident, the fraternity house was provided information by the university about rape and sexual assault on college campuses. This information placed the fraternity house on notice that such incidents could occur and what should be done to prevent future incidents (*Delta Tau Delta v. Johnson*, 1999).

Confidentiality of Records

Schools are required to maintain *confidentiality of records* with respect to materials received during the admission process and during the course of the student's studies. This includes references that may have been submitted, students' grades earned before and during the course of the program, and clinical evaluations. Students can sue for defamation if faculty inadvertently or inappropriately reveal to third parties confidential information that is false and that is damaging to their reputation or career.

Because of the possibility of sensitive information, medical records of students should be placed apart from their academic files and access to medical records restricted. Such confidentiality of medical records further ensures that information will not be revealed except to a few individuals.

STANDARD OF CARE

The *standard of care* owed by nursing students to patients for whom they care is identical to the standard of care owed the patient by the registered nurse. This applies even though the nursing faculty has assigned the patient to the student, not a member of the clinical facility. The rationale underlying this standard of care is that the patient has the right to expect that professional services supplied by the hospital or health care facility will be provided by persons with the prerequisite degree of professional skill and competence.

LIABILITY FOR NEGLIGENCE BY STUDENTS

Nursing students have the ultimate responsibility for their own actions and may be liable for their own negligence. *Student liability* holds true even if the student is not an adult under state law. The often quoted adage that students practice on their instructor's license is not a true or valid statement because only the individual rewarded the license practices on the license. The individual student always retains accountability, and nurse practice acts allow nursing students to perform professional actions without being awarded a license to practice professional nursing. If it were any other way, nursing students could not be allowed to learn their profession until after graduation and licensure.

The licensure exception places great accountability on the nursing student, since the same competent care that the reasonably prudent nurse would give must be the standard of care of the professional nursing student also. The student as well as the faculty must know hospital policies and procedures and remain current in medical and nursing knowledge. The licensure exception further requires that unprepared nursing students or students who need additional supervision inform the faculty instructor of their special needs or inadequate preparation for clinical practice.

Nursing students remain accountable for their knowledge and skills, and faculty or staff may become accountable for individual student incompetence or unpreparedness. For example, in *Blanding v. Richland Memorial Hospital* (1988), an 18-year-old patient suffered a cardiac arrest and died following a simple skin graft surgery. The nursing student who was caring for him at the time of the arrest had failed to place his head in a position so that he could breathe and also failed to notice that he was not breathing. There was student liability in the case, plus liability to the instructor and nursing staff at the institution.

A more recent case further illustrates the accountability of nursing students. In *Dimora v. Cleveland Clinic Foundation* (1996), an elderly patient was harmed because of the failure of a nursing student to ensure the patient's safety. Mrs. Dimora's chart clearly indicated that she had serious difficulty with balance, making it necessary for her to have assistance when standing or walking with a walker or when transferring. The patient had fallen backward six days prior to the current incident, but was caught and lowered gently to the floor. She was afraid of falling and needed not only physical assistance, but also encouragement to take steps without her walker.

Prior to caring for the patient, the nursing student had read the patient's chart and knew of the patient's weakness and unsteady gait. Nonetheless, the student helped Mrs. Dimora up from the toilet, then walked away and left her standing with the walker in the bathroom, while the student propped the door open and adjusted the patient's wheelchair, expecting the patient to walk to the wheelchair on her own to transfer with assistance. Mrs. Dimora took a step forward, fell backward, and was injured.

Expert witnesses at trial testified that a nursing student at this student's level of education should have been able to safely care for this patient. The student testified that she had received training to assist patients with ambulation and transfer and had successfully passed those skills tests. Finally, the nursing student's preceptor testified that the patient needed someone close to her at a safe distance at all times when ambulating. Thus, liability was assessed in this case against the defendants.

Students are also charged with following hospital policy and procedure. Faculty must ensure that students understand and are aware of hospital policy. If students then exceed their student role and a patient suffers harm because of their actions, they are more likely to incur sole responsibility since no liability will be imputed to the faculty or the hospital staff member.

Hospital liability may be decreased by an existing contract between the clinical institution and the educational institution. Usually, the hospital agrees to accept a predetermined number of clinical nursing students in its various departments, and the educational institution agrees to prescreen the nursing students prior to their clinical assignments. Only nursing students whose academic and clinical records meet the standard of care of the reasonable prudent nursing student will be allowed to practice under close faculty supervision.

Thus, a duty arises for the faculty and educational institution to allow only competent students the right to practice in the clinical setting. A duty also arises for the clinical institution to maintain safe, competent, clinical sites. Both have an equal duty to monitor the other, and both parties may incur liability for allowing substandard conditions or substandard care to persist. *Dustin v. DHCI Home Health Services, Inc.* (1996) illustrates this concept. In *Dustin*, a male student at a commercial vocational school specializing in the training and placement of medical support personnel was placed in the emergency department of an acute care medical center as one of his clinical assignments. According to the record, it was the instructor at the school who made the clinical assignment.

Shortly after arriving on his first clinical day, Dustin was asked to assist with restraining a violent patient. The student was not aware that the patient was human immunodeficiency virus (HIV) positive and had acquired immune deficiency syndrome (AIDS), nor was he aware of standard universal precautions. While the patient was being restrained, his blood and saliva (from the patient's lacerated lip) were "projected into the student's eyes and mouth" (at 358). Shortly after the incident, the student tested positive for HIV, and this suit was filed against both the school and the hospital for damages.

The court upheld the student's right to sue, finding that the student's training in universal bloodborne pathogen precautions and restraint techniques was inadequate and that he should not have been placed in the emergency department as part of his clinical experience nor should he have been involved in restraining the patient. Thus, the court allowed damages against both the school and the hospital for failure to ensure that students are taught basic skills technique, including Occupational Safety and Health Act (OSHA) standards.

Students also have potential liability for course materials that they have mastered and passed successfully. These skills and competencies should be evaluated and documented by faculty as the student completes the skills and competencies. Documentation of competencies can be done by meeting skills objectives, test scores, and evaluation performances, both in the clinical facility and in the skills laboratory. This documentation can then be used to attest to the fact that the faculty delegated appropriately should a subsequent patient injury occur.

Much of the early case law concerning negligence and accountability of nursing students centered on whether the student is an employee of the hospital or of the educational institution. Today, in a collegiate atmosphere in which the nursing student receives no compensation from the clinical institution but rather pays for the right to attend classes, it would seem that the nursing student has more of a relationship with the institution of higher education. This is especially true because the school has a duty to adequately supervise and teach its students, and incurs potential liability for failure to prevent unsafe nursing practices by its students.

■ EXERCISE 19–1

You are a junior nursing student on a busy surgical unit. It is your third clinical day and, while you are well prepared to take care of the patient assigned to you, your clinical experience is limited. The nurse-manager stops you, hands you a posey belt and soft wrist restraints, telling you to go "Restrain that maniac in 502!" You have never cared for a patient who was restrained nor have you ever seen a posey belt in use. How do you handle this situation? Do you restrain the patient? How do you later report the incident to your clinical instructor?

Aside from the legal issues involved, what are ethical principles that guide the care of patients in such instances? Should individuals consider ethical principles when confronted with situations in which physical harm may be involved? Are the ethical issues related to this scenario different for the student as opposed to a staff member who might restrain the patient?

NURSING FACULTY

Several issues concern *nursing faculty,* their employer institutions, and the hospitals or health care settings in which they supervise students. Probably the most important factor

GUIDELINES: NURSING STUDENTS' CLINICAL PERFORMANCE

1. Understand the institution's policies and procedures prior to undertaking any clinical assignment. Prepare adequately for clinical settings, ensuring that you are knowledgeable about the patient's condition, interventions, medications, and treatment.
2. If you are unprepared for the clinical setting, inform the clinical instructor. Never undertake to perform skills or procedures or give medications for which you are unprepared. Remember, the patient's ultimate safety is the first priority.
3. When unsure of a procedure or skill, ask for help before beginning the skill or procedure, even if this delays the intervention. If the instructor is not readily available, allow the staff nurse to complete the intervention. Again, the patient's ultimate safety is the primary goal.
4. Never allow yourself to be bullied into performing skills or procedures with which you are unfamiliar or are not listed by the institution as those that nursing students may perform. Staff members may be hurried and ask you to assist them. That is appropriate so long as you are knowledgeable about the skill and the skill is approved by the institution as one that students can perform. You may want to volunteer to assist in another way, rather than refusing entirely. For example, you might volunteer to give the patient's bath so that the staff member is free to perform other interventions.

to remember is that the individual faculty member is licensed to practice professional nursing within the given jurisdiction and as such owes the same duty of care to the patients or clients that he or she encounters as would any professional nurse.

Since the primary responsibilities of nursing faculty are to teach and supervise students, faculty owe themselves and those they encounter the duty of remaining current in nursing and medical matters such as diagnoses, etiologies, therapies, current treatments, and innovative interventions and of continually reevaluating and reassessing students in the clinical area. Not all faculty will be interesting lecturers or outstanding role models, but all faculty should teach current concepts and be competent practitioners. Many nursing schools are now encouraging nursing faculty to have a *concurrent clinical practice*, as technologies and interventions are continuously being upgraded and updated. A concurrent clinical practice allows the instructor to remain knowledgeable in his or her clinical field.

The faculty's role is critical in the education of nursing students. The individual faculty member determines the nursing students' capabilities and skills and ultimately determines if the patients' needs can be entrusted to a particular nursing student. Thus, faculty must know the given hospital's policies and procedures, teach necessary skills to the students, and evaluate student performance on a continuing basis. Faculty must also be willing to counsel students and/or fail students who fail to meet clinical expectations or who fail to follow safe nursing practices. The patient's safety is the ultimate goal of both faculty and students.

Education must be conducted in an environment that is free from discrimination and bias. A recent finding by the Montana Department of Labor and Industry illustrates this point. Scott Dion, a student in the Montana University College of Technology at Great Falls, filed a complaint with the Montana Department of Labor and Industry alleging discrimination against male students by the female administrator of the school. The student alleged that he failed his final nursing course because of the sexual discrimination shown by Ms. Connie MacKay. She referred to men as "sperm donors," suggesting that was their only genuine use, and often made jokes about male anatomy, one of the milder references being to "the worthless male appendages." She called men "lazy," criticized them for relying on women for support, and said that men should be held accountable for the lower economic status of women.

The Department of Labor and Industry found that such remarks amounted to sexual discrimination and that "the practical nursing program allowed hostile and derogatory comments about men by its director for a period of years. This conduct rose to the level of sexual intimidation. Because of this intimidation, Dion reasonably feared that his instructors might treat him more harshly than they would a female student" (Schneider, 1999, p. 1). Though the department would not make a judgment stating that the student's failure to pass the clinical course was due solely to such harassment, the department did order that the student's failing grades be expunged from his record and that he be allowed to repeat the course, free of charge. Both sides are expected to resolve the matter at the court level (Schneider, 1999).

To foster student–faculty relationships and to keep students current in their performance grades, faculty should meet the following evaluation guidelines:

1. Specify course requirements and expectations at the onset of the course. This is best accomplished by clear and complete course syllabi that are inclusive of attendance requirements, methods of evaluation, penalties for late work, availability of faculty by phone, office hours, and times for individual and group student conferences. Refrain from changing syllabus requirements during the semester because that encourages students who are unsuccessful in the course or who make lower grades in the course to challenge the final grade.

2. Allow students the opportunity to review all evaluation data and reports that will become part of their permanent file. Ensure that evaluations are timely and that students have an opportunity to correct unsatisfactory performance. Forms signed by both the faculty member and the student ensure student review as well as the accountability of the faculty member. Students may wish to add their own account of occurrences and happenings, and they should be encouraged to do so. This further opens communications and shows the desire on the part of the faculty to work with the student.

3. Retain all graded papers, tests, case studies, and care plans. It is advisable to retain such data rather than return the papers to students during the course, though students should be able to see the graded papers. Retained data further support the faculty's assignment of grades, and the papers should be retained for a time period equal to that in which the student may appeal the grade. Allow students adequate time to review the paper data so that they can gain insight into the faculty's grading scale, methods, and areas of mastery versus areas in which they need more study.

4. Conduct regular student–faculty conferences for feedback to the student. At a minimum, there should be a midcourse and a final course evaluation conference, especially for clinical courses. These conferences allow faculty the opportunity to discover areas in which they could concentrate their efforts in assisting students to learn, and give students the opportunity to ask questions and offer explanations in a private setting.

5. Establish and publish as part of the student policies a review of the grading policy and steps in the school's grievance policy. Such policies allow students a formal recourse and prevent a charge of arbitrary treatment from occurring.
6. Maintain anecdotal notes for reference. These allow for specific examples and help to refresh the faculty member's memory should a grade be appealed or a grievance filed. These may also be used to give students examples of how they were effective in the clinical setting and examples showing their need for improvement. Anecdotal notes, because of their content, should be kept in secure, preferably locked, areas.

Academic Versus Disciplinary Dismissal

Given the subjective nature of student performance evaluations, many faculty hesitate to place students on probation or to fail them. When working with students demonstrating no or low competence, faculty may wish to consider the distinction between academic and disciplinary issues.

1. To dismiss a student for *disciplinary reasons,* such as infractions of the school's rules and regulations, students should be accorded due process. Specifically, oral or written notice of the charges against them must be made. If students deny the charges, the faculty must explain the evidence and give students an opportunity to present their side. Even in private schools where the Fourth Amendment due process rights do not attach, it is advisable to afford such rights to the student.
2. If students are to be dismissed for *academic reasons,* such as failure to pass a required course, they must be given the opportunity to present their objections before the academic body responsible for dismissal. The faculty themselves are the best judges of students' academic performance. Courts have been reluctant to override this idea of faculty's professional judgment (*Morin v. Cleveland Metro,* 1986; *Bruner v. Petersen,* 1997; and *Hernandez v. Overlook Hospital,* 1997).

Records that should be required when reviewing disputes between students and faculty include the following, as applicable:

1. School catalog
2. Attendance records
3. Grading appeals procedures and policies and/or grievance policies and procedures
4. Student papers, examinations, and written clinical care plans
5. Student handbooks
6. Clinical or student evaluations
7. Course syllabi
8. Committee minutes

It is of extreme importance for faculty to categorize whether a student dismissal is for academic or disciplinary reasons. If academic dismissal is forthcoming, the faculty may wish to counsel the student, to aid the student in pursuing other academic programs or careers, or to withdraw the student from the course with a passing grade. For disciplinary dismissal, students should still be counseled, placed on probation or informed of grade expectations for the course, and given an opportunity to present their side formally. Students may appeal through the dean of the school as well as through the president of the institution or equivalent. At all stages, written minutes and/or records of the various proceedings should be kept and signed by all concerned parties.

Evaluating noncognitive aspects of student performance is indeed difficult. Clinical competence, interpersonal relationships, and professionalism are vital components of the professional nurse. The grading of these is subjective, and students should be afforded ample safeguards. Such safeguards may be in the form of adequate conferences and unambiguous course requirements. Perhaps the most important factor for faculty to remember is that open communication lines must be maintained. Counsel students as needed when an incident occurs, give frequent evaluation conferences, and be open and constructive with students. A close family member of the student may also want to attend the conference, and faculty should make the ultimate determination to either allow or refuse such a request. Students and their parents or spouse seldom sue a faculty that is perceived as fair, impartial, and accessible. Just as adequate communications may prevent patient lawsuits, those same communications may keep a student from filing suit or may be instrumental in helping faculty prevail if a suit is tried.

Lastly, faculty should carry professional liability insurance coverage in an adequate dollar amount. Since legal action could come from either a dissatisfied student or an in-

 # GUIDELINES: FACULTY–STUDENT ACCOUNTABILITY

1. Delineate course requirements at the onset of the course. Both faculty and students should be clear on the following:
   a. Credit hours
   b. Lecture and clinical schedules
   c. Methods and tools of evaluations
   d. Assignment deadlines and penalties for late submission
   e. Course description and specific requirements
   f. Standards for students as identified in a selected style manual or in a student policy manual
   g. Conference times
2. Conduct frequent, individual student–faculty conferences. Include in each conference:
   a. Written evaluation forms
   b. Opportunity for both sides to clarify particular expectations and instances or happenings
   c. Written identification of any deficiencies
   d. Opportunity for students to respond orally or in writing to evaluator's comments or suggestions
   e. Signed conference sheet that will become part of the student's permanent file
3. Maintain current policies and procedures of the institution, and ensure that students have a mechanism to recommend new policies to faculty.
4. Maintain a permanent file of all student written work, including tests, papers, case studies, and written care plans. Students should be allowed and should take responsibility for reviewing such materials at a time convenient to both instructor and student.
5. Establish a formal grievance policy. Both students and faculty share responsibility for knowing and implementing such policy.
6. Allow sufficient time for open communications. Faculty and students alike benefit from honest and open discussions.

jured party within the clinical setting, faculty are well advised to maintain sufficient coverage, even if covered by the institution.

■ EXERCISE 19–2

The nursing instructor has decided, for the fifth time in the last month, to change the number of written care plans you are expected to do, the due dates for the care plans, and information needed to complete each care plan. How might this issue best be addressed? Can the issue be addressed so that both the students' learning and the faculty member benefit?

SUMMARY

Issues relating to student–faculty interactions can pose difficult questions for everyone concerned. The ultimate goals of such interactions are to ensure that adequately prepared students will be able to care for patients competently and to ensure future nursing professionals.

AFTER COMPLETING THIS CHAPTER, YOU SHOULD BE ABLE TO

- Describe student rights including:
  Admission requirements.
  Disciplinary and grievance procedures.
  Arbitrary treatment.
  Legal representation.
  Safe environment.
  Confidentiality of records.
- Describe the standard of care owed patients by nursing students.
- Describe areas of negligence for which nursing students may be held accountable.
- Describe faculty responsibilities in relationship to nursing students.
- Differentiate between academic and disciplinary issues in relationship to assisting students.

APPLY YOUR LEGAL KNOWLEDGE

- How should faculty react to admissions of clinical unpreparedness?
- What responsibility does a faculty member have when he or she discovers that a student is unprepared to care for a given patient in the clinical setting? To whom is this duty owed?

- What responsibilities do students have for their continual learning?
- Should students volunteer to assist staff nurses in the performance of clinical interventions? Why or why not?

YOU BE THE JUDGE

A third-year nursing student was enrolled in the childbearing course when she took a 7½-hour-old infant from the nursery at Mid-Maine Medical Center to be breast-fed by his mother. The student misread the infant's arm band and gave the newborn to the wrong mother. The error was discovered approximately three to five minutes after the infant was with the other mother, and he was immediately returned to the nursery by one of the staff registered nurses.

The infant's mother did not witness what had transpired and was informed, by the same staff nurse who had returned the infant to the nursery, of the incident about an hour later. No harm could be shown to have occurred, and the infant and his mother were discharged in excellent health on the second day postdelivery.

The mother brought this lawsuit on her behalf and on behalf of her infant son for negligence and negligent infliction of emotional distress. The trial court dismissed the lawsuit as unfounded and the mother appealed.

Legal Questions

1. What is the standard of care owed this new mother by the nursing student?
2. Do the actions of the nursing student constitute malpractice?
3. Can the cause of action "negligent infliction of emotional distress" be upheld?
4. How would you decide this case?

REFERENCES

Blanding v. Richland Memorial Hospital, No. JR 155725 (1988). *Medical Malpractice Verdicts, Settlements and Experts* 4(5), 22.

Bruner v. Petersen, 944 P.2d 43 (Alabama, 1997).

Clements v. County of Nassau, 835 F.2d 1000 (2nd Cir., 1987).

Delta Tau Delta v. Johnson, Cause #45S02-9601-CV-40 (Idaho, 1999).

Dimora v. Cleveland Clinic Foundation, 683 N.E.2d 1175 (Ohio App., 1996).

District of Columbia v. Doe, 524 A.2d 30 (District of Columbia, 1987).

Dustin v. DHCI Home Health Services, Inc., 673 So.2d 356 (La. App., 1996).

Hernandez v. Overlook Hospital, 692 A.2d 271 (New Jersey, 1997).

Morin v. Cleveland Metro, 516 N.E.2d 1257 (Ohio, 1986).

Schneider, A. (July 27, 1999). Administrator who called men "sperm donors" is found to have committed bias. *The Chronicle of Higher Education: Online.*
http://chronicle.com/daily/99/07/99072704n.htm

The University of Texas Health Science Center at Houston, School of Nursing v. Babb, 646 S.W.2d 502 (Texas, 1982).

twenty

Federal Laws: The Americans with Disabilities Act of 1990 and the Civil Rights Act of 1991

■ PREVIEW

The Americans with Disabilities Act (ADA) of 1990 and the Civil Rights Act of 1991 were both signed into legislation during the term of President George Bush. Both of these acts have significant implications for health care delivery. The ADA affects health care providers as well as consumers, with various sections of the act addressing hiring and retention of providers as well as access to health care. The Civil Rights Act of 1991 also affects both health care providers and consumers. This chapter explores both acts, defining purpose, application, expanding case law, and projected future of both.

■ KEY CONCEPTS

Americans with Disabilities Act
  of 1990 (ADA)
disability
reasonable accommodations

essential job functions
undue hardship
Civil Rights Act of 1991
sexual harrassment

quid pro quo sexual harassment
hostile work environment
preferential treatment

THE AMERICANS WITH DISABILITIES ACT OF 1990

Background of the Act

On July 26, 1990, George Bush signed the *Americans with Disabilities Act of 1990 (ADA)* into law, providing comprehensive protection to Americans with disabilities. The ADA is one of the most significant pieces of legislation since the Civil Rights Act of 1964 and was seen by its sponsors as "the Emancipation Act of disabled persons." The Act had been necessitated by the discrimination faced by human immunodeficiency virus/acquired immune deficiency syndrome (HIV/AIDS) individuals, as those persons identified loopholes not adequately addressed by previous laws, both state and federal.

Bills were originally introduced in the 100th Congress, with joint hearings on the bills occurring in September 1988. Although many senators and representatives cosponsored the legislation by the end of that Congressional term, the bills never came out of committee.

Stating that the bill was too vague as originally proposed, the 101st Congress conducted several hearings on the bill. The Senate in September 1989, and the House of Representatives in May 1990, passed the bill by overwhelming margins. A Conference Committee approved the bill on July 13, 1990, and the bill was enacted on July 26, 1990.

In enacting the ADA, Congress was faced with the challenge of combining two legal concepts—disability and equality. The aim was to ensure equality for the disabled, without undue hardships being placed on those regulated by the Act.

Covered Entities

Title I primarily covers employment provisions and is perhaps the best known portion of the ADA. The act defines a "covered entity" as an employer, employment agency, or labor organization or joint labor–management committee. While the act was originally restricted to employers of 25 or more employees, it now applies to all employers who have 15 or more employees. The United States, corporations wholly owed by the United States, Indian tribes, and bona fide tax-exempt private membership clubs are not included in the definition of employer. State governments, governmental agencies, and political subdivisions, though not specifically included in the act, were intended by Congress to be part of the ADA.

While the ADA does not exclude religious organizations, it does authorize them to give preference in employment to their own members and to require that applicants and employees conform to their religious tenets.

Definition of Disability

The ADA defines *disability* broadly. Individuals are covered if: (1) the disability is a physical or mental impairment that substantially limits one or more of the major life enjoyments of the person; (2) there is a record of such impairment; or (3) the individuals are regarded as having such an impairment.

A *physical or mental impairment* includes:

1. Any physiologic disorder or condition, cosmetic disfigurement, or anatomical loss affecting one or more of the following body systems: neurological, musculoskeletal, special sense organ, respiratory (including speech organs), cardiovascular, reproductive, digestive, genitourinary, hemic, lymphatic, skin, and endocrine.
2. Any mental or psychological disorder such as mental retardation, organic brain syndrome, emotional or mental illness, and specific learning disabilities. Conditions that would qualify under this definition include diabetes, cancer, heart diseases, and AIDS, as well as those persons recovering from alcoholism and drug abuse.

The existence of a disability is determined without regard to the availability of alleviating measures such as medicines and prosthetic devices. Thus, the fact that a physical or mental impairment may be successfully treated with a medicine or remedial device does not remove the impairment from the ADA coverage of disabilities.

The ADA does not regard advancing age as an impairment, but illnesses associated with advanced age such as hearing loss, arthritis, and impairment of gait would constitute impairments.

Major life events are defined as those fundamental acvivities that the average person in the general population can perform with little or no difficulty, such as caring for oneself, performing manual tasks, walking, seeing, hearing, speaking, breathing, learning, and working. *Substantially limits* is defined as (1) the inability to perform a major life activity that the average person in the general population can perform, or (2) a significant restriction as to the condition, manner, or duration under which a person can perform a particular major life activity as compared to the condition, manner, or duration under which the average person in the general population can perform that same major life activity.

A *record of impairment* is someone who has a history of, or has been classified as having, a mental or physical impairment that substantially limits one or more of the major life activities. This provision is intended to ensure that the covered entities do not discriminate against individuals because they have a history of a disability or because they have been misclassified as being disabled. This clause was included because Congress clearly intended to prohibit discrimination against individuals with disabilities based on society's myths and unfounded fears about disabilities.

A *qualified individual* is a person who can safely perform all aspects of the job with or without reasonable accommodations. The employer has the right to demand that individuals do not pose any threats to the safety of themselves or others.

Reasonable accommodations refer to the employer's responsibilities to provide the necessary structure, reassignment, and equipment modifications or devices; interpreters; or other reasonable needs that would allow the disabled person to perform the job satisfactorily. Employees and potential employees should be prepared to inform the employer of modifications or special needs that will accommodate them. Reasonable accommodations may be as simple as providing telephone devices so that a hearing-impaired person applying for the position of telephone switchboard operator can qualify for the position. Other reasonable accommodations include job restructuring, part-time or modified work, provision of qualified readers or interpreters, or reassignment to another position.

To meet the qualifications of this section, employers must also identify ***essential job functions.*** These functions are based on the employer's judgment, the job description, and amount of time performing the given function. The purpose of such a provision is to ensure that, if qualified disabled applicants apply for a job, they will not be discriminated against because of nonessential job functions that they are not able to perform. However, if there are other, more or equally qualified nondisabled applicants, the employer does not have to hire the disabled person. The issue arises when more qualified disabled applicants are passed over for less qualified, nondisabled applicants.

■ EXERCISE 20–1

Review all of the components and skills used in staff performance. What are the essential job functions you would want to include when authoring a list of staff nurses' essential job functions? What are their nonessential functions? Give the rationale for your answers. Define what you consider to be essential versus nonessential job functions? Are there areas of overlap?

Exclusions from the Definition of Disability

There are many exclusions from the definition of disability under the ADA. The ADA excludes homosexuality and bisexuality from its coverage. It further excludes transvestism, transsexualism, pedophilia, exhibitionism, voyeurism, gender identity disorders not resulting from physical impairments, and other sexual behavior disorders. The ADA does not protect compulsive gamblers, kleptomaniacs, pyromaniacs, and those who currently use illegal drugs. Moreover, the employer may hold alcoholics to the same qualifications and job performance standards as other employees even if the unsatisfactory behavior or performance is directly related to the alcoholism.

PROVISIONS OF THE ADA

The ADA is closely related to the Civil Rights Act of 1964 and incorporates the antidiscrimination principles established in Section 504 of the Rehabilitation Act of 1973. There are five titles in the Act.

Title I

Title I of the ADA prohibits employment discrimination, adopting the remedies and procedures provided by Title VII of the Civil Rights Act of 1964. This title also incorporates the concepts of reasonable accommodation and undue hardship that were established in parts of the Rehabilitation Act.

The purpose of this section is to ensure that people with disabilities are not excluded from job opportunities or adversely affected in any other aspect of employment unless they are not qualified or otherwise unable to perform the job. This protects qualified and disabled individuals in regard to application, salary, promotions, discharge, transfer, and all other aspects of work.

The ADA's prohibition against employment discrimination extends to medical examinations and inquiries on applications. The employer is not allowed to ask about disabilities or about the extent of obvious disabilities. The employer may make inquiries into the ability of the applicant to fulfill the job requirements. A medical examination may be conducted after a job offer has been extended to the disabled person and provided that all applicants for the position are subjected to the same examinations. Drug testing to determine the illegal use of drugs may be performed because such screens are not considered medical examinations. Depending on the job, employers may make inquiries about disabilities if the inquiry is job-related and consistent with business necessity. Employers may also conduct voluntary medical examinations that are part of an employee health program made available to all employees at the worksite.

Defenses that the employer has to the ADA include ***undue hardship.*** This provision is available if the accommodation to be made is extremely expensive or difficult to implement. The act provides that the employer must investigate the required accommodations and offer data proving this hardship. Undue hardships are based on cost, numbers of employees, and type of business enterprise.

Other possible defenses include public safety defense and health and safety defense. Under these two defenses, the employer must show that reasonable accommodation cannot prevent potential compromised safety and health hazards to others in the workplace. For example, health care institutions have requirements that persons with contagious diseases may not work in the facility during the active phase of the illness. As stated earlier, religious employers may give preference to individuals of the same religious sect.

Title II

Title II of the ADA prohibits discrimination against disabled individuals by any state or local government entity without regard to the receipt of federal funds and includes comprehensive provisions designed to ensure access to and use of public transportation by disabled persons. Title II incorporates the remedies and procedures set forth by the Rehabilitation Act.

Title III

Title III prohibits discrimination by public accommodations against individuals on the basis of disability in the full and equal enjoyment of the entity's goods, services, facilities, privileges, advantages, or accommodations. Title III mandates the removal of architectural and structural barriers and the provision of auxiliary aids and services in many cases. Public accommodations are required to remove barriers in existing facilities if such removal can be accomplished without substantial difficulty or expense. However, newly constructed facilities and major renovations of existing structures must be designed to be readily accessible to and usable by individuals with disabilities. Title III also includes provisions on discrimination in transportation services provided by private entities. Title III incorporates remedies and procedures from the Civil Rights Act of 1964.

Title IV

Title IV is designed to ensure that individuals with speech and hearing impairments have meaningful access to and use of telephone services. The ADA requires common carriers engaged in intrastate and interstate communications to provide telecommunications relay services to individuals with hearing and speech impairments.

Title V

Title V contains miscellaneous provisions including some construction clauses. Provisions under this section include the statement that the ADA does not invalidate or limit other federal or state laws, allows insurance carriers to continue classifying risks in the manner consistent with state laws, and prohibits retaliation against persons who file discrimination charges under the act or assist others who file such charges.

LAWSUITS UNDER THE ADA

Since its enactment, the number of cases filed under the ADA continues to be extensive. This is partly due to the what might be considered the flexibility of definitions given the act by its creators. To prevent the act from being overly narrow, explicit definitions of which individuals are "qualified individuals with a disability will of necessity . . . be done on a case to case method" (ADA, 1990, 42 U.S.C. Section 12101). The protected class is composed of employees or applicants for employment who meet three discrete provisions:

1. The individual must have a disability in the sense that he or she has a "physical or mental impairment."
2. The impairment must be such that it "substantially limits one of more of the major life activities" of the individual.
3. The qualified person must still be able to perform "the essential function of the employment position" sought or in which the individual is currently employed (ADA, 1990, 42 U.S.C. Section 12111).

Court cases have continued to challenged the definition of a qualified individual with a disability. From the first passage of the act, early challenges to the ADA concerned HIV and AIDS patients. An average of nine years passes between HIV infection and AIDS diagnosis. During that time, people with HIV infection often continue to work and engage in other activities, many times unaware of their HIV-positive status. The media has advanced the concept that persons with HIV infection can avail themselves of newer advances in treatment and live longer and healthier lives. One only has to follow the career of Magic Johnson to see that HIV-positive persons can return even to vigorous sports arenas.

Early cases presented such issues as mandatory HIV testing, whether the ADA prohibited discrimination against HIV-infected persons, or whether the asymptomatic HIV-infected person was qualified under the ADA. In *Leckelt v. Board of Commissioners* (1990), the court upheld the dismissal of a nurse for refusal to take an HIV antibody test. The court reasoned that the nurse was not otherwise qualified, because he refused to take a test that the court felt was consistent with appropriate infection control procedures. Even though the likelihood that Leckelt would transmit an HIV infection was small, the court found the hospital policy was justifiable given the hospital's need to protect and safeguard patients.

This view had been rejected by the Supreme Court in *School Board v. Arline* (1987), a pre-ADA case. In that case, the Supreme Court had rejected the claim that HIV presented a direct threat to the public, given the fact that HIV cannot, in most circumstances, be transmitted in the workplace. The *Arline* standard, though, prohibited discrimination against HIV-infected individuals who, with reasonable accommodations, could perform jobs in the workplace.

Following the *Arline* reasoning, some state courts allowed disability discrimination to be upheld if the individual bringing suit could show that the sole reason for firing an employee was his or her positive HIV status. For example, in *Raintree Health Care Center v. Human Rights Commission* (1995), the court upheld the employee's contention that the sole reason for firing him was his positive HIV status. The employee in this case was a cook working at a long-term care facility, whose sole responsibilities were confined to preparing the evening meal, placing the meal on trays, and cleaning the kitchen and storeroom areas after the evening meal. He was fired on the same day that his HIV status was reported to the administrator of the facility. Other states follow a stricter standard and disallow disability discrimination lawsuits for removing HIV-positive employees from the workplace.

A landmark 1998 Supreme Court decision has hopefully brought this issue to a final determination. The court was asked to decide in *Bragdon v. Abbott* (1998) if HIV infection was a disability under the ADA, even when the HIV-positive person was asymptomatic. In that case, Sidney Abbott went to Dr. Bragdon's office for a scheduled dental appointment. At the appointment, Ms. Abbott disclosed the fact that she was HIV positive on the patient registration form. Dr. Bragdon discovered a cavity during his examination of Abbott and informed her that he had a policy against filling cavities of HIV-infected patients. He offered to treat her at the local hospital at no extra cost for his services, but stated that she would be responsible for the hospital costs incurred in filling the cavity. This suit was then brought under provisions of the ADA, asserting that Abbott was a qualified individual with a disability even though she was totally asymptomatic. The lower court found for Abbott, noting that Bragdon had introduced no genuine issue of material fact regarding whether Abbott's HIV status would have posed a direct threat to the health or safety of others during a dental examination.

The Supreme Court applied a three-part process in finding that Abbott's infection allowed her to be qualified under the ADA. First, the justices considered whether the infection constituted a physical impairment. In finding that Abbott's asymptomatic HIV infection constituted a physical impairment, the court noted that "HIV is an impairment from the moment of infection and during every stage of the disease . . . and that it must be regarded as a physiological disorder with a constant and detrimental effect on the infected person's hemic and lymphatic systems" (at 2204).

Second, they identified the life activity on which Abbott relied (reproduction and child bearing), and determined it to be a major life activity. In this finding, the Supreme Court emphatically rejected the notion that "Congress intended the ADA to only cover those aspects of a person's life which have a public, economic, or daily character" (at 2205). The court reiterated that the ADA must be construed consistently with regulations implementing the Rehabilitation Act, and pointed out that the act's regulations provide an illustrative but not exhaustive list of major life activities, which includes functions such as caring for oneself, learning, and working, and that reproduction could not be considered less important than working and learning.

Finally, the justices determined that the impairment did substantially limit a major life activity. Relying on medical evidence, the court determined that Abbott's physical impairment limited her ability to reproduce in two ways. By trying to conceive, the HIV-positive woman imposes on her male partner a significant risk of infection, and a woman infected with HIV risks infecting her child during gestation and delivery. Thus, although conception and childbirth may not be impossible for a woman with HIV, those activities are "dangerous to the public health" and that is sufficient to meet the definition of a substantial limitation (at 2206).

Addressing the second issue presented—that Bragdon had not introduced evidence that Abbott posed a direct health threat to Bragdon and others, the court conceded that the existence of such a significant risk must be determined from Bragdon's viewpoint, but that the "risk assessment must also be based on medical or other objective evidence" (at 2210).

The impact of this ruling is far-reaching. In its broadest sense, the holding mandates that HIV is a disability, one that is protected by the ADA. Even if one limits the holding to this specific fact situation (that the major life activity is reproduction), the foundation has been laid for expanding coverage to other types of life activity in the future that are outside caring for oneself, learning, and working. The decision in Bragdon may also signal expanded protection for persons with other nontraditional disabilities, such as infertility. The second issue—the broader inference of what evidence is necessary to determine whether there is significant risk to the provider—was left open by this court and presumably will be decided in later cases. The court's decision, though, suggests that the courts will apply a relatively stringent standard of proof before upholding discriminatory acts that are allegedly necessary to protect public health and safety.

Courts across the country have held that a variety of conditions do not constitute a disability. Such examples include the finding that a nurse with a lifting disability was not qualified under ADA (*Thompson v. Holy Family Hospital*, 1997), erratic behavior does not give notice to the employer that an employee is suffering from a disabling mental impairment (*Webb v. Mercy Hospital*, 1996), depression and anxiety are not disabling mental conditions (*Cody v. Cigna Healthcare of St. Louis, Inc.*, 1998), a nurse taking medication for depression is not disabled (*Wilking v. County of Ramsey*, 1997), a nurse's inability to handle the stress of a particular job is not a disability (*Paleologos v. Rehab Consultants, Inc.*, 1998), migraine headaches and non-latex allergies are not disabilities (*Howard v. North Mississippi Medical Center*, 1996), a short-term condition (hypertension causing a one-month leave of absence) is not a disability (*McIntosh v. Brookdale Hospital Medical Center*, 1996), pregnancy is not a disability (*Jessie v. Carter Health Care Center, Inc.*, 1996), and a back injury caused by turning a patient is not a disability (*Maloney v. Barberton Citizens Hospital*, 1996).

Courts have also examined how individuals with disabilities accommodate to their disability. In *Downs v. Hawkeye Health Services, Inc.* (1998), the nurse had been infected with hepatitis C and, unable to meet the demands of his job, resigned. He filed for Social Security disability benefits, stating it was impossible for him to complete nursing tasks in a safe manner due to extreme fatigue, nausea, anxiety, and depression. He then was hired as the supervisor of home health aides and withdrew his application for Social Security benefits.

The U.S. Circuit Court of Appeals for the Eighth Circuit applauded this nurse for genuinely trying to make the most of this employment opportunity. Unfortunately, his medical condition rendered him unable to perform the duties of the supervisory role, and he was terminated by the home health agency. The nurse sued the home health agency for disability discrimination and refiled his Social Security disability application, stating he was completely unable to work because of his hepatitis C status.

The court ruled in favor of the home health agency and against the nurse, despite sympathy for the nurse's plight. They held that just because a person files for disability benefits does not mean that person cannot be a qualified individual with a disability. Theoretically, an employer can accommodate the disability and thereby make the person qualified, though it is difficult to envision how this could happen in a patient care position. The justices further noted that persons who make statements in applying for Social Security or other disability benefits must stand by those statements if they subsequently file a lawsuit for employment disability discrimination.

A nurse cannot refuse to participate in an interactive process that would result in alternative employment and be successful in a disability discrimination lawsuit. In *Webster v.*

Methodist Occupational Health Centers, Inc. (1998), a nurse desired to return to work following stroke rehabilitation. Her physician testified that she had a residual decreased inability to sustain attention and concentration at times, as well as mild decreases in visual spatial skills and scanning and occasional impulsivity. He testified that she could probably function effectively, but only in an environment in which she had close supervision and was supported by the resources of other staff members. According to his testimony, it was not appropriate for her to return to a nursing position where she had to be able to work alone.

She could have returned to occupational nursing if the facility were to hire a second nurse to work with her. But hiring a second nurse would effectively amount to paying a double salary for a one-nurse position, and the company refused to accommodate her. There were, however, other positions available through the agency that could accommodate her needs. She refused to consider any other option besides returning to her former job, on the same shift, with an extra second nurse. There were also non-nursing positions available that would use her expertise and accommodate her physical disability. The court ruled that the nurse's refusal to participate in the interactive process between employer and employee rules out her right to sue successfully for disability discrimination after her dismissal from the agency.

The Court of Appeals for the Sixth Circuit in 1998 clearly outlined the purpose of the disability act from the perspectives of both the qualified individual and the employer. In *Estate of Mauro v. Borgess Medical Center* (1998), the court was asked to rule in a case involving an HIV-positive surgical technician. The Sixth Circuit began by noting that the disability discrimination laws in employment are meant to protect persons with disabilities from discriminations based on prejudice, stereotypes, or unfounded fear, while giving appropriate weight to the legitimate goal of preventing other persons from exposure to significant health and safety risks.

Few aspects of disability discrimination give rise to the same level of public fear and misapprehension as the possibility of HIV contagion from an infected health care worker. The fact that some persons with HIV may pose a health threat to others under certain circumstances does not justify exclusion of all persons with HIV from health care employment. Persons with contagious diseases must have their individual circumstances evaluated in light of scientific evidence, rather than being victimized by discrimination based on mythology.

Whether the possibility of disease transmission is a direct threat depends on how the disease is transmitted, the severity of the risk if the disease is transmitted, and the probability that the disease will be transmitted. Where there is no direct threat of an HIV-positive health care worker transmitting an HIV infection to a patient, it is unlawful disability discrimination to exclude the worker from the position based solely on the worker's HIV status.

The Centers for Disease Control and Prevention (CDC) does not find a direct threat of HIV transmission from health care worker to patient in most medical and surgical procedures, even invasive procedures such as inserting intravenous lines. However, the court noted that the CDC has defined a class of exposure-prone invasive procedures that pose a direct threat of transmission. Exposure-prone procedures occur when fingers and a sharp object are simultaneously present in a confined or poorly visualized anatomic site. In this case, the hospital's written job description for a surgical technician stated that, on an infrequent basis, the technician could be required to assist the surgeon by holding retractors, by manually drawing back muscle tissue, and by assisting with suturing inside a body cavity. There was, the court said, a real threat of an HIV-positive worker's skin being poked or broken and the worker then bleeding unknowingly into a patient's body cavity or surgical wound. Thus, the court ruled that it was not discrimination to exclude an HIV-positive health care worker from a job that entails participation in exposure-prone procedures as defined by the CDC. As an aside, the court also noted that this same worker had been offered a position in the operating arena not involving the threat of HIV transmission but had rejected that position (*Estate of Mauro v. Borgess Medical Center*, 1998).

A second area that the courts have addressed concerns reasonable accommodation. This may include but is not limited to job restructuring, part-time or modified work schedules, reassignment or transfers to other departments that have vacant positions, acquisition or modification of equipment or devices, educational materials or policies, and the provision of qualified readers or interpreters. What constitutes reasonable accommodation is judged on a case-by-case basis.

To file suit alleging that reasonable accommodation has not been made, the employer must first know of the person's disability and be given an opportunity to accommodate the employee. The court in *Clapp v. Northern Cumberland Memorial Hospital* (1997) was asked to decide whether infertility is a dysfunction of a major life event, one that would make the individual a qualified individual under the ADA. The nurse in *Clapp* was given a 12-week leave, to which she was entitled under the Family and Medical Leave Act, to adopt a child. Although the child was healthy, the nurse asked to extend her leave. The extra time off was denied, and the nurse filed a disability discrimination lawsuit, citing infertility as the causing factor for her adoption proceedings.

The court, however, never answered the question because the nurse in this case never informed her supervisors that her request concerned her own infertility or that she considered herself to be disabled and thus was requesting reasonable accommodation. Thus, the court ruled that her infertility may or may not be a legally recognized disability. The more important point was that she had not told her employer that she was disabled, and thus they did not discriminate against her.

A similar conclusion had been reached in *Fromm-Vane v. Lawnwood Medical Center, Inc.* (1997). There, a nurse's psychologist wrote a letter to the nurse's supervisors, indicating that this individual was suffering from a severe depressive state due to marital dysfunction and job stress and that the nurse required reasonable accommodation. Such accommodation consisted of four weeks' medical leave for intensive outpatient psychotherapy. The letter further stated that the nurse would then be able to return to work. This letter was received by the facility after the decision had been made to terminate the nurse for inadequate job performance stemming from her depressive illness, but before she was actually informed of the termination. The court held that the facility had been timely notified of the disability and must make reasonable accommodations.

Often, the court must decide what is reasonable accommodation. In *Zamudio v. Patia* (1997), a nurse with asthma and obstructive lung disease was told by her physician that walking outside in very cold weather between residential cottages at a facility for the developmentally disabled where she worked greatly aggravated her condition. She was able to perform all other required functions of her job as a registered nurse.

The facility had sufficient resources to offer the nurse flexible use of her medical leave when the weather outside was too cold for her to work. The nurse, however, insisted that the facility offer her a position in which she could work indoors at all times.

The court found that the facility had made a reasonable accommodation. The facility did not have a position available in which the nurse would not be required to walk between buildings, nor was the facility obligated to create a new position or displace another employee from such a position to accommodate this nurse.

The facility would be required to inform the nurse when the type of position she wanted became available. She would be allowed to apply, but as a disabled employee seeking reasonable accommodation she did not have to be given preference over other employees without disabilities who may be better qualified or have more seniority. Thus, the court held that an employee is not necessarily entitled to the specific accommodation requested, but to accommodations that are reasonable under the circumstances and that place no undue hardships on the employer.

A similar finding occurred in *Feliciano v. State of Rhode Island* (1998). In that case, the nurse had lifting restrictions resulting from an on-the-job injury and was unable to perform the essential job functions for her position. The court ruled that a mechanical lift would not be a reasonable accommodation in this case because physically and mentally incapacitated patients often cannot position themselves correctly on a power lift to be lifted safely, nor would this nurse be able to position them correctly because of her lifting restrictions. Lifting a patient safely with such a device is basically a two-person operation, which in light of the hospital's budgeting and staffing constraints would defeat the whole purpose of the lift as an accommodation to one employee who could not perform essential lifting tasks alone. The court went on further to hold that the ADA does not mandate that a physically nondemanding position be automatically given to a disabled person. The employer's duty to reassign a disabled employee is subject to the employer's more important obligation to uphold seniority rights, rights based in collective bargaining agreements, and other nondiscriminatory job selection processes.

Neither do employers have an obligation under the ADA to tolerate frequent unpredictable absences as reasonable accommodation. In *Willett v. State of Kansas* (1996), the facility had made reasonable accommodations for a nurse with systemic lupus erythematosus. They had provided a lighter medication cart and assigned her to a portion of the building where walking distances were shorter and there were fewer floor ramps. But the reasonable accommodation standard did not extend to frequent absences because these imposed an undue hardship on the facility, on the clients it served, and on other staff members. An unscheduled absence by a professional nurse required the facility to try to provide quality patient care while short staffed, to call in other staff who were scheduled time off from work, or to force staff already on duty to stay and work overtime.

The court in *Amato v. St. Luke's Episcopal Hospital* (1997) also addressed the issue of frequent absenteeism on the part of one of its employees. In holding for the hospital and against the employee, the court stated that even if the employee has a genuine disability, a hospital is not required to accommodate sporadic and unpredictable absences. A hospital "having to retain and compensate a surplus employee to be available in the event that another employee fails to report for work is not reasonable accommodation" (at 538).

Note that an employer need not retain a disabled person unless reasonable accommodation may be made. In *Rourk v. Oakwood Hospital Corporation* (1998), a nurse wanted to return to work after more than 12 months off the job due to a shoulder injury that she had incurred in an automobile accident. The injury left her with a lifting restriction not to exceed five pounds, and the nurse herself admitted she could not return to a clinical position at the hospital as a registered nurse.

The nurse approached the facility about an open position in utilization review. She was not qualified for the position, and it was not offered to her. She then sued for disability discrimination. The court found that, as a general rule, an employee is entitled to reasonable accommodation, and that can mean considering the employee for positions compatible with the employee's disability. But the employer need not transfer the employee to a completely different position than the position for which the individual was hired, just to avoid charges of failing to make reasonable accommodation. This would create an unreasonable financial burden on the part of the employer because it would require employers to retain workers for different positions if they should become disabled. Thus, the court rejected this nurse's claim as a qualified individual with a disability.

Since these cases are decided on a case-by-case basis, the opposite outcome can also be true. In *Community Hospital v. Fail* (1998), the Colorado Supreme Court ruled that reasonable accommodation could include offering an employee a lower-paying position for which the individual was qualified. In this case, a rehabilitation aide suffered a disabling knee injury and could no longer perform the essential functions of her job because she could no longer safely lift heavy patients.

The aide was at step nine in her rehabilitation position. A clerical position was open in medical records, and the aide possessed the qualifications for that position. However, the hospital's policy stated that anyone transferring into any new position could enter the new position at no higher that a step six. That means a $2.20 per hour pay cut for this aide. It is the employee's choice whether to take the lower-paying position. The employer had met the provisions of the act in offering an employee who became disabled a reassignment to an open position for which she was qualified.

The final hurdle for such cases concerns essential job functions. These are defined by the ADA as those functions that a person must be able to perform in order to be qualified for the employment position, not qualifications that would be ideal to possess. Courts have also been involved in deciding what constitutes essential job functions. For example, the court in *Feliciano v. State of Rhode Island* (1998), noted that the essential functions for an institutional attendant included the following: performing personal hygiene; transferring and lifting patients; administering minor treatments; bathing, dressing, and grooming patients; cleaning bedpans and other equipment; exercising and walking patients to various locations; and participating in food service to patients at mealtimes. Once persons can perform all the essential functions of a position, then they can be considered qualified individuals with disabilities.

For example, the court in *Jones v. Kerrville State Hospital* (1998) held that it was an essential job function for a psychiatric nurse to be able to restrain patients. The facility in that case had a practice of allowing nurses to opt out of training in take-down and restraint procedures but still be employed in direct patient care positions. A nurse with degenerative osteoarthritis had never had the training and was taken out of direct patient care activities. The court decided that such training was an essential job skill for such a nurse and held that the facility was correct in taking this nurse out of her direct care position.

A more interesting case regarding essential job functions is *Laurin v. Providence Hospital and Massachusetts Nurses Association* (1998). In *Laurin*, the nurse had worked on the maternity unit for six years prior to suffering a seizure at home. Her neurologist determined that the seizure was fatigue-related and indicated in a report to the hospital that a day-time position was absolutely necessary for this nurse. The hospital, as part of a collective bargaining agreement, had a policy that stated in part that nurses with less than 15 years of seniority and who worked on 24-hour units must rotate shifts. This meant that the maternity nurses worked about one third of their shifts at night.

Initially, the hospital did accommodate Laurin by temporarily assigning her to a 6-week, days-only schedule. The hospital expected her to use this period to look for alternative employment, in areas that offered day positions, such as perioperative areas. After she suffered a second seizure, the hospital extended her day-only position, but informed her that her employment would be terminated if she did not return to shift work.

Reasonable accommodation does not mandate that an employer dispense with an essential job function, the court said in its opinion. Thus, the court ruled that availability for night-shift work was an essential job function on a unit that provides care on a 24-hour basis. Other nurses, the court noted, also suffered fatigue from juggling family responsibilities and night-work obligations. Although they might not have been disabled by their fatigue, the court said they had rights that their employer was not compelled to ignore in accommodating a disabled employee.

In an interesting case filed under Title III of the ADA, *Parker v. Metropolitan Life Insurance Company* (1997) defined the purpose of the ADA. The court found, in a rather complicated fact scenario, that Title III's prohibitions do not apply to employer-sponsored benefit plans. But what the court said was that "the purpose of the ADA was to prevent discrimination among nondisabled and disabled persons, not to ensure equal treatment for people with different disabilities" (at 1015).

Enforcement of the ADA

Enforcement of the ADA is done primarily through the Equal Employment Opportunity Commission. Complaints are filed with this commission and trials by jury may be a second option. The Department of Justice oversees Title III violations. Enforcement ensures one of the primary purposes of the Act—that no one, either disabled or abled, will be given a greater advantage in employment opportunities, public services, transportation, and communications.

■ EXERCISE 20–2

Imagine that a coworker of yours, also an RN, is HIV positive and works in the emergency center at your hospital. What are the essential job functions of a registered nurse in the emergency department? Do these essential job functions differ from those of nurses in other departments of the hospital? Are there special risks to the nurse as well as to potential patients? What would be reasonable accommodation for such a registered nurse?

What are the ethical duties owed by nurses who are HIV positive toward potential patients? Should they continue caring for patients in this type of setting, knowing the consequences to themselves, and potentially to their families? Are there other areas of acute care settings where nurses might be better able to be employed?

GUIDELINES: THE ADA AND HIRING PROCESSES

1. To be a qualified individual with a disability under the ADA definition, the applicant must be able to perform essential job functions. This allows employers to question individuals about their educational and experiential qualifications for the job, plus licensure and required certification if that is a prerequisite of all candidates for the position.
2. Applicants can be questioned about their ability to perform the job safely, with or without accommodation. No accommodations are necessary unless the disabled person requests such accommodations.
3. No accommodation is required if the needed accommodation would impose an undue hardship on the employer. Such undue hardships include costly or disruptive renovations to the existing facility, or costs disproportionate with the size of the employer, numbers of other employees, and nature of the business place.
4. Applicants may be questioned about their ability to perform essential job functions, and case scenarios can be devised to ascertain qualifications for clinical-based jobs. What cannot be asked are questions about disabilities, past medical problems, or previous workers' compensation claims.
5. Employment tests that would screen out disabled workers may not be used unless the test is shown to be job-related and consistent with business necessity. Tests that screen for illegal drug usage may be given, if required of all applicants for the position, not just disabled job applicants.
6. If preemployment physicals are part of the hiring process, they cannot be done until after the job is offered conditioned on the applicants passing the examination. The same medical examination requirements must be made of all persons applying for the position, and all test data must be kept confidential. Only persons with a need to know may be told of the disabled person's medical data following the examination.
7. All applicants should be queried about their qualifications for the position and have explained to them policies and procedures of the facility. Remember, the ADA does not mandate that disabled persons be hired. It mandates that all persons—the disabled as well as the abled—be given the same advantages in job opportunities.

Conclusion

The act represents an expansive vision of the capabilities of disabled individuals and rightly regards them as productive members of society. Similarly, the act holds that the societal costs of discrimination against and isolation of disabled individuals far outweigh the economic costs of accommodation. The ADA's scope is vast, and over time the act can be expected to effect major changes in the areas of employment, transportation, communications, access to public services and public accommodations, and in all other areas where the disabled have been subject to discrimination, isolation, and segregation. The ADA offers a historic opportunity to fully integrate disabled individuals into the mainstream of American society.

■ EXERCISE 20–3

Review the hiring practices of your institution by asking the nurse-manager who hires personnel on your unit. During the interview, what types of questions are asked and what information is imparted? Is there a preemployment physical and/or a mandatory drug screen for employment? What essential job functions have been developed for the positions for which applicants are interviewed? Having read this section, what advice would you give the nurse-manager?

CIVIL RIGHTS ACT OF 1991

Background of the Act

Congress, the federal courts, and numerous other courts struggled with issues of sexual discrimination and harassment during the last half of the twentieth century. The culminating factor that brought the issue to a final showdown was the Clarence Thomas Supreme Court confirmation hearings in October 1991, heightening awareness of concern about sexual harassment in the workplace. The Thomas hearings pushed sexual harassment to the top of the national agenda, and the act was signed into law on November 21, 1991.

Unlike the ADA, the *Civil Rights Act of 1991* did not have smooth sailing in committee nor in Congress. Following the Thomas hearings, Senator Danforth catalyzed the warring factions into temporary harmony, with most of the "rough edges" addressed. President Bush, in signing the act, stated "most of the Act's major provisions have been subject to bipartisan consensus" (Sacher, 1992).

Definition of Sexual Harassment

The major portion of the act definitions of *sexual harassment,* with two categories of sexual harassment being identified. Overall, sexual harassment is simply "unwelcome sexual conduct that is a term of employment" (29 CRF, Section 1604.11[a]). The two categories of sexual harassment are discussed separately.

Quid Pro Quo Sexual Harassment

Quid pro quo sexual harassment occurs when submission to or rejection of the sexual conduct by an individual is used as a basis for employment decisions affecting the individual. To show quid pro quo sexual harassment, the individual must show that:

1. The employee was subjected to unwelcome harassment in the form of sexual advances or requests for sexual favors.
2. The harassment complained of was based on sex.
3. The employee's submission to the unwelcome advances was an expressed or implied condition for receiving job benefits or that the employee's refusal to submit to the supervisor's sexual demands resulted in tangible job detriment.
4. The individual is a member of a protected class (an employee in a lower position in the power chain of command).

Additionally, employers are strictly liable for the conduct of supervisory personnel in quid pro quo harassment suits.

Hostile Work Environment

The majority of the cases brought under the act concern *hostile work environment* sexual harassment. In these instances, there are no tangible job benefits or detriment. Here, the employee is subjected to sexual innuendos, remarks, and physical acts so offensive as to "alter the conditions of the employee's employment and create an abusive work environment" (*Meritor Savings Bank v. Vinson,* 1986). Elements that must be shown in this type of case include (1) establishing that the harassment unreasonably interfered with work performance and (2) that the harassment would affect a reasonable person's work environment. The employer is not strictly liable in such a suit, but becomes liable when the individual alleging the harassment files complaints with the employer or when the harassment is so pervasive that knowledge can be inferred.

Because most issues in this area affect women, the court addressed the issue of a "reasonable woman standard." In *Robinson v. Jacksonville Shipyards, Inc.* (1991), the court concluded that:

> ". . . the cumulative, corrosive effect of their work environment over time affects the psychological well-being measured by the impact of the work environment on a reasonable woman's work performance or more broadly by the impact of the stress inflicted on her by the continuing presence of the harassing behavior. The fact that some female employees did not complain of the work environment or find some behaviors objectionable does not affect this conclusion concerning the objective offensiveness of the work environment as a whole" (at 1492).

The *Robinson* case was the first to carve out the "reasonable woman standard" in dealing with sexual harassment cases since there is a gender issue in this area of perception. *Ellison v. Brady* (1991) had concluded that a complete understanding of the victim's views requires an analysis of the different perspectives between men and women, and what men may consider unobjectionable may offend many women.

In hostile work environment sexual harassment cases, the conduct need not be directed at the individual who files the complaint. It is enough that the behavior or condition was observed or known by the individual and that the behavior affected the psychological well-being of the individual. For example, hostile work environment sexual harassment may be triggered by posting of pornography in the office, displaying lewd cartoons labeled with a worker's name, making sexually demeaning comments or jokes, touching or attempting to touch the individual, and sexual propositions. A hostile work environment can originate from sexually discriminatory verbal intimidation, ridicule, or insults, if "sufficiently severe or pervasive as to alter the conditions of the victim's employment and create an abusive working environment" (*Farpella-Crosby v. Horizon Health Care,* 1996, at 805). The conduct/behavior complained of must be unwelcome, and the victim's perspective is what is relevant.

Conduct akin to that of a quid pro quo sexual harassment case may also exist in this type of suit, but the offending employee has no direct supervision over the individual or there is no corresponding job benefit or detriment connected with the harassment. For example, in *Hamm v. Lakeview Community Hospital* (1996), the U.S. District Court for the Middle District of Alabama ruled that an emergency department nurse's suit for quid pro quo sexual harassment was without merit. Title VII of the Civil Right Act outlaws acts of sexual harassment on the job between an employee and an employer. In this case, the physician was the employee of a separate corporation that had a contract with the hospital (also the nurse's employer) to provide emergency department physician's services, and the court was unwilling to infer that the physician was the hospital's designated agent in supervising the nurse. The nurse more likely would have prevailed if she had brought this suit as a hostile environment suit, since it was conceivable that she could show the hospital knew of the hostile environment and chose to allow the situation to continue.

Employees who feel that there is some type of hostile environment sexual harassment should notify superiors or the employer directly, depending on the size of the facility/place of employment and organizational chart. The employer has a duty to investigate the report, maintaining confidentiality, and reporting back to the initiating complainant. Documentation should be made of the investigation, maintaining professionalism, but speaking with the alleged victim as well as the alleged harasser and other potential witnesses. Consider what action needs to be taken and communicate the results of the investigation back to all parties involved.

Two separate cases serves as examples of the preceding statements. In *Farpella-Crosby v. Horizon Health Care* (1996), the nurse bringing a sexual harassment suit was employed as a treatment nurse, responsible for monitoring and treating decubitus ulcers and other skin-related conditions in the nursing home's residents.

The director of nursing made numerous inappropriate sexual comments to the nurse, asking about her sexual habits and asking others about the nurses' sexual habits, both in apparent seriousness and in apparent jest. He also joked in the presence of others that she must not know how to use condoms as she was the mother of seven children. The nurse repeatedly asked the director of nursing to stop making such remarks about her and to her.

The nurse complained to the human resources director about the nursing director's offensive remarks, as did another nurse in the nursing home who was subjected to similar treatment. Neither nurse specifically said that they were being sexually harassed, nor did they need to, said the court. In upholding the sexual harassment claim against the nursing home, the court found that the human resources director had made no effort to investigate and did essentially nothing about the issue except tell Farpella-Crosby to "hang in there." The court ruled that this provided substantial evidence that the nurse's employer had failed to take prompt remedial action upon the employee's justifiable complaint of sexually hostile treatment on the job, as required by law.

"An employer can be sued for the discriminatory acts of an employee only if the employer knew or should have known of the employee's offensive conduct and failed to take steps to repudiate that conduct and eliminate the hostile environment" (at 806).

The second case, *Grodzdanich v. Leisure Hills Health Center* (1998) shows how prompt action can prevent finding for the complainant. In *Grodzdanich*, a female staff member brought a charge of hostile working environment against her employer after a male charge nurse had fondled her. While the court concurred that sexual harassment had occurred, there was no liability for damages on the part of the nursing home as employer.

Following notification by the staff nurse that she has been sexually harassed, the nursing home followed its already disseminated policy exactly. The policy defined sexual harassment and promised that would-be perpetrators would be dealt with harshly. Within minutes of the complaint, management talked to witnesses whom the nurse had identified. The nurse was immediately given the choice to work in another area, away from the perpetrator, once the witnesses had corroborated the nurse's charges. Then, when the victim was fully validated by complete internal disciplinary process against the perpetrator, the perpetrator was fired.

The court in this case could not stress often enough the importance of an employer's taking the victim seriously and acting speedily, for the victim's sake and to avoid or minimize legal liability. Such a ruling contrasts with the holding in *Smith v. St. Louis University* (1997), in which the employer took four months to speak with the alleged perpetrator. Four months, that court held, did not meet the employer's legal requirement of prompt remedial action reasonably calculated to end the harassment.

Interestingly, a health care institution may also be held liable if the source of the harassment is a patient and nothing is done to protect potential victims. In *Crist v. Focus Homes, Inc.* (1997), female caregivers at a facility for developmentally disabled adolescents and adults complained to management that they were being accosted and fondled by a 17-year-old resident. The resident stood over six feet tall and weighted over 200 pounds, but had the functional capacity of a 2- to 5-year-old child.

The court found that management was incorrect for not heeding their complaints. While the resident's conduct sprang from his inability to control impulses due to profound mental retardation, the facility still had a responsibility for a harassment-free environment and could still be help accountable in a suit for sexual harassment.

The facility should have conducted a sexuality assessment. Such an assessment, the court concluded, would have prompted the facility to assign male caregivers who would not be taken as sexual objects and to bring in caregivers of either gender capable of physically restraining the resident.

Termination of the alleged harasser is not mandatory, and other remedial action may be taken, such as a transfer of the offender to other units or worksites and disciplinary warnings. Generally, courts have held that for serious physical harassment, termination may be required, whereas less serious verbal harassment may justify lesser discipline. Most importantly, some action must be taken if a potential lawsuit is to be avoided.

Additionally, there is some evidence to support that courts may hold independent contractors—those with no direct employee–employer relationship—liable under this act. Thus, physicians and agency personnel, who have no direct employer–employee relationship with health care facilities, may make health care facilities liable for their actions or comments within these facilities.

Preferential Treatment or Sexual Favoritism

An employer may also be liable for unlawful sexual discrimination when an employee is denied a job opportunity or benefit due to the *preferential treatment* of another employee who submits to the employer's sexual advances. Additionally, there may be liability when employers promote employees who give sexual favors to supervisors, rather than other, better qualified employees.

■ EXERCISE 20–4

For the following examples, state whether there are grounds for a sexual harassment claim and what type of sexual harassment claim could be brought—quid pro quo or hostile environment.

GUIDELINES: AVOIDING SEXUAL HARASSMENT CLAIMS

1. Try to prevent the harassment from occurring since this is the most effective and cost effective means to deal with the reality of workplace relationships.
2. Take affirmative action to prevent harassment, such as educational programs to alert persons about how to react to such advances and hostile environments, expressing strong disapproval, informing persons of their right to raise sexual harassment issues, and sensitizing all concerned.
3. Develop policies prohibiting either type of sexual harassment. The policy should include strong language prohibiting such actions and stating that such actions will not be tolerated; a procedure for reporting complaints; notice that violators will be subject to stern disciplinary procedures, including discharge; identification of an employee representative to whom complaints should be directed; and a statement that all complaints and investigations will be treated in a confidential manner.
4. Effectively communicate the policy, including placement in policy manuals, bulletin boards, interoffice memoranda, and employee handbooks.
5. Conduct training programs for supervisory personnel.

1. John rejects a homosexual advance by David, a nurse-manager, and is subsequently fired by the unit manager.
2. William, the hospital chief operating officer, asks Judy, the assistant director of nursing, for a date.
3. During a conference sponsored by the institution, Paul makes remarks and sexual physical contact with a female coworker, Judy. Judy complains to her direct supervisor, and 12 hours later, the hospital director of nursing tells her that she needs to stay at the conference, but will no longer be required to work with Paul after the conference.
4. Marilyn and Jeff, both employed by the same institution, are having an affair. They are both upper-level managers, but work in different departments.
5. During a trip, Rita makes sexual innuendos and tells lewd jokes to a male coworker, Richard. After Richard complains, the company transfers Richard and reprimands Rita.

SUMMARY

The ADA is a significant enactment because it affects health care employers, health care personnel, potential employees, and consumers of the health care delivery system. Hiring practices should be changed to accommodate the new restrictions when interviewing potential employees, and necessary accommodations made for disabled persons—employees or patients.

Although it is virtually impossible to eliminate sexual harassment from the workplace, an employer can implement policies and practices that will significantly limit its practice. An employer should have a written sexual harassment policy, promptly respond to allegations of sexual harassment, and take remedial actions as warranted.

AFTER COMPLETING THE CHAPTER, YOU SHOULD BE ABLE TO

- Describe the conditions within the United States that caused both the ADA and the Civil Rights Act of 1991 to be written and implemented.
- Describe the various sections of the two acts, necessary definitions, and intended purposes.
- Describe how the acts affect the health care delivery system in terms of consumers and providers.
- Analyze the ever-expanding number of cases filed under both of these acts.

APPLY YOUR LEGAL KNOWLEDGE

- How do staff nurses comply with these two acts in providing competent care to patients?
- Have these two laws had the effect that their drafters intended?
- What revisions or redefinitions to the original laws have been created by the number of legal cases filed concerning these two acts?
- What would you advise employers to implement or change to prevent further cases from being filed under these two acts?

YOU BE THE JUDGE

On September 6, 1992, Denise Dupre was hired to work as a nurse in the neonatal intensive care unit at Ben Taub Hospital. Shortly thereafter, she requested a "compressed weekend schedule," which meant working eight hours or more on consecutive days. Her request was granted, resulting in Dupre's shifts regularly lasting about 16 hours. Dupre generally worked Fridays, Saturdays, and Sundays, although occasionally she worked other days. While employed at Ben Taub, she was first supervised by Pippa Andrews and subsequently by Felicia King. During that period, the director of nursing was Lella Thomas.

In December 1994, Dupre took time off from work for treatment of depression. She was treated by Dr. Fallace, who prescribed Klonopin, Paxil, and lithium and advised her to rest. She was also diagnosed with bipolar disorder by Dr. Fallace. Dupre provided the hospital with a return-to-work form, signed by Dr. Fallace, dated December 15, 1994, which stated in part that she had been under treatment since December 8, 1994, and that she be allowed to return to work, starting December 16, 1994.

According to Dupre, she informed King and Thomas of her bipolar disorder about this same time. Dupre also alleged that her coworkers were aware of her disability, while Thomas stated in her deposition that she was only "aware that Dupre had an attendance problem." Dupre contends that she specifically informed King that her disability restricted the amount of stress she could endure on the job. Further, she purportedly told King that the physical fatigue associated with her condition and her medication also limited her ability to work a 16-hour shift. Dupre alleges that she requested accommodation of her condition in the form of a transfer to a low-risk nursery or a shorter shift. Dupre maintains that King refused her request and told her that no other positions were available. Dupre maintains that others were transferred to positions that were less stressful than hers during the same time intervals that Dupre asked for a transfer.

The deposition of the director of human resources for the institution confirms that another nurse was transferred from the neonatal intensive care unit to the newborn nursery, but that the transfer did not occur until October 21, 1995, nine months after Dupre was terminated. There is evidence to also show that two "potentially less stressful" positions were posted and became available on December 26, 1994, and January 2, 1995, but there is no evidence that Dupre ever applied for either of these positions.

Throughout Dupre's employment at the hospital, nurses in the neonatal intensive care area were responsible for the care of two to three infants. On January 13, 1995, King filed an employee report concerning an allegation that Dupre was negligent and conducted unsafe nursing practices with respect to one of the infants under her care. A second employee report was filed on January 13, 1995, alleging unsafe practices in regard to a second patient who was under her care. Both reports concerned negligent care that occurred on January 8, 1995. Dupre acknowledged that she was made aware of both of these reports. Dupre was placed on 90 days' probation, purportedly based on these two reports. Dupre contends that her disability and absences from work were the true reason that she was placed on probation.

Dupre's probationary period was to be from January 24, 1995, to April 23, 1995. Dupre stated that she understood that any incidents of neglect during this time frame would result in further disciplinary action, including termination. On January 25, 1995, King filed another employee report form alleging that Dupre and a second coworker had failed to do the 24-hour chart check on January 22, 1995. Because of an error in transcribing a physician's orders from the chart to the kardex, a patient was given an incorrect amount of feeding and required additional corrective actions, including a chest x-ray, administration of oxygen, and a diuretic. This discrepancy would have been noted, alleges King, if the chart check had been performed as stated in the hospital policy.

After this last report was filed, Dupre met with King and Thomas to discuss the incident. Dupre was terminated on January 30, 1995, purportedly for her failure to perform the required 24-hour chart check. She was also reported to the Board of Nurse Examiners for the State of Texas. The second nurse involved in the failure to perform the 24-hour chart check received a less severe discipline—suspension for three days and 90 days' probation—purportedly because she was not already on probation. Dupre asserts that, were it not for her disability, she "would not have been terminated when another nurse had mistranscribed the feeding order."

Following her termination, Dupre filed a grievance with Harris County, the operator of Ben Taub Hospital, which was upheld by Harris County. On April 14, 1995, Harris County informed Dupre that it was terminating any further action in regard to the grievance because Dupre had filed a charge of discrimination with the Equal Employment Opportunity Commission (EEOC), per policy as stated in the Harris County Hospital District Employee Handbook.

Since leaving Ben Taub Hospital, Dupre held five different nursing positions from April 1995 to November 1997, including traveling nurse, school nurse, maternity nurse, neonatal intensive care nurse, and pediatric nurse. She alleges that none of these employers have ever complained about the quality of her work. She filed a discrimination charge with the EEOC on March 20, 1995, alleging discrimination as well as retaliation against the hospital district. She filed a second charge of discrimination on May 26, 1995, alleging retaliation due to Harris County's decision to end the internal review of her grievance. On October 2, 1996, she filed this action, seeking recovery for discrimination and retaliation under the ADA as well as intentional infliction of emotional distress under Texas law.

Legal Questions

1. Is Dupre a protected individual under the provisions of the ADA?
2. Does Dupre have a qualifying disability as defined by the ADA?
3. Does the hospital have a legitimate, nondiscriminatory reason for her termination?
4. How should this case have been resolved?

REFERENCES

Amato v. St. Luke's Episcopal Hospital, 987 F. Supp. 523 (S.D. Tex., 1997).
Bragdon v. Abbott, 118 S. Ct. 2196 (1998).
Clapp v. Northern Cumberland Memorial Hospital, 964 F. Supp. 503 (D. Me., 1997).
Crist v. Focus Homes, Inc., 122 F.3d 1107 (8th Cir., 1997).
Cody v. Cigna Healthcare of St. Louis, Inc., 139 F.3d 595 (8th Cir., 1998).
Community Hospital v. Fail, 969 P.2d 667 (Colorado, 1998).
Downs v. Hawkeye Health Services, Inc., 148 F.3d 948 (8th Cir., 1998).
Ellison v. Brady, 924 F.2d 872 (9th Cir., 1991).
Estate of Mauro v. Borgess Medical Center, 137 F.3d 398 (6th Cir., 1998).
Farpella-Crosby v. Horizon Health Care, 97 F.3d 803 (5th Cir., 1996).
Feliciano v. State of Rhode Island, 160 F.3d 780 (1st Cir., 1998).
Fromm-Vane v. Lawnwood Medical Center, Inc., 995 F. Supp. 1471 (S.D. Fla., 1997).
Grodzdanich v. Leisure Hills Health Center, Inc., 25 F. Supp.2d 953 (D. Minn., 1998).
Hamm v. Lakeview Community Hospital, 950 F. Supp. 330 (M.D. Ala., 1996).
Howard v. North Mississippi Medical Center, 939 F. Supp. 505 (N.D. Miss., 1996).
Jessie v. Carter Health Care Center, Inc., 926 F. Supp. 613 (E. D. Ky., 1996).
Jones v. Kerrville State Hospital, 142 F.3d 263 (5th Cir., 1998).
Laurin v. Providence Hospital and Massachusetts Nurses Association, 150 F.3d 52 (1st Cir., 1998).
Leckelt v. Board of Commissioners, 909 F.2d 820 (5th Cir., 1990).
Maloney v. Barberton Citizens Hospital, 672 N.E. 223 (Ohio App., 1996).
McIntosh v. Brookdale Hospital Medical Center, 942 F. Supp. 813 (E.D. N.Y., 1996).
Meritor Savings Bank v. Vinson, 477 U.S. 57 (1986).
Paleologos v. Rehab Consultants, Inc., 990 F. Supp. 1460 (N.D. Ga., 1998).
Parker v. Metropolitan Life Insurance Company, 121 F.3d 1006 (6th Cir., 1997).
Raintree Health Care Center v. Human Rights Commission, 655 N.E.2d 944 (Ill. App., 1995).
Robinson v. Jacksonville Shipyards, Inc., 760 F. Supp. 1486 (M.D. Fla., 1991).
Rourk v. Oakwood Hospital Corporation, 580 N.W.2d 397 (Michigan, 1998).
Sacher, J. (1992). *Sexual Harassment in the Workplace*. Houston, TX: South Texas College of Law.
School Board v. Arline, 480 U.S. 273 (1987).

Smith v. St. Louis University, 109 F.3d 1261 (8th Cir., 1997).

Thompson v. Holy Family Hospital, 122 F.3d 537 (9th Cir., 1997).

29 *CRF,* Section 1604.11(A), 1991.

Webb v. Mercy Hospital, 102 F.3d 958 (8th Cir., 1996).

Webster v. Methodist Occupational Health Centers, Inc., 141 F.3d 1236 (7th Cir., 1998).

Wilking v. County of Ramsey, 983 F. Supp. 848 (D. Minn., 1997).

Willett v. State of Kansas, 942 F. Supp. 1387 (D. Kan., 1996).

Zamudio v. Patia, 956 F. Supp. 803 (N.D. Ill., 1997).

Index